At a Glance...

The book is divided into six main sections. The color-coded reference guide on the first page will help you find what you need.

The aspects of each pathogen are covered systematically, using the following order wherever practicable:

- Classification
- Localization
- Morphology and Culturing
- Developmental Cycle
- Pathogenesis and Clinical Picture
- Diagnosis
- Therapy
- Epidemiology and Prophylaxis

■ A **summary** at the beginning of a chapter or section provides a quick overview of what the main text covers. Students can use the summaries to obtain a quick recapitulation of the main points. ■

The Main Sections at a Glance

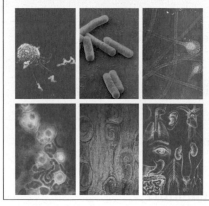

a The many **colored illustrations** serve to clarify complex topics or provide definitive impressions of pathogen morphology.

b The **header caption** above each illustration gives the reader the essence of what is shown.

c The **detailed legends** explain the illustrations independently of the main text.

Additional information

In-depth expositions and supplementary knowledge are framed in boxes interspersed throughout the main body of text. The headings outline the topic covered, enabling the reader to decide whether the specific material is needed at the present time.

Medical Microbiology

Fritz H. Kayser, M.D.
Emeritus Professor of Medical Microbiology
Institute of Medical Microbiology
University of Zurich
Zurich, Switzerland

Kurt A. Bienz, Ph.D.
Emeritus Professor of Virology
Institute of Medical Microbiology
University of Basle
Basle, Switzerland

Johannes Eckert, D.V.M.
Emeritus Professor of Parasitology
Institute of Parasitology
University of Zurich
Zurich, Switzerland

Rolf M. Zinkernagel, M.D.
Professor
Institute of Experimental Immunology
Department of Pathology
Zurich, Switzerland

177 illustrations
97 tables

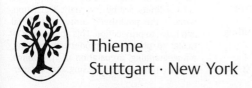

Thieme
Stuttgart · New York

Library of Congress Cataloging-in-Publication Data is available from the publisher

1st German edition 1969
2nd German edition 1971
3rd German edition 1974
4th German edition 1978
5th German edition 1982
6th German edition 1986
7th German edition 1989
8th German edition 1993
9th German edition 1998

1st Greek edition 1995

1st Italian edition 1996

1st Japanese edition 1980

1st Spanish edition 1974
2nd Spanish edition 1982

1st Turkish edition 2001

This book is an authorized and updated translation of the 10th German edition published and copyrighted 2001 by Georg Thieme Verlag, Stuttgart, Germany. Title of the German edition: Medizinische Mikrobiologie

© 2005 Georg Thieme Verlag,
Rüdigerstraße 14, 70469 Stuttgart,
Germany
http://www. thieme.de
Thieme New York, 333 Seventh Avenue,
New York, NY 10001 USA
http://www.thieme.com

Cover design: Cyclus, Stuttgart
Typesetting by Mitterweger & Partner
GmbH, 68723 Plankstadt
Printed in Germany by Appl, Wemding

ISBN 3-13-131991-7 (GTV)
ISBN 1-58890-245-5 (TNY)   1 2 3 4 5

Important note: Medicine is an ever-changing science undergoing continual development. Research and clinical experience are continually expanding our knowledge, in particular our knowledge of proper treatment and drug therapy. Insofar as this book mentions any dosage or application, readers may rest assured that the authors, editors, and publishers have made every effort to ensure that such references are in accordance with **the state of knowledge at the time of production of the book.**

Nevertheless, this does not involve, imply, or express any guarantee or responsibility on the part of the publishers in respect to any dosage instructions and forms of applications stated in the book. **Every user is requested to examine carefully** the manufacturers' leaflets accompanying each drug and to check, if necessary in consultation with a physician or specialist, whether the dosage schedules mentioned therein or the contraindications stated by the manufacturers differ from the statements made in the present book. Such examination is particularly important with drugs that are either rarely used or have been newly released on the market. Every dosage schedule or every form of application used is entirely at the user's own risk and responsibility. The authors and publishers request every user to report to the publishers any discrepancies or inaccuracies noticed.

Preface

Medical Microbiology comprises and integrates the fields of immunology, bacteriology, virology, mycology, and parasitology, each of which has seen considerable independent development in the past few decades. The common bond between them is the focus on the causes of infectious diseases and on the reactions of the host to the pathogens. Although the advent of antibiotics and vaccines has certainly taken the dread out of many infectious diseases, the threat of infection is still a fact of life: New pathogens are constantly being discovered; strains of „old" ones have developed resistance to antibiotics, making therapy more and more difficult; incurable infectious diseases (AIDS, rabies) are still with us.

The objective of this textbook of medical microbiology is to instill a broad-based knowledge of the etiologic organisms causing disease and the pathogenetic mechanisms leading to clinically manifest infections into its users. This knowledge is a necessary prerequisite for the diagnosis, therapy, and prevention of infectious diseases. This book addresses primarily students of medicine, dentistry, and pharmacy. Beyond this academic purpose, its usefulness extends to all medical professions and most particularly to physicians working in both clinical and private practice settings.

This book makes the vast and complex field of medical microbiology more accessible by the use of four-color graphics and numerous illustrations with detailed explanatory legends. The many tables present knowledge in a cogent and useful form. Most chapters begin with a concise summary, and in-depth and supplementary knowledge are provided in boxes separating them from the main body of text.

This textbook has doubtless benefited from the extensive academic teaching and the profound research experience of its authors, all of whom are recognized authorities in their fields.

The authors would like to thank all colleagues whose contributions and advice have been a great help and who were so generous with illustration material. The authors are also grateful to the specialists at Thieme Verlag and to the graphic design staff for their cooperation.

Zurich, fall of 2004   On behalf of the authors
                                                         Fritz H. Kayser

Abbreviations

ABC:	antigen-binding cell	CCC:	covalently closed circular (DNA)
ABS:	antigen-binding site		
ADA:	adenosine deaminase	CD:	cluster of differentiation/ cluster determinant
ADCC:	antibody-dependent cellular cytotoxicity		
		CDR:	complementarity-deter-mining regions
ADE:	antibody-dependent enhancement (of viral infection)		
		CE:	cystic echinococcosis
		CEA:	carcinoembryonic antigen
AE:	alveolar echinococcosis	CFA:	colonizing factor antigen
AFC:	antibody-forming cell	CFT:	complement fixation test
AFP:	alpha-fetoprotein	CFU:	colony forming units
AIDS:	acquired immune deficiency syndrome	CJD:	Creutzfeldt-Jakob disease
		CLIP:	class II-inhibiting protein
ANA:	antinuclear antibodies	CMI:	cell-mediated immunity
APC:	antigen-presenting cell	CMV:	cytomegaly virus (cytomegalovirus)
APO:	apoptosis antigen		
aPV:	acellular pertussis vaccine	CNS:	central nervous system/ coagulase-negative staphylococci
ASL titer:	antistreptolysin titer		
AZT:	azidothymidine		
		Con A:	concanavalin A
BAL:	bronchoalveolar lavage	CPE:	cytopathic effect
BALT:	bronchus-associated lymphoid tissue	CPH:	chronic persistent hepatitis
BCG:	bacillus Calmette-Guerin	CR:	cistron region
BCGF:	B-cell growth factor	CSF:	colony-stimulating factor
Bcl2:	B-cell leukemia 2 antigen	CTA:	cholera toxin A
BSE:	bovine spongiform ence-phalopathy	CTB:	cholera toxin B
		CTL:	cytotoxic CD8+ T cell
		CTX:	cholera toxin (element)
C:	complement		
CAH:	chronic aggressive hepatitis	DAF:	decay accelerating factor
		DAG:	diacyl glycerol
CAM:	cell adhesion molecules	DARC:	Duffy antigen receptor for chemokines
CAPD:	continuous ambulant peritoneal dialysis		
		DC:	dendritic cells

DHF: dengue hemorrhagic fever

DHPG: dihydroxy propoxy-methyl guanine

D vaccine: diphtheria toxoid vaccine

DNA: deoxyribonucleic acid

DNP: dinitrophenol

DR: direct repeats

ds: double-stranded nucleic acid

DSS: dengue shock syndrome

DTH: delayed type hypersensitivity

DtxR: diphtheria toxin repressor

■ EA: early antigen

EAE: experimental allergic encephalitis

EAF: EPEC adhesion factor

EaggEC: enteroaggregative *Escherichia coli*

EB: elementary body

EBNA: Epstein-Barr nuclear antigen

EBV: Epstein-Barr virus

EDTA: ethylene diamine tetra-acetic acid

eEF2: eucaryotic elongation factor 2

EF: edema factor in spotted fevers

EHEC: enterohemorrhagic *E. coli*

EIA: enzyme immunoassay

EIEC: enteroinvasive *E. coli*

EITB: enzyme-linked immuno-electrotransfer blot

ELISA: enzyme-linked immuno-sorbent assay

EM: electron microscopy

EMB: ethambutol

EMCV: encephalomyocarditis virus

EPEC: enteropathogenic *E. coli*

EPS: extracellular polymer substance

ETEC: enterotoxic *E. coli*

EU: European Union

■ F factor: fertility factor

FA: Freund's adjuvant

FACS: fluorescence-activated cell sorter

Fas: F antigen

FcR: Fc receptor

FDC: follicular dendritic cell

FHA: filamentous hemagglutin

FITC: fluorescein isothiocyanate

FTA-ABS: fluorescent treponemal antibody absorption test

■ G6PDD: glucose-6-phosphate dehydrogenase deficiency

GAE: granulomatous amebic encephalitis

gag: group-specific antigen

GALT: gut-associated lymphoid tissue

GC: guanine-cytosine/gas chromatography

GM-CSF: granulocyte-macrophage colony-stimulating factor

GP: glycoprotein

GSS: Gerstmann-Sträussler-Scheinker (syndrome)

GVH: graft-versus-host (reaction)

■ H: heavy chain

HACEK: *Haemophilus, Actinobacillus, Cardiobacterium, Eikenella, Kingella*

HAT: hypoxanthine, aminopterin, thymidine

Hb: hemoglobin

HBs: hepatitis B surface antigen
HBV: hepatitis B virus
HB vaccine: hepatitis B vaccine
HCC: hepatocellular carcinoma
HCV: hepatitis C virus/
          (human corona virus)
HDCV: human diploid cell
          vaccine
HDV: hepatitis D virus
HEV: hepatitis E virus/high
          endothelial venules
Hfr: high frequency of recom-
          bination
HGE: human granulocytic
          ehrlichiosis
HGV: hepatitis G virus
HHV: human herpes virus
HI: hemagglutination
          inhibition
Hib: *Haemophilus influenzae*,
          type b serovar
HIV: human immunodefi-
          ciency virus
HME: human monocytic
          ehrlichiosis
HPLC: high-pressure liquid
          chromatography
HPS: hantavirus pulmonary
          syndrome
HRF: homologous restriction
          factor (also histamine
          releasing factor)
HFRS: hemorrhagic fever with
          renal syndrome
hsp70:   heat shock protein 70
HSV: herpes simplex virus
HTLV: human T cell leukemia
          virus
HuCV: human calicivirus
HUS: hemolytic-uremic
          syndrome
HVG: host-versus-graft
          (reaction)

■ IB: initial body
IEP: immunoelectrophoresis
IFAT: indirect immunofluores-
          cent antibody test
IFN: interferon
Ig: immunoglobulin
IHA: indirect hemagglutina-
          tion
(I)IF: (indirect) immunofluor-
          escence
IL: interleukin
In: integron
INH: isoniazid (isonicotinic
          acid hydrazide)
IP_3:   inositol trisphosphate
IPV: inactivated polio vaccine
IR: inverted repeats
Ir genes: immune response genes
IS: insertion sequence/inter-
          cistron space

■ K cells: killer cells

■ L: light chain
LA: latex agglutination
lac operon: lactose operon
LAK: lymphokine-activated
          killer cells
LB: leprosy bacterium
LCA: leukocyte common
          antigen
LCM(V):   lymphocytic chorio-
          meningitis (virus)
LE: lupus erythematosus
LFA: lymphocyte function
          antigen
LGL: large granular
          lymphocyte
LIF: leukemia inhibitory
          factor
LL: lepromatous leprosy
LM: light microscopy
LMC: larva migrans cutanea

LMV: larva migrans visceralis
LOS: lipo-oligosaccharide
LPS: lipopolysaccharide
LT: heat-labile *E. coli* enterotoxin
LTR: long terminal repeats

■ MAC: membrane attack complex
MAF: macrophage activating factor
MALT: mucosa-associated lymphoid tissue
MBC: minimal bactericidal concentration
MBP: major basic protein/myelin basic protein
MCP: membrane cofactor protein
M-CSF: macrophage colony-stimulating factor
MF: merthiolate-formalin
Mf: microfilaria
MHC: major histocompatibility complex
MIC: minimal inhibitory concentration
MIF: migration inhibitory factor/microimmunefluorescence
MLC: mixed lymphocyte culture
MLR: mixed lymphocyte reaction
MMR: live, attenuated, trivalent measles, mumps, and rubella vaccine
MMTV: murine mammary tumor virus
MOMP: major outer membrane protein
MOTT: mycobacteria other than TB (see NTM)

MZM: marginal zone macrophages

■ NANB: nonA, nonB hepatitis
NCVP: noncapsidic viral protein
NE: *Nephropathica epidemica*
Nfa: nonfimbrial adhesin
NGU: nongonococcal urethritis
NIDEP: German study on assessment and prevention of nosocomial infections
NK cells: natural killer cells
NTM: nontuberculous (atypical) mycobateria (see MOTT)
NTR: nontranslated region

■ OC: open circular (DNA)
OM: opportunistic mycosis
OMP, Omp: outer membrane protein
OPV: oral polio vaccine
OSP, Osp: outer surface protein

■ P: promoter
PAE: postantibiotic effect
PAIR: puncture, aspiration, injection, respiration
PAS: para-aminosalicylic acid/periodic acid-Schiff stain
PAM: primary amebic meningoencephalitis
PAP: pyelonephritis-associated pili
PBL: peripheral blood lymphocytes
PC: phosphoryl choline/primary (tuberculous) complex, Ghon's complex
PCA: passive cutaneous anaphylaxis
PCR: polymerase chain reaction

PEG:	polyethylene glycol
PFC:	plaque-forming cell
PHA:	phytohemagglutinin
PI:	pathogenicity island
p.i.:	post infection
PIP_2:	phosphatidylinositol bisphosphate
PKC:	protein kinase C
PLC:	phospholipase C
PMA:	pokeweed mitogen
PML:	progressive multifocal leukoencephalopathy
PMN:	polymorphonuclear neu-trophilic granulocytes
PNP:	purine nucleoside phos-phorylase
PPD:	purified protein derivative
PRP:	polyribosylribitol phos-phate
PrP:	prion protein
Ptx:	pertussis toxin
PZA:	pyrazinamide
■ QBC:	quantitative buffy coat analysis
■ R:	rubella vaccine
RAST:	radioallergosorbent test
RES:	reticuloendothelial system
RF:	rheumatoid factor
RFFIT:	rapid fluorescent focus inhibition test
Rh antigen:	rhesus antigen
RIA:	radioimmunoassay
RIBA:	recombinant immuno-blot assay
RIG:	rabies immunoglobulin
RIST:	radioimmunosorbent test
RMP:	rifampicin
RMSF:	Rocky Mountain spotted fever

RNA:	ribonucleic acid
RNP:	ribonucleoprotein
RS:	respiratory syncytial virus
RT:	reverse transcriptase
RT-PCR:	reverse transcriptase-polymerase chain reaction
RTI:	respiratory tract infection
RVF:	Rift Valley fever
■ SAF:	sodium acetate-acetic acid-formalin
SALT:	skin-associated lymphoid tissue
SCF:	stem cell factor
SCID:	severe combined immuno-deficiency disease
SDS:	sodium (Na^+) dodecyl sulfate
SEA-E:	staphylococcal entero-toxins A-E
SEM:	scanning electron micro-scopy
SEP:	sepsis
SEPEC:	septic *E. coli* pathovar
SFT:	Sabin-Feldman test
SLE:	systemic lupus erythe-matosus
SPE:	streptococcal pyrogenic exotoxin
SRBC:	sheep red blood cells
SRSV:	small round-structured virus
ss:	single-stranded (nucleic acids)
SSME:	spring-summer meningo-encephalitis
SSPE:	subacute sclerosing panencephalitis
ST:	heat-stable *E. coli* entero-toxin

sp.:	species		Tra:	transfer
spp.:	species (plural)		TSE:	transmissible spongiform encephalopathy
SV:	simian virus			
SWI:	surgical wound infection		TSS:	toxic shock syndrome
			TSST-1:	toxic shock syndrome toxin-1
■ TATA:	tumor-associated transplantation antigen		TU:	tuberculin units
TB:	tuberculosis bacterium			
Tc:	cytotoxic T cell		■ UPEC:	uropathogenic *E. coli*
TCGF:	T cell growth factor		UTI:	urinary tract infection
TCP:	toxin coregulated pili			
TCR:	T cell receptor		■ VacA:	vacuolating cytotoxin
Td:	tetanus/low-dose diphtheria toxoids		var.:	variety
			VCA:	viral capsid antigen
T-dep:	thymus dependent antigens		VCAM:	vascular cell adhesion molecule
T-DTH:	delayed type hypersensitivity (T cells)		VDRL:	Venereal Disease Research Laboratory
TEM:	transmission electron microscopy		VLA:	very late antigen
			vmp:	variable major protein
Th, TH:	T helper cell		VPv:	viral protein
T-ind:	thymus-independent antigens		VPg:	genome-linked viral protein
TL:	tuberculoid leprosy		VSA:	variant surface antigen
TME:	transmissible mink encephalopathy		VSV:	vesicular stomatitis virus
			VTEC:	verocytotoxin-producing *E. coli*
Tn:	transposon			
TNF:	tumor necrosis factor		VZV:	varicella zoster virus
TPHA:	*Treponema pallidum* hemagglutination assay			
			■ WB:	Western blot
TPI test:	*Treponema pallidum* immobilization test		WHO:	World Health Organization
TPPA:	*Treponema pallidum* particle agglutination assay			

Contents

2   **Basic Principles of Immunology**   43
   R. M. Zinkernagel

II   Bacteriology

3   General Bacteriology
F. H. Kayser

4 Bacteria as Human Pathogens ▬▬▬▬▬▬▬▬▬▬ 229
F. H. Kayser

III Mycology

5 General Mycology 348
F. H. Kayser

6 Fungi as Human Pathogens 358
F. H. Kayser

IV   Virology

7   General Virology   376
K. A. Bienz

8 **Viruses as Human Pathogens** 412
K. A. Bienz

V Parasitology

11 Arthropods 606
J. Eckert

VI   Organ System Infections

12   Etiological and Laboratory Diagnostic Summaries in Tabular Form ▬▬▬▬ 630
F. H. Kayser, J. Eckert, K. A. Bienz

I
Basic Principles of
Medical Microbiologie
and Immunology

Dr. Karl Thomae GmbH

Macrophage hunting bacteria

1 General Aspects of Medical Microbiology

F. H. Kayser

■ Infectious diseases are caused by subcellular infectious entities (prions, viruses), prokaryotic bacteria, eukaryotic fungi and protozoans, metazoan animals, such as parasitic worms (helminths), and some arthropods. Definitive proof that one of these factors is the cause of a given infection is demonstrated by fulfillment of the three Henle-Koch postulates. For technical reasons, a number of infections cannot fulfill the postulates in their strictest sense as formulated by R. Koch, in these cases a modified form of the postulates is applied. ■

The History of Infectious Diseases

The Past

Infectious diseases have been known for thousands of years, although accurate information on their etiology has only been available for about a century. In the medical teachings of Hippocrates, the cause of infections occurring frequently in a certain locality or during a certain period (epidemics) was sought in "changes" in the air according to the theory of miasmas. This concept, still reflected in terms such as "swamp fever" or "malaria," was the predominant academic opinion until the end of the 19th century, despite the fact that the Dutch cloth merchant A. van Leeuwenhoek had seen and described bacteria as early as the 17th century, using a microscope he built himself with a single convex lens and a very short focal length. At the time, general acceptance of the notion of "spontaneous generation"—creation of life from dead organic material—stood in the way of implicating the bacteria found in the corpses of infection victims as the cause of the deadly diseases. It was not until Pasteur disproved the doctrine of spontaneous generation in the second half of the 19th century that a new way of thinking became possible. By the end of that century, microorganisms had been identified as the causal agents in many familiar diseases by applying the Henle-Koch postulates formulated by R. Koch in 1890.

The Henle–Koch Postulates

The postulates can be freely formulated as follows:

■ The microorganism must be found under conditions corresponding to the pathological changes and clinical course of the disease in question.

■ It must be possible to cause an identical (human) or similar (animal) disease with pure cultures of the pathogen.

■ The pathogen must not occur within the framework of other diseases as an "accidental parasite."

These postulates are still used today to confirm the cause of an infectious disease. However, the fact that these conditions are not met does not necessarily exclude a contribution to disease etiology by a pathogen found in context. In particular, many infections caused by subcellular entities do not fulfill the postulates in their classic form.

The Present

The frequency and deadliness of infectious diseases throughout thousands of years of human history have kept them at the focus of medical science. The development of effective preventive and therapeutic measures in recent decades has diminished, and sometimes eliminated entirely, the grim epidemics of smallpox, plague, spotted fever, diphtheria, and other such contagions. Today we have specific drug treatments for many infectious diseases. As a result of these developments, the attention of medical researchers was diverted to other fields: it seemed we had tamed the infectious diseases. Recent years have proved this assumption false. Previously unknown pathogens causing new diseases are being found and familiar organisms have demonstrated an ability to evolve new forms and reassert themselves. The origins of this reversal are many and complex: human behavior has changed, particularly in terms of mobility and nutrition. Further contributory factors were the introduction of invasive and aggressive medical therapies, neglect of established methods of infection control and, of course, the ability of pathogens to make full use of their specific genetic variability to adapt to changing conditions. The upshot is that physicians in particular, as well as other medical professionals and staff, urgently require a basic knowledge of the pathogens involved and the genesis of infectious diseases if they are to respond effectively to this dynamism in the field of infectiology. The aim of this textbook is to impart these essentials to them.

Table 1.**1** provides an overview of the causes of human infectious diseases.

Table 1.1 Human Pathogens

Subcellular biological entities	Prokaryotic microorganisms	Eukaryotic microorganisms	Animals
Prions (infection proteins)	Chlamydiae (0.3–1 μm)	Fungi (yeasts 5–10 μm, size of mold fungi indeterminable)	Helminths (parasitic worms)
Viruses (20–200 nm)	Rickettsiae (0.3–1 μm)	Protozoa (1–150 μm)	Arthropods
	Mycoplasmas		
	Classic bacteria (1–5 μm)		

Pathogens

Subcellular Infectious Entities

■ **Prions (proteinaceous infectious particles).** The evidence indicates that prions are protein molecules that cause degenerative central nervous system (CNS) diseases such as Creutzfeldt-Jakob disease, kuru, scrapie in sheep, and bovine spongiform encephalopathy (BSE) (general term: transmissible spongiform encephalopathies [TSE]).

Viruses. Ultramicroscopic, obligate intracellular parasites that:

— contain only one type of nucleic acid, either DNA or RNA,
— possess no enzymatic energy-producing system and no protein-synthesizing apparatus, and
— force infected host cells to synthesize virus particles.

Prokaryotic and Eukaryotic Microorganisms

According to a proposal by Woese that has been gaining general acceptance in recent years, the world of living things is classified in the three domains *bacteria*, *archaea*, and *eucarya*. In this system, each domain is subdivided into kingdoms. Pathogenic microorganisms are found in the domains bacteria and eucarya.

Bacteria, Archaea, Eucarya

Bacteria. This domain includes the kingdom of the heterotrophic eubacteria and includes all human pathogen bacteria. The other kingdoms, for instance that of the photosynthetic cyanobacteria, are not pathogenic. It is estimated that bacterial species on Earth number in the hundreds of thousands, of which only about 5500 have been discovered and described in detail.

Archaea. This domain includes forms that live under extreme environmental conditions, including thermophilic, hyperthermophilic, halophilic, and methanogenic microorganisms. The earlier term for the archaea was archaebacteria (ancient bacteria), and they are indeed a kind of living fossil. Thermophilic archaea thrive mainly in warm, moist biotopes such as the hot springs at the top of geothermal vents. The hyperthermophilic archaea, a more recent discovery, live near deep-sea volcanic plumes at temperatures exceeding 100 °C.

Eucarya. This domain includes all life forms with cells possessing a genuine nucleus. The plant and animal kingdoms (animales and plantales) are all eukaryotic life forms. Pathogenic eukaryotic microorganisms include fungal and protozoan species.

Table 1.2 lists the main differences between prokaryotic (bacteria and archaea) and eukaryotic pathogens.

Bacteria

■ **Classic bacteria.** These organisms reproduce asexually by binary transverse fission. They do not possess the nucleus typical of eucarya. The cell walls of these organisms are rigid (with some exceptions, e.g., the mycoplasma).

■ **Chlamydiae.** These organisms are obligate intracellular parasites that are able to reproduce in certain human cells only and are found in two stages: the infectious, nonreproductive particles called elementary bodies (0.3 µm) and the noninfectious, intracytoplasmic, reproductive forms known as initial (or reticulate) bodies (1 µm).

■ **Rickettsiae.** These organisms are obligate intracellular parasites, rod-shaped to coccoid, that reproduce by binary transverse fission. The diameter of the individual cell is from 0.3–1 µm.

Table 1.2 Characteristics of Prokaryotic (Eubacteria) and Eukaryotic (Fungi, Protozoans) Microorganisms

Characteristic	Prokaryotes (bacteria)	Eukaryotes (fungi, protozoans)
Nuclear structure	Circular DNA molecule not covered with proteins	Complex of DNA and basic proteins
Localization of nuclear structure	Dense tangle of DNA in cytoplasm; no nuclear membrane; nucleoid or nuclear equivalent	In nucleus surrounded by nuclear membrane
DNA	Nucleoid and plasmids	In nucleus and in mitochondria
Cytoplasm	No mitochondria and no endoplasmic reticulum, 70S ribosomes	Mitochondria and endoplasmic reticulum, 80S ribosomes
Cell wall	Usually rigid wall with murein layer; exception: mycoplasmas	Present only in fungi: glucans, mannans, chitin, chitosan, cellulose
Reproduction	Asexual, by binary transverse fission	In most cases sexual, possibly asexual

■ **Mycoplasmas.** Mycoplasmas are bacteria without rigid cell walls. They are found in a wide variety of forms, the most common being the coccoid cell (0.3–0.8 μm). Threadlike forms also occur in various lengths.

Fungi and Protozoa

■ **Fungi.** Fungi (*Mycophyta*) are nonmotile eukaryotes with rigid cell walls and a classic cell nucleus. They contain no photosynthetic pigments and are carbon heterotrophic, that is, they utilize various organic nutrient substrates (in contrast to carbon autotrophic plants). Of more than 50 000 fungal species, only about 300 are known to be human pathogens. Most fungal infections occur as a result of weakened host immune defenses.

■ **Protozoa.** Protozoa are microorganisms in various sizes and forms that may be free-living or parasitic. They possess a nucleus containing chromosomes and organelles such as mitochondria (lacking in some cases), an endoplasmic reticulum, pseudopods, flagella, cilia, kinetoplasts, etc. Many parasitic protozoa are transmitted by arthropods, whereby multiplication and transformation into the infectious stage take place in the vector.

Animals

■ **Helminths.** Parasitic worms belong to the animal kingdom. These are metazoan organisms with highly differentiated structures. Medically significant groups include the trematodes (flukes or flatworms), cestodes (tapeworms), and nematodes (roundworms).

■ **Arthropods.** These animals are characterized by an external chitin skeleton, segmented bodies, jointed legs, special mouthparts, and other specific features. Their role as direct causative agents of diseases is a minor one (mites, for instance, cause scabies) as compared to their role as vectors transmitting viruses, bacteria, protozoa, and helminths.

Host–Pathogen Interactions

■ The factors determining the genesis, clinical picture and outcome of an infection include complex relationships between the host and invading organisms that differ widely depending on the pathogen involved. Despite this variability, a number of general principles apply to the interactions between the invading pathogen with its aggression factors and the host with its defenses. Since the pathogenesis of bacterial infectious diseases has been researched very thoroughly, the following summary is based on the host–invader interactions seen in this type of infection.

The determinants of bacterial pathogenicity and virulence can be outlined as follows:

■ Adhesion to host cells (adhesins).

■ Breaching of host anatomical barriers (invasins) and colonization of tissues (aggressins).

■ Strategies to overcome nonspecific defenses, especially antiphagocytic mechanisms (impedins).

■ Strategies to overcome specific immunity, the most important of which is production of IgA proteases (impedins), molecular mimicry, and immunogen variability.

■ Damage to host tissues due to direct bacterial cytotoxicity, exotoxins, and exoenzymes (aggressins).

■ Damage due to inflammatory reactions in the macroorganism: activation of complement and phagocytosis; induction of cytokine production (modulins).

The above bacterial pathogenicity factors are confronted by the following host defense mechanisms:

■ Nonspecific defenses including mechanical, humoral, and cellular systems. Phagocytosis is the most important process in this context.

■ Specific immune responses based on antibodies and specific reactions of T lymphocytes (see chapter on immunology).

The response of these defenses to infection thus involves the correlation of a number of different mechanisms. Defective defenses make it easier for an infection to take hold. Primary, innate defects are rare, whereas acquired, secondary immune defects occur frequently, paving the way for infections by microorganisms known as "facultative pathogens" (opportunists). ■

Basic Terminology of Infectiology

Tables 1.**3** and 1.**4** list the most important infectiological terms together with brief explanations.

The terms **pathogenicity** and **virulence** are not clearly defined in their relevance to microorganisms. They are sometimes even used synonymously. It has been proposed that pathogenicity be used to characterize a particular species and that virulence be used to describe the sum of the disease-causing properties of a population (strain) of a pathogenic species (Fig. 1.**1**)

Pathogenicity and virulence in the microorganism correspond to **susceptibility** in a host species and **disposition** in a specific host organism, whereby an individual may be anywhere from highly disposed to resistant.

Determinants of Bacterial Pathogenicity and Virulence

Relatively little is known about the factors determining the pathogenicity and virulence of microorganisms, and most of what we do know concerns the disease-causing mechanisms of bacteria.

Table 1.3 Basic Infectiological Terminology I (Pathogen)

Term	Explanation
Saprophytes	These microorganisms are nonpathogenic; their natural habitat is dead organic matter
Parasites	Unicellular or metazoan organism living in or on an organism of another species (host) on the expense of the host
– Commensals	Normal inhabitants of skin and mucosa; the normal flora is thus the total commensal population (see Table 1.7, p. 25)
– Pathogenic microorganisms	Classic disease-causing pathogens
– Opportunists or facultatively pathogenic microorganisms	Can cause disease in immunocompromised individuals given an "opportune" situation; these are frequently germs of the normal flora or occasionally from the surrounding environment, animals, or other germ carriers
Pathogenicity	Capacity of a pathogen species to cause disease
Virulence	Sum of the disease-causing properties of a strain of a pathogenic species
Incubation period	Time between infection and manifestation of disease symptoms; this specific disease characteristic can be measured in hours, days, weeks, or even years
Prepatency	A parasitological term: time between infection and first appearance of products of sexual reproduction of the pathogen (e.g., worm eggs in stool of a host with helminthosis)
Infection spectrum	The totality of host species "susceptible" to infection by a given pathogen
Minimum infective dose	Smallest number of pathogens sufficient to cause an infection
Mode of infection	Method or pathway used by pathogen to invade host

Tab 1.4 Basic Infectiological Terminology II (Host)

Term	Explanation
Contamination	Microbiological presence of microorganisms on objects, in the environment, or in samples for analysis
Colonization	Presence of microorganisms on skin or mucosa; no penetration into tissues; typical of normal flora; pathogenic microorganisms occasionally also show colonization behavior
Infection	Invasion of a host organism by microorganisms, proliferation of the invading organisms, and host reaction
Inapparent (or subclinical) infection	Infection without outbreak of clinical symptoms
Infectious disease (or clinical infection)	Infection with outbreak of clinical symptoms
Probability of manifestation	Frequency of clinical manifestation of an infection in disposed individuals (%)
Endogenous infection	Infection arising from the colonizing flora
Exogenous infection	Infection arising from invasion of host by microorganisms from sources external to it
Nosocomial infection	Infection acquired during hospitalization (urinary tract infections, infections of the respiratory organs, wound infection, sepsis)
Local infection	Infection that remains restricted to the portal of entry and surrounding area
Generalized infection	Lymphogenous and/or hematogenous spread of invading pathogen starting from the portal of entry; infection of organs to which pathogen shows a specific affinity (organotropism); three stages: incubation, generalization, organ manifestation
Sepsis	Systemic disease caused by microorganisms and/or their toxic products; there is often a localized focus of infection from which pathogens or toxic products enter the bloodstream continuously or in intermittent phases
Transitory bacteremia/viremia/parasitemia	Brief presence of microorganisms in the bloodstream
Superinfection	Occurrence of a second infection in the course of a first infection
Relapses	Series of infections by the same pathogen
Reinfection	Series of infections by different pathogens

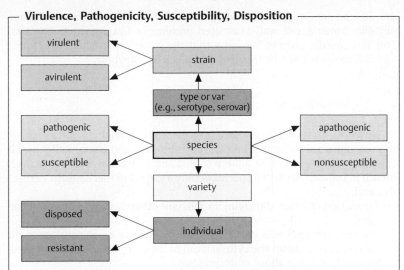

Virulence, Pathogenicity, Susceptibility, Disposition

Fig. 1.**1** Pathogenicity refers to pathogens, susceptibility to host species. The term virulence refers to individual strains of a pathogen species. The terms disposition and resistance are used to characterize the status of individuals of a susceptible host species.

There are five groups of potential bacterial contributors to the pathogenesis of infectious diseases:

1. **Adhesins.** They facilitate adhesion to specific target cells.
2. **Invasins.** They are responsible for active invasion of the cells of the macroorganism.
3. **Impedins.** These components disable host immune defenses in some cases.
4. **Aggressins.** These substances include toxins and tissue-damaging enzymes.
5. **Modulins.** Substances that induce excess cytokine production (i.e., lipopolysaccharides of Gram-negative bacteria, superantigens, murein fragments).

Adhesion

When pathogenic bacteria come into contact with intact human surface tissues (e.g., mucosa), they contrive to adhere to receptors on the surface of the target cells by means of various surface structures of their own (attachment pili, attachment fimbriae, adhesion proteins in the outer membrane of Gram-negative bacteria, cell wall-associated proteins in Gram-positive bacteria). This is a specific process, meaning that the adhesion structure (or ligand) and the receptor must fit together like a key in a keyhole.

Invasion and Spread

■ **Invasion.** Bacteria may invade a host passively through microtraumata or macrotraumata in the skin or mucosa. On the other hand, bacteria that invade through intact mucosa first adhere to this anatomical barrier, then actively breach it. Different bacterial species deploy a variety of mechanisms to reach this end:
— Production of tissue-damaging exoenzymes that destroy anatomical barriers.
— Parasite-directed endocytosis, initiated by invasins on the surface of the bacterial cells, causes the cytoskeleton of the epithelial cell to form pseudopods that bring about endocytosis.
— Phagocytosis of enteropathogenic bacteria by M cells in the intestinal mucosa (cells that can ingest substances from the intestinal lumen by way of phagocytosis).

■ **Spread.**
— Local tissue spread beginning at the portal of entry, helped along by tissue-damaging exoenzymes (hyaluronidase, collagenase, elastase, and other proteases).
— Cell-to-cell spread. Bacteria translocated into the intracellular space by endocytosis cause actin to condense into filaments, which then array at one end of the bacterium and push up against the inner side of the cell membrane. This is followed by fusion with the membrane of the neighboring tissue cell, whereupon the bacterium enters the new cell (typical of *Listeria* and *Shigella*).
— Translocation of macrophage-resistant bacteria with macrophages into intestinal lymphoid tissue following their ingestion by M cells.
— Lymphogenous or hematogenous generalization. The bacteria then invade organs for which they possess a specific tropism.

Strategies against Nonspecific Immunity

Establishment of a bacterial infection in a host presupposes the capacity of the invaders to overcome the host's nonspecific immune defenses. The most important mechanisms used by pathogenic bacteria are:

1

■ **Antiphagocytosis** (see also Fig. 1.**6**, p. 23).
- *Capsule*. Renders phagocytosis more difficult. Capsule components may block alternative activation of complement so that C3b is lacking (ligand for C3b receptor of phagocytes) on the surface of encapsulated bacteria. Microorganisms that use this strategy include *Streptococcus pneumoniae* and *Haemophilus influenzae*.
- *Phagocyte toxins*. Examples: leukocidin from staphylococci, streptolysin from streptococci.
- Macrophages may be disabled by the type III secretion system (see p. 17) of certain Gram-negative bacteria (for example salmonellae, shigellae, yersiniae, and coli bacteria). This system is used to inject toxic proteins into the macrophages.
- *Inhibition of phagosome-lysosome fusion*. Examples: tuberculosis bacteria, gonococci, *Chlamydia psittaci*.
- *Inhibition of the phagocytic "oxidative burst."* No formation of reactive O_2 radicals in phagocytes. Examples: *Legionella pneumophilia*, *Salmonella typhi*.

■ **Serum resistance.** Resistance of Gram-negative bacteria to complement. A lipopolysaccharide in the outer membrane is modified in such a way that it cannot initiate alternative activation of the complement system. As a result, the membrane attack complex (C5b6789), which would otherwise lyse holes in the outer membrane, is no longer produced (see p. 86ff.).

■ **Siderophores.** Siderophores (e.g., enterochelin, aerobactin) are low-molecular-weight iron-binding molecules that transport Fe^{3+} actively into the intracellular space. They complex with iron, thereby stealing this element from proteins containing iron (transferrin, lactoferrin). The intricate iron transport system is localized in the cytoplasmic membrane, and in Gram-negative bacteria in the outer membrane as well. To thrive, bacteria require 10^{-5} mol/l free iron ions. The free availability of only about 10^{-20} mol/l iron in human body fluids thus presents a challenge to them.

Strategies against Specific Immunity

■ **Immunotolerance.**
- *Prenatal infection*. At this stage of development, the immune system is unable to recognize bacterial immunogens as foreign.
- *Molecular mimicry*. Molecular mimicry refers to the presence of molecules on the surface of bacteria that are not recognized as foreign by the immune system. Examples of this strategy are the hyaluronic acid capsule of *Streptococcus pyogenes* or the neuraminic acid capsule of *Escherichia coli* K1 and serotype B *Neisseria meningitidis*.

1

Mechanism of Molecular Variation of Pilin in Gonococci

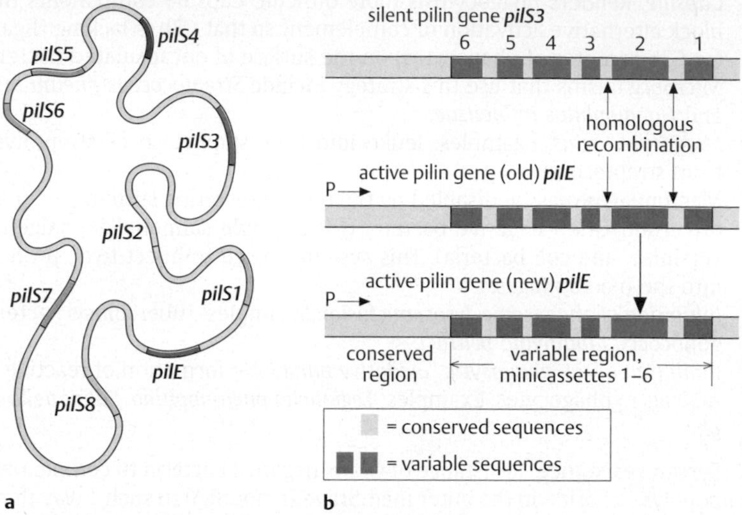

Fig. 1.2 The structural element of the attachment pili of gonococci is the polypeptide monomer pilin. Mucosal immunity to gonococci depends on antibodies in the secretions of the urogenital mucosa that attach to the immunodominant segment of the pilin, thus blocking adhesion of gonococci to the target cells.

a Model of the gonococcal genome. The primary structure of the pilin is determined by the expressed gene *pilE*. The gonococcal genome has many other *pil* genes besides the *pilE* without promoters, i.e., "silent" genes that are not transcribed (*pilS1, pilS2, pilS3*, etc.).

b *pil* genes have both a conserved and a variable region. The variable region of all *pil* genes has a mosaic structure, i.e., it consists of minicassettes. Minicassette 2 codes for the most important immunodominant segment of the pilin. Intracellular homologous recombination of conserved regions of silent *pil* genes and corresponding sequences of the expressed gene results in *pilE* genes with changed cassettes. These code for a pilin with a changed immunodominant segment. Therefore, antibodies to the "old" pilin can no longer bind to the "new" pilin.

■ **Antigen variation.** Some bacteria are characterized by a pronounced variability of their immunogens (= immune antigens) due to the genetic variability of the structural genes coding the antigen proteins. This results in production of a series of antigen variants in the course of an infection that no longer "match" with the antibodies to the "old" antigen. Examples: gonococci can modify the primary structure of the pilin of their attachment pili at a high rate (Fig. 1.**2**). The borreliae that cause relapsing fevers have the capacity to change the structure of one of the adhesion proteins in their outer membrane (vmp = variable major protein), resulting in the typical "recurrences" of fever. Similarly, meningococci can change the chemistry of their capsule polysaccharides ("capsule switching").

■ **IgA proteases.** Mucosal secretions contain the secretory antibodies of the $sIgA_1$ class responsible for the specific local immunity of the mucosa. Classic mucosal parasites such as gonococci, meningococci and *Haemophilus influenzae* produce proteases that destroy this immunoglobulin.

Clinical Disease

The clinical symptoms of a bacterial infection arise from the effects of damaging noxae produced by the bacteria as well as from excessive host immune responses, both nonspecific and specific. Immune reactions can thus potentially damage the host's health as well as protect it (see Immunology, p. 103ff.).

■ **Cytopathic effect.** Obligate intracellular parasites (rickettsiae, chlamydiae) may kill the invaded host cells when they reproduce.

■ **Exotoxins.** Pathogenic bacteria can produce a variety of toxins that are either the only pathogenic factor (e.g., in diphtheria, cholera, and tetanus) or at least a major factor in the unfolding of the disease. One aspect the classification and nomenclature of these toxins must reflect is the type of cell affected: **cytotoxins** produce toxic effects in many different host cells; **neurotoxins** affect the neurons; **enterotoxins** affect enterocytes. The structures and mechanisms of action of the toxins are also considered in their classification (Table 1.**5**):

— *AB toxins.* They consist of a binding subunit "B" responsible for binding to specific surface receptors on target host cells, and a catalytic subunit "A" representing the active agent. Only cells presenting the "B" receptors are damaged by these toxins.

— *Membrane toxins.* These toxins disrupt biological membranes, either by attaching to them and assembling to form pores, or in the form of phospholipases that destroy membrane structure enzymatically.

— *Superantigens* (see p. 72). These antigens stimulate T lymphocytes and macrophages to produce excessive amounts of harmful cytokines.

■ **Hydrolytic exoenzymes.** Proteases (e.g., collagenase, elastase, nonspecific proteases), hyaluronidase, neuraminidase (synonymous with sialidase), lecithinase and DNases contribute at varying levels to the pathogenesis of an infection.

Table 1.**5**   Examples of Bacterial Toxins; Mechanisms of Action and Contribution to Clinical Picture

Toxin	Cell specificity	Molecular effect	Contribution to clinical picture
AB toxins			
Diphtheria toxin (*Corynebacterium diphtheriae*)	Many different cell types	ADP-ribosyl transferase. Inactivation of ribosomal elongation factor eEF2 resulting from ADP-ribosylation during protein synthesis; leads to cell death.	Death of mucosal cells. Damage to heart musculature, kidneys, adrenal glands, liver, motor nerves of the head.
Cholera toxin (*Vibrio cholerae*)	Enterocytes	ADP-ribosyl transferase. ADP-ribosylation of regulatory protein G_s of adenylate cyclase, resulting in permanent activation of this enzyme and increased levels of cAMP (second messenger) (see Fig. 4.**20**, p. 298). Result: increased secretion of electrolytes.	Massive watery diarrhea; severe loss of electrolytes and water.
Tetanus toxin (*Clostridium tetani*)	Neurons (synapses)	Metalloprotease. Proteolytic cleavage of protein components from the neuroexocytosis apparatus in the synapses of the anterior horn that normally transmit inhibiting impulses to the motor nerve terminal.	Increased muscle tone; cramps in striated musculature.
Membrane toxins			
Alpha toxin (*Clostridium perfringens*)	Many different cell types	Phospholipase.	Cytolysis, resulting tissue damage.
Lysteriolysin (*Listeria monocytogenes*)	Many different cell types	Pore formation in membranes.	Destruction of phagosome membrane; intracellular release of phagocytosed listeriae.

Table 1.**5** *Continued: Examples of Bacterial Toxins*

Toxin	Cell specificity	Molecular effect	Contribution to clinical picture
Superantigen toxins			
Toxic shock syndrome toxin-1 (TSST-1) (*Staphylococcus aureus*)	T lymphocytes; macrophages	Stimulation of secretion of cytokines in T cells and macrophages.	Fever; exanthem; hypotension.

■ **Secretion of virulence proteins.** Proteins are synthesized at the ribosomes in the bacterial cytoplasm. They must then be secreted through the cytoplasmic membrane, and in Gram-negative bacteria through the outer membrane as well. The secretion process is implemented by complex protein secretion systems (I-IV) with differing compositions and functional pathways. The type III (virulence-related) secretion system in certain Gram-negative bacteria (*Salmonella, Shigella, Yersinia, Bordetella, Escherichia coli, Chlamydia*) is particularly important in this connection (see Fig. 1.**3**).

Needle Complex of Type III Secretion System

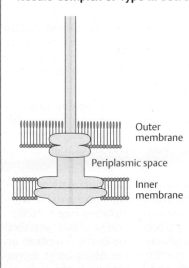

Outer membrane

Periplasmic space

Inner membrane

Fig. 1.**3** When certain Gram-negative rod bacteria make contact with eukaryotic target cells, a sensor molecule interacts with a receptor on the target cells. This interaction results in the opening of a secretion channel of the so-called "needle complex" (extending through both the cytoplasmic membrane and outer membrane) and in formation of a pore in the membrane of the target cell. Through the pore and channel, cytotoxic molecules are then translocated into the cytosol of the target cell where they, for example, inhibit phagocytosis and cytokine production (in macrophages), destroy the cytoskeleton of the target cell, and generally work to induce apoptosis.

■ **Cell wall.** The endotoxin of Gram-negative bacteria (lipopolysaccharide) plays an important role in the manifestation of clinical symptoms. On the one hand, it can activate complement by the alternative pathway and, by releasing the chemotactic components C3a and C5a, initiate an inflammatory reaction at the infection site. On the other hand, it also stimulates macrophages to produce endogenous pyrogens (interleukin 1, tumor necrosis factor), thus inducing fever centrally. Production of these and other cytokines is increased, resulting in hypotension, intravasal coagulation, thrombocyte aggregation and stimulation of granulopoiesis. Increased production of cytokines by macrophages is also induced by soluble murein fragments and, in the case of Gram-positive bacteria, by teichoic acids.

■ **Inflammation.** Inflammation results from the combined effects of the nonspecific and specific immune responses of the host organism. Activation of complement by way of both the classic and alternative pathways induces phagocyte migration to the infection site. Purulent tissue necrosis follows. The development of typical granulomas and caseous necrosis in the course of tuberculosis are the results of excessive reaction by the cellular immune system to the immunogens of tuberculosis bacteria. Textbooks of general pathology should be consulted for detailed descriptions of these inflammatory processes.

Regulation of Bacterial Virulence

Many pathogenic bacteria are capable of living either outside or inside a host and of attacking a variety of host species. Proliferation in these differing environments demands an efficient regulation of virulence, the aim being to have virulence factors available as required. Four different regulatory mechanisms have been described:

■ **DNA changes.** The nucleotide sequences of virulence determinants are changed. Examples of this include pilin gene variability involving intracellular recombination as described above in gonococci and inverting a leader sequence to switch genes on and off in the phase variations of H antigens in salmonellae (see p. 284).

■ **Transcriptional regulation.** The principle of transcriptional control of virulence determinants is essentially the same as that applying to the regulation of metabolic genes, namely repression and activation (see p. 169f.):
— *Simple regulation.* Regulation of the diphtheria toxin gene has been thoroughly researched. A specific concentration of iron in the cytoplasm activates the diphtheria toxin regulator (DtxR). The resulting active repressor prevents transcription of the toxin gene by binding to the promoter

region. Other virulence genes can also be activated by regulators using this mechanism.

— *Complex regulation, virulence regulon*. In many cases, several virulence genes are switched on and off by the same regulator protein. The virulence determinants involved are either components of the same operon or are located at different genome sites. Several vir (virulence) genes with promoter regions that respond to the same regulator protein form a so-called vir regulon. Regulation of the virulence regulon of *Bordetella pertussis* by means of gene activation is a case in point that has been studied in great detail. This particular regulon comprises over 20 virulence determinants, all controlled by the same vir regulator protein (or BvgA coding region) (Fig. 1.**4**).

■ **Posttranscriptional regulation.** This term refers to regulation by mRNA or a posttranslational protein modification.

■ **Quorum sensing.** This term refers to determination of gene expression by bacterial cell density (Fig. 1.**5**). Quorum sensing is observed in both

Regulation of Bacterial Virulence: Two-Component Regulator System

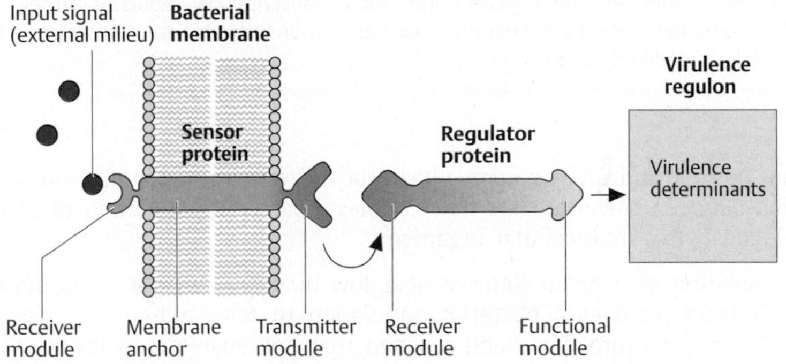

Fig. 1.4 A sensor protein integrated in the cytoplasmic membrane receives signals from a receiver module extending into the external milieu, activating the transmitter module. These signals from the external milieu can carry a wide variety of information: pH, temperature, osmolarity, Ca^{2+}, CO_2, stationary-phase growth, hunger stress, etc. The transmitter module effects a change in the receiver module of the regulator protein, switching the functional module of the regulator to active status, in which it can then repress or activate the various virulence determinants of a virulence regulon by binding to the different promoter regions. Phosphorylation is commonly used to activate the corresponding sensor and regulator modules.

1

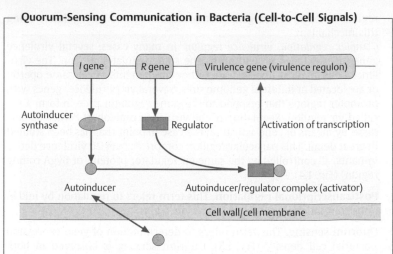

Quorum-Sensing Communication in Bacteria (Cell-to-Cell Signals)

Fig. 1.5 Cell-to-cell signaling is made possible by activation of two genes. The *I* gene codes for the synthase responsible for synthesis of the autoinducer. The autoinducer (often an *N*-acyl homoserine lactone) can diffuse freely through the cell membrane. The *R* gene codes for a transcriptional regulator protein that combines with the autoinducer to become an activator for transcription of various virulence genes.

Gram-positive and Gram-negative bacteria. It denotes a mode of communication between bacterial cells that enables a bacterial population to react analogously to a multicellular organism.

Accumulation of a given density of a low-molecular-weight pheromone (autoinducer) enables a bacterial population to sense when the critical cell density (quorum) has been reached that will enable it to invade the host successfully, at which point transcription of virulence determinants is initiated.

The Genetics of Bacterial Pathogenicity

The virulence genes of pathogenic bacteria are frequently components of mobile genetic elements such as plasmids, bacteriophage genomes, or conjugative transposons (see p. 170ff.). This makes lateral transfer of these genes between bacterial cells possible. Regions showing a high frequency of virulence genes in a bacterial chromosome are called pathogenicity islands (PI).

PIs are found in both Gram-positive and Gram-negative bacteria. These are DNA regions up to 200 kb that often bear several different vir genes and have specific sequences located at their ends (e.g., IS elements) that facilitate lateral translocation of the islands between bacterial cells. The role played by lateral transfer of these islands in the evolutionary process is further underlined by the fact that the GC contents in PIs often differ from those in chromosomal DNA.

Defenses against Infection

A macroorganism manifests defensive reactions against invasion by microorganisms in two forms: as **specific, acquired immunity** and as **nonspecific, innate resistance** (see also Chapter 2, Basic Principles of Immunology, p. 43).

Nonspecific Defense Mechanisms

Table 1.**6** lists the most important mechanisms.

■ **Primary defenses.** The main factors in the first line of defense against infection are mechanical, accompanied by some humoral and cellular factors. These defenses represent an attempt on the part of the host organism to prevent microorganisms from colonizing its skin and mucosa and thus stave off a generalized invasion.

■ **Secondary defenses.** The second line of defense consists of humoral and cellular factors in the blood and tissues, the most important of which are the professional phagocytes.

■ **Phagocytosis.** "Professional" phagocytosis is realized by polymorphonuclear, neutrophilic, eosinophilic granulocytes—also known as microphages— and by mononuclear phagocytes (macrophages). The latter also play an important role in antigen presentation (see p. 62). The total microphage cell count in an adult is approximately 2.5×10^{12}. Only 5% of these cells are located in the blood. They are characterized by a half-life of only a few hours. Microphages contain both primary granules, which are lysosomes containing lysosomal enzymes and cationic peptides, and secondary granules. Both microphages and macrophages are capable of ameboid motility and chemotactic migration, i.e., directed movement along a concentration gradient toward a source of chemotactic substances, in most cases the complement components C3a and C5a. Other potentially chemotactic substances include secretory products of lymphocytes, products of infected and damaged cells or the N-formyl peptides (fMet-Phe and fMet-Leu-Phe).

Table **1.6** The Most Important Mechanisms in Nonspecific Defenses Against Infection

a Mechanical factors

Anatomical structure of skin and mucosa

Mucus secretion and mucus flow from mucosa

Mucociliary movement of the ciliated epithelium in the lower respiratory tract

Digestive tract peristalsis

Urine flow in the urogenital tract

b Humoral factors

Microbicidal effect of the dermal acidic mantle, lactic acid from sweat glands, hydrochloric acid in the stomach, and the unsaturated fatty acids secreted by the sebaceous glands

Lysozyme in saliva and tear fluid: splitting of bacterial murein

Complement (alternative activation pathway)

Serum proteins known as acute phase reactants, for example C-reactive protein, haptoglobin, serum amyloid A, fibrinogen, and transferrin (iron-binding protein)

Fibronectin (a nonspecific opsonin); antiviral interferon

Mannose-binding protein: binds to mannose on the outer bacterial surface, thus altering the configuration and triggering alternative activation of complement

c Cellular factors

Normal flora of skin and mucosa

Natural killer cells (large, granulated lymphocytes; null cells)

Professional phagocytes: microphages (neutrophilic and eosinophilic granulocytes); mononuclear phagocytes (macrophages, monocytes, etc.)

Phagocytes are capable of ingestion of both particulate matter (phagocytosis) and solute matter (pinocytosis). Receptors on the phagocyte membrane initiate contact (Fig. 1.**6**). Particles adhering to the membrane are engulfed, ingested and deposited in a membrane-bound vacuole, the so-called phagosome, which then fuses with lysosomes to form the phagolysosome. The bacteria are killed by a combination of lysosomal factors:

— *Mechanisms that require no oxygen.* Low pH; acid hydrolases, lysozyme; proteases; defensins (small cationic peptides).

Phagocytosis of Bacteria

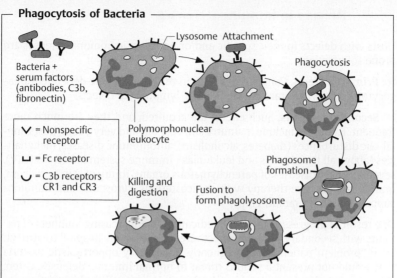

Bacteria +
serum factors
(antibodies, C3b,
fibronectin)

Lysosome Attachment

Phagocytosis

∨ = Nonspecific
    receptor

⊔ = Fc receptor

∪ = C3b receptors
    CR1 and CR3

Polymorphonuclear
leukocyte

Killing and
digestion

Fusion to
form phagolysosome

Phagosome
formation

Fig. 1.6   Encapsulated bacteria can only be effectively phagocytosed if IgG-class antibodies (Fc ligand) or the complement component C3b, or both, are located on their surfaces. The Fc and C3b ligands bind to their specific receptors on the phagocyte surface.

— *Mechanisms that require oxygen.* Halogenation of essential bacterial components by the myeloperoxidase-H_2O_2–halide system; production of highly reactive O_2 radicals (oxidative burst) such as superoxide anion (O_2^-), hydroxyl radical (•OH), and singlet oxygen ($^1O_2$).

Specific Defense Mechanisms

Specific immunity, based on antibodies and specifically reactive T lymphocytes, is acquired in a process of immune system stimulation by the corresponding microbial antigens. Humoral immunity is based on antitoxins, opsonins, microbicidal antibodies, neutralizing antibodies, etc. Cellular immunity is based on cytotoxic T lymphocytes (T killer cells) and T helper cells. See Chapter 2 on the principles of specific immunity.

Defects in Immune Defenses

Hosts with defects in their specific and/or nonspecific immune defenses are prone to infection.

■ **Primary defects.** Congenital defects in the complement-dependent phagocytosis system are rare, as are B and T lymphocyte defects.

■ **Secondary defects.** Such effects are acquired, and they are much more frequent. Examples include malnutrition, very old and very young hosts, metabolic disturbances (diabetes, alcoholism), autoimmune diseases, malignancies (above all lymphomas and leukemias), immune system infections (HIV), severe primary diseases of parenchymatous organs, injury of skin or mucosa, immunosuppressive therapy with corticosteroids, cytostatics and immunosuppressants, and radiotherapy.

One result of progress in modern medicine is that increasing numbers of patients with secondary immune defects are now receiving hospital treatment. Such "problem patients" are frequently infected by opportunistic bacteria that would not present a serious threat to normal immune defenses. Often, the pathogens involved ("problem bacteria") have developed a resistance to numerous antibiotics, resulting in difficult courses of antibiotic treatment in this patient category.

Normal Flora

Commensals (see Table 1.**3**, p. 9) are regularly found in certain human microbiotopes. The normal human microflora is thus the totality of these commensals. Table 1.**7** lists the most important microorganisms of the normal flora with their localizations.

Bacteria are the predominant component of the normal flora. They proliferate in varied profusion on the mucosa and most particularly in the gastrointestinal tract, where over 400 different species have been counted to date. The count of bacteria per gram of intestinal content is 10^1–10^5 in the duodenum, 10^3–10^7 in the small intestine, and 10^{10}–10^{12} in the colon. Over 99% of the normal mucosal flora are obligate anaerobes, dominated by the Gram-neg. anaerobes. Although life is possible without normal flora (e.g., pathogen-free experimental animals), commensals certainly benefit their hosts. One way they do so is when organisms of the normal flora manage to penetrate into the host through microtraumas, resulting in a continuous **stimulation of the immune system**. Commensals also compete for living space with overtly pathogenic species, a function known as **colo-**

Table 1.7 Normal Microbial Flora in Humans

Microorganisms	Microbiotopes				
	Skin	Oral cavity	Intes- tine	Upper re- spiratory tract	Genital tract
Staphylococci	+++	+	+	++	++
Enterococci			++		+
α-hemolytic streptococci	+	+++	+	+	+
Anaerobic cocci		+	+		+
Pneumococci		+		+	
Apathogenic neisseriae		+		+	+
Apathogenic corynebacteria	++	+	+	+	+
Aerobic spore-forming bacteria	(+)				
Clostridia			+++		(+)
Actinomycetes		+++			+
Enterobacteriaceae	(+)	(+)	+++	(+)	+
Pseudomonas			+		
Haemophilus		+		++	(+)
Gram-neg. anaerobes		+++	+++	+++	+++
Spirochetes		++		+	(+)
Mycoplasmas		++	+	+	++
Fungi (yeast)	++	+	+	+	+
Entamoeba, Giardia, Trichomonas		+		+	

+++ = numerous, ++ = frequent, + = moderately frequent, (+) = occasional occurrence

nization resistance. On the other hand, a potentially harmful effect of the normal flora is that they can also cause infections in immunocompromised individuals.

General Epidemiology

■ Within the context of medical microbiology, epidemiology is the study of the occurrence, causality, and prevention of infectious diseases in the populace. Infectious diseases occur either sporadically, in epidemics or pandemics, or in endemic forms, depending on the time and place of their occurrence. The frequency of their occurrence (morbidity) is described as their *incidence* and *prevalence*. The term *mortality* is used to describe how many deaths are caused by a given disease in a given population. *Lethality* is a measure of how life-threatening an infection is. The most important sources of infection are infected persons and carriers. Pathogens are transmitted from these sources to susceptible persons either directly (person-to-person) or indirectly via inert objects or biological vectors. Control of infectious diseases within a populace must be supported by effective legislation that regulates mandatory reporting where required. Further measures must be implemented to prevent exposure, for example isolation, quarantine, disinfection, sterilization, use of insecticides, and dispositional prophylaxis (active and passive immunization, chemoprophylaxis). ∎

Epidemiological Terminology

Epidemiology investigates the distribution of diseases, their physiological variables and social consequences in human populations, and the factors that influence disease distribution (World Health Organization [WHO] definition). The field covered by this discipline can thus be defined as medical problems involving large collectives. The rule of thumb on infectious diseases is that their characteristic spread depends on the virulence of the pathogen involved, the susceptibility of the threatened host species population, and environmental factors. Table 1.**8** provides brief definitions of the most important epidemiological terms.

Transmission, Sources of Infection

Transmission

Pathogens can be transmitted from a source of infection by direct contact or indirectly. Table 1.**9** lists the different direct and indirect transmission pathways of pathogenic microorganisms.

Person-to-person transmission constitutes a **homologous chain of infection**. The infections involved are called **anthroponoses**. In cases in which the pathogen is transmitted to humans from other vertebrates (and occasionally the other way around) we have a **heterologous chain of infection** and the infections are known as **zoonoses** (WHO definition) (Table 1.**10**).

Table 1.8 Epidemiological Terminology

Term	Definition
Sporadic occurrence	Isolated occurrence of an infectious disease with no apparent connections between localities or times of occurrence
Endemic occurrence	Regular and continuing occurrence of infectious diseases in populations with no time limit
Epidemic occurrence	Significantly increased occurrence of an infectious disease within given localities and time periods
Pandemic occurrence	Significantly increased occurrence of an infectious disease within a given time period but without restriction to given localities
Morbidity	Number of cases of a disease within a given population (e.g., per 1000, 10 000 or 100 000 inhabitants)
Incidence	Number of new cases of a disease within a given time period
Prevalence	Number of cases of a disease at a given point in time (sampling date)
Mortality	Number of deaths due to a disease within a given population
Lethality	Number of deaths due to a disease in relation to total number of cases of the disease
Manifestation index	Number of manifest cases of a disease in relation to number of infections
Incubation period	Time from infection until occurrence of initial disease symptoms
Prepatency	Time between infection and first appearance of products of sexual reproduction of the pathogen (e.g., worm eggs in stool)

Tab. 1.**9** Transmission Pathways of Pathogenic Microorganisms

Direct transmission	Indirect transmission
Fecal-oral (smear infection)	Transmission via food
Aerogenic transmission (droplet infection)	Transmission via drinking water
Genital transmission (during sexual intercourse)	Transmission via contaminated inanimate objects or liquids
Transmission via skin (rare)	Transmission via vectors (arthropods)
Diaplacental transmission	Transmission via other persons (e.g., via the hands of hospital medical staff)
Perinatal transmission (in the course of birth)	

Tab. 1.**10** Examples of Zoonoses Caused by Viruses, Bacteria, Protozoans, Helminths, and Arthropods

Zoonoses	Pathogen	Reservoir hosts	Transmission
Viral zoonoses			
Rabies	*Rhabdoviridae*	Numerous animal species	Bite of diseased animals
Tickborne encephalitis (TBE)	*Flaviviridae*	Wild animals	Ticks
Bacterial zoonoses			
Brucellosis	*Brucella* spp.	Cattle, pig, goat, sheep, (dog)	Contact with tissues or secretions from diseased animals; milk and dairy products
Lyme disease	*Borrelia burgdorferi*	Wild rodents; red deer, roe deer	Ticks
Plague	*Yersinia pestis*	Rodents	Contact with diseased animals; bite of rat flea
Q fever	*Coxiella burnetii*	Sheep, goat, cattle	Dust; possibly milk or dairy products
Enteric salmonellosis	*Salmonella enterica* (enteric serovars)	Pig, cattle, poultry	Meat, milk, eggs

Tab. 1.**10** *Continued: Examples of Zoonoses*

Zoonoses	Pathogen	Reservoir hosts	Transmission
Protozoan zoonoses			
Toxoplasmosis	*Toxoplasma gondii*	Domestic cat, sheep, pigs, other slaughter animals	Postnatal toxoplasmosis: oral; prenatal toxoplasmosis: diaplacental
Cryptosporidiosis	*Cryptosporidium hominis*; *C. parvum*	Cattle (calves), domestic animals	Ingestion of oocysts
Helminthic zoonoses			
Echinococcosis	*Echinococcus granulosus, Echinococcus multilocularis*	Dog, wild canines, fox	Ingestion of eggs
Taeniosis	*Taenia saginata, Taenia solium, Taenia asiatica*	Cattle, buffalo, pigs Pigs, cattle, goat	Ingestion of metacestodes with meat
Zoonoses caused by arthropods			
Pseudo scabies	*Sarcoptes* spp.; mite species from domestic animals	Dog, cat, guinea pig, domestic ruminants, pig	Contact with diseased animals

Other Zoonoses

(For details see the corresponding chapters)

Viral zoonoses	Hantavirus and other bunyavirus infections; infections by alphavirus, flavivirus, and arenavirus.
Bacterial zoonoses	Ehrlichiosis; erysipeloid; campylobacteriosis; cat scratch disease; leptospirosis; anthrax; ornithosis; rat-bite fever; rickettsioses (variety of types); tularemia; gastroenteritis caused by *Vibrio parahaemolyticus*; gastroenteritis caused by *Yersinia enterocolitica*.
Protozoan zoonoses	African trypanosomosis (sleeping sickness); American trypanosomosis (Chagas disease); babesiosis; balantidosis; cryptosporidosis; giardiosis; leishmaniosis; microsporidosis; sarcocystosis; toxoplasmosis. ▶

■ *Continued:* **Other Zoonoses** ■

Helminthic zoonoses	Cercarial dermatitis; clonorchiosis; cysticercosis; dicrocoeliosis; diphyllobothriosis; echinococcosis; fasciolosis; hymenolepiosis; larva migrans interna; opisthorchiosis; paragonimosis; schistosomosis (bilharziosis); taeniosis; toxocariosis; trichinellosis.
Zoonoses caused by arthropods	Flea infestation; larva migrans externa; mite infestation; sand flea infestation.

Sources of Infection

Every infection has a source (Table 1.**11**). The **primary source of infection** is defined as the location at which the pathogen is present and reproduces. **Secondary sources of infection** are inanimate objects, materials, or third persons contributing to transmission of pathogens from the primary source to disposed persons.

Table 1.**11**   Primary Sources of Infection

Source of infection	Explanation
Infected person	The most important source; as a rule, pathogens are excreted by the organ system through which the infection entered; there are some exceptions
Carriers during incubation	Excretion during incubation period; typical of many viral diseases
Carriers in convalescence	Excretion after the disease has been overcome; typical of enteric salmonelloses
Chronic carriers	Continued excretion for three or more months (even years) after disease has been overcome; typical of typhoid fever
Asymptomatic carriers	They carry pathogenic germs on skin or mucosa without developing "infection"
Animal carriers	Diseased or healthy animals that excrete pathogenic germs
Environment	Soil, plants, water; primary source of microorganisms with natural habitat in these biotopes

The Fight against Infectious Diseases

Legislation

Confronting and preventing infectious diseases can sometimes involve substantial incursions into the private sphere of those involved as well as economic consequences. For these reasons, such measures must be based on effective disease control legislation. In principle, these laws are similar in most countries, although the details vary.

The centerpiece of every disease prevention system is provision for reporting outbreaks. Basically, reporting is initiated at the periphery (individual patients) and moves toward the center of the system. Urgency level classifications of infections and laboratory findings are decided on by regional health centers, which are in turn required to report some diseases to the WHO to obtain a global picture within the shortest possible time.

Concrete countermeasures in the face of an epidemic take the form of prophylactic measures aimed at interrupting the chain of infection.

Exposure Prophylaxis

Exposure prophylaxis begins with *isolation* of the source of infection, in particular of infected persons, as required for the disease at hand. *Quarantine* refers to a special form of isolation of healthy first-degree contact persons. These are persons who have been in contact with a source of infection. The quarantine period is equivalent to the incubation period of the infectious disease in question (see International Health Regulations, www.who.int/en/).

Further measures of exposure prophylaxis include *disinfection* and *sterilization*, use of insecticides and pesticides, and eradication of animal carriers.

Immunization Prophylaxis

Active immunization. In active immunization, the immune system is stimulated by administration of vaccines to develop a disease-specific immunity. Table 1.**12** lists the vaccine groups used in active immunization. Table 1.**13** shows as an example the vaccination schedule recommended by the Advisory Committee on Immunization Practices of the USA (www.cdc.gov/nip). Recommended adult immunization schedules by age group and by medical conditions are also available in the National Immunization Program Website mentioned above. The vaccination calendars used in other countries deviate from these proposals in some details. For instance, routine varicella and

Table 1.**12**   Vaccine Groups Used in Active Immunization

Vaccine group	Remarks
Killed pathogens	Vaccination protection often not optimum, vaccination has to be repeated several times
Living pathogens with reduced virulence (attenuated)	Optimum vaccination protection; a single application often suffices, since the microorganisms reproduce in the vaccinated person, providing very good stimulation of the immune system; do not use in immunocompromised persons and during pregnancy (some exceptions)
Purified microbial immunogens	
– Proteins	Often recombinant antigens, i.e., genetically engineered proteins; well-known example: hepatitis B surface (HBs) antigen
– Polysaccharides	Chemically purified capsular polysaccharides of pneumococci, meningococci, and *Haemophilus influenzae* serotype b; problem: these are T cell-independent antigens that do not stimulate antibody production in children younger than two years of age
– Conjugate vaccines	Coupling of bacterial capsular polysaccharide epitopes to proteins, e.g., to tetanus toxoid, diphtheria toxoid, or proteins of the outer membranes of meningococci; children between the ages of two months and two years can also be vaccinated against polysaccharide epitopes
Toxoids	Bacterial toxins detoxified by formaldehyde treatment that still retain their immunogen function
Experimental vaccines	DNA vaccines. Purified DNA that codes for the viral antigens (proteins) and is integrated in plasmid DNA or nonreplicating viral vector DNA. The vector must have genetic elements—for example a transcriptional promoter and RNA-processing elements—that enable expression of the insert in the cells of various tissues (epidermis, muscle cells)
	Anti-idiotype-specific monoclonal antibodies
	Vaccinia viruses as carriers of foreign genes that code for immunogens

Table 1.**13** Recommended Childhood and Adolescent Immunization Schedule—
United States, 2004

1. Hepatitis B vaccine (HepB).
   Infants born to HBs-Ag-positive mothers should receive HepB and 0.5 ml HepB
   Immune Globulin within 12 h of birth at separate sites.

2. Diphtheria (D) and tetanus (T) toxoids and acellular pertussis (aP) vaccine (DTaP).
   The term "d" refers to a reduced dose of diphtheria toxoid.

3. Haemophilus influenzae type b conjugate vaccine (see Table 1.**12**).

4. Measles, mumps, and rubella vaccine (MMR).
   Attenuated virus strains.

5. Varicella vaccine.
   Varicella vaccine is recommended for children who lack a reliable history of
   chickenpox.

6. Pneumococcal vaccine.
   The heptavalent conjugate vaccine (PCV) is recommended for all children age
   2–23 months. Pneumococcal polysaccharide vaccine (PPV) can be used in elder
   children.

7. Hepatitis A vaccine.
   The "killed virus vaccine" is recommended in selected regions and for certain
   high-risk groups. Two doses should be administered at least six months apart.

8. Influenza vaccine.
   Influenza vaccine is recommended annually for children with certain risk factors
   (for instance asthma, cardiac disease, sickle cell disease, HIV, diabetes etc.). Children aged ≤ eight years who are receiving influenza vaccine for the first time
   should receive two doses separated at least four weeks.

Vaccine ▾ Age ▶	Birth	1 mo	2 mo	4 mo	6 mo	12 mo	15 mo	18 mo	24 mo	4–6 y	11–12 y	13–18 y
Hepatitis B	HepB #1		HepB #2			HepB #3					HepB Series	
Diphtheria, Tetanus, Pertussis			DTaP	DTaP	DTaP		DTaP			DTaP	Td	Td
Haemophilus influenzae type b			Hib	Hib	Hib	Hib						
Inactivated Poliovirus			IPV	IPV		IPV				IPV		
Measles, Mumps, Rubella						MMR #1				MMR #2	MMR #2	
Varicella						Varicella					Varicella	
Pneumococcal		Vaccines below red line are for selected populations	PCV	PCV	PCV	PCV			PCV		PPV	
Hepatitis A										Hepatitis A Series		
Influenza					Influenza (Yearly)							

pneumococcal vaccinations are not obligatory in Germany, Austria, and Switzerland (see www.rki.de). To simplify the application of vaccines, licensed combination vaccines may be used whenever any components of the combination are indicated and the vaccine's other components are not contraindicated. Providers should consult the manufacturers' inserts for detailed information.

Passive immunization. This vaccination method involves administration of antibodies produced in a different host. In most cases, homologous (human) hyperimmune sera (obtained from convalescent patients or patients with multiple vaccinations) are used. The passive immunity obtained by this method is limited to a few weeks (or months at most).

Principles of Sterilization and Disinfection

■ Sterilization is defined as the killing or removal of all microorganisms and viruses from an object or product. Disinfection means rendering an object, the hands or skin free of pathogens. The term asepsis covers all measures aiming to prevent contamination of objects or wounds. Disinfection and sterilization makes use of both physical and chemical agents. The killing of microorganisms with these agents is exponential. A measure of the efficacy of this process is the D value (decimal reduction time), which expresses the time required to reduce the organism count by 90%. The sterilization agents of choice are hot air (180 °C, 30 minutes; 160 °C, 120 minutes) or saturated water vapor (121 °C, 15 minutes, 2.02×10^5 Pa; 134 °C, three minutes, 3.03×10^5 Pa). Gamma rays or high-energy electrons are used in radiosterilization at a recommended dose level of 2.5×10^4 Gy.

Disinfection is usually done with chemical agents, the most important of which are aldehydes (formaldehyde), alcohols, phenols, halogens (I, Cl), and surfactants (detergents). ■

Terms and General Introduction

Terms

Sterilization is the killing of all microorganisms and viruses or their complete elimination from a material with the highest possible level of certainty.

An object that has been subjected to a sterilization process, then packaged so as to be contamination-proof, is considered **sterile**.

Killing of Prions and Thermophilic Archaea

The standard sterilization methods used in medical applications (see below) are capable of causing irreversible damage to medically relevant microorganisms such as bacteria, protozoans, fungi, and helminths including worm eggs. Much more extreme processes are required to inactivate prions, such as autoclaving at 121 °C for 4.5 hours or at 134 °C for 30 minutes. Hyperthermophilic archaea forms have also been discovered in recent years (see p. 5) that proliferate at temperatures of 100 °C and higher and can tolerate autoclaving at 121 °C for one hour. These extreme life forms, along with prions, are not covered by the standard definitions of sterilization and sterility.

Disinfection is a specifically targeted antimicrobial treatment with the objective of preventing transmission of certain microorganisms. The purpose of the disinfection procedure is to render an object incapable of spreading infection.

Preservation is a general term for measures taken to prevent microbe-caused spoilage of susceptible products (pharmaceuticals, foods).

Decontamination is the removal or count reduction of microorganisms contaminating an object.

The objective of **aseptic measures and techniques** is to prevent microbial contamination of materials or wounds.

In antiseptic measures, chemical agents are used to fight pathogens in or on living tissue, for example in a wound.

The Kinetics of Pathogen Killing

Killing microorganisms with chemical agents or by physical means involves a first-order reaction. This implies that no pathogen-killing method kills off all the microorganisms in the target population all at once and instantaneously. Plotting the killing rate against exposure time in a semilog coordinate system results in a straight-line curve (Fig. **1.7**).

Sigmoid and asymptotic killing curves are exceptions to the rule of exponential killing rates. The steepness of the killing curves depends on the sensitivity of the microorganisms to the agent as well as on the latter's effectiveness. The survivor/exposure curve drops at a steeper angle when heat is applied, and at a flatter angle with ionizing radiation or chemical disinfectants. Another contributing factor is the number of microorganisms contaminating a product (i.e., its *bioburden*): when applied to higher organism concentrations, an antimicrobial agent will require a longer exposure time to achieve the same killing effect.

Bacterial Death Kinetics

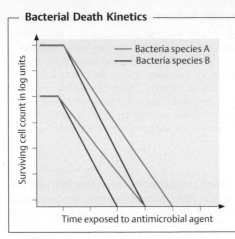

Bacteria species A
Bacteria species B

Surviving cell count in log units

Time exposed to antimicrobial agent

Fig. 1.7 The death rate varies among bacterial species. The higher the initial concentration of a bacterial culture, the longer an applied antimicrobial agent will require to achieve the same effect.

Standard sterilization methods extend beyond killing all microorganisms on the target objects to project a theoretical reduction of risk, i.e., the number of organisms per sterilized unit should be equal to or less than 10^{-6}.

The D value (decimal reduction time), which expresses the time required to reduce the organism count by 90%, is a handy index for killing effectiveness.

The concentration (c) of chemical agents plays a significant role in pathogen-killing kinetics. The relation between exposure time (t) and c is called the *dilution coefficient* (n): $t \cdot c^n$ = constant. Each agent has a characteristic coefficient n, for instance five for phenol, which means when c is halved the exposure time must be increased by a factor of 32 to achieve the same effect.

The *temperature coefficient* describes the influence of temperature on the effectiveness of chemical agents. The higher the temperature, the stronger the effect, i.e., the exposure time required to achieve the same effect is reduced. The coefficient of temperature must be determined experimentally for each combination of antimicrobial agent and pathogen species.

Mechanisms of Action

When microorganisms are killed by heat, their proteins (enzymes) are irreversibly denatured. Ionizing radiation results in the formation of reactive groups that contribute to chemical reactions affecting DNA and proteins. Exposure to UV light results in structural changes in DNA (thymine dimers) that prevent it from replicating. This damage can be repaired to a certain extent by light (photoreactivation). Most chemical agents (alcohols, phenols, aldehydes, heavy metals, oxidants) denature proteins irreversibly. Surfactant compounds (amphoteric and cationic) attack the cytoplasmic membrane. Acridine derivatives bind to DNA to prevent its replication and function (transcription).

Physical Methods of Sterilization and Disinfection

Heat

The application of heat is a simple, cheap and effective method of killing pathogens. Methods of heat application vary according to the specific application.

■ **Pasteurization.** This is the antimicrobial treatment used for foods in liquid form (milk):
— Low-temperature pasteurization: 61.5 °C, 30 minutes; 71 °C, 15 seconds.
— High-temperature pasteurization: brief (seconds) of exposure to 80–85 °C in continuous operation.
— Uperization: heating to 150 °C for 2.5 seconds in a pressurized container using steam injection.

■ **Disinfection.** Application of temperatures below what would be required for sterilization. Important: boiling medical instruments, needles, syringes, etc. does not constitute sterilization! Many bacterial spores are not killed by this method.

■ **Dry heat sterilization.** The guideline values for hot-air sterilizers are as follows: 180 °C for 30 minutes, 160 °C for 120 minutes, whereby the objects to be sterilized must themselves reach these temperatures for the entire prescribed period.

■ **Moist heat sterilization.** Autoclaves charged with saturated, pressurized steam are used for this purpose:
— 121 °C, 15 minutes, one atmosphere of pressure (total: 202 kPa).
— 134 °C, three minutes, two atmospheres of pressure (total: 303 kPa).

In practical operation, the heating and equalibriating heatup and equalizing times must be added to these, i.e., the time required for the temperature in the most inaccessible part of the item(s) to be sterilized to reach sterilization level. When sterilizing liquids, a cooling time is also required to avoid boiling point retardation.

The significant heat energy content of steam, which is transferred to the cooler sterilization items when the steam condenses on them, explains why it is such an effective pathogen killer. In addition, the proteins of microorganisms are much more readily denatured in a moist environment than under dry conditions.

Radiation

■ **Nonionizing radiation.** Ultra-violet (UV) rays (280–200 nm) are a type of nonionizing radiation that is rapidly absorbed by a variety of materials. UV rays are therefore used only to reduce airborne pathogen counts (surgical theaters, filling equipment) and for disinfection of smooth surfaces.

■ **Ionizing radiation.** Two types are used:
— Gamma radiation consists of electromagnetic waves produced by nuclear disintegration (e.g., of radioisotope ^{60}Co).
— Corpuscular radiation consists of electrons produced in generators and accelerated to raise their energy level.

Radiosterilization equipment is expensive. On a large scale, such systems are used only to sterilize bandages, suture material, plastic medical items, and heat-sensitive pharmaceuticals. The required dose depends on the level of product contamination (bioburden) and on how sensitive the contaminating microbes are to the radiation. As a rule, a dose of 2.5×10^4 Gy (Gray) is considered sufficient.

One Gy is defined as absorption of the energy quantum one joule (J) per kg.

Filtration

Liquids and gases can also be sterilized by filtration. Most of the available filters catch only bacteria and fungi, but with ultrafine filters viruses and even large molecules can be filtered out as well. With membrane filters, retention takes place through small pores. The best-known type is the membrane filter made of organic colloids (e.g., cellulose ester). These materials can be processed to produce thin filter layers with gauged and calibrated pore sizes. In conventional depth filters, liquids are put through a layer of fibrous material (e.g., asbestos). The effectiveness of this type of filter is due largely to the principle of adsorption. Because of possible toxic side effects, they are now practically obsolete.

Chemical Methods of Sterilization and Disinfection

1

Ethylene oxide. This highly reactive gas (C_2H_4O) is flammable, toxic, and a strong mucosal irritant. Ethylene oxide can be used for sterilization at low temperatures (20–60 °C). The gas has a high penetration capacity and can even get through some plastic foils. One drawback is that this gas cannot kill dried microorganisms and requires a relative humidity level of 40–90 % in the sterilizing chamber. Ethylene oxide goes into solution in plastics, rubber, and similar materials, therefore sterilized items must be allowed to stand for a longer period to ensure complete desorption.

Aldehydes. *Formaldehyde* (HCHO) is the most important aldehyde. It can be used in a special apparatus for gas sterilization. Its main use, however, is in disinfection. Formaldehyde is a water-soluble gas. *Formalin* is a 35 % solution of this gas in water. Formaldehyde irritates mucosa; skin contact may result in inflammations or allergic eczemas. Formaldehyde is a broad-spectrum germicide for bacteria, fungi, and viruses. At higher concentrations, spores are killed as well. This substance is used to disinfect surfaces and objects in 0.5–5 % solutions. In the past, it was commonly used in gaseous form to disinfect the air inside rooms ($5\,g/m^3$). The mechanism of action of formaldehyde is based on protein denaturation.

Another aldehyde used for disinfection purposes is *glutaraldehyde*.

Alcohols. The types of alcohol used in disinfection are *ethanol* (80 %), *propanol* (60 %), and *isopropanol* (70 %). Alcohols are quite effective against bacteria and fungi, less so against viruses. They do not kill bacterial spores. Due to their rapid action and good skin penetration, the main areas of application of alcohols are surgical and hygienic disinfection of the skin and hands. One disadvantage is that their effect is not long-lasting (no depot effect). Alcohols denature proteins.

Phenols. Lister was the first to use phenol (carbolic acid) in medical applications. Today, phenol derivatives substituted with organic groups and/or halogens (alkylated, arylated, and halogenated phenols), are widely used. One common feature of phenolic substances is their weak performance against spores and viruses. Phenols denature proteins. They bind to organic materials to a moderate degree only, making them suitable for disinfection of excreted materials.

Halogens. Chlorine, iodine, and derivatives of these halogens are suitable for use as disinfectants. Chlorine and iodine show a generalized microbicidal effect and also kill spores.

Chlorine denatures proteins by binding to free amino groups; hypochlorous acid (HOCl), on the other hand, is produced in aqueous solutions, then

Surfactant Disinfectants

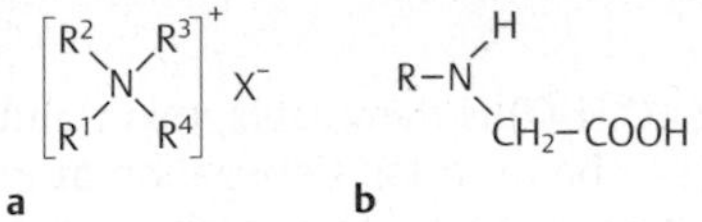

Fig. 1.8 Quaternary ammonium compounds (**a**) and amphoteric substances (**b**) disrupt the integrity and function of microbial membranes.

disintegrates into HCl and $^1/_2\,O_2$ and thus acts as a powerful oxidant. Chlorine is used to disinfect drinking water and swimming-pool water (up to 0.5 mg/l). Calcium hypochlorite (chlorinated lime) can be used in nonspecific disinfection of excretions. Chloramines are organic chlorine compounds that split off chlorine in aqueous solutions. They are used in cleaning and washing products and to disinfect excretions.

Iodine has qualities similar to those of chlorine. The most important iodine preparations are the solutions of iodine and potassium iodide in alcohol (tincture of iodine) used to disinfect skin and small wounds. Iodophores are complexes of iodine and surfactants (e.g., polyvinyl pyrrolidone). While iodophores are less irritant to the skin than pure iodine, they are also less effective as germicides.

Oxidants. This group includes ozone, hydrogen peroxide, potassium permanganate, and peracetic acid. Their relevant chemical activity is based on the splitting off of oxygen. Most are used as mild antiseptics to disinfect mucosa, skin, or wounds.

Surfactants. These substances (also known as surface-active agents, tensides, or detergents) include anionic, cationic, amphoteric, and nonionic detergent compounds, of which the cationic and amphoteric types are the most effective (Fig. 1.**8**).

The bactericidal effect of these substances is only moderate. They have no effect at all on tuberculosis bacteria (with the exception of amphotensides), spores, or nonencapsulated viruses. Their efficacy is good against Gram-positive bacteria, but less so against Gram-negative rods. Their advantages include low toxicity levels, lack of odor, good skin tolerance, and a cleaning effect.

Practical Disinfection

The objective of **surgical hand disinfection** is to render a surgeon's hands as free of organisms as possible. The procedure is applied after washing the hands thoroughly. Alcoholic preparations are best suited for this purpose, although they are not sporicidal and have only a brief duration of action.

Alcohols are therefore often combined with other disinfectants (e.g., quaternary ammonium compounds). Iodophores are also used for this purpose.

The purpose of **hygienic hand disinfection** is to disinfect hands contaminated with pathogenic organisms. Here also, alcohols are the agent of choice.

Alcohols and/or iodine compounds are suitable for **disinfecting patient's skin** in preparation for surgery and injections.

Strong-smelling agents are the logical choice for **disinfection of excretions** (feces, sputum, urine, etc.). It is not necessary to kill spores in such applications. Phenolic preparations are therefore frequently used. Contaminated hospital sewage can also be thermally disinfected (80–100 °C) if necessary.

Surface disinfection is an important part of hospital hygiene. A combination of cleaning and disinfection is very effective. Suitable agents include aldehyde and phenol derivatives combined with surfactants.

Instrument disinfection is used only for instruments that do not cause injuries to skin or mucosa (e.g., dental instruments for work on hard tooth substance). The preparations used should also have a cleaning effect.

Laundry disinfection can be done by chemical means or in combination with heat treatment. The substances used include derivatives of phenols, aldehydes and chlorine as well as surfactant compounds. Disinfection should preferably take place during washing.

Chlorine is the agent of choice for **disinfection of drinking water and swimming-pool water**. It is easily dosed, acts quickly, and has a broad disinfectant range. The recommended concentration level for drinking water is 0.1–0.3 mg/l and for swimming-pool water 0.5 mg/l.

Final room disinfection is the procedure carried out after hospital care of an infection patient is completed and is applied to a room and all of its furnishings. Evaporation or atomization of formaldehyde (5 g/m^3), which used to be the preferred method, requires an exposure period of six hours. This procedure is now being superseded by methods involving surface and spray disinfection with products containing formaldehyde.

Hospital disinfection is an important tool in the prevention of cross-infections among hospital patients. The procedure must be set out in written form for each specific case.

2 Basic Principles of Immunology

R. M. Zinkernagel

Introduction

■ Resistance to disease is based on **innate mechanisms** and adaptive or **acquired immunity**. Acquired immune mechanisms act in a specific manner and function to supplement the important **nonspecific** or **natural resistance mechanisms** such as physical barriers, granulocytes, macrophages, and chemical barriers (lysozymes, etc.). The **specific immune mechanisms** constitute a combination of less specific factors, including the activation of macrophages, complement, and necrosis factors; the early recognition of invading agents, by cells exhibiting a low level of specificity, (natural killer cells, γδ [gamma-delta] T cells); and systems geared toward highly specific recognition (antibodies and αβ [alpha-beta] T cells).

Many components of the specific immune defenses also contribute to nonspecific or natural defenses such as natural antibodies, complement, interleukins, interferons, macrophages, and natural killer cells. ■

In the strict sense, "immunity" defines an acquired resistance to infectious disease that is specific, i.e., resistance against a particular disease-causing pathogen. For example, a person who has had measles once will not suffer from measels a second time, and is thus called immune. However, such specific or acquired immune mechanisms do not represent the only factors which determine resistance to infection. The canine distemper virus is a close relative of the measles virus, but never causes an infection in humans. This kind of resistance is innate and nonspecific. Our immune system recognizes the pathogen as foreign based on certain surface structures, and eliminates it. Humans are thus born with resistance against many microorganisms (**innate immunity**) and can acquire resistance to others (**adaptive or acquired immunity**; Fig. 2.**1**). Activation of the mechanisms of innate immunity, also known as the primary immune defenses, takes place when a pathogen breaches the outer barriers of the body. Specific immune defense factors are mobilized later to fortify and regulate these primary defenses. Responses of the adaptive immune system not only engender immunity in the strict sense, but can also contribute to pathogenic processes. The terms **immunopathology, autoimmunity,** and **allergy** designate a group of immune

The Components of Anti-Infection Defense

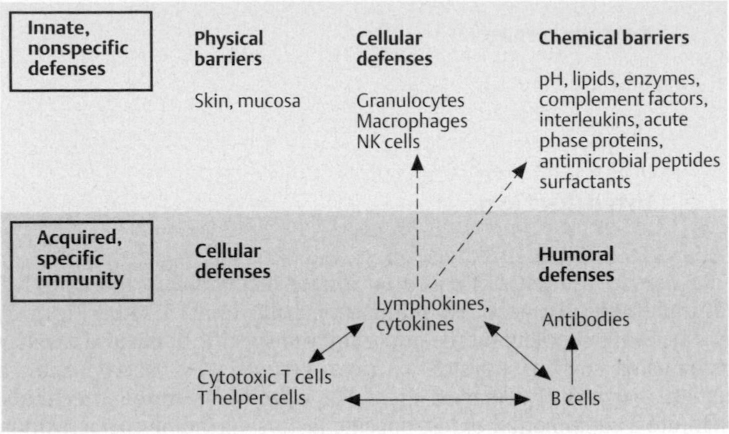

| Innate, nonspecific defenses | Physical barriers | Cellular defenses | Chemical barriers |

Fig. 2.1 The innate immune defense system comprises nonspecific physical, cellular, and chemical mechanisms which are distinct from the acquired immune defense system. The latter comprises cellular (T-cell responses) and humoral (antibodies) components. Specific T cells, together with antibodies, recruit non-specific effector mechanisms to areas of antigen presence.

phenomena causing mainly pathological effects, i.e., tissue damage due to inadequate, misguided, or excessive immune responses. However, a failed immune response may also be caused by a number of other factors. For instance, certain viral infections or medications can suppress or attenuate the immune response. This condition, known as **immunosuppression**, can also result from rare genetic defects causing congenital immunodeficiency.

The inability to initiate an immune response to the body's own self antigens (also termed autoantigens) is known as immunological **tolerance**.

Anergy is the term used to describe the phenomenon in which cells involved in immune defense are present but are not functional.

An immune response is a reaction to an immunological stimulus. The stimulating substances are known as **antigens** and are usually proteins or complex carbohydrates. The steric counterparts of the antigens are the **antibodies**, i.e., immunoreceptors formed to recognize segments, roughly 8–15 amino acids long, of the folded antigenic protein. These freely accessible structural elements are known as **epitopes** when present on the antigens, or as **antigen-binding sites** (ABS) from the point of view of the immunoreceptors. Presented alone, an epitope is not sufficient to stimulate an immunological response. Instead responsiveness is stimulated by epitopes constituting part of a macromolecule. This is why the epitope component of an antigen is terminologically distinguished from its macromolecular carrier; together they form an **immunogen**. B lymphocytes react to the antigen stimulus by producing antibodies. The T lymphocytes (T cells) responsible for cellular immunity are also activated. These cells can only recognize protein antigens that have been processed by host cells and presented on their surface. The T-cell receptors recognize antigen fragments with a length of 8–12 sequential amino acids which are either synthesized by the cell itself or produced subsequent to phagocytosis and presented by the cellular transplantation antigen molecules on the cell surface. The T cells can then complete their main task—recognition of infected host cells—so that infection is halted.

Our understanding of the immune defense system began with studies of infectious diseases, including the antibody responses to diphtheria, dermal reactions to tuberculin, and serodiagnosis of syphilis. Characteriztion of pathological antigens proved to be enormously difficult, and instead erythrocyte antigens, artificially synthesized chemical compounds, and other more readily available proteins were used in experimental models for more than 60 years. Major breakthroughs in bacteriology, virology, parasitology, biochemistry, molecular biology, and experimental embryology in the past 30–40 years have now made a new phase of intensive and productive research possible within the field of immune defenses against infection. The aim of this chapter on immunology, in a compact guide to medical microbiology, is to present the **immune system** essentially as a system of **defense against infections** and to identify its strengths and weaknesses to further our understanding of pathogenesis and prevention of disease.

The Immunological Apparatus

■ The immune system is comprised of various continuously circulating cells (T and B lymphocytes, and antigen-presenting cells present in various tissues). T and B cells develop from a common stem cell type, then mature in the thymus (T cells) or the bone marrow (B cells), which are called **primary (or central) lymphoid organs**. An antigen-specific differentiation step then takes places within the specialized and highly organized **secondary (or peripheral) lymphoid organs** (lymph nodes, spleen, mucosa-associated lymphoid tissues [MALT]). The antigen-specific activation of B and/or T cells involves their staggered interaction with other cells in a contact-dependent manner and by soluble factors.

B cells bear antibodies on their surfaces (cell-bound **B-cell receptors**). They secrete antibodies into the blood (**soluble antibodies**) or onto mucosal surfaces once they have fully matured into plasma cells. Antibodies recognize the three-dimensional structures of complex, folded proteins, and hydrocarbons. Chemically, B-cell receptors are globulins ("immunoglobulins") and comprise an astounding variety of specific types. Despite the division of immunoglobulins into classes and subclasses, they all share essentially the same structure. Switching from one Ig class to another generally requires T-cell help.

T cells recognize peptides presented on the cell surface by major histocompatibility (gene) complex (MHC) molecules. A T-cell response can only be initiated within organized lymphoid organs. Naive T cells circulate through the blood, spleen, and other lymphoid tissues, but cannot leave these compartments to migrate through peripheral nonlymphoid tissues and organs unless they are activated. Self antigens (autoantigens), presented in the thymus and lympoid tissues by mobile lymphohematopoietic cells, induce T-cell destruction (so-called **negative selection**). Antigens that are expressed only in the periphery, that is outside of the thymus and secondary lymphoid organs, are ignored by T cells; potentially autoreactive T cells are thus directed against such self antigens. T cells react to peptides that penetrate into the organized lymphoid tissues. New antigens are first localized within few lymphoid tissues before they can spread systemically. These must be present in lymphoid tissues for three to five days in order to elicit an immune response. An immune response can be induced against a previously ignored self antigen that does not normally enter lymphoid tissues if its entry is induced by circumstance, for instance, because of cell destruction resulting from chronic peripheral infection. It is important to remember that induction of a small number of T cells will not suffice to provide immune protection against a pathogen. Such protection necessitates a certain minimum sum of activated T cells.

The function of the immunological apparatus is based on a complex series of interactions between humoral, cellular, specific, and nonspecific mechanisms. This can be better understood by examining how the individual components of the immune response function.

The human immunological system can be conceived as a widely distributed organ comprising approximately 10^{12} individual cells, mainly **lymphocytes**, with a total weight of approximately 1 kg. Leukocytes arise from pluripotent stem cells in the bone marrow, then differentiate further as two distinct lineages. The **myeloid lineage** constitutes granulocytes and monocytes, which perform important basic defense functions as phagocytes ("scavenger cells"). The **lymphoid lineage** gives rise to the effector cells of the specific immune response, **T** and **B** lymphocytes. These cells are constantly being renewed (about 10^6 new lymphocytes are produced in every minute) and destroyed in large numbers (see Fig. 2.**17**, p. 88). T and B lymphocytes, while morphologically similar, undergo distinct maturation processes (Table 2.**1**, Fig. 2.**2**). The antigen-independent phase of lymphocyte differentiation takes place in the so-called **primary lymphoid organs**: T lymphocytes mature in the **t**hymus and B lymphocytes in the **b**ursa fabricl (in birds). Although mammals have no bursa, the term B lymphocytes (or B cells) has been retained to distinguish these cells, with their clearly distinct functions and maturation in the **b**one marrow, from T lymphocytes, which mature in the thymus (Table 2.**1**). B cells mature in the fetal liver as well as in fetal and adult **b**one marrow. In addition to their divergent differentia-

---

Maturation of B and T cells

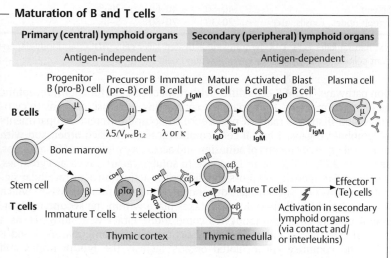

Fig. 2.**2**   All lymphoid cells originate from pluripotent stem cells present in the bone marrow which can undergo differentiation into B or T cells. Stem cells that remain in the bone marrow develop into mature B cells via several antigen-independent stages; including the λ5Vpre-B cell stage, and pre-B cells with a special λ5 precursor chain. Antigen contact within secondary lymphoid organs can then activate these cells, finally causing them to differentiate into antibody-secreting plasma cells.

T cells mature in the thymus; pTα is a precursor α chain associated with TCRβ chain surface expression. The pTα chain is later replaced by the normal TCRα chain. Immature CD4$^+$ CD8$^+$ double-positive thymocytes are localized within the cortical region of the thymus; some autoreactive T cells are deleted in the cortex, whilst some are deleted in the medulla as mature single-positive T cells. The remaining T cells mature within the medulla to become CD4$^+$ CD8$^-$ or CD4$^-$ CD8$^+$ T cells. From here, these single positive T cells can emigrate to peripheral secondary lymphoid organs, where they may become activated by a combination of antigen contacts, secondary signals, and cytokines.

Table 2.**1** Distribution of Lymphocyte Subpopulations and APCs in Various Organs (% of All Mononuclear Cells)

	B	T	NK, LAK, ADCC	APC
Peripheral blood	10–15	70–80	5–10	<1
Lymph	5	95–100	?	?
Thoracic duct	5–10	90–95	?	?
Thymus	1	95–100	?	0
Bone marrow	15–20	10–15	?	0
Spleen	40–50	40–60	20–30	1
Lymph nodes, tonsils, etc.	20–30	70–80	5–8	1

NK: natural killer cells; LAK: lymphokine-activated killer cells, ADCC: antibody-dependent cellular toxicity, APC: antigen-presenting cells

tion pathways, T and B cells differ with respect to their functions, receptors, and surface markers. They manifest contrasting response patterns to cytokines, and display a marked preference to occupy different compartments of lymphoid organs. T and B cells communicate with each other, and with other cell types, by means of adhesion and accessory molecules (CD antigens, see Table 2.**13**, p. 137) or in response to soluble factors, such as cytokines, which bind to specific receptors and induce the activation of intracellular signaling pathways. The antigen-dependent differentiation processes which leads to T and B cell specialization, takes place within the **secondary lymphoid organs** where lymphocytes come into contact with antigens. As a general rule the secondary lymphoid organs contain only mature T and B cells, and comprise encapsulated organs such as the **lymph nodes** and **spleen**, or non-encapsulated structures which contain lymphocytes and are associated with the skin, mucosa, gut, or bronchus (i.e. **SALT**, **MALT**, **GALT**, and **BALT**). Together, the primary and secondary lymphoid organs account for approximately 1–2% of body weight.

The B-Cell System

■ B lymphocytes produce antibodies in two forms; a membrane-bound form and a secreted form. Membrane-bound antibody forms the B-cell antigen receptor. Following antigen stimulation, B lymphocytes differentiate into **plasma cells**, which secrete antibodies exhibiting the same antigen specificity as the B-cell receptor. This system is characterized as **humoral immunity,** due to this release of receptors into the "humoral" system which constitutes vascular contents and mucous environments. The humoral

Table 2.**2**   Characteristics of the Various Immunoglobulin Classes

	IgM	IgD	IgG	IgE	IgA
Svedberg unit	19 S	7 S	7 S	8 S	7 S, 9 S, 11 S
Molecular weight	900 kDa	185 kDa	150 kDa	200 kDa	160 kDa
Number of dimeric units	5	1	1	1	1, 2, 3
H chain (constant domains)	μ (4)	δ (3)	γ (3)	ε (4)	α (3)
L chain			← κ or λ →		
Antigen-binding sites (ABS)	10	2	2	2	2, 4, 6
Concentration in normal serum (g/l)	0.5–2	0–0.4	8–16	0.02–0.50	1.4–4
% of Ig	6	0–1	80	0.002	13
Half-life (days)	1–2	?	7–21	1–2 in serum >200 on mast cells	3–6
Complement (C) activation:					
Classic	+	–	+	–	–
Alternative	–	–	–	–	+
Placental passage	–	–	+	+	–
Binding to mast cells and basophils	–	–	–	+	–
Binding to macrophages, granulocytes, and thrombocytes	–	–	(+)	–	(+)
Subclasses	–	–	+ (4)	–	+ (2)

IgG subclasses	IgG1	IgG2	IgG3	IgG4
% of total IgG	60–70	14–20	4–8	2–6
Reaction to *Staphlococcus* protein A	+	+	–	+
Placental passage	+	(+)	+	+
Complement (C) activation:	+++	++	++++	(+)
Binding to monocytes/macrophages	+++	+	+++	(+)
Blocks IgE binding	(–)	–	–	+
Half-life (days)	21–23	21–23	7–9	21–23

2

system also contains non-specific defense mechanisms, including the complement system (see "Immune response and effector mechanisms," p. 66ff.). In chemical terms, B-cell receptors are globulins (Ig or immunoglobulins). These immunoglobulins comprise a number of classes and subclasses, as well as numerous different specificities, but share a common structure (Fig. 2.**3a**). ∎

Immunoglobulin Structure

All immunoglobulin monomers have the same basic configuration, in that they consist of two identical light chains (L) and two identical heavy chains (H). The light chains appear as two forms; **lambda** (λ) or **kappa** (κ). There are five main heavy chain variants; μ, δ, γ, α, and ε. The five corresponding immunoglobulin classes are designated as **IgM**, **IgD**, **IgG**, **IgA**, or **IgE**, depending on which type of heavy chain they use (Fig. 2.**3b**). A special characteristic of the immunoglobulin classes IgA and IgM is that these comprise a basic monomeric structure that can be doubled or quintupled (i.e., these can exist in a dimeric or pentameric form). Table 2.**2** shows the composition, molecular weights and serum concentrations of the various immunoglobulin classes (p. 49).

Fig. 2.**3   a Immunoglobulin monomers.** The upper half of the figure shows the intact monomer consisting of two L and two H chains. The positions of the disulfide bonds, the variable N-terminal domains, and the antigen-binding site (ABS) are indicated. The lower half of the figure shows the monomers of the individual polypeptide chains as seen following exposure to reducing conditions (which break the disulfide bonds) and denaturing conditions; note that the ABS is lost. Papain digestion produces two monovalent Fab fragments, and one Fc fragment. Following pepsin digestion (right), the Fc portion is fragmented, but the Fab fragments remain held together by disulfide bonds. The F(ab')$_2$ arm is bivalent (with two identical ABS). Fv fragments comprise a single-chain ABS formed by recombinant technology. These consist of the variable domains of the H and L chains, joined covalently by a synthetic linker peptide.
b Classes of immunoglobulins. IgM, IgD, IgG, IgA, and IgE are differentiated by their respective heavy chains (μ, δ, γ, α, ε). IgA (α chain) forms dimers held together by the J (joining) chain; the secretory (S) piece facilitates transport of secretory IgA across epithelial cells, and impairs its enzymatic lysis within secretions. IgM (μ chain) forms pentamers with 10 identical ABS; the IgM monomers are held together by J chains. The light chains (λ and κ) are found in all classes of immunoglobulins. ▶

Immunoglobulins contain numerous domains, as illustrated by the structure of IgG. In monomeric IgG each domain consists of a protein segment which is approximately 110 amino acids in length. Both light chains possess two such domains, and each heavy chain possesses four or five domains. The domain structure was first revealed by comparison of the amino acid sequence derived from many different immunoglobulins belonging to the

2

Basic Immunoglobulin Structures

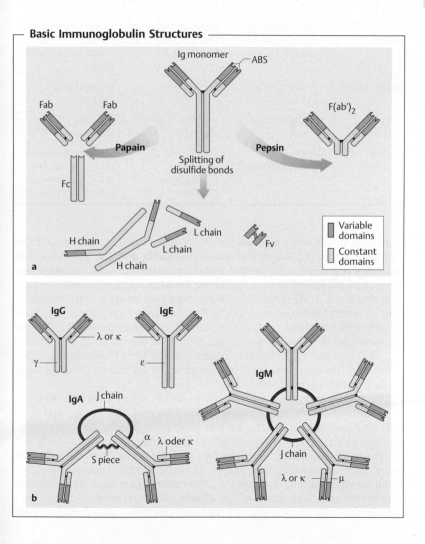

Table 2.**3** Antigen Recognition by B and T Cells

	B lymphocytes	T helper cells (CD4$^+$)	Cytotoxic T cells (CTL; CD8$^+$)
Recognition structure of B or T cell	Surface Ig (BCR)	TCR	TCR
Recognized epitope	Conformational epitopes (no MHC restriction)	Linear epitopes only (10–15 amino acids) + MHC class II	Linear epitopes (peptides) (8)–9–(10) amino acids + MHC class I
Antigen type	Proteins/carbohydrates	Peptides only	Peptides only
Antigen presentation	Not necessary	Via MHC class II structures	Via MHC class I structures
Effectors	Antibodies (+/– complement)	Signals induced by contact (T/B help) or cytokines	Cytotoxicity mediated by contact (perforin, granzyme), or release of cytokines

same class. In this way a high level of sequence variability was revealed to be contained within the N-terminal domain (**variable domain, V**), whilst such variability was comparably absent within the other domains (**constant domains, C**). Each light chain consists of one variable domain (V_L) and one constant domain (C_L). In contrast, the heavy chains are roughly 440–550 amino acids in length, and consist of four to five domains. Again, the heavy chain variable region is made up of one domain (V_H), whereas the constant region consists either of three domains (γ, α, δ chains), or four domains (μ, ϵ chains) (C_{H1}, C_{H2}, C_{H3}, and C_{H4}). Disulfide bonds link the light chains to the heavy chains and the heavy chains to one another. An additional disulfide bond is found within each domain.

The three-dimensional form of the molecule forms a letter Y. The two short arms of this 'Y' consist of four domains each (V_L, C_L, V_H, and C_{H1}), and this structure contains the antigen-binding fragments—hence its designation as **Fab** (**f**ragment **a**ntigen **b**inding). The schematic presented in Fig. 2.**3** is somewhat misleading, since the two variable domains of the light and heavy chains are in reality intertwined. The binding site—a decisive structure for an epitope reaction—is formed by the combination of variable domains from both chains. Since the two light chains, and the two heavy chains, contain identical amino acid sequences (this includes the variable domains), each immunoglobulin monomer has two identical **antigen-binding sites** (**ABS**), and these form the ends of the two short arms of the 'Y'. An area within the antibody consisting of 12–15 amino acids contacts the peptide region contained within the antigen and consisting of approximately 5–800 $Å^2$ (Table 2.**3**). The trunk of the 'Y' is called the **Fc** fragment (named, "**f**raction **c**rystallizable" since it crystallizes readily) and is made up of the constant domains of the heavy chains (C_{H2} and $C_{H3,}$ and sometimes C_{H4}).

Diversity within the Variable Domains of the Immunoglobulins

The specificity of an antibody is determined by the amino acid sequence of the variable domains of the H and L chains, and this sequence is unique for each corresponding cell clone. How has nature gone about the task of producing the needed diversity of specific amino acid sequences within a biochemically economical framework? The genetic variety contained within the B-cell population is ensured by a process of continuous diversification of the genetically identical B-cell precursors. The three gene segments (variable, diversity, joining) which encode the variable domain (the VDJ region for the H chain, and the VJ region for the L chain) are capable of undergoing a process called recombination. Each of these genetic segments are found as a number of variants (Fig. 2.**4**, Table 2.**4**). B-cell maturation involves a process of genetic re-

Table 2.**4** Organization of the Genetic Regions for the Human Immunoglobulins and T-Cell Receptors (TCR)

	Immunoglobulins		TCRαβ		TCRγδ	
	H	L	α	β	γ	δ
V segments	95	150	50–100	75–100	9	6
D segments	23	–	–	2	–	3
J segments	9	12	60–80	13	5	3
Nucleotide additions	VD, DJ	VJ	VJ	VD, DJ	VJ	VD
Number of potential combinations for V (H + L)	15 000		8000		54	
Theoretical upper limit of all combinations	>10^{12}		>10^{12}		>10^{12}	

2

combination resulting in a **rearrangement** of these segments, such that one V_H, one D_H, and one J_H segment become combined. Thus the germ line does not contain *one gene* governing the variable domain, but rather gene segments which each encode fragments of the necessary information. Mature B cells contain a functional gene which, as a result of the recombination process, is comprised of one $V_H D_H J_H$ segment. The diversity of T-cell receptors is generated in a similar manner (see p. 57).

Fig. 2.4 explains the process of genetic recombination using examples of an immunoglobulin H chain and T-cell receptor α chain.

The major factors governing immunoglobulin diversity include:

- Multiple V gene segments encoded in the germ lines.
- The process of VJ, and VDJ, genetic recombination.
- Combination of light and heavy chain protein structures.
- Random errors occurring during the recombination process, and inclusion of additional nucleotides.
- Somatic point mutations.

In theory, the potential number of unique immunoglobulin structures that could be generated by a combination of these processes exceeds 10^{12}, however, the biologically viable and functional range of immunoglobulin specificities is likely to number closer to 10^4.

The Different Classes of Immunoglobulins

Class switching. The process of genetic recombination results in the generation of a functional VDJ gene located on the chromosome upstream of those

---

Fig. 2.4 **a Heavy chain of human IgG.** The designations for the gene segments in the variable part of the H chain are V (variable), D (diversity), and J (joining). The segments designated as μ, δ, γ, α, and ε code for the constant region and determine the immunoglobulin class. The V segment occurs in several hundred versions, the D segment in over a dozen, and the J segment in several forms. V, D, and J segments combine randomly to form a sequence (VDJ) which codes for the variable part of the H chain. This rearranged DNA is then transcribed, creating the primary RNA transcript. The non-coding intervening sequences (introns) are then spliced out, and the resulting mRNA is translated into the protein product. **b α chain of mouse T-cell receptor.** Various different V, D, and J gene segments (for β and δ), V and J gene segments (for α and γ) are available for the T-cell receptor chains. The DNA loci for the δ chain genes are located between those for the α chain. ►

Rearrangement of the B- and T-Cell Receptor Genes

a Heavy Ig chain

Germ line DNA

| V_1 | V_2 | V_3 | V_n | D_1 D_2 D_3 | D_n | J_1 | J_2 | J_3 | J_n | μ | δ | γ_1 | γ_2 | ε | α_1 |

1. Rearrangement
- → D_H–J_H -rearrangement
- → V_H–$D_H J_H$ -rearrangement

Exon   Intron

B cell DNA

| V_1 | $V_2 D_3 J_1$ | μ | δ | γ_1 | γ_2 | ε | α_1 |

2. Transcription
- → Primary RNA

| $V_2 D_3 J_1$ | μ |

3. Splicing
- → mRNA

| $V_2 D_3 J_1$ μ |

4. Translation
- → Protein (H chain)

V_H μ

b TCR-α-chain

Germ line DNA

β | $V_{\beta(1-20)}$ | $D_{\beta1}$ | $J_{\beta1}$ | $C_{\beta1}$ | $D_{\beta2}$ | $J_{\beta2}$ | $C_{\beta2}$ |

γ | V_γ | $J_{\gamma1}$ $C_{\gamma1}$ | V_γ | $J_{\gamma3}$ $C_{\gamma3}$ | V_γ | $J_{\gamma2}$ $C_{\gamma2}$ |

α | $V_{\alpha(1-100)}$ | $V_{\delta(1-?)}$ | D_δ J_δ C_δ | J_α | C_α |

1. Rearrangement
- → No D region
- → V_α–J_α -rearrangement

T lymphocyte DNA

| $V_{\alpha1}$ $V_{\alpha2}$ J_α | C_α |

2. Transkription
- → Primary RNA

| $V_{\alpha2}$ J_α | C_α |

3. Splicing
- → mRNA

| V J C |

4. Translation
- → Protein (α chain)

regions encoding the H chain segments Cμ, Cδ, Cγ, Cα, and Cε, in consecutive order. Thus all immunoglobulin production begins with the synthesis of IgM and IgD (resulting from transcription of the VDJ and the Cμ or Cδ gene segments). This occurs without prior antigen stimulus and is transitional in nature. Antigen stimulation results in a second gene rearrangement—during which the VDJ gene is relocated to the vicinity of Cγ, Cα, or Cε by a process of recombination involving deletion of the intervening regions. Following this event, the B cell no longer produces H chains of the IgM or IgD classes, but is instead committed to the production of IgG, IgA, or IgE—thus allowing secretion of the entire range of immunoglobulin types (Table 2.**2**). This process is known as class switching, and results in a change of the Ig class of an antibody whilst allowing its antigen specificity to be retained.

Variability types. The use of different heavy or light chain constant regions results in new immunoglobulin classes known as **isotypes**. Individual Ig classes can also differ, with such genetically determined variations in the constant elements of the immunoglobulins (which are transmitted according to the Mendelian laws) are known as **allotypes**. Variation within the variable region results in the formation of determinants, known as **idiotypes**. The idiotype determines an immunoglobulins antigenic specificity, and is unique for each individual B-cell clone.

Functions. Each different class of antibody has a specific set of functions. IgM and IgD act as B-cell receptors in their earlier transmembrane forms, although the function of **IgD** is not entirely clear. The first antibodies produced in the primary immune response are **IgM** pentamers, the action of which is directed largely against micro-organisms. IgM pentamers are incapable of crossing the placental barrier. The immunoglobulin class which is most abundant in the serum is **IgG**, with particularly high titers of this isotype being found following secondary stimulation. IgG antibodies pass through the placenta and so provide the newborn with a passive form of protection against those pathogens for which the mother exhibits immunity. In certain rare circumstances such antibodies may also harm the child, for instance when they are directed against epitopes expressed by the child's own tissues which the mother has reacted against immunologically (the most important clinical example of this is rhesus factor incompatibility). High concentrations of **IgA** antibodies are found in the intestinal tract and contents, saliva, bronchial and nasal secretions, and milk—where they are strategically positioned to intercept infectious pathogens (particularly commensals) (Fig. 2.**5**). **IgE** antibodies bind to high-affinity Fcε receptors present on basophilic granulocytes and mast cells. Cross-linking of mast cell bound IgE antibodies by antigen results in cellular degranulation and causes the release of highly active biogenic amines (histamine, kinines). IgE antibodies are produced in large quantities following parasitic infestations of the intestine, lung or skin, and play a significant role in the local immune response raised against these pathogens.

The Mucosa-Associated Lymphoid Tissue (MALT) Immune System and "Homing"

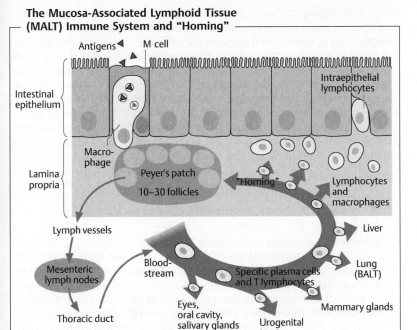

Fig. 2.**5** Specialized APCs (M cells in the intestinal wall or pulmonary macrophages in the lung) take up antigens in mucosa and present them in the Peyer's patches or local lymph nodes. This probably enhances T cell-dependent activation of IgA-producing B cells, which are preferentially recruited to the mucosal regions ("homing") via local adhesion molecules and antigen depots, resulting in a type of geographic specificity within the immune response.

The T-Cell System

T-Cell Receptors (TCR) and Accessory Molecules

Like B cells, T cells have receptors that bind specifically to their steric counterparts on antigen epitopes. The diversity of **T-cell receptors** is also achieved by means of genetic rearrangement of V, D, and J segments (Fig. 2.**4b**). However, the T-cell receptor is never secreted, and instead remains membrane-bound.

Each T-cell receptor consists of **two transmembrane chains,** of either the α and β forms, or the γ and δ forms (not to be confused with the heavy

2

chains of Ig bearing the same designations). Both chains have two extracellular domains, a transmembrane anchor element and a short intracellular extension. As for Ig, the terminal domains are variable in nature (i.e., Vα and Vβ), and together they form the antigen binding site (see Fig. 2.**9**, p. 65). T-cell receptors are associated with their so-called co-receptors—other membrane-enclosed proteins expressed on the T cell surface—which include the multiple-chain **CD3 complex,** and **CD4 or CD8 molecules** (depending on the specific differentiation of the T cell). CD stands for "cluster of differentiation" or "cluster determinant" and represents differentiation antigens defined by clusters of monoclonal antibodies. (Table 2.**13**, p. 135f., provides a summary of the most important CD antigens.)

T-Cell Specificity and the Major Histocompatibility Complex (MHC)

T-cell receptors are unable to recognize free antigens. Instead the T-cell receptor can only recognize its specific epitope once the antigen has been cleaved into shorter peptide fragments by the presenting cell. These fragments must then be embedded within a specific molecular groove and presented to the T-cell receptor (a process known as MHC-restricted **T-cell recognition or MHC restriction**). This "binding groove" is located on the MHC molecule. The MHC encodes for the powerful histocompatibility or transplantation antigens (also known in humans as HLA, human leukocyte antigen molecules, Fig. 2.**6**).

The designation "MHC molecule" derives from the initial discovery of the function of the complex as a cell surface structure, responsible for the

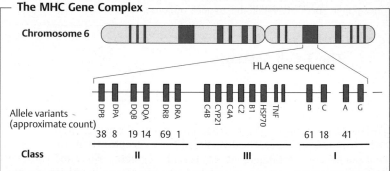

The MHC Gene Complex

Chromosome 6

HLA gene sequence

Allele variants (approximate count)

DPB	DPA	DQB	DQA	DRB	DRA	C4B	CYP21	C4A	C2	B1	HSP70	TNF	B	C	A	G
38	8	19	14	69	1								61	18	41	

Class   II   III   I

Fig. 2.**6** The human major histocompatibility gene complex (HLA genes) is located on chromosome 6. There are three different classes of MHC molecules.

immunological rejection of cell transfusions or tissue and organ transplants. Its true function as a peptide-presenting molecule was not discovered until the seventies, when its role became apparent whilst testing the specificity of virus-specific cytotoxic T cells. During these experiments it was observed that immune T cells were only able to destroy infected target cells if both cell types were derived from the same patient or from mice with identical MHC molecules. The resulting conclusion was that a T-cell receptor not only recognizes the corresponding amino acid structure of the presented peptide, but additionally recognizes certain parts of the MHC structure. It is now known that this contact between MHC on the APC and the T-cell receptor is stabilized by the co-receptors CD4 and CD8.

MHC classes. Molecules encoded by the MHC can be classified into three groups according to their distribution on somatic cells, and the types of cells by which they are recognized:

■ **MHC class I molecules.** These molecules consist of a heavy α chain with three Ig-like polymorphic domains (these are encoded by 100–1000 alleles, with the α1 and α2 domains being much more polymorphic than the α3 domain) and a nonmembrane-bound (soluble) single-domain β_2 microglobulin (β_2M, which is encoded by a relatively small number of alleles). The α chain forms a groove that functions to present antigenic peptides (Fig. 2.**7**). Human HLA-A, HLA-B, and HLA-C molecules are expressed in varying densities on all somatic cells (the relative HLA densities for fibroblasts and hepatic cells, lymphocytes, or neurons are 1x, 100x and 0.1×, respectively). Additional, nonclassical, class I antigens which exhibit a low degree of polymorphism are also present on lymphohematopoietic cells and play a role in cellular differentiation.

■ **MHC class II molecules.** These are made up by two different polymorphic transmembrane chains that consist of two domains each (α_1 is highly polymorphic, whilst β_1 is moderately polymorphic, and β_2 is fairly constant). These chains combine to form the antigen-presenting groove. Class II molecules are largely restricted to *lymphohematopoetic cells, antigen-presenting cells* (APC), *macrophages*, and so on. (see Fig. 2.**9a**, p. 65) In humans, but not in mice, they are also found on some epithelial cells, neuroendocrine cells, and T cells. The products of the three human gene regions HLA-DP, HLA-DQ and HLA-DR can additionally form molecules representing combinations of two loci—thus providing additional diversity for peptide presentation.

■ **MHC class III molecules.** These are not MHC antigens in the classical sense, but are encoded within the MHC locus. These include complement (C) components C4 and C2, cytokines (IL, TNF), heat shock protein 70 (hsp70), and other products important for peptide presentation.

Protein Structure of MHC Class I Molecules

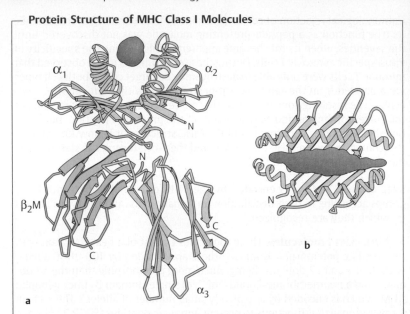

Fig. 2.7 MHC class I translation antigen: **a** lateral view, **b** vertical view. The presenting peptide is shown in violet. The three domains of the heavy chain are α_1, α_2, and α_3. β_2 microglobulin (β_2M) functions as a light chain, and is not covalently bound to the heavy chain.

Functions of MHC molecules. MHC class I and II molecules function mainly as molecules capable of presenting peptides (Figs. 2.**7**–2.**9**). These two classes of MHC molecules present two different types of antigens:
— **Intracellular antigens**; these are cleaved into peptides within the proteasome and are usually associated with MHC class I molecules via the endogenous antigen processing pathway (Fig. 2.**8**, left side).
— **Antigens taken up from exogenous sources;** these are processed into peptides within phagolysosomes, and in most cases are then presented on MHC class II molecules on the cell surface (Fig. 2.**8**, right side). Within the phagolysosome, a fragment called the invariant chain (CLIP, class II-inhibiting protein) is replaced by an antigen fragment. This CLIP fragment normally blocks the antigen-binding site of the MHC class II dimer, thus preventing its occupation by other intracellular peptides.

The presentation groove of MHC class I molecules is closed at both ends, and only accommodates peptides of roughly 8–10 (usually 9) amino acids in

Presentation of Endogenous and Exogenous Antigens

Endogenous pathway | Exogenous pathway

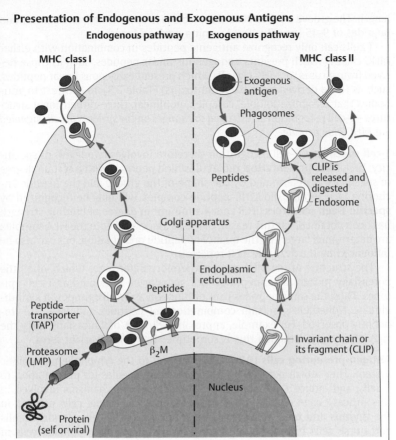

MHC class I

MHC class II

Exogenous antigen

Phagosomes

Peptides

CLIP is released and digested

Endosome

Golgi apparatus

Endoplasmic reticulum

Peptides

Peptide transporter (TAP)

Proteasome (LMP)

$\beta_2 M$

Invariant chain or its fragment (CLIP)

Nucleus

Protein (self or viral)

Fig. 2.**8** Intracellularly synthesized endogenous antigen peptides (left side) are bound to MHC class I molecules within the endoplasmic reticulum, fixed into the groove by $\beta_2 M$, and presented on the cell surface. Antigens taken up from exogenous sources (right) are cleaved into peptides within phagosomes. The phagosome then merges with endosomes containing MHC class II molecules, the binding site of which had been protected by the so-called CLIP fragment. These two presentation pathways functionally separate MHC class I restricted CD8+ T cells from MHC class II restricted CD4+ T cells.

2

length. The groove of MHC class II molecules is open-ended, and can contain peptides of 9–15 (usually 10–12) amino acids in length.

T cells can only recognize antigenic peptides in combination with either MHC class I (which presents endogenous linear peptides, such as those derived from viruses) or MHC class II (which present exogenous linear peptides, such as those derived from bacterial toxins) (Table 2.3). In contrast to antibodies that recognize soluble, complex, nonlinear, three-dimensional structures—T-cell recognition is *restricted to changes on the surfaces of cells signaled via MHC plus peptide.*

T-cell specificity. T-cell recognition therefore involves two levels of specificity: first, **MHC presentation molecules** bind peptides with a certain degree of specificity as determined by the shape of the groove and the peptide anchoring loci. Second, the MHC-peptide complex will only be recognized by **specific T-cell receptors** (TCR) once a minimum degree of binding strength has been obtained. For this reason diseases associated with the HLA complex are determined largely by the quality of peptide presentation, but can also be influenced by the available TCR repertoire.

The structure of the MHC groove therefore determines which, of all the potentially recognizable, peptides will actually be presented as T-cell epitopes. Thus, the same peptides cannot function as T-cell epitopes in all individuals. Nonetheless, certain combinations of peptides and MHC are frequently observed. For example, approximately 50% of Caucasians carry the HLA-A2 antigen, although this is sometimes found in a variant form.

Antigen-presenting cells (APC). APCs belong to the lymphohematopoietic system. They attach peptides to MHC class II molecules for presentation to T cells, and induce T-cell responses. The complex mechanisms involved in this process have not yet been fully delineated. *Stromal cells* present in the **thymus and bone marrow** (i.e., connective tissue cells, dendritic cells and nurse cells in both thymus and bone marrow, plus *epithelial cells* in the thymus) can also function as APCs. The following cell types function as APCs in **peripheral secondary lymphoid organs**:

- Circulating monocytes.

- Sessile macrophages in tissues, microglia in the central nervous system.

- Bone marrow derived dendritic cells with migratory potential—these occur as cutaneous Langerhans cells, as veiled cells during antigen transfer into the afferent lymph vessels, as interdigitating cells in the spleen and lymph nodes, and as interstitial dendritic cells or as M cells within MALT.

- Follicular dendritic cells (FDC)—these are found within the germinal centers of the secondary lymph organs, do not originate in the bone marrow, and do not process antigens but rather bind antigen-antibody complexes via Fc receptors and complement (C3) receptors.

■ B lymphocytes—these serve as a type of APC for T helper cells during T-B collaborations.

The consequences of MHC variation. Because every individual differs with regard to the set of polymorphic MHC molecules and self antigens expressed (with the exception of monozygotic twins and inbred mice of the same strain), the differences between two given individuals are considerable. The high degree of variability in MHC molecules—essential for the presentation of a large proportion of possible antigenic peptides for T-cell recognition—results in these molecules becoming targets for T cell recognition following cellular or organ transplantation resulting in **transplant rejection**. The term "transplantation antigens" is therefore a misnomer, and is only used because their real function was not discovered until a later time. Normally antigens are only recognized by T cells if they are associated with MHC-encoded self-structures. Transplant recognition, which apparently involves the imitation of the combination of a non-self antigen plus a self-MHC molecule, can therefore be considered an exception. The process probably arises from T-cell receptor cross-reactivity between host self-MHC antigens plus foreign peptides on the one hand, and non-self transplantation antigens associated with self-peptides from the donor on the other hand (for example, the T-cell receptor for HLA-A2 peptide X cross-reacts with HLA-A13 peptide Y). Transplant rejection is therefore a consequence of the enormous variety of combinations of antigenic peptide plus MHC, which is exhibited by each individual organism.

T-Cell Maturation: Positive and Negative Selection

Maturation of T cells occurs largely within the **thymus**. Fig. 2.**2** (p. 47) shows a schematic presentation of this process. Because the MHC-encoded presentation molecules are highly polymorphic, and are also subject to mutation, the **repertoire of TCRs is not genetically pre-determined**. One prerequisite for an optimal repertoire of T-cells is therefore the **positive selection** of T cells such that these preferentially recognize peptides associated only with self transplantation (MHC) antigens. A second prerequisite is **negative selection**, which involves the deletion of T cells that react too strongly against self MHC plus self peptide. The random processes governing the genetic generation of an array of T-cell receptors results $\alpha\beta$ or $\gamma\delta$ receptor chain combinations which are in the majority of cases are non-functional. Those T cells preserved through to maturity represent cells carrying receptors capable of effectively recognizing self-MHC molecules (positive selection). However, the T cells within this group which express too high an affinity for self-MHC plus self-peptides are deleted (negative selection).

The process of positive selection was demonstrated in experimental mice expressing MHC class I molecules of type b (MHC classI^b) from which the thymus had been removed (and which therefore had no T cells). Implantation of a new thymus with MHC class I molecules of type a (MHC class I^a) into the MHC class I^b mice resulted in the maturation of T cells which only recognized peptides presented by MHC class I^a molecules, and not peptides presented by MHC class I^b molecules. However, recent experiments have shown that this is probable an experimental artefact and that it is not (or not solely) the thymic epithelial cells that determine the selection process, but that this process is driven by cells formed in the bone marrow. Positive selection is generally achieved by weak levels of binding affinity between the T-cell receptor and the self-MHC molecules, whereas negative selection eliminates those T cells exhibiting the highest levels of affinity (namely the self-or auto-reactive T cells) and absence of binding causes death by neglect. Thus, only T cells with moderate binding affinities are allowed to mature and exit the thymus. These T cells can potentially react to non-self (foreign) peptides presented by self MHC molecules. The enormous proliferation of immature thymocytes is paralleled by continuous cell death of large numbers of thymocytes (apoptosis, see summary in Fig. 2.**17**, p. 88). In general, the maturation and survival of lymphocytes is considered to be dependent on a continuous, repetitive, signaling via transmembrane molecules, and cessation of these signals is usually taken as a reliable indicator of cell death.

T-Cell Subpopulations

In order to recognize the presented antigen, T cells require the specific T-cell receptor and a molecule which functions to recognize the appropriate MHC molecules (i.e. CD4 or CD8 which recognize MHC class II and MHC class I, respectively). Thus T cells are classified into different subpopulations based on the CD4 or CD8 surface molecules:

CD4$^+$ T cells. These T cells recognize only MHC class II-associated antigens. They are also called **T helper cells** due to their important role in **T-B cell collaboration** (Fig. 2.**9a**), although they exhibit many other additional functions. CD4$^+$ cells can produce, or induce, the production *of cytokines* by which means they can activate macrophages and exercise a regulatory effect on other lymphocytes (see p. 75f.). Although these cells sometimes demonstrate an ability to cause cytotoxic destruction in vitro, this does not hold true in vivo.

CD8$^+$ T cells. Only MHC class I-associated antigens are recognized by the CD8$^+$ molecule. These cells are also known as **cytotoxic T cells** due to their ability to destroy histocompatible virus-infected, or otherwise altered, target cells as well as allogeneic cells. This effect can be observed both in vitro and in vivo (Fig. 2.**9b**). Costimulatory molecules are not required for this lytic

Interactions in T-Cell Antigen Recognition

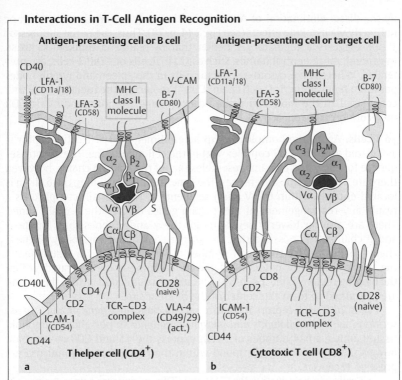

Fig. 2.**9** **a** The interactions of APCs or B cells with CD4+ T cells (T helper cells) are mediated by MHC class II molecules (heterodimers). **b** Interactions between CD8+ T cells (cytotoxic T cells) and their target cells are mediated by MHC class I molecules. The presenting peptide is shown in violet. "S" indicates a superantigen, named after its capacity to activate many different T helper cells through its ability to bind to the constant regions of both the MHC and TCR molecules (naive = non-activated T cells, act. = activated T cells).

effector function. However, cytotoxicity is only one of several important functions expressed by CD8+ T cells. They also have many other non-lytic functions which they execute via the production, or induction of, cytokine release. The designation (CD8+) T suppressor cell is misleading and should not be used. It was originally coined to distinguish these cells from the function of T helper cells, mentioned above. However, plausible documentation of a suppressor effect by CD8+ T cells has only been obtained in a very small number of cases. In most cases, this suppressive effect can in fact be explained by the direct elimination of APC (i.e., by changing the antigen kinetics), or indirectly via cytokine effects (see Fig. 2.**14**, p. 78). Thus, the name suppressor T cell suggests a regulatory function that in reality is unlikely to exist. In general, more neutral names, such as CD4$^+$ T cells or CD8$^+$ T cells, are preferable. Whereas the cytotoxic effector cells in the spleen and lymph nodes possess a heterodimeric ($\alpha + \beta$ chain) CD8$^+$ T molecule, the function of CD8$^+$ T cells found in the intestinal wall and expressing the α-homodimeric CD8 molecule remains unclear.

$\gamma\delta$ **T cells.** As for the homologous $\alpha\beta$ heterodimer, the $\gamma\delta$ T-cell receptor is associated with the CD3 complex within the cell membrane. The genetic sequence for the γ and δ chains resembles that of the α and β chains, however, there are a few notable differences. The gene complex encoding the δ chain is located entirely within the V and J segments of the α chain complex. As a result, any rearrangement of the α chain genes deletes the δ chain genes. There are also far fewer V segments for the γ and δ genes than for the α and β chains. It is possible that the increased binding variability of the δ chains makes up for the small number of V segments, as a result nearly the entire variability potential of the $\gamma\delta$ receptor is concentrated within the binding region (Table 2.**4**, p. 53). The amino acids coded within this region are presumed to form the center of the binding site.

T cells with $\gamma\delta$ receptors recognize certain *class I-like gene products in association with phospholipids and phosphoglycolipids*. In peripheral lymphoid tissues, only a small number of T cells express the $\gamma\delta$ and CD3 co-receptor, however, many of the T cells found within the mucosa and submucosa express $\gamma\delta$ receptors.

$\gamma\delta$ T cells can be negative for CD4$^+$ and CD8$^+$, or express two α chains (but no β chain) of the CD8$^+$ molecule. Although it is assumed that $\gamma\delta$ T cells may be responsible for early, low-specificity, immune defense at the skin and mucosa, their specificities and effector functions are still largely unknown.

Immune Responses and Effector Mechanisms

■ The effector functions of the immune system comprise antibodies and complement-dependent mechanisms within body fluids and the mucosa, as well as tissue-bound effector mechanisms executed by T cells and monocytes/macrophages. B cells are characterized by antigen specificity. Following antigen stimulation, specific B cells proliferate and differentiate into plasma cells that secrete antibodies into the surroundings. The type of B-cell response induced is determined by the amount and type of bound antigen recognized. Induction of an IgM response in response to antigens which are lipopolysaccharides—or which exhibit an highly organized, crystal-like structure containing identical and repetitively arranged determinants—is a highly efficient and T cell-independent process which involves direct cross-linking of the B-cell receptor. In contrast to this process, antibody responses against monomeric or oligomeric antigens are less efficient and strictly require T cell help, for both non-self and self antigens.

Some forms of T-cell responses involve the release of soluble mediators (cytokines), which effectively expands the field of T cell function beyond individual cell-to-cell contacts to an ability to regulate the function of large numbers of surrounding cells. Other T-cell effector mechanisms are mediated in a more precise manner through cell-to-cell contacts. Examples of this include perforin-dependent cytolysis and induction of the signaling pathways involved in B-cell differentiation or Ig class switching.　　■

B Cells

B-Cell Epitopes and B-Cell Proliferation

Burnet's **clonal selection theory**, formulated in 1957, states that every B-cell clone is characterized by an unique antigen specificity, i.e., it bears a specific antigen receptor. Accordingly, once rearrangement of the Ig genes has taken place, the corresponding protein will be expressed as a surface receptor. At the same time further rearrangement is stopped. Thus, only one ABS, or **one specificity** (one V_H plus V_L [either κ or λ]), derived from a single allele can be expressed on a single cell. This phenomenon is called **allelic exclusion**. The body faces a large number of different antigens in its lifetime, necessitating that a correspondingly large number of different receptor specificities, and therefore different B cells, must continuously be produced. When a given antigen enters an organism, it binds to the B cell which exhibits the correct receptor specificity for that antigen. One way to describe this process is to say that the antigen selects the corresponding B-cell type to which it most efficiently binds. However, as long as the responding B cells do not proliferate, the specificity of the response is restricted to a very small number of cells. For an effective response, **clonal** proliferation of the responsive B cells must be induced. After several cell divisions B cells differentiate into **plasma cells** which release the specific receptors into the surroundings in the form of soluble antibodies. B-cell stimulation proceeds with, or without, T cell help depending on the structure and amount of bound antigen.

Antigens. Antigens can be divided into two categories; those which stimulate B cells to secrete antibodies without any T-cell help, and those which require additional T-cell signals for this purpose.

2

■ **Type 1 T-independent antigens (TI1).** These include paracrystalline, identical epitopes arranged at approximately 5–10 nm intervals in a repetitive two-dimensional pattern (e.g., proteins found on the surface of viruses, bacteria, and parasites); and antigens associated with lipopolysaccharides (LPS). Thus TI1 antigens represent structures with a repetitive arrangement, which allows the engagement of several antigen receptors at one time and results in optimal Ig receptor cross-linking; or structures which result in sub-optimal cross-linking, but which are complemented by an LPS-mediated activation signal. Either type of antigen can induce B cell activation in the absence of T cell help.

■ **Type 2 T-independent antigens (TI2).** These antigens are less stringently arranged, and are usually flexible or mobile on cell surfaces. They can cross-link Ig receptors, but to a lesser extent than TI1 antigens. TI2 antigens require a small amount of indirectly associated T help in order to elicit a B-cell response (e.g., hapten-Ficoll antigens or viral glycoproteins on infected cell surfaces).

■ **T help-dependent antigens.** These are monomeric or oligomeric (usually soluble) antigens that do not cause Ig cross-linking, and are unable to induce B-cell proliferation on their own. In this case an additional signal, provided by contact with T cells, is required for B-cell activation (see also B-cell tolerance, p. 93ff.).

Receptors on the surface of B cells and soluble serum antibodies usually recognize epitopes present on the surface of native antigens. For protein antigens, the segments of polypeptide chains involved are usually spaced far apart when the protein is in a denatured, unfolded, state. A **conformational** or **structural epitope** is not formed unless the antigen is present in its native configuration. So-called **sequential** or **linear epitopes**—formed by contiguous segments of a polypeptide chain and hidden inside the antigen—are largely inaccessible to B cell receptors or antibodies, as long as the antigen molecule or infectious agent retains its native configuration. These epitopes therefore contribute little to biological protection. The specific role of linear epitopes is addressed below in the context of T cell-mediated immunity. B cells are also frequently found to be capable of specific recognition of sugar molecules on the surface of infectious agents, whilst T cells appear to be incapable of recognizing such sugar molecules.

Proliferation of B cells. As mentioned above, contact between one, or a few, B-cell receptors and the correlating antigenic epitope does not in itself suffice for the induction of B-cell proliferation. Instead proliferation requires either a high degree of B cell receptor cross-linking by antigen, or additional T cell-mediated signals.

Proliferation and the rearrangement of genetic material—a continuous process which can increase cellular numbers by a million-fold—occasionally result in errors, or even the activation of oncogenes. The results of this process may therefore include the generation of **B-cell lymphomas and leukemia's**. Since the original error occurs in a single cell, such tumors are *monoclonal*. Uncontrolled proliferation of differentiated B cells (plasma cells) results in the generation of **monoclonal plasma cell tumors** known as multiple myelomas or plasmocytomas. Occasionally, myelomas produce excessive amounts of the light chains of the monoclonal immunoglobulin, and these proteins can then be detected in the urine as **Bence-Jones proteins**. Such proteins represented some of the first immunoglobulin components accessible for chemical analysis and they revealed important early details regarding immunoglobulin structure.

Monoclonal Antibodies

A normal immune response usually involves the response and proliferation of numerous B cell clones, bearing ABS with varying degrees of specificity for the different epitopes contained within the antigen. Thus the immune response is normally **polyclonal.** It is possible to isolate a single cell from such a polyclonal immune response in an experimental setting. Fusing this cell with an "immortal" proliferating myeloma cell results in generation of a **hybridoma**, which then produces chemically uniform immunoglobulins of the original specificity, and in whatever amounts are required. This method was developed by Koeler and Milstein in 1975, and is used to produce **monoclonal antibodies** (Fig. 2.**10**), which represent important tools for experimental immunology, diagnostics, and therapeutics. Many monoclonal antibodies are still produced in mouse and rat cells, making them xenogeneic for humans. Attempts to avoid the resulting rejection problems have involved the production of antibodies by human cells (which remains difficult), or the "humanization" of murine antibodies by recombinant insertion of the variable domains of a murine antibody adjacent to the constant domains of a human antibody. The generation of a transgenic mice, in which the Ig genes have been replaced by human genes, has made the production of hybridoma's producing completely human antibodies possible.

T-Independent B Cell Responses

B cells recognize antigens via the Ig receptor. However, if the antigen is in a monomeric, or oligomeric, soluble form the B cell can only mount a response if it undergoes the process of T-B collaboration. Many infectious pathogens carry surface antigens with **polyclonal activation properties** (e.g., lipopolysaccharide [LPS]) and/or crystal-like identical determinants, which are often

Production of Monoclonal Antibodies

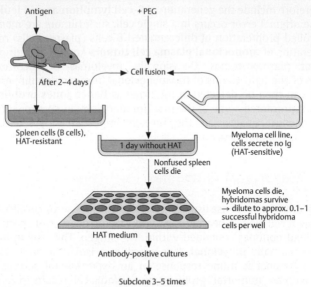

Fig. 2.**10** Monoclonal antibodies are produced with the help of cell lines obtained from the fusion of a B lymphocyte to an immortal myeloma cell. In the first instance, mice are immunized against an antigen. They then receive a second, intravenous, dose of antigen two to four days before cell fusion. Then spleen cells are removed and fused to the myeloma cell line using polyethylene glycol (PEG). Those spleen cells that fail to fuse to a myeloma cell die within one day of culture. Next, the fused cells are subjected to selection using HAT medium (hypoxanthine, aminopterin, thymidine). Aminopterin blocks specific metabolic processes, but with the help of the intermediary metabolites (hypoxanthine and thymidine) spleen cells are able to complete these processes using auxiliary pathways. The myeloma cells, on the other hand, have a metabolic defect which prevents them from utilizing such alternative pathways and resulting in the death of those cells cultured in HAT medium. However, once a spleen cell has fused with a myeloma cell, the fused spleen-myeloma product (hybridoma) is HAT-resistant. In this way only the successfully fused cells will be able to survive several days of culture on HAT medium. After this time, the cell culture is diluted such that there is, ideally, only one hybridoma within each well. Individual wells are then tested for the presence of the desired antibody. If the result is positive, the hybridoma cells are subcloned several times to ensure clonality; with the specificity of the produced antibody being checked following each round to subcloning. Production of purely human monoclonal antibodies is carried out using mice whose Ig genes have been completely replaced by human Ig genes.

repeated in a *regular pattern* (linear e.g., flagella, or two-dimensional e.g., viruses) with intervals of 5–10 nm. These paracrystalline-patterned antigens are capable of inducing B-cell responses without contact-dependent T cell help. This probably occurs by means of *maximum Ig receptor cross-linking*. Such B-cell responses are usually of the **IgM type**, since switching to different isotype classes is either impossible or very inefficient in the absence of T cell help. The IgM response is of a relatively brief duration (exhibiting a half-life of about 24 h), but can nonetheless be highly efficient. Examples of this efficiency include IgM responses induced by many viral envelope antigens which bear neutralizing ("protective") determinants accessible to the corresponding antibodies, and responses to bacterial surface antigens (e.g., flagellae, lipopolysaccharides) or parasites.

T Cells

T-Cell Activation

There are two classes of T cells; T helper cells (CD4+) and cytotoxic T cells (CD8+). Table 2.5 summarizes the reliance of T-cell responses on the dose, localization, and duration of presence of antigen. T-cell stimulation via the TCR, accessory molecules and adhesion molecules results in the activation

Table 2.**5**   Dependence of T-Cell Response on Antigen Localization, Amount, and Duration of Presence

	Antigen		T-cell response
Localization	**Amount**	**Duration of presence**	
Thymus	Small-large	Always	Negative selection by deletion
Blood, spleen, lymph nodes (secondary lymphoid organs)	Small	Short (1 day)	No induction
	Small	Long (7 days)	Induction
	Large	Short	No induction
	Large	Long (>10 days)	Exhaustive induction/ deletion (anergy?)
Peripheral non lymphoid tissue	Large or small	Always or short	Ignorance, indifference

of various tyrosine kinases (Fig. 2.**11**) and mediates stringent and differential regulation of several signaling steps. T-cell induction and activation result from the activation of two signals. In addition to *TCR activation (signal 1 = antigen)*, a *costimulatory signal (signal 2)* is usually required. Important costimulatory signals are delivered by the binding of B7 (B7.1 and B7.2) proteins (present on the APC or B cell) to ligands on the T cells (CD28 protein, CTLA-4), or by CD40–CD40 ligand interactions. T-cell expansion is also enhanced by IL-2.

T-Cell Activation by Superantigens

In association with MHC class II molecules, a number of bacterial and possibly viral products can efficiently stimulate a large repertoire of $CD4^+$ T cells at one time. This is often mediated by the binding of the bacterial or viral product to the constant segment of certain $V\beta$ chains (and possibly $V\alpha$ chains) with a low level of specificity (see Fig. 2.**9a**, p. 65). Superantigens are categorized as either exogenous or endogenous. **Exogenous superantigens** mainly include *bacterial* toxins (staphylococcus enterotoxin types A–E [SEA, SEB, etc.]), toxic shock syndrome toxin (TSST), toxins from *Streptococcus pyogenes*, and certain retroviruses. **Endogenous superantigens** are derived from components of certain retroviruses found in mice, and which display superantigen-like behavior (e.g., murine mammary tumor virus, MMTV). The function of superantigens during T cell activation can be compared to the effect of bacterial lipopolysaccharides on B cells, in that LPS-induced B cell activation is also polyclonal (although it functions by way of the LPS receptors instead of the Ig receptors (see below)).

Interactions between Cells of the Immune System

T Helper Cells (CD4$^+$ T Cells) and T-B Cell Collaboration

Mature T cells expressing CD4 are called T helper (Th) cells (see also p. 64f.), reflecting their role in co-operating with B cells. Foreign antigens, whose three-dimensional structures are recognized by B cells, also contain linear peptides. During the **initial phase** of the T helper cell response, these antigens are taken up by APCs, processed, and presented as peptides in association with **MHC class II molecules**—allowing their recognition by Th cells (see Fig. 2.**8**, p. 61 and Fig. 2.**13**, p. 76). Prior to our understanding of MHC restriction, B-cell epitopes were known as **haptens,** whilst those parts of the antigens which bore the T-cell epitope were known as **carriers**. In order

T-Cell Activation

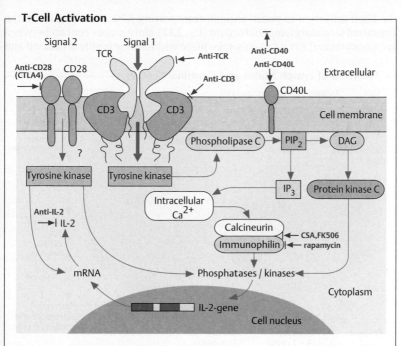

Fig. 2.**11**   Regulation of T-cell activation is controlled by multiple signals, including costimulatory signals (Signal 2). Stimulation of the T cell via the T-cell receptor (TCR; Signal 1) activates a tyrosine kinase, which in turn activates phospholipase C (PLC). PLC splits phosphatidylinositol bisphosphate (PIP$_2$) into inositol trisphosphate (IP$_3$) and diacyl glycerol (DAG). IP$_3$ releases Ca^{2+} from intracellular depots, whilst DAG activates protein kinase C (PKC). Together, Ca^{2+} and PKC induce and activate the phosphoproteins required for *IL-2* gene transcription within the cell nucleus. Stimulation of a T cell via the TCR alone results in production of only very small amounts of IL-2. Increased IL-2 production often requires additional signals (costimulation, e.g., via CD28). Costimulation via CD28 activates tyrosine kinases, which both sustain the transcription process and ensure post-transcriptional stabilization of IL-2 mRNA. Immunosuppressive substances (in red letters) include cytostatic drugs, anti-TCR, anti-CD3, anti-CD28 (CTLA4), anti-CD40, cyclosporine A and FK506 (which interferes with immunophilin-calcineurin binding, thus reducing IL-2 production), and rapamycin (which binds to, and blocks, immunophilin and hardly reduces IL-2 at all). Anti-interleukins (especially anti-IL-2, or a combination of anti-IL-2 receptor and anti-IL-15) block T-cell proliferation.

for T cell activation to occur, antigen-transporting APCs must first reach the *organized secondary lymphoid organs* (Fig. 2.**12**), since proper contact between lymphocytes and APCs can only take place within these highly organized and

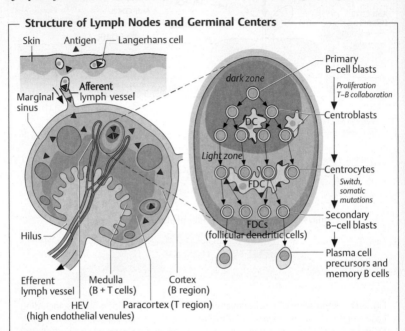

Structure of Lymph Nodes and Germinal Centers

Skin — Antigen — Langerhans cell

Marginal sinus

Afferent lymph vessel

Hilus

Efferent lymph vessel | Medulla (B + T cells) | Cortex (B region)

HEV (high endothelial venules) | Paracortex (T region)

dark zone

DC

Light zone

FDCA

FDCs (follicular dendritic cells)

Primary B–cell blasts

Proliferation T–B collaboration

Centroblasts

Centrocytes

Switch, somatic mutations

Secondary B–cell blasts

Plasma cell precursors and memory B cells

Fig. 2.**12**   Antigen carried by antigen-presenting cells (e.g., Langerhans cells in the skin which have taken up local antigens), or soluble antigens enter the marginal sinus of the lymph node through afferent lymphatic vessels. In the spleen, blood-borne antigens are taken up by specialized macrophages present in the marginal zone (marginal zone macrophages, MZM). Each lymph node has its own arterial and venous vascularization. T and B cells migrate from blood vessels, through specialized venules with a high endothelium (HEV: high endothelial venules), into the paracortex which is largely comprised of T cells. Clusters of B cells (so-called primary follicles) are located in the cortex, where following antigen-stimulation, secondary follicles with germinal centers develop (right side). Active B-cell proliferation occurs at this site. Differentiation of B cells begins with the proliferation of the primary B-cell blasts within the dark zone and involves intensive interaction with antigen-presenting dendritic cells (DC). Antibody class switching and somatic mutation follows and takes place in the light zone, where FDC (follicular dendritic cells) stimulate B cells and store the antigen-antibody complexes that function to preserve antibody memory. Secondary B-cell blasts develop into either plasma cells or memory B cells. Lymphocytes can only leave the lymph nodes through efferent lymph vessels.

compartmentalized organs. The cytokines IFNγ, IL-1, IL-2, IL-4, and IL-12 play an important role in this process—as do various other factors.

During the **second phase** (Fig. 2.**13**), *activated T helper cells* recognize the same MHC class II peptide complex, but on the surface of a **B cell**. Prior to this event, the B cell must have responded to the same antigen (by virtue of its Ig surface receptor recognizing a conformational antigenic epitope), then internalized the antigen, processed it, and finally presented parts of it in the form of linear peptides bound to MHC class II molecules on the cell surface for recognition by the T helper cell. The resulting B-T cell contact results in further interactions mediated by CD4, CD40, and CD28 (see Fig. 2.**9**, p. 65)—and sends a signal to the B cell which initiates the switch from IgM to IgG or other Ig classes. It also allows induction of a process of somatic mutation, and probably enhances the survival of the B cell in the form of a memory B cell.

Subpopulations of T Helper Cells

Soluble signaling substances, cytokines (interleukins), released from T helper cells can also provide an inductive stimulus for B cells. Two subpopulations of T helper cells can be differentiated based on the patterns of cytokines produced (Fig. 2.**14**). Infections in general, but especially those by intracellular parasites, induce cytokine production by natural killer (NK) cells in addition to a strong **T helper 1 (TH1) response**. The response by these cells is characterized by early gamma interferon (IFNγ) production, increased levels of phagocyte activity, elimination of the antigen by IFNγ-activated macrophages, production of IgG2a and other complement-binding (opsonizing) antibodies (see the complement system, pp. 86ff.), and induction of cytotoxic T-cell responses. IL-12 functions as the most important promoter of TH1 cell function and additionally acts as an inhibitor of TH2 cells.

In contrast, worm infections or other parasitic diseases induce the early production of IL-4, and result in the development of a **TH2 response**. TH2 cells, in turn, recruit eosinophils and induce production of *IgG1* and *IgE* antibodies. Persons suffering from allergies and atopic conditions show a pathologically excessive TH2 response potential. IL-4 not only promotes the TH2 response but also inhibits TH1 cells.

Cytotoxic T Cells (CD8+ T Cells)

Mature CD8+ T cells perform the biologically important function of lysing target cells. Target cell recognition involves the association of **MHC class I** structures with peptides normally derived from endogenous sources, i.e., originating in the cells themselves or synthesized within them by intracellular parasites. Induction of cytotoxic CD8+ T cell response often does not require helper

2

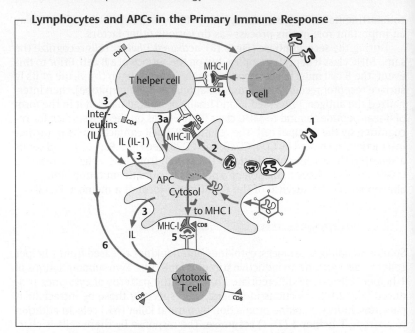

Lymphocytes and APCs in the Primary Immune Response

cells—or only requires these cells indirectly. However, should the antigen stimulus and the accompanying inflammation be of a low-level nature, the quantity of cytokines secreted by the cytotoxic T cells themselves may not suffice, in which case the induction of a CD8+ T cell response will be reduced unless additional cytokines are provided by helper T cells. The cytotoxic activity of CD8+ T cells is mediated via *contact and perforin release* (perforin renders the membrane of the target cell permeable resulting in cellular death). CD8+ T cells also function in *interleukin release* (mainly of IFNγ) by which they mediate non-cytotoxic effector functions (Fig. 2.**15**). The role of **perforin** in **contact-dependent direct cytolysis** by natural killer (NK) cells and cytotoxic T cells (see also Fig. 2.**17**, p. 88) has been investigated in gene knockout mice. In these animals the *perforin* gene has been switched off by means of homologous recombination, and as a result they can no longer produce perforin. Perforin-dependent cytolysis is important for the control of *noncytopathic viruses, tumors,* and *transformed cells,* but also plays a large role in the control of highly virulent viruses that produce syncytia (e.g., the smallpox virus). Release of **noncytolytic effector molecules** by CD8+ cells, mostly IFNγ, plays a major role in control of *cytopathic viruses* and *intracellular bacteria.* Cytolytic effector mechanisms may also contribute to release of intracellular micro-organisms and parasites (e.g., tuberculosis) from cells that only express MHC class I.

◄ Fig. 2.**13** For the sake of simplicity, the principles illustrated here are based on an antigen (1) which only contains a single B epitope and a single T epitope. As an example, the structural B epitope (blue) is present on the surface of the antigen; whilst the linear T epitope (red) is hidden inside it. An antigen-presenting cell (APC), or macrophage, takes up the antigen and breaks it down in a nonspecific manner. The T-cell epitope is thus released and loaded onto MHC class II molecules which are presented on the cell surface (2). A T helper cell specifically recognizes the T epitope presented by the MHC class II molecule. This recognition process activates the APC (3a) (or the macrophages). T cells, APC, and macrophages all produce cytokines (Fig. 2.**14**), which then act on T cells, B cells, and APCs (causing up-regulation of CD40, B7)(3). This in turn stimulates the T cells to proliferate, and encourages the secretion of additional signaling substances (IL-2, IFNγ, IL-4, etc.). A B cell whose surface Ig has recognized and bound a B epitope present on the intact antigen, will present the antigenic T cell epitope complexed to MHC class II on its cell surface, in a manner similar to that described for the APC (4). This enables direct interaction between the T helper cell and the specific B cell, resulting in induction of proliferation, differentiation, and B-cell class switching from IgM to other Ig classes. The B cell finally develops into an antibody-producing plasma cell. The antibody-binding site of the produced antibody thus fits the B epitope on the intact antigen. The induction of cytotoxic effector cells by peptides presented on MHC class I molecules (violet) is indicated in the lower part of the diagram (5). The cytotoxic T cell precursors do not usually receive contact-mediated T help, but are rather supported by secreted cytokines (mainly IL-2) (6). (Again, in the interest of simplicity, the CD3 and CD4 complexes and cytokines are not shown in detail; see Fig. 2.**8**, p. 61 for more on antigen presentation.)

Cytokines (Interleukins) and Adhesion

Cytokines are bioactive hormones, normally glycoproteins, which exercise a wide variety of biological effects on those cells which express the appropriate receptors (Table 2.**6**). Cytokines are designated by their cellular origin such that **monokines** include those interleukins produced by macrophages/monocytes, whilst **lymphokines** include those interleukins produced by lymphocytes. The term **interleukins** is used for cytokines which mostly influence cellular interactions. All cytokines are cyto-regulatory proteins with molecular weights under 60 kDa (in most cases under 25 kDa). They are produced locally, have very short *half-lives* (a matter of seconds to minutes), and are effective at *picomolar concentrations*. The effects of cytokines may be *paracrine* (acting on cells near the production locus), or *autocrine* (the same cell both produces, and reacts to, the cytokine). By way of interaction with highly specific cell surface receptors, cytokines can induce cell-specific or more general effects (including mediator release, expression of differen-

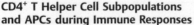

CD4⁺ T Helper Cell Subpopulations and APCs during Immune Responses

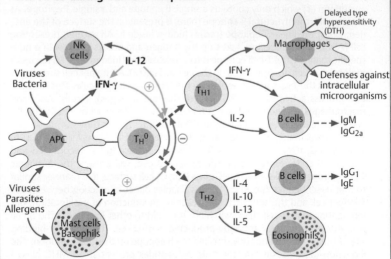

Fig. 2.**14** TH1 and TH2 cells are derived from a TH0 cell, and undergo differentiation in the presence of help derived from cytokines, DC, macrophages, and other cell types. TH1 cells are activated by IL-12 and IFNγ and inhibited by IL-4; whilst for TH2 cells the reverse is true. Viruses and bacteria (particularly intracellular bacteria) can induce a TH1 response by activating natural killer cells. In contrast, allergens and parasites induce a TH2 response via the release of IL-4. However, the strong in-vitro differentiation of CD4+ T cells into TH1–TH2 subsets is likely to be less sharply defined in vivo.

tiation molecules and regulation of cell surface molecule expression). The functions of cytokines are usually *pleiotropic*, in that they display a number of effects of the same, or of a different, nature on one or more cell types. Below is a summary of cytokine functions:

- Promotion of inflammation: IL-1, IL-6, TNFα, chemokines (e.g., IL-8).
- Inhibition of inflammation: IL-10, TGFβ.
- Promotion of hematopoiesis: GM-CSF, IL-3, G-CSF, M-CSF, IL-5, IL-7.
- Activating B cells: CD40L, IL-6, IL-3, IL-4.
- Activating T cells: IL-2, IL-4, IL-10, IL-13, IL-15.
- Anti-infectious: IFNα, IFNβ, IFNγ, TNFα.
- Anti-proliferative: IFNα, IFNβ, TNFα, TGFβ.

Antiviral Protection by T Cells

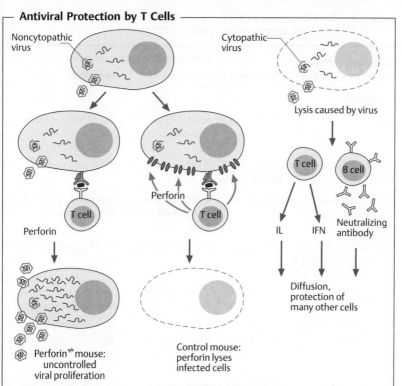

Fig. 2.**15** Certain viruses destroy the infected host cells (right), others do not (left). Cytotoxic T cells can destroy freshly infected cells by direct contact (with the help of perforin), thus inhibiting viral replication (middle). Whether the result of this lysis is clinically desirable depends on the balance between protection from viral proliferation, and the damage caused by immunologically mediated cell destruction. In perforin knockout mice (perforin$^{o/o}$), T cells are unable to produce perforin and therefore do not destroy the infected host cells. Replication of non-cytopathic viruses thus continues unabated in these mice. Soluble anti-viral interleukins (especially IFNγ and TNFα), and neutralizing antibodies, combat cytopathic viruses (which replicate comparatively rapidly) more efficiently than do cytolytic T cells; this is because interleukin and antibody molecules can readily diffuse through tissues and reach a greater number of cells, more rapidly, than can killer T cells.

Table 2.**6** The Most Important Immunological Cytokines and Costimulators plus Their Receptors and Functions

Cytokines/costimulators/chemokines	Receptor	Cytokines/cytokine receptors produced by	Functions
Interleukins			
IL-1	CD121 (α)β	Macrophages Endothelial cells	Hypothalamic fever, NK cell activation, T and B stimulation
IL-2 (T-cell growth factor)	CD25 (α) CD122 (β), γc	T cells	T-cell proliferation
IL-3 (multicolony stimulating factor)	CD123, βc	T cells, B cells, thymic epithelial cells	Synergistic effect in hematopoiesis
IL-4 (BCGF-1, BSF-1) (B-cell growth factor, B-cell stimulating factor)	CD124, γc	T cells, mast cells	B-cell activation, switch to IgE
IL-5 (BCGF-2)	CD125, βc	T cells, mast cells	Growth and differentiation of eosinophilis
IL-6 (interferon/IFNβ_2, BSF-2, BCDF)	CD126, CD$_w$130	T cells, macrophages	Growth and differentiation of T and B cells, acute-phase immune response
IL-7	CD$_w$127, γc	Bone marrow stroma	Growth of pre-B and pre-T cells
IL-10		T cells	Macrophages, reduction of TH1 cytokines
IL-9	IL-9R, γc	T cells	Effect on mast cells
IL-10		T helper cells (especially mouse TH2), macrophages, Epstein-Barr virus	Efficient inhibitor for macrophage functions, inhibits inflammatory reactions
IL-11	IL-11R, CD$_w$130	Stromal fibroblasts	Synergistic effect with IL-3 and IL-4 in hematopoiesis

Table 2.6 *Continued: The Most Important Immunological Cytokines...*

Cytokines/costimulators/chemokines	Receptor	Cytokines/cytokine receptors produced by	Functions
IL-12		B cells, macrophages	Activates natural killer cells, induces differentiation of CD4$^+$ T cells into TH1-like cells, encourages IFNγ production
IL-13	IL-13R, γc	T cells	Growth and differentiation of B cells, inhibits production of inflammatory cytokines by means of macrophages
IL-15	IL-15R, γc	T cells, placenta, muscle cells	IL-2-like, mainly intestinal effects
GM-CSF (granulocyte macrophage colony stimulating factor)	CD$_w$116, βc	Macrophages, T cells	Stimulates growth and differentiation of the myelomonocytic lineage
LIF (leukemia inhibitory factor)	LIFR, CD$_w$130	Bone marrow stroma, fibroblasts	Maintains embryonal stem cells; like IL-6, IL-11
Interferons (IFN)			
IFNγ	CD119	T cells, natural killer cells	Activation of macrophages, enhances MHC expression, antiviral
IFNα	CD118	Leukocytes	Antiviral, enhances MHC class I expression
IFNβ	CD118	Fibroblasts	Antiviral, enhances MHC class I expression
Immunoglobulin superfamily			
B7.1 (CD80)	CD28 (promoter); CTLA-4 (inhibitor)	Antigen-presenting cells	Costimulation of T cell responses
B7.2 (CD86)	CD28; CTLA-4	Antigen-presenting cells	Costimulation of T cell responses

2

Table 2.6 *Continued: The Most Important Immunological Cytokines. . .*

Cytokines/costimulators/chemokines	Receptor	Cytokines/cytokine receptors produced by	Functions
TNF (tumor necrosis factor) family			
TNFα (cachexin)	p55, p75, CD120a, CD120b	Macrophages, natural killer cells	Local inflammations, endothelial activation
TNFβ (lymphotoxin, LT, LTα)	p55, p75, CD120a, CD120b	T cells, B cells	Endothelial activation, organization of secondary lymphoid tissues
LTβ		T cells, B cells	Organization of secondary lymphoid tissues
CD40 ligand (CD40-L)	CD40	T cells, mast cells	B-cell activation, class switching
Fas ligand	CD95 (Fas)	T cells	Apoptosis, Ca^{2+}-independent cytotoxicity
Chemokines			
IL-8 (prototype) CXCL8	CXCR1, CXCR2	Activated endothelium, activated fibroblasts	Attraction of neutrophils, degranulation of neutrophils
MCP-1 (monocyte chemoattractant protein) CCL2	CCR2	Activated endothelium, tissue macrophages, synovial cells	Inflammation
MIP-1α (macrophage inflammatory protein) CCL3	CCR5, CCR1	T cells, activated Mφ	Proinflammatory HIVα receptor
MIP-1β CCL4	CCR5	T cells, activated Mφ	Proinflammatory HIVα receptor
RANTES (regulated on activation, normal T cell expressed and secreted) CCL5	CCR5, CCR1, CCR3	T cells, blood platelets	Inhibits cellular entry by M-trophic HIV, proinflammatory
IP-10 (interferon gamma-inducible protein) CXCL10	CXCR3	Inflamed tissue due to effects of IFNγ	Proinflammatory

Table 2.**6** *Continued: The Most Important Immunological Cytokines...*

Cytokines/costimulators/chemokines	Receptor	Cytokines/cytokine receptors produced by	Functions
Chemokines			
MIG (monokine induced by interferon gamma) CXCL11	CXCR3	Inflamed tissue, due to effects of IFNγ	Proinflammatory
Eotaxin CCL22	CCR3	Endothelium, epithelial cells	Buildup of infiltrate in allergic diseases, e.g., asthma
MDC (macrophage-derived chemokine)	CCR4	T-cell zone DCs, activated B cells, monocytes	Supports T-B cell collaboration during humoral immune responses
Fractalkine CXCL1	CX₃CR1	Intestinal epithelium, endothelium	Endothelial cells activation of thrombocytes
Constitutive chemokines			
LARC (liver and activation-regulated chemokine) MIP-3α	CCR6	Intestinal epithelia, Peyer's patches	Participation in mucosal immune responses
SLC (secondary lymphoid organ chemokine)	CCR7	High endothelial lymph nodes, T-cell zone	Facilitates entry of naive T cells, contact between T cells and DCs
TECK (thymus-expressed chemokine)	CCR9	Thymic and intestinal epithelia	Presumed role in T-cell selection
SDF-1α (stromal cell-derived factor)	CXCR4 (also known as fusin)	Stromal cells of bone marrow	Involved in hematopoiesis, inhibits cellular entry by T-trophic HIV
BCA-1 (B-cell attractant)	CXCR5	Follicular DCs (?)	Contact between TH and B cells, and between TH and follicular DCs
Others:			
TGFβ (transforming growth factor β)		Many cells, including monocytes and T cells	Inhibits cell growth, inhibits macrophages and production of IL-1 and TNFα, represents a switching factor for IgA

Cell adhesion molecules often play an essential role in cell-to-cell interactions. Two lympho-hematopoietic cells can only establish contact if one of them expresses surface molecules that interact with ligands expressed on the surface of the other cell. As for APC and T cell interactions, the result of such contact may be that a signal capable of inducing differentiation and functional changes will be induced. Adhesion proteins are usually comprised of several chains which can induce different effects when present in various combinations. Interaction of several cascades is often required for the final differentiation of a cell. Cell adhesion molecules normally form part of the Ig superfamily (e.g., ICAM, VCAM, CD2), integrin family (lymphocyte function antigen, LFA-1), selectin family, cadherin family, or various other families. Selectins and integrins also play an important role in interactions between leukocytes and the vascular wall, and thus mediate the migration of leukocytes from the bloodstream into inflamed tissues, or the entry of recirculating lymphocytes into the lymph node parenchyma through high endothelial venules (HEV).

Chemokines (*chemo*attractant cyto*kines*) comprise a family of over 30 small (8–12 kDa) secreted proteins. These contribute to the recruitment of "inflammatory cells" (e.g., monocytes) into inflamed tissues, and influence the recirculation of all classes of leukocytes (Table 2.**6**). Some chemokines result in the activation of their target cell in addition to exerting chemotatic properties. Chemokines can be classified into three families based on their N terminus structure: *CC chemokines* feature two contiguous cysteine residues at the terminus; *CXC chemokines* have an amino acid between the two residues; and *CX3C* and *C chemokines* thus far comprise only one member each (fractalkine and lymphotactin, respectively). Although the N terminus carries bioactive determinants, using a chemokines amino acid sequence to predict its biological function is not reliable. The chemokine system forms a redundant network, or in other words, a single chemokine can often act upon a number of receptors, and the same receptor may recognize a number of different chemokines. Many of the chemokines also overlap in terms of biological function.

Chemokines can be grouped in two functional classes: *inflammatory chemokines* which are secreted by inflamed or infected tissues as mediators of the nonspecific immune response; and *constitutive chemokines* which are produced in primary or secondary lymphoid organs. Together with endothelial adhesion molecules, inflammatory chemokines determine the cellular composition of the immigrating infiltrate. In contrast, the function of constitutive chemokines is to direct lymphocytes to precise locations within lymphoid compartments. Thus, chemokines play a major role in the establishment of inflammatory and lymphoid microenvironments. Chemokine receptors are G protein-coupled membrane receptors with seven transmembrane sequences. In keeping with the above nomenclature, they are designated as CCR, CXCR, or CX3CR plus consecutive numbering. Some viruses, for instance the cytomegaly virus, encode proteins that are functionally analogous to chemokine receptors. This allows a rapid neutralization of locally induced chemokines, and may offer an advantage to the virus. The Duffy antigen receptor for chemokines, DARC, is expressed on endothelial cells and is capable of a high-affinity binding interaction with various chemokine types. Since this receptor has no downstream signaling cascade, it is assumed to function in the presentation of chemokines to leukocytes as they flow past. DARC also functions as a receptor for *Plasmodium vivax*. CCR5 and CXCR4 are co-receptors for HIV infection of CD4+ T cells.

Antibody-Dependent Cellular Immunity and Natural Killer Cells

Lymphocytes can nonspecifically bind IgG antibodies by means of Fc receptors, then specifically attack targets cells (e.g., infected or transformed cells) using the bound antibody. This phenomenon, known as **antibody-dependent cellular cytotoxicity (ADCC)**, has been demonstrated in vitro—however its in-vivo function remains unclear. **Natural killer (NK) cells** also play a role in ADCC. The genesis of NK cells appears to be mainly thymus-independent. These cells can produce IFNγ very early following activation and do not require a specific receptor. These cells are therefore early contributors to the IFNγ-oriented TH1 immune response. NK cells can respond to cells that *do not express MHC class I* molecules, and are inactivated by contact with MHC molecules. This recognition process functions via special receptors that are not expressed in a clonal manner. NK cells probably play an important role in the *early defensive* stages of infectious diseases, although the exact nature of their role remains to be clarified (virus-induced IFNα and IFNβ promote NK activation). NK cells also appear to contribute to rejection reactions, particularly the rejection of stem cells.

Humoral, Antibody-Dependent Effector Mechanisms

The objectives of the immune response include: the inactivation (neutralization) and removal of foreign substances, microorganisms, and viruses; the rejection of exogenous cells; and the prevention of proliferation of pathologically altered cells (tumors). The systems and mechanisms involved in these effector functions are largely non-specific. Specific immune recognition by B and T cells directs these effector mechanisms to specific targets. For instance, immunoglobulins opsonize microbes (e.g., pneumococci) which are equipped with polysaccharide capsules enabling them to resist phagocyte digestion. **Opsonization** involves the coating of such microbes with Fc-expressing antibodies which facilitates their phagocytosis by granulocytes. Many cells, particularly phagocytes (and interestingly enough also some bacteria like staphylococci), bear surface Fc receptors that interact with different Ig classes and subclasses. Mast cells and basophils bear IgE molecules, and undergo a process of degranulation following interaction with allergens against which the IgE molecules are directed. This induces the release of pharmacologically active biogenic amines (e.g., histamine). In turn, these amines represent the causative agent for physiological and clinical symptoms observed during allergic reactions (see also types I-IV, p. 108ff.).

The Complement System

The complement system (C system, Fig. 2.**16**) represents a non-specific defense system against pathogens, but can also be directed toward specific targets by antibodies. It is made up of a co-operative network of plasma proteins and cellular receptors, and is largely charged with the following tasks:

■ **Opsonization** of infectious pathogens and other foreign substances, with the aim of more efficient pathogen elimination. Bound complement factors can: enhance the binding of microbes to phagocytozing cells; result in the activation of inflammatory cells; mediate chemotaxis; induce release of inflammatory mediators; direct bactericidal effects; and induce cell lysis (Fig. 2.**17**, p. 88).

Fig. 2.**16** The classic activation pathway is initiated by antigen-antibody complexes, the alternative pathway by components of microbial pathogens. The production of a C3 convertase, which splits C3 into C3a and C3b, is common to both pathways. C3b combines with C3 convertase to generate C5 convertase. C5b, produced by C5 convertase, binds to the complement factors 6–9 to form a membrane attack complex (MAC). C3b degradation products are recognized by receptors on B lymphocytes; they stimulate the production of antibodies as well as pathogen phagocytosis. The cleavage products C3a and C4a are chemotactic in their action, and stimulate expression of adhesion molecules.

Nomenclature: the components of the alternative pathway (or *cascade*) are designated by capital letters (B, D, H, I; P for properdin), those of the classical pathway (or *cascade*) plus terminal lysis are designated by "C" and an Arabic numeral (1–9). Component fragments are designated by small letters, whereby the first fragment to be split off (usually of low molecular weight) is termed "a" (e.g., C3a), the remaining (still bound) part is called "b" (e.g., C3b), the next split-off piece "c," and so on. Molecules often group to form complexes; in their designations the individual components are lined up together and are usually topped by a line. ▶

■ **Solubilization** of otherwise insoluble antigen-antibody complexes.

■ **Promotion of the transport** of immune complexes, and their elimination and degradation.

■ **Regulation of the immune response**, achieved via their influence on antigen presentation and lymphocyte function.

Over 20 proteins of the complement system have been identified to date, and are classified as either activation or control proteins. These substances account for about 5% of the total plasma proteins (i.e., 3–4 g/l). C3 is not only present in the largest amount, but also represents a central structure for complement activation. A clear difference exists between "classic"

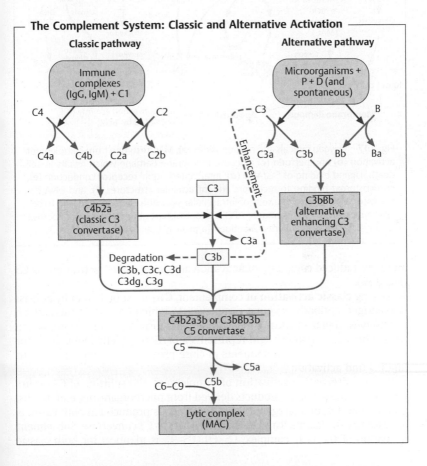

The Complement System: Classic and Alternative Activation

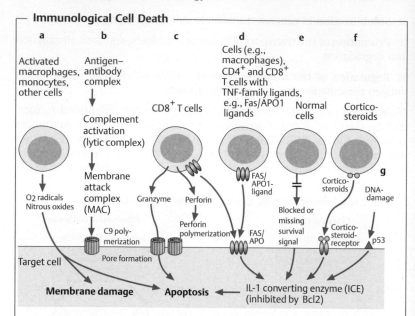

Fig. 2.**17** Oxygen radicals and nitrous oxides (**a**), MAC resulting from complement activation (**b**) and perforin (**c**) all cause membrane damage which results in cell death. Ligand binding of Fas/APO (**d**), interrupted signal receptor conduction (**e**), corticosteroid binding to receptors and intracellular structures (**f**), and DNA damage (**g**) all result in alterations of intracellular signaling cascades and lead to cellular apoptosis. (Fas = F antigen; APO = apoptosis antigen; TNF = tumor necrosis factor; Bcl2 = B-cell leukemia-2 antigen [a protein that inhibits apoptosis].)

antibody-induced complement activation and "alternative" activation via C3 (Fig. 2.**16**).

During **classic activation** of complement, C1q must be bound by at least two antigen-antibody immune complexes, to which C4 and C2 then attach themselves. Together, these three components form a C3 convertase, which then splits C3. Pentameric IgM represents a particularly efficient C activator since at least two Ig Fc components in close proximity are required for C1q binding and activation.

During **alternative activation** of complement, the splitting of C3 occurs directly via the action of products derived from microorganisms, endotoxins, polysaccharides, or aggregated IgA. C3b, which is produced in both cases, is activated by the factors B and D, then itself acts as C3 convertase. Subsequent formation of the lytic complex, C5–C9 (C5–9), is identical for both classic and alternative activation, but is not necessarily essential since the released chemotaxins and opsonins are often alone enough to mediate the functions of microbe neutralization and elimination. Some viruses can activate the complement system without the intervention of antibodies by virtue of their ability to directly bind C1q. This appears to be largely restricted to retro-viruses (including HIV). Importantly, without a stringent control mechanism complement would be activated in an uncontrolled manner, resulting in the lysis of the hosts own cells (for instance erythrocytes).

2

Complement Control Proteins

The following regulatory proteins of the complement system have been character-ized to date:

C1 inhibitor, prevents classic complement activation.

DAF (decay accelerating factor), prevents the association of C3b with factor B, or of C4b with C2, on the cell surface. DAF can also mediate the dissolution of existing complexes, and is responsible for the regulation of classic and alternative C activities.

MCP (membrane cofactor protein), enhances the activity of the factor which de-grades C3b to iC3b. Factor H and CR1 (complement receptor 1) have similar effects.

HRF (homologous restriction factor). Synonyms: MAC (membrane attack complex), inhibitory protein, C8-binding protein. HRF protects cells from C5-9-mediated lysis. This protein is lacking in patients suffering from paroxysmal nocturnal hemoglobinuria.

CD59. Synonyms: HRF20, membrane attack complex (MAC)-inhibiting factor, protec-tin. This is a glycolipid anchored within the cell surface which prevents C9 from binding to the C5b-8 complex, thus protecting the cell from lysis.

Those complement components with the most important biological effects include:

■ **C3b**, results in the opsonization of microorganisms and other antigens, either directly or in the form of immune complexes. "C-marked" microorgan-isms then bind to the appropriate receptors (R) (e.g., CRI on macrophages and erythrocytes, or CR2 on B cells).

■ **C3a and C5a**, contribute to the degranulation of basophils and mast cells and are therefore called anaphylatoxins. The secreted vasoactive amines (e.g., histamine) raise the level of vascular permeability, induce contraction of the smooth musculature, and stimulate arachidonic acid metabolism. C5a initi-ates the chemotactic recruitment of granulocytes and monocytes, promotes their aggregation, stimulates the oxidative processes, and promotes the re-lease of the thrombocyte activating factor.

■ **"Early" C factors,** in particular **C4**, interact with immune complexes and inhibit their precipitation.

■ **Terminal components (C5–9),** together form the so-called membrane at-tack complex, MAC, which lyses microorganisms and other cells.

Some components mediate general regulatory functions on B-cell responses, especially via **CR1** and **CR2**.

Immunological Cell Death

Fig. 2.**17** summarizes the mechanisms of cell death resulting from immunological cell interactions and differentiation processes, as they are understood to date.

Immunological Tolerance

■ **T-cell tolerance**, as defined by a lack of immune reactivity can be due to a number of processes: Firstly, Negative selection in the thymus (referred to as deletion); secondly a simple lack of reactivity to antigen (self or nonself) as a result of the antigen having not been present in the secondary lymphoid organs in a sufficient quantity or for a sufficient amount of time; and thirdly an excessive stimulation of T-cells resulting from the ubiquitous presence of sufficient antigen resulting in T cell exhaustion. Finally, it may also be possible that T cells can become temporarily "anergized" by partial or incomplete antigen stimulation. As a general rule, self-reactive (autoimmune) **B cells** are not generally deleted by negative selection and can therefore be present in the periphery. Exceptions to this rule include B cells specific for membrane-bound self-determinants, some of which are deleted or anergized. B cells react promptly to antigens, even self-antigens, which are arranged repetitively. However, they only react to soluble monomeric antigens if they additionally receive T cell help. Thus, B-cell non-reactivity largely results from a lack of patterned antigen presentation structures or as a result of T-cell tolerance. ■

Immunological tolerance describes the concept that the immune system does not normally react to autologous structures, but maintains the ability to react against foreign antigens. Tolerance is acquired, and can be measured as the selective absence of immunological reactivity against specified antigens.

T-Cell Tolerance

A distinction can be made between **central tolerance**, which develops in the thymus and is based on the *negative selection* (deletion) of T cells recognizing self antigens present in the thymus, and **peripheral tolerance**. Peripheral tolerance results in the same outcome as central tolerance, however, this form of tolerance involves antigen recognition by antigen-reactive peripheral T cells, followed by a process of clonal cell proliferation, end differentiation and death. The following mechanisms have been postulated, and in some cases confirmed, to account for a lack of peripheral T-cell responsiveness (Table 2.**5**, p. 71):

■ **T-cell indifference or ignorance.** Both host and foreign antigens present only within peripheral epithelial, mesenchymal or neuroectodermal cells and tissues—and which do not migrate, or are not transported by APCs, in sufficient amounts to the organized lymphoid organs—are simply ignored by T and B cells. Most self-antigens, not present in the serum or in lymphohematopoietic cells, belong to this category and are ignored despite the fact that they are potentially immunogenic. Certain viruses, and their antigens, actually take advantage of this system of ignorance. For instance, the immune system ignores the rabies virus when it is restricted to axons, and papilloma viruses as long as the antigens are restricted to keratinocytes (warts). The main reason why many self antigens, and some foreign antigens, are ignored by T cells is that immune responses can only be induced within the spleen or in lymph nodes, and non-activated (or naive) T cells do not migrate into the periphery. It has also been postulated that those naive T and B cells which do encounter antigens in the periphery will become anergized, or inactivated, due to a lack of the so-called costimulatory or secondary signals at these sites. However, the evidence supporting this theory is still indirect. Experiments seeking to understand the "indifference" of T cells are summarized in the box on p. 92f. In all probability, a great many self-antigens (as well as peripheral tumors) are ignored by the immune system in this way. These self-antigens represent a potential target for autoimmunity.

■ **Complete, exhaustive T-cell induction.** When an antigen, self or non-self, enters a lymphoid organ it encounters many APCs and T cells, resulting in the extremely efficient activation those T cells carrying the appropriate TCR. During such a scenario the responding T cells differentiate into short-lived effector cells which only survive for two to four days. This induction phase may actually correspond to the postulated phenomenon of anergy (see Table 2.**5**, p. 71). Should this be the case, anergy—defined as the inability of T cells to react to antigen stimulation in vitro—may in fact be explained by the responding cells having already entered a pathway of cell death (apoptosis) (see Fig. 2.**17**, p. 88). Once all the terminally differentiated effector T cells have died, immune reactivity against the stimulating antigen ends. Tolerance is hereafter maintained, as should the responsible antigen have entered into the thymus those newly maturing thymocytes will be subjected to the process of negative selection (e.g., as seen in chronic systemic (viremic) infections with noncytopathic viruses). Moreover, those newly matured T cells which may have escaped negative selection and emigrated into the periphery will continuously be induced to undergo activation and exhaustion within the secondary lymphoid organs.

Exhaustive T-cell induction most likely occurs in responses to hepatitis C virus and HIV, and has been observed in mice experimentally infected with the noncytopathic virus causing lymphocytic choriomeningitis. Successful establishment of lymphocyte chimerism following liver transplants appears to based on the same principle. For example, a relatively short period of immunosuppression following transplantation may allow the establishment of numerous dendritic cells from the transplanted organ within the secondary lymphoid organs of the recipient, resulting in the subsequent elimination of those recipient T cells which react against the foreign MHC molecules.

Two Important Experiments addressing the induction of Immune Responses

APCs transport antigens to the peripheral lymphoid organs via the lymph vessels. *Skin flap experiment.* To prove that antigens contacted at peripheral localizations (e.g. the skin) must first be transported on APCs *through the lymph vessels* into the local lymph node, in order to induce an immune response—an experiment was performed in which a guinea pig skin flap was prepared such that the supply vessels (lymph vessel, vein and artery) remained intact and functional.

Following sensitization of the skin flap with a contact antigen the animal reacted to a second antigenic exposure of the remaining (intact) skin with accelerated kinetics. When the lymph vessel leading from the prepared skin flap to the lymph node was interrupted, or the draining lymph node was destroyed prior to the initial sensitization, the typical secondary response was not observed—leading to the conclusion that *no T cell response was induced*. Following an initial sensitization at any other location on the skin the secondary response was observed, even on the skin flap regardless of interruption of the lymph vessel or destruction of the draining lymph node. This result indicated that the antigen-experienced effector lymphocytes reached the site of antigen via the bloodstream.

Many self antigens are ignored by CD8[+] cells. *A Transgenic mouse encoding a viral glycoprotein gene.* As a comparison to the many self-antigens present in the peripheral non-lymphoid organs and cells, a gene encoding a viral glycoprotein (GP) was incorporated into mice, under the control of a regulatory gene which allowed GP expression only within the pancreatic insulin-producing β cells. This artificially integrated "self antigen" was ignored by the host's immune system, as indicated by the absence of β cell destruction or autoimmunity (diabetes). When the GP expressing transgenic mouse was infected with a virus encoding the *GP* gene, which infects lymphoid organs, GP-specific cytotoxic T cells were induced and these cells destroyed the transgenic islet cells, resulting in the onset of diabetes.

This model demonstrated that many self-antigens are ignored by the immune system simply because they are only present outside of the lymphatic system. However, should such antigens enter the immune system in a suitable form (in this case by viral infection) the host will produce an autoimmune T-cell response.

In summary, the non-responsiveness of T-cells can be achieved by: *negative selection in the thymus*; by *excessive induction in the periphery;* or by *sequestration* of the antigen outside the lymphoid organs. Persistence of the antigen within the lymphoid tissues is a prerequisite for the first two mechanisms. For the third mechanism, it is the absence of antigen within lymphatic organs which guarantees non-responsiveness. There is also a necessary role for 'second'- or 'costimulatory'-signals in the activation of T cells within lymphoid tissues, however, their role in T-cell responsiveness within solid organs remains unclear.

2

B-Cell Tolerance

In contrast to classic central T-cell tolerance, B cells capable of recognizing self-antigens appear *unlikely to be subjected to negative selection* (Table 2.**7**). B-cell regeneration in the bone marrow is a very intensive process, during which antigen selection probably does not play an important role. Although negative selection of bone marrow B cells can be demonstrated experimentally for highly-expressed membrane-bound MHC molecules (in antibody-transgenic mice)—this apparently does not occur for more rare membrane-bound antigens, or for most soluble self-antigens. As a general rule, these potentially self-reactive B cells are not stimulated to produce an immune response because the necessary T helper cells are not present as a result of having being subjected to negative selection in the thymus. B cell and antibody tolerance is therefore largely a result of T cell tolerance which results in the *absence of T help.*

The finding that a certain antigenic structures and sequences can activate B cells in the absence of T help indicates that autoreactive B cells which are present could be prompted to produce an IgM autoantibody response via Ig cross-linking by paracrystalline multimeric antigens. However, since self-antigens are not normally accessible to B cells in such *repetitive paracrystalline patterns*, the induction of IgM autoantibody responses is not normally observed. It is interesting to note that DNA and collagen, which often contribute to chronic autoantibody responses, exhibit repetitive antigen structures. These structures become accessible to B cells within inflamed lesions, and may therefore induce autoantibody responses in certain circumstances. A chronic autoantibody response of the IgG type, however, always requires T help arising from the presentation of self-peptides by MHC class II molecules. Ignored self-peptides, and in all likelihood infectious agents, may play a role in providing such T help. (For instance *Klebsiella* or *Yersinia* in rheumatic diseases, *Coxsackie* virus infections in diabetes, or other chronic parasitic infections.)

Table **2.7** B Cells Do Not Differentiate between Self and Nonself Antigens, but Rather Distinguish Repetitive (Usually Nonself) from Monomeric (Usually Self) Antigens

Antigen			B cells present	IgM response		
				T cell-independent	T help present	T cell-dependent
On cell membranes in the bone marrow	High concentration	Self	Unclear –	–	–	–
	Low concentration	Self	+[1]	+[1]	–	+[1]
Monomeric antigen	High concentration	Self	+[1]	not applicable	–	–
	Low concentration	Nonself	+	not applicable	+	+
Repetitive, identical 5–10 nm intervals, paracrystalline	Self (very rare)[2]		+	(+)[2]	(+)	(+)
	Nonself ("always" infectious)		+	+	+	++

[1] B cells are present and are stimulated by antigen arranged in a repetitive and paracrystalline pattern (T helper-independent type I). B-cell responses to poorly organized or monomeric antigens are not directly induced; in such cases, indirect (T helper-independent type II) or conventionally coupled T help is required.

[2] Such self antigens are not normally accessible to B cells; however collagens presents in lesions, or acetylcholine receptors, may stimulate and possibly activate B cells. When combined with T help, this activation can result in an autoimmune response.

Immunological Memory

Immunological memory is usually defined by an earlier and better immune response, mediated by increased frequencies of specific B or T cells as determined by in vitro or adoptive transfer experiments. **B-cell** immunological memory is more completely described as the ability to mediate protective immunity by means of increased antibody concentrations. Higher frequencies of specific B and T lymphocytes alone, appears to only provide limited or no protection. Instead, immunological protection requires **antigen-dependent activation of B and T cells**, which then produce antibodies continuously or can rapidly mediate effector T functions and can rapidly migrate into peripheral tissues to control virus infections.

Usually the second time a host encounters the same antigen its immune response is both accelerated and augmented. This **secondary immune response** is certainly different from the **primary response**, however, it is still a matter of debate as to whether these parameters alone correlate with immune protection. It is not yet clear whether the difference between a primary and secondary immune response results solely from the increased numbers of antigen-specific B and T cells and their acquisition of "memory qualities", or whether immune protection is simply due to continuous antigen-induced activation (Table 2.**8**).

Table 2.**8** Characteristics of T- and B-Cell Memory

| | **Memory T cells** | | **Memory B cells** | |
	Resting	Activated	Resting	Activated
Localization and migration	Blood, spleen, lymph nodes	Blood, spleen, lymph nodes, and solid tissues	Blood, spleen, lymph nodes	Germinal centers in local lymph nodes, bone marrow
Function	Secondary T-cell response	Immediate target cell lysis and interleukin release	Secondary B-cell response	Sustained IgG response
Time lapse to protective response	Slow	Fast	Slow	Immediate
Proliferation and location of proliferation	In secondary lymphoid organs	Only in secondary lymphoid organs with antigen residues	Blood, spleen	Germinal centers with antigen-IgG complexes
Antigen dependence	No	Yes	No	Yes

There is no surface marker which can unequivocally differentiate between memory T and B cells and "naive" (never before activated) cells. Instead, immunological memory is normally taken to correlate with an increased number of specific precursor T and B cells. Following an initial immunization with antigen, this increased precursor frequency of specific cells is thought to be maintained by an antigen-independent process. Yet the precursor cells can only be activated (or re-activated) by antigen, and only *activated T cells* can provide immediate protection against re-infection outside the lymphoid organs, e.g., in the solid peripheral organs. Similarly, *only antigen activated B cells can mature to become plasma cells* which maintain the increased blood antibody titers responsible for mediating protection. This indicates that residual antigen must be present to maintain protective immunological memory. As a general rule, the level of protective immunity mediated by the existence of memory T and B cells per se is minimal. Highly effective immunity and resistance to re-infection are instead provided by migratory T cells which have been recently activated (or re-activated) by antigen, and by antibody-secreting B cells. **B-cell and antibody memory** is maintained by re-encounters with antigen, or by antigen-IgG complexes which by virtue of their Fc portions or by binding to C3b are captured by-, and maintained for long periods on-, *follicular dendritic cells* present in germinal centers. **Memory T cells**, and in some cases **B cells**, can be re-stimulated and maintained in an active state by: persistent infections (e.g., tuberculosis, hepatitis B, HIV); antigen deposits in adjuvants; periodic antigen re-exposure; peptide-loaded MHC molecules with long half-lives; or possibly (but rarely) by cross-reactive antigens. Thus, secondarily activated (protective) memory T and B cells cannot easily be distinguished from primarily activated T and B cells. The antigen-dependent nature of immunological protection indeed questions the relevance of a specialized "memory quality" of B and T cells.

B-Cell Memory

It is important to differentiate between the characteristics of memory T and B cells as detected in vitro, and the salient in-vivo attributes of improved immune defenses. Following a primary immune response, increased numbers of memory B cells can of course be detected using in vitro assays or by murine experiments involving the transfer of cells into naive recipients. However, these increased B cell frequencies do not necessarily ensure immune protection against, for instance, viral re-infection. Such protection requires the existence of an increased titer of protective antibodies within the host.

Why is Immunological Memory Necessary?

A host which does not survive an initial infection obviously does not require further immunological memory. On the other hand, survival of the initial infection proves that the host's immune system can control or defeat the infection, once again apparently negating the need for immunological memory. Even assuming that better immune defenses provide a clear evolutionary advantage, especially during pregnancy, the idea of immunological memory must be understood as protection within a developmental framework:

1. Due to MHC restriction of T-cell recognition, it is not possible for a mother to pass on T-cell immunological experience to her progeny as the histoincompatibility reaction would induce mutual cellular rejection. For the same reason, a child's T cells apparently cannot mature until relatively late in its development (usually around the time of birth). This explains why newborns are almost entirely lacking in active immune defenses (Fig. 2.**18**). Newborn mice require about three to four weeks (humans three to nine months) before the T-cell immune response and the process of T-B cell collaboration which results in the generation of antibody responses become fully functional. During this period passive immune protection is essential. This type of protection is mediated by the transfer of protective, largely IgG, antibodies from mother to child through the placenta during pregnancy, and to some extent within the mother's milk. An example of this is provided by cattle where the acquisition of colostral milk by the calf is essential to its survival. Calves can only access protective IgG through the colostral milk delivered during the first 24 hours after birth (fetal calf serum contains no Ig). During the first 18 hours post partum, the calf's intestine expresses Fc receptors which allow the uptake of undigested antibodies from the mothers milk into the bloodstream. How can comprehensive, transferable, antibody-mediated protection be ensured under these conditions? During a three-week murine or 270-day human pregnancy, mothers do not normally undergo all of the major types of infection (indeed infection can be potentially life-threatening for both the embryo/fetus and the mother), and so the array of antibodies required for comprehensive protection cannot be accumulated during this period alone. Instead, an accumulation of the immunological protective antibody levels representing the **immunological life experience of infections in the mother's serum** is necessary. The female sex hormones also encourage Ig synthesis, correlating with women's higher risk level (about fivefold) for developing autoantibody diseases (e.g., lupus), and for autoimmune diseases in general.

2. Reproduction requires a relatively **good level of health** and a good nutritional status **of the mother**. However, it also requires an effective immune defense status within the population (herd), including males, since all would otherwise be threatened by repeated and severe infections. The increased frequency of specific precursor B and T cells improves immune defenses against such infections. However, this relative protection is in clear contrast to the absolute protection an immunoincompetent newborn requires to survive.

Ig Serum Concentration Curve

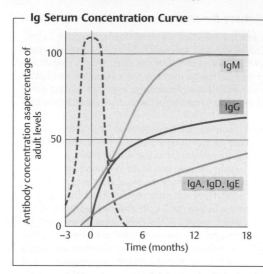

Fig. 2.**18** Synthesis of significant amounts of immunoglobulins only begins during the perinatal period (uninterrupted lines). IgG from the mother is therefore the child's main means of protective immunity before the age of three to six months (dotted line). Infections encountered during this early period are attenuated by maternal antibodies, rendering such infections vaccine-like.

T-Cell Memory

As with B cells and antibodies, enhanced defenses against intracellular pathogens (especially viruses and intracellular bacteria) does not solely depend on increased numbers of specific T cells, but rather is determined by the *activation status* of T cells. Here again it must be emphasized that protective immunological memory against most bacteria, bacterial toxins, and viruses, is mediated by *antibodies*! *Memory T cells* are nonetheless important in the *control of intracellular bacterial infections* (e.g., tuberculosis [TB], leprosy), as well as persistent *noncytopathic viruses* such as hepatitis B and HIV (see also p. 106). It has been demonstrated, at least in mouse models, that a higher number of T cells alone is often insufficient for the protection of the host against the immunopathological consequences of a defensive CD8+ T-cell response. Yet such T cell responses must be activated in order to provide immunity. In the case of *tuberculosis,* sustained activation of a controlled T-cell response by minimal infection foci was postulated, and confirmed, in the 1960s as constituting **infection immunity**—i.e. the lifelong, and usually effective, immune control of the disease by an ongoing localized low-level of infection. A similar situation is observed for cell-mediated immune responses against leprosy, salmonellae, and numerous parasitic diseases (often together with antibodies). The existence of infection-immunity explains why apparently controlled, minimal, infections tend to *flare up* when the immune system is *compromised* by cytostatic drugs, age, or HIV infection. Delayed type (dermal) hypersensitivity (DTH, see below and p. 114f.) can be applied diagnostically to determine infection immunity (for example against tuberculosis and leprosy), since the existence of continued infection continuously activates those T cells required for both pathogen control and DTH reactions.

Delayed Dermal Hypersensitivity Reaction

The classic example of a **delayed type hypersensitivity (DTH)** reaction is the **tuberculin reaction** (Mantoux test in humans). It was one of the first specific cell-mediated immune responses to be identified—as early as the 1940s in guinea pigs. The response is specific for MHC class II antigens and is CD4$^+$ T cell-dependent. In some cases, especially during active viral infections, a DTH reaction is transiently observed and is mediated by CD8$^+$ T cells. The simplest way to elicit a DTH reaction is to introduce a diagnostic protein, obtained from the pathogen, into the skin. The test reaction will only develop should continuously activated T cells be present within the host, since only these cells are capable of migrating to dermal locations within 24–48 hours. If no activated T cells are present, re-activation within the local lymph nodes must first take place, and hence migration into the dermis will require more time. By this time the small amount of introduced diagnostic peptide, or protein, will have been digested or will have decayed and thus will no longer be present at the injection site in the quantity required for induction of a local reaction.

A positive delayed hypersensitivity reaction is, therefore, an indicator of the presence of activated T cells. The absence of a reaction indicates either that the host had never been in contact with the antigen, or that the host no longer possesses activated T cells. In the case of tuberculosis, a negative skin test can indicate that; no more antigen or granuloma tissue is present, or that the systemic immune response is massive and the pathogen is spread throughout the body. In the latter case, the amount of diagnostic protein used is normally insufficient for the attraction of responsive T cells to the site of injection, and as a consequence no measurable reaction becomes evident (so that the Mantoux test may be negative in Landouzy sepsis or miliary tuberculosis). DTH reactions provide a diagnostic test for **tuberculosis** (Mantoux test), **leprosy** (lepromin test), and **Boeck's sarcoid** (Kveim test). However, these dermal reactions may disappear in those patients that are immunosuppressed or infected with measles or AIDS.

Immune Defenses against Infection and Tumor Immunity

■ Protection against infections can be mediated by either; non-specific defense mechanisms (interferons, NK cells), or specific immunity in the form of antibodies and T cells which release cytokines and mediate contact- and perforin-dependent cell lysis. Control of cytopathic viruses requires soluble factors (antibodies, cytokines), whilst control of noncytopathic viruses and tumors is more likely to be mediated via perforins and cytolysis. However, cytotoxic immune responses can also cause disease, especially during noncytopathic infections. Development of an evolutionary balance between infectious agents and immune responses is an ongoing process, as reflected by the numerous mechanisms employed by pathogens and tumors to evade immune-mediated defenses.

All immune defense mechanisms (see Fig. 2.1, p. 44) are important in the battle against infections. Natural humoral mechanisms (antibodies, complement, and cytokines) and cellular mechanisms (phagocytes, natural killer cells, T cells) are deployed by the immune system in different relative amounts, during different phases of infection, and in varying combinations. Gross simplifications are not very helpful in the immunological field, but a small number of tenable rules can be defined based on certain model infections. Such models are mainly based on experiments carried out in mice, or on clinical experience with immunodeficient patients (Fig. 2.19).

General Rules Applying to Infection Defenses

■ **Non-specific defenses** are very important (e.g., Toll-like receptors, IFNα/β), and 'natural immunity' (meaning not intentionally or specifically induced) represented by natural antibodies, direct complement activation, NK cell and phagocytes, plays a significant role in all infections. However, much remains to be learned about their roles.

■ **Antibodies** represent potent effector molecules against acute bacterial infections, bacterial toxins, viral re-infections, and in many cases against acute cytopathic primary viral infections (e.g., rabies and influenza). Antibodies are also likely to make a major contribution to the host-parasite balance occurring during chronic parasitic infections. IgA is the most important defense mechanism at mucosal surfaces (Fig. 2.5, p. 57).

■ **Perforin-dependent cytotoxicity in CD8$^+$ T cells** is important for defense against noncytopathic viruses, for the release of chronic intracellular bacteria, and for protection against intracellular stages of certain parasites.

■ **Nonlytic T-cell responses** provide protection in the form of cytokines (very important cytokines include IFNγ and TNFα), which promote the enhanced digestion and destruction of intracellular bacteria and parasites (e.g., listeria, leishmania, etc.), and in some situations enhance immunity against complex viruses (e.g., the smallpox virus) (Fig. 2.15, p. 79). Infectious agents apparently induce cytokines within a matter of hours (for instance IFNγ, IL-12 , and IL-4), and this early cytokine production in turn functions to define the ensuing T cell response as type 1 or type 2 (see p. 75 and Fig. 2.14, p. 78).

2

General Schemes of Infectious Diseases

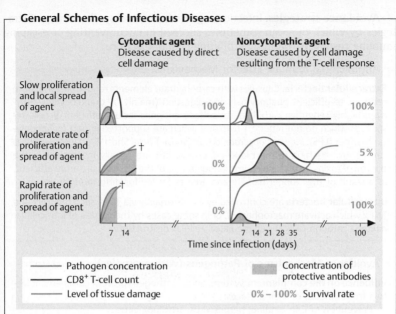

Fig. 2.**19** The degree of host survival depends on both the rate of proliferation, and the extent of spread, of an infectious agent – as well as the intensity of the host's cytotoxic T-cell response. Infection by cytopathic pathogens can only be controlled if pathogenic proliferation is slow and the pathogen remains localized; otherwise the outcome is usually fatal. In the case of noncytopathic pathogens, the cytotoxic T-cell response is the critical parameter. Pathogens which proliferate slowly are quickly eradicated. The T-cell response can be halted by pathogens which proliferate rapidly and spread widely due to the deletion of responding T cells. The degree of survival for hosts is high in both of these cases. For pathogens which exhibit moderate rates of proliferation and spread, the T-cell response may cause extensive immunopathological damage, and thus reduce the proportion of surviving hosts, some of which will controll virus, some not.

A weakened immune defense system may not progress beyond an unfavorable virus-host balance, even when confronted with a static or slowly replicating pathogen which represents an initially favorable balance.

■ **IgE-mediated defense** is important, along with IgA, in enhancing the elimination of gastrointestinal, pulmonary, and dermal parasites. Although details of the process are still sketchy, IgE-dependent basophil and eosinophil defense mechanisms have been described for model schistosomal infections.

■ **Avoidance strategies.** Infectious agents have developed a variety of strategies by which they can sometimes succeed in circumventing or escaping immune responses, often by inhibiting cytokine action.

Antibacterial Immune Effector Mechanisms

Extracellular bacteria. Capsules with carbohydrate elements render bacteria more resistant to efficient phagocytosis and digestion (mainly by granulocytes)—however, highly repetitive carbohydrate surface antigens induce efficient B cells responses which do not require T help and which are supported in part by lipopolysaccharides (LPS). *Pure carbohydrates do not induce T help!* Short-lived IgM responses can control bacteria in the blood effectively, but are usually insufficient in the control of toxins. In such cases, immunoglobulins of the IgG class are more efficient, as a result of their longer half-life and greater facility for diffusing into tissues.

Intracellular bacteria are controlled by T cells (mainly via T cell secreted IFNγ and TNFα which activate macrophages), or in some cases by the release of intracellular bacteria through CD8$^+$ T cell mediated cellular destruction.

Avoidance Mechanisms of Pathogens (with examples)

Influence on the complement system. Some pathogens prevent complement factors from binding to their surfaces:
- Prevention of C4b binding; herpes virus, smallpox virus.
- Prevention of C3b binding; herpes simplex virus (imitates DAF, see p. 86), trypanosomes.

Compartmentalization in non-lymphoid organs. Viruses can avoid confrontation with the immune defenses by restricting their location to peripheral cells and organs located outside of lymphoid tissues:
- Papilloma viruses; infect keratinocytes.
- Rabies virus; infects neurons.

Modulation and down-regulation of surface antigens. Infection agents can avoid immune defenses by mutating or reducing their expression of T- or B-cell epitopes.
- Influenza viruses; antigenic shift caused by rearrangement of genetic elements or drift resulting from mutation of hemagglutinin (at the population level).
- Gonococci; recombination of pili genes.
- Schistosoma; mutation of envelope proteins or masking by adoption of host MHC antigens.

Interference with phagocytosis and digestion. *Mycobacterium tuberculosis* uses CR1, CR2, or fibronectin as a receptor for cell entry; it does not induce efficient oxidative mechanisms in macrophages.
- Components of bacterial cell walls can impede phagosome-lysosome fusion and are resistant to digestion.
- Heat shock proteins (hsp60 and hsp70) or superoxidedismutase aid resistance.

▬ *Continued:* **Avoidance Mechanisms of Pathogens (with examples)** ▬▬▬

Influence on lymphocytes and immunosuppression.
▪ Direct destruction of lymphocytes, or negative regulation of their function (HIV?).
▪ Induction of immunopathological T-cell responses (in some cases these can be immunosuppressive, e.g. HIV).
▪ Induction of immunosuppressive autoantibodies.

Influence on selection, induction, and deletion of T cells.
▪ Negative selection of T cells; if viral antigens are present in the thymus responsive T cells will be deleted.
▪ Exhaustive activation, and subsequent deletion, of peripheral T cells; in some overwhelming peripheral virus infections all of the responding T cells are deleted (HBV, HCV).

Interference with cytokines, cytokine and chemotaxin receptors (R), etc. Many viruses produce substances that block or inhibit receptors for the humoral components of the immune defense system, for instance:
▪ IL-1βR, TNFαR, IFNγR; herpesvirus, smallpox virus.
▪ Chemotaxin receptor; cytomegalovirus.
▪ IL-10R; the Epstein-Barr virus produces B-cell receptor factor I, which binds to the IL-10R thus preventing activation of TH2 cells.
▪ Viral-induced inhibition of interleukin production.

Impairment of MHC antigen expression. Down-regulation of MHC class I and/or class II expression:
▪ Adenovirus; E19 protein reduces expression of MHC class I on infected cells.
▪ Murine cytomegalovirus; prevents transport of MHC class I to the Golgi apparatus.

Immune Protection and Immunopathology

Whether the consequences of an immune response are protective or harmful depends on the balance between infectious spread and the strength of the ensuing immune response. As for most biological systems, the immune defense system is optimized to succeed in 50–90% of cases, not for 100% of cases. For example, immune destruction of virus-infested host cells during the eclipse phase of a virus infection represents a potent means of preventing virus replication (Fig. 2.**15**, p. 79). From this point of view, **lytic CD8+ T-cell responses** make good sense as the host will die if proliferation of a *cytopathic virus* is not halted early on. If a *noncytopathic virus* is not brought under immediate control, the primary illness is not severe—however, the delayed cytotoxic response may then lead to the destruction of very large numbers of infected host cells and thus exacerbate disease (Tables 2.**9** and 2.**10**). Since an infection with noncytopathic viruses is not in itself life-threatening to the

Table 2.**9**   Balance between Infection and Host Immunity: Effect on the Disease

Infectious agent	Cytopatho-genicity of agent	Efficiency of immune response		
		Early start	*Later start*	*No immune response*
Extracellular bacteria				
Meningococci Staphylococci	High	Recovery	Death	Death
Facultatively intracellular bacteria				
Listeria	High	Recovery	Death	Death
Tuberculosis bacilli	Moderate	Recovery	Immuno-pathological inflamma-tion	Miliary tuberculo-sis (early death) Landouzy sepsis (very early death)
Leprosy bacilli	Very low	Recovery	Tuberculoid leprosy	Lepromatous leprosy (late death)
Viruses				
Smallpox virus	High	Recovery	Death	Death (early)
LCMV (lymphocytic choriomeningitis)	Very low	Recovery	Immuno-pathological disease	Healthy carrier
Hepatitis B virus	Very low	Recovery	Aggressive hepatitis	Carrier (very late liver carcinoma)
HIV	Low (?)	Recovery	AIDS	Healthy carrier (occult infection) (?)
Unrecognized and unknown infections, viruses, bacteria, and endogenous retroviruses	Low	?	Auto-immunity	"Healthy" or occult carrier (although infec-tious agent is unknown)
Clinical symptoms		None	Chronic disease	Variable disease symptoms, some-times delayed or asymptomatic

Table 2.**10** Hepatitis B Virus (HBV) Infection. Inter-relations between Efficient Antigen Presentation by MHC Molecules, T-Cell Responses, Course of Infection, and Clinical Picture. Decreased Immunocompetence or Enhanced HBV Proliferation Shifts the Balance Towards an Unfavorable Outcome; Vaccination Shifts the Balance Towards a Favorable Outcome

Presentation of HBV antigen by MHC	T-cell response	Kinetics of infection	Clinical phenotype
+++	*Early*	HBV proliferation is halted	Acute hepatitis with or without icterus, due to hepatocyte damage being minimal
+/–	*Late*	HBV proliferation is halted too late. Liver cells are lysed by CD8+ T cells	Acute to chronic aggressive hepatitis
–	*None*	HBV proliferation is not halted, but there is no immunopathology	Healthy HBV carrier (late liver cell carcinoma)

host, it is paradoxically the immune response that is responsible for pathology and illness due to its ability to destroy infected host tissue.

Hepatitis B viral infections in humans (Table 2.**10**), and LCMV infections (lymphocytic choriomeningitis) in mice, are amongst the most thoroughly studied examples of this potentially negative consequence of protective immune responses. A similar situation is also observed for the cellular immune response against facultative intracellular tuberculosis and leprosy bacilli which themselves have relatively low levels of pathogenicity (Table 2.**9**). A healthy immune system will normally bring such infectious agents under control efficiently, and the immunological cell and tissue damage (which occurs in parallel with the elimination of the pathogen) will be minimal, ensuring that there is little by way of pathological or clinical consequence. However, should the immune system allow these agents to spread further, the result will be a chronic immunopathological response and resultant tissue destruction—as seen during hepatitis B as *chronic or acute aggressive hepatitis* and in leprosy as the *tuberculoid form*. Should a rapidly spreading infection result in exhaustion of the T cell response, or should an insufficient level of immunity be generated, the infected host will become a carrier. This carrier state, which only occurs during infections characterized by an absent or low-level of cytopathology, is convincingly demonstrated in hepatitis B carriers and sufferers of lepromatous leprosy.

Immunopathological Damage and AIDS

Could it be that immunopathological damage resulting from T cell immune responses play a role in AIDS?

The general assumption at the present time is that the causal HIV virus destroys those T helper cells it infects, yet no unequivocal in-vivo proof of this assumption has been obtained. T helper cells do disappear, but how and why they disappear remains unclear. Animal models employing viruses similar to HIV suggest that AIDS might also develop by alternative means:

Assuming that HIV is a *noncytopathic, or only mildly cytopathic*, virus—infection of macrophages, dendritic cells, and/or T helper cells will not cause an immediate outbreak of disease. Soon, however, the virus-infected macrophages and T helper cells will be destroyed by specifically reacting cytotoxic $CD8^+$ T cells. Because the immune response also acts to inhibit virus proliferation, the process of cellular destruction is generally a gradual process. However, over time the immune system itself may become damaged and weakened. Paradoxically, the process of immunological cell destruction would help the virus survive for longer periods in the host and hence facilitate its transmission. From the point of view of the virus this would be an astounding, and highly advantageous, strategy—but one with tragic consequences for the host following, in most cases, a lengthy illness. If proliferation of HIV could be slowed or even halted, the virus would infect fewer lymphocytes, and thus fewer cells would be destroyed by the cytotoxic T-cell response. Prevention or reduction of HIV proliferation, either by pharmacological means or by bolstering the early immune defenses through other means, therefore represents an important objective despite the likelihood that HIV is not very cytopathic.

Influence of Prophylactic Immunization on the Immune Defenses

Vaccines provide protection from diseases, but in most cases cannot entirely prevent re-infection. Vaccination normally results in a limited infection by an attenuated pathogen, or induces immunity through the use of killed pathogens or toxoids. The former type of vaccine produces a very *mild infection or illness* capable of inducing an immune response and which subsequently protects the host against re-infection. The successful eradication of smallpox in the seventies so far represents the greatest success story in the history of vaccination. The fact is that vaccinations never offer absolute security, but instead improve the chances of survival by a factor of 100 to 10 000. A special situation applies to infections with noncytopathic agents in which disease results from the immune response itself (see above). Under certain circumstances, and in a small number of vaccinated persons, the vaccination procedure may therefore shift the balance between immune defense and infection towards an unfavorable outcome, such that the vaccination will actually *strengthen the disease*. Rare examples of this phenomenon may include the use of inactivated vaccines against the respiratory syncytial virus (RSV) in the sixties, and experience with certain so-called subunit vaccines and recombinant vaccines against noncytopathic viral infections in rare model situations. Generally, it should be kept in mind that most of the successful immunization programs developed to date have mediated *protection via antibodies*. This particularly applies to the classic protective vaccines listed in Table 1.**13** (p. 33) for children, and explains why antibodies not only are responsible for the protection of neonates during the immuno-incompetent early postnatal period where immunological experience is passed on from the mother via antibodies, but also attenuate early childhood infections to become vaccine-like. This explains why successful vaccines all protect via neutralizing antibodies, because this pathway has been selected by co-evolution. As mentioned earlier, with regard to immunological memory, memory T cells appear to be essential to host immune protection, particularly in those situations when antigen persistence is controlled efficiently by means of infection-immunity (e.g., tuberculosis, HIV).

2

Tumor Immunity

Our knowledge concerning the immune control of tumors is still modest. Some tumor types bear defined tumor-associated, or tumor-specific, antigens. However this is apparently not sufficient for induction of an efficient immune defense. There is also the problem of tumor diagnosis; the presence of tumors is sometimes confirmed using a functional or immunological basis, yet the tumor cannot be located because conventional examinations are often unable to discover them until they reach a size of about 10^9 cells (i.e., about 1 ml) of tumor tissue.

Factors important in immune defense reactions include the location and rate of proliferation, vascularization or the lack thereof, and necrosis with phagocytosis of disintegrating tumor tissue. We never actually get to see those rare tumors against which immune control might have been successfully elicited, instead we only see those clinically relevant tumors that have unfortunately become successful tumors which have escaped immune control.

Evidence of the immune system's role in tumor control includes:

■ Greater than 85% of all tumors are carcinomas and sarcomas, that is nonlymphohematopoietic tumors which arise in the periphery, outside of organized lymphoid tissues. The immune system, in a manner similar to that seen for many strictly extra-lymphatic self antigens, ignores such tumors at first.

■ Lymphohematopoietic tumors often present immunological oddities such as unusually low, or entirely absent, MHC and/or low tumor antigen concentrations, plus they frequently lack accessory molecules and signals.

■ Congenital or acquired immunodeficiency—whether caused by anti-lymphocytic sera, cytostatic drugs, gamma irradiation, UV irradiation, or infection—usually encourages tumor growth, especially for lymphohematopoietic tumors. Carcinomas and sarcomas show little or no increased susceptibility. Interestingly, experimental carcinogens are frequently also immunosuppressive.

■ Surgical removal of a large primary tumor may result in the disappearance (or rarely in rapid growth) of metastases within the lymph nodes.

■ Tumor cells often display modulated MHC expression—some tumors lack MHC class I molecules entirely—or in some cases tumors selectively down-modulate the only MHC allele capable of presenting a specific tumor-associated peptide (e.g., the colon adenocarcinomas). Other tumors side-step immune defenses by down-regulating tumor-specific antigens.

■ The immune response may fail if tumor differentiation antigens are expressed, against which the host exhibits an immunological tolerance (e.g., carcinoembryonic antigen [CEA], T-cell leukemia antigen).

■ Blockade of the reticuloendothelial system may encourage the development of lymphohematopoietic tumors. For instance, chronic parasitic infections or infection by malaria can result in the development of Burkitt lymphoma, a B-cell malignancy.

The Pathological Immune Response

■ An immune response can also cause disease. Such responses can be classified into the following types: **Type I:** allergic IgE-dependent diseases; **Type II:** antibody-dependent responses to cell membranes, blood group antigens or other auto-antigens; **Type III:** immune complex-initiated diseases whereby surplus antigen-antibody complexes are deposited on basement membranes, resulting in development of chronic disease via complement activation and inflammatory reactions; **Type IV:** cellular immunopathology resulting from excessive T-cell responses against infections that otherwise exhibit low cytopathogenicity, or against allogenic organ transplants. ■

Type I: IgE-Triggered Anaphylaxis

This type of immediate hypersensitivity reaction occurs within minutes in allergically sensitized individuals. Although serum IgE has a short half-life (one to two days), IgE antibodies bound to the Fc_ε receptor on basophils and mast cells have a half-life of several months and when bound by the specific allergen mediate cellular degranulation and the release of biogenic amines (e.g., histamine, serotonin). These mediators can influence the smooth musculature, and mainly result in the constriction of the pulmonary- and broncho-postcapillary venules, together with arteriole dilation. The local manifestations of IgE-triggered anaphylaxis include whealing of the skin (urticaria), diarrhea for food allergies, rhinitis or asthma for pollen allergies, or a generalized anaphylactic shock. IgE reactions are usually measured in vitro using RIA (radioimmunoassay), RIST (radioimmunosorbent test) or RAST (radioallergosorbent test) (see Fig. 2.**28** and Fig. 2.**29**, p. 131f.) Frequent causal agents of IgE allergies in humans include pollen, animal hair, house dust (mites), insect bites and stings, penicillin, and foods. Examples of allergic diseases include local allergic rhinitis and conjunctivitis, allergic bronchial asthma, systemic anaphylactic shock, insect toxin allergies, house dust (mite) and food allergies, urticaria, and angioedemas.

Degranulation of mast cells and basophils can be induced by factors other than the cross-linking of specific IgE antibodies. Such factors include the complement factors C3a and C5a, and pharmacological inducers ("pseudo-allergy!").

Atopic patients suffer severely from allergies. Atopia is genetically conditioned, with a child exhibiting a 50% risk of developing atopy if both parents are allergic, or a 30% risk if only one parent is allergic. The incidence level of atopy within the general population is roughly 10–15%. Atopia correlates with high levels of IgE production, and desensitization refers to attempts to change a TH2 (IgE-producing) response into a TH1 (IgG-favoring) response by means of repeated inoculations or oral doses of allergens (see Fig. 2.**14**, p. 78). It is likely that increased production of IgG—as opposed to IgE—antibodies plays a major role in the success of desensitization. IgE no doubt has an important biological function, probably against ectoparasites, with allergic reactions representing nothing more than an unfortunate side effect of this biological system. Little research has been performed on the nature of the protective function of IgE during parasitic infections (or on the role of eosinophils). However, we do know that mediators released by IgE-triggering of mast cells and basophils cause the smooth intestinal musculature to contract, and in this way facilitate the elimination of intestinal parasites.

Type II: Cytotoxic Humoral Immune Responses

These are pathological immune responses induced by the binding of IgM or IgG antibodies to antigens present on a cell surface (including viral products or haptens), or within tissue components. The mediators responsible for such tissue damage are usually components of the complement system,

Table 2.**11**   Examples of Antibody–Related Type II Immunopathologies

Antibody	Autoimmune pathology or immunopathology
Anti-cell membrane	– Rhesus incompatibility – Blood transfusion complications – Autoimmune hemolytic anemia – Immune neutropenia, idiopathic thrombocytopenia
Anti-basement membrane	– Goodpasture syndrome
Anti-collagen	– Sclerodermia – Pemphigoid (anti-epidermal basal membrane)
Anti-desmosome	– Pemphigus vulgaris
Anti-receptor	– Anti-acetylcholine receptors: myasthenia gravis – Anti-TSH receptors: Basedow disease
Anti-hormone	– Anti-thyroid hormone (Hashimoto thyroiditis) – Anti-intrinsic factor (pernicious anemia)
Anti-medication	– Chemical groups (haptens) bound to cell surface (cytolysis, agranulocytosis)
Anti-cell component	– Anti-DNA (lupus erythematosus, LE) – Anti-mitochondrial (LE, Hashimoto thyroiditis)

or granulocytic digestive enzymes. The most important diseases resulting from cytotoxic humoral immune responses are listed in Table 2.**11**.

Autoantibody Responses

Some clinically important autoantibodies are directed against hormone receptors, for example thyrotoxicosis in Basedow's disease is caused by autoantibodies that stimulate the TSH receptor, and myasthenia gravis is caused by blockage of the acetylcholine receptor by specific autoantibodies. Other antibody-induced diseases mediated by antibodies, directed against hormones and other cellular self antigens, include Hashimoto thyroiditis (induced by anti-thyroglobulin and anti-mitochondrial autoantibodies), pernicious anemia (anti-intrinsic factor), pemphigus vulgaris (anti-desmosome) Guillain-Barré syndrome (ascending paralysis caused by specific myelin autoantibodies), and scleroderma (involving anti-collagen antibodies). Other immunopathologies involving autoantibodies include transplant rejection as a result of endothelial damage (especially in xenogeneic transplants), and tumor rejection caused by antibodies against tumor-associated antigens present on neoplastic cells (especially relevant for lymphohematopoietic

Table 2.**12** Mechanisms Of Autoantibody Induction

Possible mechanisms	Autoimmune pathology or immunopathology
Polyclonal B-cell activation	Lipopolysaccharides, viruses, chronic parasitic infection
Molecular mimicry (overall very rare)	Anti-tat (HTLV-1), anti-H. pylori, or anti-streptococcus crossreacting with self-antigens
Exposure of hidden autoantigens	Cytopathic effects of infectious agents
Adjuvant effects	In the presence of granuloma formation and chronic inflammatory reactions lymphoid tissue may form in peripheral organs (e.g., during Hashimoto's thyroiditis)
Breakdown of tolerance	Due to coupling of T helper epitopes to autoantigens, possible in connection with virus infections of cells

2

tumors). However, in general the detection of autoantibodies does not necessarily correlate with evidence of pathological changes or processes. In fact, our detection methods often measure low-avidity autoantibodies that may have no direct disease-causing effects.

Exactly how autoantibody responses are induced remains to be clarified. As explained earlier (in the discussion of immunological tolerance) such IgG responses cannot be induced without T help. Thus, intensive research is currently focused on those mechanisms by which T cell help for autoreactive B cells is regulated; Table 2.**12** sums up some of the possible mechanisms.

Anti-blood Group Antibody Reactions

ABO system. These B-cell epitopes consist of *sugar groups present in the membranes of red blood cells.* The four classic blood groups are determined by one gene with three alleles. This gene controls glycosylation. The O allele codes only for a basic cell surface structure (H substance) with the terminal sugars galactose and fucose. The A allele adds *N*-acetylgalactosamine to this basic structure, the B allele adds galactose. This results in epitopes, which are also seen frequently in nature largely as *components of intestinal bacteria.* Individuals who carry the A allele are tolerant to the A-coded epitope, whilst individuals with the B allele are tolerant to the B epitope. Individuals who carry both of these alleles (genotype AB) are tolerant to both epitopes, whereas persons who are homozygotes for the O allele are not tolerant to either A or B. Following birth, the intestinal tract is colonized by bacteria containing large numbers of epitopes similar to the A and B epitopes. During the first months of life, people with blood group O (homozygous for the O allele) produce both anti-A and anti-B antibodies, people with blood group A (genotype AO or AA) produce only anti-B antibodies, people with blood group B (genotype BO or BB) produce only anti-A antibodies, and people with blood group AB produce neither anti-A or anti-B antibodies.

These so-called "natural" antibodies (meaning these antibodies are produced without a recognizable immunization process) are of the IgM class; there is usually no switch to IgG, probably resulting from a lack of necessary helper T-cell epitopes. The presence of the blood group antibodies makes blood transfusions between non-matched individuals extremely risky, necessitating that the blood group of both the donor and recipient is determined before the blood transfusion takes place. Nevertheless, the *antibodies in the donor blood are not so important* because they are diluted. The O genotype is therefore a universal donor. Note that IgM antibodies to blood groups present no danger to the fetus since they cannot pass through the placental barrier.

Rhesus factor. This system is also based on genetically determined antigens present on red blood cells, although as a general rule there is no production of "natural" antibodies against these. IgM and IgG antibodies are not induced unless an *immunization* (resulting from blood transfusion or pregnancy) takes place. During the birth process, small amounts of the child's blood often enter the mother's bloodstream. Should the child's blood cells have paternal antigens, which are lacking in the mother's blood, his or her blood will effectively 'immunize' the mother. Should IgG antibodies develop they will represent a potential risk during *subsequent pregnancies* should the fetus once again present the same antigen. The resulting clinical picture is known as *morbus hemolyticus neonatorum* or *erythroblastosis fetalis* ("immune hydrops fetalis").

Once immunization has occurred, *thus endangering future pregnancies*, genetically at risk children can still be saved by means of cesarean section and exchange blood transfusions. Should the risk of rhesus immunization be recognized at the end of the first pregnancy, immunization of the mother can be prevented by means of a *passive infusion* of antibodies against the child's antigen, immediately following the birth. This specific immunosuppressive procedure is an empirical application of immunological knowledge, although the precise mechanism involved is not yet been completely understood.

Other blood group systems. There are other additional blood group systems against which antibodies may be produced, and which can present a risk during transfusions. Thus, the crossmatch test represents an important measure in the avoidance of transfusion problems. Immediately prior to a planned transfusion, serum from the prospective recipient is mixed with erythrocytes from the prospective donor, and serum from the prospective donor is mixed with erythrocytes from the prospective recipient. To ensure no reaction following transfusion, there should be no agglutination present in either mixture. Some potentially dangerous serum antibodies may bind to the erythrocytes causing opsonization, but not necessarily inducing agglutination. To check for the presence of such antibodies, anti-human immunoglobulin serum is added and should it crosslink such antibodies agglutination will result.

Type III: Diseases Caused by Immune Complexes

Pathologies initiated by immune complexes result from the deposition of **small, soluble, antigen-antibody complexes** within tissues. The main hallmark of such reactions is *inflammation* with the involvement of complement. Normally, large antigen-antibody complexes (that is, those produced in equivalence) are readily removed by the phagocytes of the reticuloendothelial system. Occasionally, however—especially in the presence of *persistent bacterial, viral, or environmental, antigens* (e.g., fungal spores, vegetable or animal materials), or during *autoimmune diseases* directed against autoantigens (e.g., DNA, hormones, collagen, IgG) where autoantibodies to the body's own antigens are produced continuously—deposition of antigen-antibody complexes may become widespread often being present on active secretory membranes and within smaller vessels. Such processes are mainly observed within infected organs, but can also occur within kidneys, joints, arteries, skin and lung, or within the brain's plexus choroideus. The resulting inflammation causes local tissue damage. Most importantly, activation of complement by such complexes results in production of inflammatory C components (C3a and C5a). Some of these *anaphylatoxins* cause the release of vasoactive amines which increase vascular permeability (see also p. 103f.). Additional chemotactic activities attracts *granulocytes* which attempt to phagocytize the complexes. When these phagocytes die, their lysosomal hydrolytic enzymes are released and cause further tissue damage. This process can result in long-term chronic inflammatory reactions.

There are two basic patterns of immune complex pathogenesis:

■ **Immune complexes in the presence of antigen excess.** The acute form of this disease results in *serum sickness*, the chronic form leads to the development of arthritis or glomerulonephritis. Serum sickness often resulted from serum therapy used during the pre-antibiotic era, but now only occurs rarely. Inoculation with equine antibodies directed against human pathogens, or bacterial toxins, often induced the production of host (human) antibodies against the equine serum. Because relatively large amounts of equine serum were administered for such therapeutic purposes, such therapy would result in the induction of antigen-antibody complexes—some of which were formed in the presence of antigen excess—and occasionally induced a state of shock.

■ **Immune complexes in the presence of antibody excess.** The so-called *Arthus reaction* is observed when an individual is exposed to repeated small doses of an antigen over a long period of time, resulting in the induction of complexes and an antibody excess. Further exposure to the antigen, particularly dermal exposure, induces a typical reaction of edema and erythema which peaks after three to eight hours and disappears within 48 hours, but which sometimes leads to necrosis. Arthus-type reactions often represent occupational diseases in people exposed to repeated doses of environmental antigens: farmer's lung (thermophilic *Actinomyces* in moldy hay), pigeon breeder's lung (protein in the dust of dried feces of birds), cheese worker's lung (spores of *Penicillium casei*), furrier's lung (proteins from pelt hairs), malt-worker's lung (spores of *Aspergillus clavatus* and *A. fumigatus*).

Type IV: Hypersensitivity or Delayed Type, Cell-Mediated Hypersensitivity

Intracutaneous injection of a soluble antigen derived from an infectious pathogen induces a delayed dermal thickening reaction in those people who have suffered a previous infection. This *delayed skin reaction* can serve as a test to confirm immunity against intracellular bacteria or parasites.

For most cases, the time between administration of the antigen and the swelling reaction is 48–72 hours—as described above for cellular delayed type hypersensitivity (DTH) reactions in the skin (p. 99). As observed for antibody-dependent hyper-reactions of types I-III, the type IV response is pathogenic and *differs from protective immune responses only in terms of the extent and consequences of the tissue damage, but not in terms of the mechanism of action.* The balance between autoimmune disease and type IV immunopathology in such cases is readily illustrated by type IV reactions (e.g., aggressive hepatitis in humans or lymphocytic choriomeningitis in mice). Should the causal infectious pathogen be known, the response is termed a type IV reaction, if the causal agent is unknown (or not yet determined) the same condition may be termed "autoimmune disease." The reader is referred to the many examples of type IV responses already discussed within various chapters (DTH [p. 99], immune protection and immunopathology [Tables 2.**9** and 2.**10**, pp. 104 and 105], transplantation immunology [see below], and autoimmunity [p. 110ff.]).

Autoimmune T cells are usually directed against autoantigens that would otherwise be ignored (since they are only expressed in the extralymphatic periphery). Autoaggressive CD4$^+$ T cells apparently respond against myelin basic protein in *multiple sclerosis*, against collagen determinants in *poly-arthritis*, and against islet cell components in *diabetes*.

Transplantation Immunity

2

■ Transplant rejection within the same species is largely a consequence of MHC-restricted T-cell recognition of foreign MHC antigens. Interspecies rejection is additionally contributed to by antibodies, and intolerance between complement activation mechanisms. Methods for reducing, or preventing, rejection include general immunosuppression, tolerance induction by means of cell chimerism, and sequestering of the transplanted cells or organ. ■

The *strong* transplantation antigens are *encoded within the MHC complex* (see p. 58ff.), whilst the *weak* antigens constitute the MHC-presented allelic differences of *non MHC-encoded host proteins or peptides.* It is possible to differentiate between the **host-versus-graft** (HVG) reaction of the recipient against a genetically foreign tissue or organ, and the **graft-versus-host** (GVH) reaction.

The GVH reaction. This type of reaction results when *immunologically responsive donor T cells* are transferred to an allogeneic recipient who is unable to reject them (e.g., following a bone marrow transplant into an immuno-incompetent or immuno-suppressed recipient). The targets against which the transplanted T cells generate an immune response include the MHC class I and II molecules of the recipient. The recipient's transplantation antigens also present allelic variants of recipient self-peptides, which can be recognized by donor T cells as weak transplantation antigens when presented by common MHC alleles (it is conceivable that strong recipient transplantation antigens could be accepted and processed by donor APCs, however even if this did occur it would be of limited functional consequence as they would not be presented by the recipient APC in the correct antigen configuration). Weak histocompatibility antigens—for instance those peptide variants recognized as nonself when presented in combination with essentially histocompatible MHC molecules—play a more significant role in bone marrow transplants. The existence, and pathological role, of weak transplantation antigens has only been demonstrated in completely histocompatible siblings or within inbred animal strains with identical MHC. The *wide variety of alloreactive T cells* can be explained by cross-reactivity, as well as by the enormous number of different combinations of MHC molecules and cellular peptides. It must be emphasized that allogeneic MHC antigens on APCs and lymphocytes (so-called passenger lymphocytes) derived from the donor organ are particularly immunogenic since they express high levels of antigens and can traffic to secondary lymphatic organs. Indeed the same foreign transplantation antigens are hardly immunogenic when expressed on fibroblasts or on epithelial or neuroendocrine cells, unless these cells are able to reach local lymphoid tissue.

To avoid a GVH reaction in immunoincompetent or suppressed bone marrow recipients, immunocompetent T cells must first be eliminated from the transplanted bone marrow. This can be achieved by using anti-T-cell antibodies, anti-lymphocyte antisera, and complement or magnetic bead cell-separation techniques. However, it is noteworthy that complete elimination of mature T cells leads to a reduction in the acceptance rate for bone marrow transplants, and that it may also weaken the anti-tumor effect of the transplant (desirable in leukemia). It seems that the small number of T cells transplanted with the bone marrow can mediate a subclinical GVH reaction, thus preventing rejection of the transplant but retaining the ability to destroy the recipient's leukemia cells and preventing tumor re-emergence.

Bone Marrow Transplants Today

- Reconstitution of immune defects involving B and T cells
- Reconstitution of other lymphohematopoietic defects
- Gene therapy via insertion of genes into lymphohematopoietic stem cells
- Leukemia therapy with lethal elimination of tumor cells and reconstitution with histocompatible, purified stem cells, either autologous or allogenic.

HVG reactions, that is immune responses of the recipient against transplanted cells or organs, are not generated in autotransplants (for instance transplantation of skin from one part of the body to another on the same individual). This also applies to transplants between monozygotic twins or genetically identical animals (**syngeneic transplants**). However, transplants between non-related or non-inbred animals of the same species (**allogeneic transplants**), and transplants between individuals of different species (**xenogeneic transplants**) are immunologically rejected. Because T cells recognition is subject to MHC restriction, cellular rejection within a species is even more pronounced than between different species, although the latter procedure involves other transplantation complications. These include the occurrence of natural *cross-reactive antibodies,* and a *lack of complement inactivation* by anti-complement factors (which are often species-incompatible and therefore absent in xenogeneic transplants), which together often results in hyperacute rejection within minutes, hours, or a few days—that is before any specific immune responses can even be induced.

Three types of transplant rejection have been characterized:

Hyperacute rejection of vascularized transplants, occurring within minutes to hours and resulting from preformed recipient antibodies reacting against antigens present on the donor endothelium, resulting in coagulation, thromboses, and infarctions with extensive necrosis.

■ **Acute rejection**, occurring within days or weeks. This is accompanied by a perivascular and prominent occurrence of T lymphocyte infiltrates. Acute rejection can be prevented by immunosuppression.

■ **Chronic rejection,** occurring within months to years. This is caused by low-level chronic T-cell responses, and can be mediated by cellular and humoral mechanisms. This can include obliterative vascular intima proliferation, vasculitis, toxic, and immune complex glomerulonephritis.

Antigenicity and Immunogenicity of MHC in Organ Transplants

A thyroid gland from donor "a," freshly transplanted under the renal capsule of an MHC (H-2)-incompatible recipient mouse "b" is acutely rejected (within seven to nine days). If the organ is treated in such a way as to kill the migratory APCs and leukocytes before it is transplanted, then transplant "a" will be accepted by recipient "b" (often permanently). However, should fresh spleen cells (APCs) from donor "a" be transferred by infusion 100 days later into the recipient "b," the previously accepted transplant "a," can sometimes be acutely rejected (i.e., within 10 days).

This experiment demonstrates that it is not the MHC antigens per se that are potently immunogenic, but rather that they only show this immunogenicity when they are located on cells capable of migration to local lymph nodes. Methods of implanting foreign tissue cells or small organs strictly extralymphatically, without inducing immune responses, are currently undergoing clinical trials (i.e., with islet cells in diabetes and neuronal cells in parkinsons disease).

Methods of measurement. The main methods used for follow-up analysis of HVG and GVH reactions are biopsies and histological evaluation, evaluation of blood cells and in-vitro mixed lymphocyte reactions (p. 132).

Immune Defects and Immune Response Modulation

■ **Immune defects** are frequently acquired by therapy or viral infections, or as a consequence of advanced age. In rare cases immune defects can also result from congenital defects, these include severe combined immunodeficiency's (SCID) or transient partial immune defects (mainly involving IgA responses). **Immunomodulation** can be attempted using interleukins or monoclonal antibodies directed against lymphocyte surface molecules or antigenic peptides. **Immunostimulation** is achieved using adjuvants or the genetically engineered insertion of costimulatory molecules into tumor cells. **Immunosuppression** can be induced globally using drugs, or specifically using antibodies, interleukins or soluble interleukin receptors; this can also be achieved by means of tolerance induction with proteins, peptides, or cell chimerism.

Immune Defects

The most important and frequent immune defects are *acquired*, e.g., iatrogenic (cytostatics, cortisone, irradiation, etc.), age-induced, or the result of viral infections (above all HIV). *Congenital defects* are rare; examples include Bruton's X-chromosome-linked B-cell defect, thymic hypoplasia (DiGeorge), and combined T- and B-cell deficiency resulting from MHC defects (bare lymphocyte syndrome) or from enzyme defects (adenosine deaminase [ADA] deficiency or purine nucleoside phosphorylase [PNP] deficiency). These defects can also be repaired by reconstitution (thymic transplants), or in some cases through the use of stem cells (gene therapy; one of the very first successful gene therapies was the treatment of ADA deficiency). More frequent congenital defects involve selective deficiencies, for example a relative-to-absolute IgA deficiency, normally being more prominent in infants than later in life. Children with such deficiencies are more susceptible to infection with *Haemophilus influenzae*, pneumococci, and meningococci. *General consequences of immune defects* include recurring and unusual infections, eczemas, and diarrhea.

Immunoregulation

This area of immunology is difficult to define and remains elusive. Antigens represent the most important positive regulator of immunity; since there is simply no immune stimulation when antigens have been eliminated or are absent. Other important regulators include interferon gamma (IFNγ) for TH1 responses, and IL-4 for TH2 responses. Further IL-dependent regulatory functions are in the process of being defined. The existence of specific CD8$^+$ T suppressor cells, capable of downregulating immune responses, has been postulated and their role was assumed to be that of counteracting the inflammatory CD4$^+$ T cell response. However, to date there has been no convincing proof of their existence. The term CD8$^+$ T suppressor cells, which is used frequently, is therefore misleading and inaccurate. In relatively rare cases, cytotoxic CD8$^+$ T cells do exercise a regulatory effect by lysing infected APCs or B cells (see also p. 106). It is unclear whether CD4$^+$ T cells could have similar effects. Regulation via *idiotypic/anti-idiotypic antibody networks* (i.e., antibodies directed against the ABS of other antibodies), or anti-TCR networks, have also been postulated—but remain hypothetical. Although attractive hypothesis, for most cases such regulatory pathways have only proved disappointing theoretical concepts, and as such should no longer be employed in the explanation of immunoregulation. In isolated cases, anti-idiotypic, or anti-TCR peptide-specific feedback, mechanisms can be modeled under forced experimental conditions. However such conditions probably fail to model normal situations, therefore they cannot accurately indicate whether these feedback mechanisms have a role in regulating the immune system as a whole.

Immunostimulation

The aim of immunological treatment of infections and tumors is to enhance immune responsiveness via the use of thymic hormones (thymopoietin, pentapeptides), leukocyte extracts, or interferons. Derivatives or synthetic analogs of microorganisms such as BCG, components of *Corynebacterium parvum* and peptidoglycans (e.g., muramyl peptide), or oligonucleic acids (CpG), are used as *adjuvants*. Components of streptococci and *Streptomyces*, eluates and fractions of bacterial mixtures, and the related synthetic substance levamisole are also used. The role of Toll-like receptors in these adjuvant effects is becoming increasingly understood, with a major role of these molecules being to link non-specific innate resistance to specific immunity. .

Recently developed immune therapy strategies aim to improve antigen presentation. For instance *interleukins,* or *costimulatory molecules* such as B7 or CD40, have been inserted into tumor cells by means of transfection. Hybrid antibodies have been constructed in an attempt to improve antigen recognition and phagocytosis (one such example is the coupling of an anti-CD3 antibody with tumor antigen-specific antibodies). Other ideas tested successfully in model experiments include systemic treatment with interleukins (this presents with frequent toxicity problems) or targeted insertion of GM-CSF, TNF, or IL-2. Alternatively, the production of IFNγ or IFNβ by cells, or the use of molecules capable of polyclonal T- and B-cell stimulation has been employed. This concept utilizes local chronic or acute infections with the aim of achieving inflammation surrounding, or direct infection of, tumor cells resulting in their cytolytic destruction. Such concepts have also been used to force phagocytosis and uptake of antigens by APCs with the aim of inducing or enhancing tumor immunity (e.g., BCG infections in bladder carcinoma treatment).

2

Immunosuppression

Various methods are employed to inhibit, or suppress, the immune response:

■ Generalized immunosuppression; glucocorticoids (inhibition of inflammatory cells), cytostatic drugs (endoxan, DNA alkylating agents, methotrexate, antimetabolites), and more specific immunosuppressants, e.g., cyclosporine A, FK506, rapamycin (inhibition of signal transduction in T cells, see Fig. 2.11, p. 73).

■ Immunosuppression by antibodies, soluble cytokine receptors, deletion of T cells or T-cell sub-populations (anti-CD4, anti-CD8, anti-CD3, anti-Thy1, etc.). Administration of monoclonal antibodies directed against adhesion molecules and accessory molecules or cytokines and cytokine receptors. Administration of soluble cytokine receptors, or soluble CTLA4, in order to block B7-1 and B7-2 (important costimulators, see p. 71ff.).

■ Specific tolerance induction or "negative immunization." Massive and depletive T-cell activation brought about by systemic administration of large amounts of peptides, proteins (risk of immunopathology), or cells (chimerism).

■ Complete neutralization and elimination of the antigen with the purpose of preventing induction of an antibody response. Example; rhesus prophylaxis with hyperimmune serum.

Adaptive Immunotherapy

This involves in-vitro antigen stimulation, and consequent proliferation, of patient T-cell effector clones or populations (CD8+ T cells or less specific **lymphokine-activated killer cells, LAK cells**), followed by transfusion of these cells back into the patient. This method is sometimes used as a means of limiting cytomegaly or Epstein-Barr virus infection of bone marrow recipients. The LAK cells also include less specific NK-like cells, which can be expanded with IL-2 in the absence of antigen stimulation.

Toxic antibodies are monoclonal antibodies to which toxins have been coupled. These are used as specific toxin transporters, administered directly, or with liposomes bearing anchored antibodies and containing a toxin or cytostatic drug.

Immunological Test Methods

Antigen and Antibody Assays

Immunoprecipitation in Liquids and Gels

Immunoprecipitate. Maximum precipitation results when both reaction partners are present in an approximately *equivalent ratio* (Fig. 2.**20**). In antibody excess, or antigen excess, the amount of precipitate is considerably reduced.

Double diffusion according to Ouchterlony. This technique allows for a *qualitative* evaluation of whether certain antibodies or antigens are present or not, plus determination of the degree of relationship between antibodies and antigens. It also provides information on whether different antigenic de-

---

Immunoprecipitation

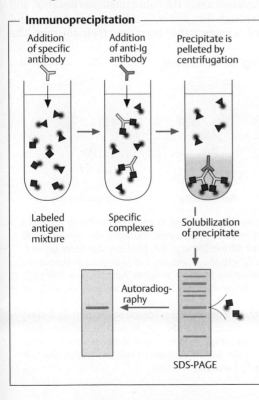

Addition of specific antibody

Addition of anti-Ig antibody

Precipitate is pelleted by centrifugation

Labeled antigen mixture

Specific complexes

Solubilization of precipitate

Autoradiography

SDS-PAGE

Fig. 2.**20** To identify the unknown antigen, a known specific antibody is added to an antigen mixture which is radio-, or otherwise-, labeled. The immune complexes are precipitated with the help of co-precipitating reagents (e.g., anti-immunoglobulin antibodies). The precipitate is thoroughly washed to remove unbound antigen, then dispersed into solution once again (e.g., in SDS), after which the components are separated using SDS polyacrylamide gel electrophoresis (SDS-PAGE). The labeled antigen is then rendered visible by means of autoradiography.

terminants are localized on the same, or on different, antigens; or whether different antibodies can bind to the same antigen (Fig. 2.**21**).

Radial immunodiffusion according to Mancini. This is a *quantitative* antigen assay based on a predetermined standard curve (Fig. 2.**22**).

Nephelometry. This method measures the amount of light scatter as a quantification of precipitation turbidity.

Immunoprecipitation Combined with Electrophoresis. Antigens are separated in an agarose gel by applying an electric current. The antibodies react by migrating in the gel, either without an electric field, or simultaneously within the electric field; and either in the same dimension as the antigens or in a second vertical step ("rocket" electrophoresis).

Immunoelectrophoresis according to Grabar and Williams. In the first instance serum proteins are electrophoretically separated within a thin agarose gel layer. A trough is then cut into the agar, next to the separated sample and parallel to the direction of migration along the entire migration distance, and anti-serum is applied to the trough. The antibodies diffuse into the gel, and precipitation lines are formed wherever they encounter their antigens. The

Double Diffusion According to Ouchterlony

a   **Identity**   b   **Non-identity**   c   **Partial Identity**

Fig. 2.**21**   This technique facilitates assignment of antigens (violet) to a certain test antibody (yellow), or vice versa. The antigens and antibodies are pipetted into troughs within the gel and diffuse through this medium (the numbers designate the epitopes present). Where they meet lines of precipitation (known as precipitin bands) develop, indicating immune complex formation. **a** The antibodies precipitate identical epitopes (epitope 1) of both antigens, resulting in formation of precipitin bands which flow together to form an arch, mutually inhibiting their migration. In **b**, three independent precipitin bands form, indicating that the antibodies differentiate three different epitopes on three different antigens. **c** Epitope 1 of both antigen samples forms precipitin bands which flow together. Anti-2 migrates beyond the line of confluence into the area in which it precipitates with free antigen 1, 2 and forms a spur.

Radial Immunodiffusion According to Mancini

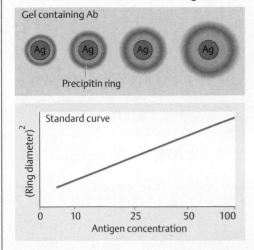

Fig. 2.**22** Quantitative assay of an antigen using a monospecific anti-serum which is mixed with agar and poured into a plate. The antigen is then diluted to different concentrations, and pipetted into wells that have been previously punched into the plate. Antigen-antibody complexes precipitate in the form of a ring around the well, the diameter of which is proportional to the antigen concentration. The result is a standard curve from which unknown test antigens can be quantified. Analogously, antibodies can also be quantified by mixing antigens into the gel.

precipitate can then be stained and evaluated. This older method is still used to identify paraproteins, monoclonal immunoglobulins, etc. (Fig. 2.**23**).

Electrophoresis plus antibody reaction: Western blotting. This method involves electrophoresis of proteins in a gel, coupled with detection by specific antibodies. The separated proteins are transferred to nitrocellulose, where they are identified with the help of specific antibodies (Fig. 2.**24**). Polyclonal sera is normally used for this purpose as monoclonal antibodies only rarely bind to denatured and separated proteins.

Agglutination Reaction

Antibodies can agglutinate antigen-loaded particles (Fig. 2.**25**), whilst antigens can agglutinate antibody-loaded particles. Application: agglutination of bacteria or erythrocytes (e.g., blood group tests).

2

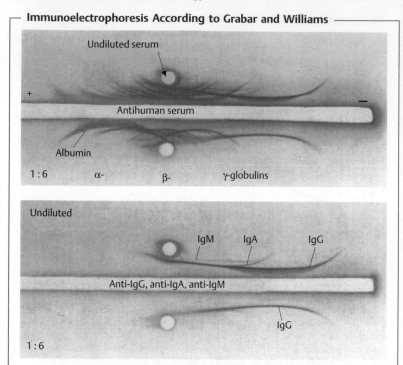

Immunoelectrophoresis According to Grabar and Williams

Undiluted serum

+

Antihuman serum

−

Albumin

1:6   α-   β-   γ-globulins

Undiluted

IgM   IgA   IgG

Anti-IgG, anti-IgA, anti-IgM

IgG

1:6

Fig. 2.**23** Serum is separated within agarose by an electric field, and rendered visible with anti-serum directed against human serum (above), or with selected specific antibodies (below).

■ **Indirect hemagglutination.** An antigen is fixed on the surface of erythrocytes and the antigen-loaded erythrocytes are then agglutinated using specific antibodies.

■ **Hemagglutination inhibition test.** The ability of a sample containing antigen to inhibit hemagglutination between antigen-loaded erythrocytes and antiserum is measured. This test is frequently used to quantify antibodies against hemagglutinating viruses (mainly influenza and parainfluenza viruses).

■ **Antiglobulin tests according to Coombs.** The direct Coombs test determines antibody binding directly to erythrocytes (e.g., anti-Rh antibodies agglutinate Rh^+ erythrocytes of neonates). The indirect Coombs test is suitable for detection of antibodies that have already bound to the Rh^+ erythrocytes of newborns (second pregnancy or sensitized mother), or which have been in-

Western Blotting

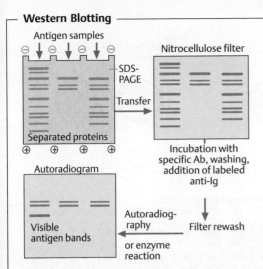

Fig. 2.**24** Antigen samples separated in a gel are transferred to nitrocellulose. Non-specific binding of the antibodies to the filter is then prevented with serum albumin or irrelevant proteins that do not cross-react with any of the antibodies used. Antibodies specific for the antigens being sought are then added. Once immune complexes have formed, the unbound antibodies are thoroughly washed away and the remaining bound antibodies are labeled using anti-immunoglobulin antibodies. These are in turn rendered visible by the autoradiographic procedure.

cubated in vitro with erythrocytes or antigenic particles. In all cases agglutination is detected using anti-Ig antibodies. Antigens can also be adsorbed to latex.

Complement Fixation Test (CFT)

CFT was formerly used to measure complement consumption by preformed antigen-antibody complexes. The unused complement is then detected by addition of a known amount of antibody-loaded erythrocytes. Should all of the erythrocytes be lysed, this indicates that no complement had been consumed and the CFT is negative. This method is no longer used very frequently, with the newer immunosorbent tests being preferred (RIA, ELISA, RAST, see below).

Direct and Indirect Immunofluorescence

Direct immunofluorescence. Immunofluorescence can be used for in-vivo detection of antibodies, complement, viruses, fungi, bacteria, or other im-

Hemagglutination

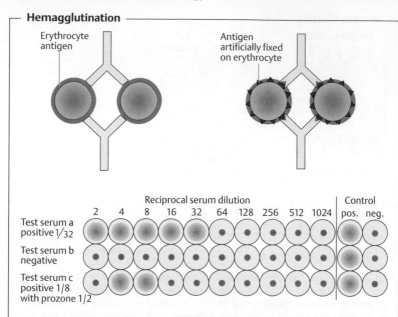

Fig. 2.**25** The hemagglutination test is based on the principle that erythrocytes cross-linked by antibodies settle to the bottom of the microtiter plate wells in mat-like aggregates (test sera **a** and **c**), whereas non-agglutinated erythrocytes collect at the lowest point of the wells to form a single "button" in the middle (test serum **b**). The test sera are first pipetted into the wells at the indicated dilutions, then the erythrocyte suspension is added. Non-specific agglutination is prevented by addition of an irrelevant protein. The test can be carried out using erythrocyte antigens (above left). Alternatively, other antigens can be fixed to the erythrocyte surface and the agglutination monitored (above right). The so-called "prozone" phenomenon results from non-specific blocking mechanisms present in sera which has not been sufficiently diluted.

mune factors present within patient cells and tissues. For this purpose tissue sections, or cell preparations, are treated with specific antibodies (anti-sera) which have been labeled with a fluorochrome (Fig. 2.**26a**). Antigen-antibody reactions can thus be detected using a fluorescence microscope. The fluorochrome absorbs light of a certain wavelength (e.g., UV light), and emits the light energy in the form of light at a different (visible) wavelength. The fluorochrome fluorescein isothiocyanate (FITC), which absorbs UV light and emits it as green light, is used most frequently (caution: bleaches out quickly!).

Antigen Detection Methods

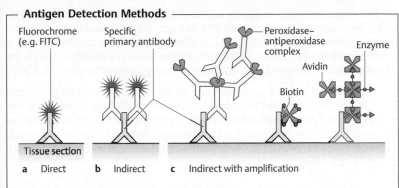

| a | Direct | b | Indirect | c | Indirect with amplification |

Fig. 2.**26**   Immunofluorescence (**a**, **b**) is particularly suitable for the detection of antigens, or specific antibodies, fixed on plastic (solid phase) (ELISA) or present within a tissue section (immunohistology). For direct immunofluorescence (**a**) the specific primary antibody is labeled with a fluorochrome, or an enzyme (ELISA = enzyme-linked immunosorbent assay). The term indirect immunofluorescence is used when it is not the primary antibody being detected, but a secondary antibody which is directed against the unlabeled primary antibody and has also been labeled with a fluorochrome or enzyme (**b**). In most cases, this method achieves a certain degree of amplification. However, an even higher level of amplification can be achieved using preformed complexes of secondary antibody and enzyme (**c**). For the peroxidase method the detector enzyme is bound directly to the secondary antibody (peroxidase catalyzes a color reaction). In the biotin-avidin method the detector enzymes are coupled to either biotin or avidin.

Indirect immunofluorescence and enzyme histology. In this technique the specific or "first" antibody can be unlabeled. The antigen–antibody complexes that form are then detected using a labeled or "second" antibody, directed against the first antibody (Fig. 2.**26b**). Instead of fluorochromes, enzyme-labeled antibodies are now frequently used for tissue sections. The enzyme catalyzes the formation of a color signal following addition of a previously colorless detector substance. This color precipitate allows the direct observation of signals using a light microscopic, and exhibits little bleaching.

Indirect immunofluorescence can be used for the qualitative and quantitative analysis of antibodies directed against particular microbial antigens, or self-tissue antigens, within a patients serum. In the quantitative test, the antigen is fixed in a well or to a tissue section on a slide. The patient sample is repeatedly diluted by a factor of two and added to the antigen or section then rendered visible with a labeled anti–antibody.

There are two main methods of amplifying the immunohistological color signal:

2

■ The direct 'primary' antibody, or the detected 'secondary' antibody, is labeled with peroxidase. Following the antigen-antibody reaction, large preformed peroxidase-antiperoxidase complexes are added to the tissue section; these complexes can attach to the peroxidase-labeled antibodies, which are already specifically bound, thus amplifying the signal considerably (Fig. 2.**26c**).

■ Similarly, biotinylated antibodies can be used. The vitamin biotin is bound with strong affinity by avidin, a basic glycoprotein. Various colorants or enzymes coupled to avidin thus facilitate the color reactions. Such reactions can be amplified on the tissue section by adding preformed biotin-avidin-peroxidase complexes that bind to those biotin-coupled antibodies which have already been bound.

Radioimmunological and Enzyme Immunological Tests

Radioimmunoassay (RIA) and enzyme immunoassay (EIA), also known as ELISA (enzyme-linked immunosorbent assay) (Fig. 2.**28**), are now used very frequently to test for antigens and antibodies. All absorbency tests involve the fixation of antigens or antibodies to a plastic surface. The lower detection limit is a few nanograms. This method forms the basis of modern hepatitis serology, HIV tests, and tests for autoantibodies, lymphokines, cytokines, etc. All of these assays can be performed in a direct form (different sandwich combinations of antigen, antibody and anti-antibody, Fig. 2.**27**)

Fig. 2.**27**   For solid phase tests both the antigen and antibody are bound to a solid phase (e.g., plastic surface). Various methods are then used to detect any interaction between the antigen and antibody. In the direct test (**a**) an immobilized, unknown, antigen can be detected using a fluorescent-labeled antibody. If the immobilized antigen is known, this test method can also be used to detect an antibody bound to the antigen. In the sandwich method (**b**) a known antibody is immobilized. Detection of antibody-antigen binding is then performed using a second, labeled antibody which interacts with the antigen at a different site. The capture method (**c**) can be used to detect any antigen, for instance IgM antibodies. First, anti-IgM antibodies are immobilized, then serum containing IgM is added to them. The bound IgM can then bind a foreign antigen (e.g., a virus). The detection procedure next makes use of either the labeled foreign antigen or a specific, additionally labeled, antibody which binds to the bound antigen but not to the plastic bound antibody. In the competition or competitive inhibition test (**d**) antibodies are immobilized, and labeled antigens are then bound to them. An unlabeled (unknown) antigen is added, which competes with the labeled antigen. The level of interaction between the antibody and the unknown antigen is then determined by measuring attenuation of the signal.   ▶

or as competition assays. Fig. 2.**28** illustrates the quantitative IgE assay, Fig. 2.**29** the procedure for detection of specific IgE in patient sera. Analogous procedures are used to detect specific antibody-binding cells or cytokine-releasing T cells (Fig. 2.**30**).

In-Vitro Cellular Immunity Reactions

Isolation of Lymphocytes

The methods used to measure cellular immunity are experimentally complex. The first step is to isolate human lymphocytes from blood, which can be achieved using Ficoll density gradient centrifugation. Certain lymphocyte

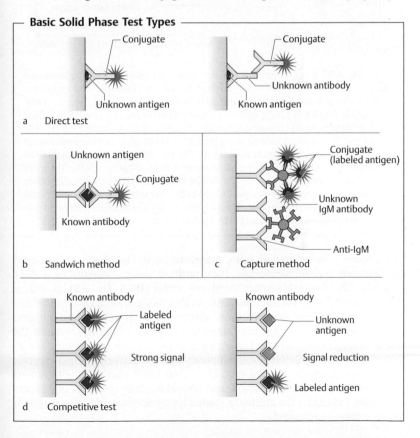

Basic Solid Phase Test Types

a Direct test
— Conjugate
— Unknown antigen
— Conjugate
— Unknown antibody
— Known antigen

b Sandwich method
Unknown antigen
— Conjugate
Known antibody

c Capture method
Conjugate (labeled antigen)
Unknown IgM antibody
Anti-IgM

d Competitive test
Known antibody
Labeled antigen
Strong signal

Known antibody
Unknown antigen
Signal reduction
Labeled antigen

2

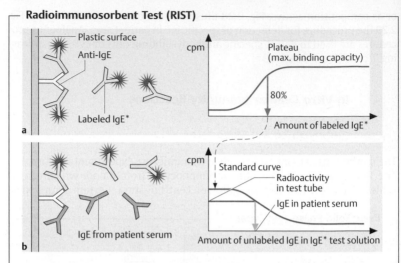

── **Radioimmunosorbent Test (RIST)** ────────────────

Fig. 2.**28** RIST is a competitive radioimmunoassay (RIA) used for quantitative measurement of antibodies of any given Ig class (in this example total IgE) within patient serum. Anti-IgE antibodies are allowed to adsorb to the solid phase (plastic surface). In the first instance, defined concentrations of radiolabeled IgE (IgE*) are used to determine the maximum binding capacity of these antibodies (**a**). The actual test (**b**) is then performed using the IgE* concentration determined to result in 80% saturation of the fixed antibodies: The IgE* test solution is added to the fixed anti-IgE antibodies and the patient serum is then added by pipette. The more IgE the serum contains, the more IgE* will be displaced by the patients antibodies, and the lower the radioactivity level will be in the test tube. The IgE concentration in the patient serum is then calculated based on a standard curve established previously by progressively "diluting" the IgE* test solution with unlabeled IgE.

populations can be coated with magnetic beads, or sheep erythrocytes loaded with specific antibodies, then purified using a magnet or a Ficoll gradient. The fluorescence-activated cell sorter (FACS, Fig. 2.**31**, p. 133) is now regularly used for this purpose. In this assay, monoclonal antibodies labeled with various fluorochromes directed against cell surface antigens (such as CD4, CD8), or against intracellular cytokines (which involves the use of detergents to increase the permeability of the cell membrane), are incubated with the isolated blood lymphocytes. Alternatively, antigen-specific T lymphocytes can be labeled with MHC class I or II plus peptide tetramers (see below). Following incubation, and several washing steps, the equipment identifies and counts the antibody-loaded lymphocytes, employing magnetic pulse sorting as required.

Radioallergosorbent Test (RAST)

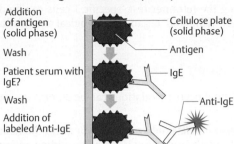

Addition
of antigen
(solid phase)

Cellulose plate
(solid phase)

Wash

Antigen

Patient serum with
IgE?

IgE

Wash

Anti-IgE

Addition of
labeled Anti-IgE

2

Fig. 2.**29** This test is a highly sensitive detection method for the presence of specific IgE in patient serum. Antigen is bound covalently to a cellulose plate (solid phase). Any IgE in the serum that binds to the antigen is then detected using radiolabeled anti-IgE antibodies.

Tetramer test for detection of specific T cells (Fig. 2.**32**, p. 134): recombinant MHC class I antigen coupled to biotin, labeled with avidin, and correctly folded together with peptide and β_2 microglobulin, forms tetramers; which are recognized by specific TCRs. Subsequent analysis of tetramer binding using FACS equipment is based on the color indicator of the avidin (fluorescein, phycoerythrin, etc.). Tetramers specific for MHC class II antigens plus

ELISPOT Assay

Fig. 2.**30** In the ELISPOT assay antigens, or specific anti-IL antibodies, are applied to the plastic surface. It is then possible to determine the number of immune cells releasing antibodies specific for the applied antigen, or releasing interleukins that are recognized by the applied anti-IL antibodies. Following incubation at 37 °C, the immune complexes which form around these cells can be visualized using a covering agarose layer which includes an enzyme-coupled antibody. These enzymes catalyze a color reaction, resulting in the formation of color spots, each of which will correspond to a single cell producing the specific antibody or interleukin.

peptide can theoretically be used to assay specific CD4[+] T cells, but are still difficult to manufacture. Using the tetramer test, specific T cells can be detected directly from blood or lymphoid organs. Histological applications are feasible, but still difficult.

Lymphocyte Function Tests

Certain functions of isolated lymphocyte populations can be determined by a number of methods:

■ Determination of the *number of cells producing antibodies*, e.g., the hemolytic plaque assay in which antibody production is tested by adding antigen-coupled erythrocytes. In the vicinity of antibody-secreting cells, the erythrocytes are covered with antibodies and can be lysed by addition of complement. Today, ELISA methods are more often used than erythrocytes (ELISPOT).

■ *ELISPOT ASSAY*: used to measure antibody-producing, or IL-releasing, lymphocytes. The antigen or anti-IL antibody is fixed on a plastic surface. Lymphocytes are then placed over this, within a thin layer of agar medium. When the cells are incubated at 37 °C, they may secrete the antibodies or IL recognized by the corresponding test substances. After a certain period of time, the cell layer is shaken off and the preparation is thoroughly washed. The bound material can then be developed using an overlaid semisolid agar, as for the ELISA method. The enzyme reaction generates spots of color, each of which corresponds to a cell, and which can be counted (Fig. 2.**30**).

■ Measurement of the *release capacity of cytokines*, or detection of mRNA, is also possible with the ELISPOT assay.

■ *Lymphocyte stimulation assay*: isolated lymphocytes are incubated with antigen in culture medium. Measuring the ^{3}H-thymidine incorporation,

Fig. 2.**31** This device analyzes cells by means of fluorescent-labeled antibodies directed against cell surface antigens – or for permeabilized cells, directed against internal cell antigens. In the example shown, peripheral blood lymphocytes (PBL) are incubated with monoclonal antibodies specific for CD4 or CD8, resulting in the distribution of fluorescence intensity as indicated in **a**. In **b** the labeling of different cell populations with anti-CD4 or anti-CD8 is shown. By this means, the percentages of the subpopulations in the total population can be determined. The fluorescence-activated cell sorter shown in (**c**) makes use of this data. By means of vibration, the cell stream is broken up into fine droplets which, depending on the fluorescence and sorting settings used, are charged just before they are separated and ideally contain one cell each. Certain parameters are measured for each cell with the help of a laser beam, where-upon the droplets are deflected into the intended containers by the + and − plate fields. ▶

interleukin release, or a pH transition, can determine whether antigen-specific lymphocytes are present or whether polyclonal T-cell responses (concanavalin [ConA], phytohemagglutinin [PHA]) or B-cell responses (lipopolysaccharide [LPS], pokeweed mitogen [PMA]) were induced.

■ Mixed lymphocyte reactions are used to measure *alloreactivity* (proliferation, cytotoxicity), mainly between recipients and donors of organ or bone

2

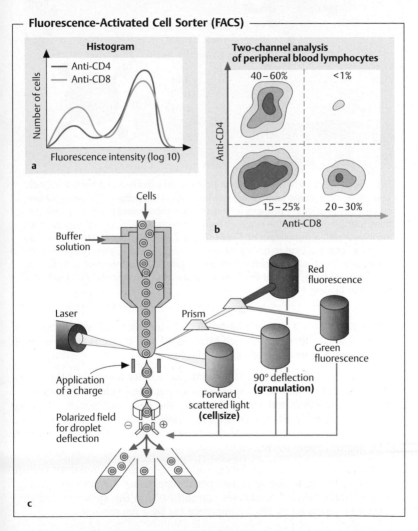

Fluorescence-Activated Cell Sorter (FACS)

Histogram

Anti-CD4
Anti-CD8

Number of cells

Fluorescence intensity (log 10)

a

Two-channel analysis of peripheral blood lymphocytes

40 – 60%   <1%

Anti-CD4

15 – 25%   20 – 30%

Anti-CD8

b

Cells

Buffer solution

Laser

Prism

Red fluorescence

Application of a charge

Forward scattered light **(cell size)**

90° deflection **(granulation)**

Green fluorescence

Polarized field for droplet deflection

⊖   ⊕

c

2

Tetramer Assay

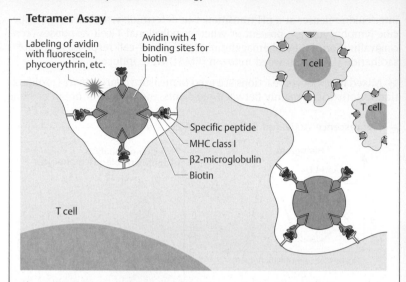

Labeling of avidin with fluorescein, phycoerythrin, etc.

Avidin with 4 binding sites for biotin

T cell

T cell

Specific peptide

MHC class I

β2-microglobulin

Biotin

T cell

Fig. 2.**32** The tetramer assay is an antigen-specific binding test for living T cells. Complexes comprising biotin-coupled MHC class I heavy chains, β_2 microglobulin, and specific peptide are properly folded, washed, then bound to avidin (which contains four binding sites for biotin). The resulting tetrameric complexes are then incubated with a population of T cells. Those T cells expressing the appropriate T-cell receptor will bind to two or three of the exposed MHC class I-peptide complexes present on each tetramer. Labeling of the avidin component with fluorescein, phycoerythrin, or other fluorescent substances then permits FACS analysis of tertramer binding T cells.

marrow transplants. This test is based on the principle that T lymphocytes are stimulated to proliferate by nonself MHC class I or II antigens and to develop into cytotoxic T cells directed against class I.

■ Chromium release assay measures *cytolytic activity*, mainly by CD8[+] T cells, directed against allogeneic, virus-infected, or peptide-loaded target cells. The target cells are incubated with ^{51}Cr which the cells incorporate. They are then cultivated with effector cells for 4–6 hours. When the target cells are lysed chromium is released into the culture medium, following which it can be quantitatively measured.

■ Assay of intracellular cytokines. Following a brief stimulatory culture (six hours), the cells are rendered permeable using a mild detergent so that specifically labeled antibodies can diffuse into the cells. Labeled cells can then be analyzed by FACS equipment (or by a microscope).

Table 2.**13**   Important CD Antigens

Designation (alternatives)	Cells which express the antigen	Functions
CD1	Cortical thymocytes, Langerhans cells, dendritic cells, B cells, intestinal epithelium	MHC class I-like molecule, associated with β_2 microglobulin. Possible special significance in specialized antigen presentation
CD2 (LFA-2)	T cells, thymocytes, natural killer cells	Adhesion molecule which binds to CD58 (LFA-3) and can activate T cells (LFA = lymphocyte function antigen)
CD3	Thymocytes, T cells	Associated with the antigen receptor of T cells, and is necessary for T-cell receptor surface expression and signal transduction
CD4	Several groups of thymocytes, T helper cells, and inflammatory T cells (about two-thirds of the peripheral T cells), monocytes, macrophages	Co-receptor for MHC class II molecules. Binds signal transducers via cytoplasmic portion. Receptor for gp120 in HIV-1 and HIV-2
CD5	Thymocytes, T cells, a subgroup of B cells	Binds to CD72
CD8	Several groups of thymocytes, cytotoxic T cells (about one-third of the peripheral T cells)	Co-receptor for MHC class I molecules, binds signal transducer via cytoplasmic portion
CD10	B and T precursor cells, bone marrow stroma cells	Zinc metal proteinase, and marker for acute lymphoid leukemia of pre-B cells
CD11a (α chain)	Lymphocytes, granulocytes, monocytes, and macrophages	α subunit of β_2 integrin LFA-1 (associated with CD18). Binds to CD54 (ICAM-1), CD102 (ICAM-2), and ICAM-3 (CD50)
CD19	B cells	Forms a complex with CD21 (CR2) and CD81 (TAPA-1), Co-receptor for B cells

2

Table 2.**13** *Continued: Important CD Antigens*

Designation (alternatives)	Cells which express the antigen	Functions
CD21 (CR2)	Mature B cells, follicular dendritic cells	Receptor for the complement components (CR) C3d and the Epstein-Barr virus. Forms a co-receptor for B cells together with CD19 and CD81
CD22	Mature B cells	Adhesion of B cells to monocytes and T cells
CD23 (FcεRII)	Mature B cells, activated macrophages, eosinophils, follicular dendritic cells, blood platelets	Low-affinity receptor for IgE, and ligand for the CD19:CD21:CD81 coreceptor
CD25 (Tac)	Activated T cells, B cells, and monocytes	α chain of the IL-2 receptor, associated with CD122 and the IL-2Rγ chain
CD26	Activated B and T cells, macrophages	A protease which may be involved in HIV entry into host cells
CD28	Subgroup of T cells, activated B cells	Activation of naïve T cells. A receptor for costimulatory signal (signal 2); binds CD80 (B7.1) and B7.2
CD29	Leukocytes	β_1 subunit of γ_1 integrins, associated with CD49a in VLA-1 integrin
CD34	Hematopoietic precursor cells, capillary endothelium	Ligand for CD62L (L-selectin)
CD35 (CR1)	Erythrocytes, B cells, monocytes, neutrophils and eosinophils, follicular dendritic cells	Complement receptor 1; binds C3b and C4b. Also mediates phagocytosis
CD38	Early B and T cells, activated T cells, germinal center B cells, plasma cells	B-cell proliferation?
CD39	Activated B cells, activated natural killer cells, macrophages, dendritic cells	Unknown fuction, but may mediate adhesion of B cells

Table 2.**13**   *Continued: Important CD Antigens*

Designation (alternatives)	Cells which express the antigen	Functions
CD40	B cells, monocytes, dendritic cells	Receptor for the costimulatory signal for B cells; binds CD40 ligand (CD40-L)
CD40L	Activated CD4 T cells	Ligand for CD40
CD44 (Pgp-1)	Leukocytes, erythrocytes	Binds hyaluronic acid and mediates adhesion of leukocytes
CD45, RO, RA, RB (leukocyte common antigen, LCA), T200, B220	Leukocytes	A tyrosine phosphatase which enhances signal mediation via the antigen receptors of B and T cells; alternative splicing results in many isoforms (see below)
CD54	Hematopoietic and nonhematopoietic cells	Intercellular adhesion molecule (ICAM-1); binds the CD11a/CD18 integrin (LFA-1) and the CD11b/CD18 integrin (MAC-1); receptor for rhinoviruses
CD55 (DAF)	Hematopoietic and nonhematopoietic cells	Decay accelerating factor (DAF); binds C3b and cleaves C3/C5 convertase
CD62E (ELAM-1, E-selectin)	Endothelium	Endothelial leukocyte adhesion molecule (ELAM); binds sialyl-Lewis x and mediates rolling of neutrophilic cells along endothelium
CD64 (FcγRI)	Monocytes, macrophages	High-affinity receptor for IgG
CD80 (B7.1) CD86 (B7.2)	Subgroup of B cells	Costimulators which act as ligands for CD28 and CTLA-4
CD88	Polymorphonuclear leukocytes, macrophages, mast cells	Receptor for the complement component C5a
CD89	Monocytes, macrophages, granulocytes, neutrophils cells, subgroups of B and T cells	IgA receptor?
CD95 (APO-1, Fas)	Many different cell lines; unclear distribution in vivo	Binds TNF-like Fas ligands; induces apoptosis

Table 2.**13** *Continued: Important CD Antigens*

Designation (alternatives)	Cells which express the antigen	Functions
CD102 (ICAM-2) (intercellular cell adhesion molecule)	Resting lymphocytes, monocytes, endothelial cells (in which expression is most pronounced)	Binds CD11a/CD18 (LFA-1), but not CD11b/CD18 (MAC-1)
CD106 (VCAM-1) (vascular cell adhesion molecule)	Endothelial cells	Adhesion molecule; ligand for VLA-4 (very late antigen)
CD115	Monocytes, macrophages	Receptor for the macrophage colony-stimulating factor (M-CSF)
CD116	Monocytes, neutrophils, and eosinophils, endothelium	α chain of the receptor for the granulocyte-macrophage colony-stimulating factor (GM-CSF)
CD117	Hematopoietic precursor cells	Receptor for stem cell factor (SCF)
CD118	Widespread	Receptor for alpha/beta interferons (IFNα/β)
CD119	Macrophages, monocytes, B cells, endothelium	Receptor for gamma interferon (IFNγ)
CD120a	Hematopoietic and nonhematopoietic cells	Most pronounced on epithelial cells

Acknowledgment
The expert editing and translating help of Nicola Harris PhD is gratefully acknowledged.

Glossary

ABC: Antigen-binding cell.

ABS: Antigen-binding site on an antibody.

ADCC: Antibody-dependent cell-mediated cytotoxicity.

Adjuvant: A substance which intensifies the immune response against an antigen, in a immunologically non-specific manner.

AFC: Antibody-forming cell.

Affinity: A measure of binding strength between an antigen determinant (epitope) and the binding site of an antibody (paratope).

Affinity maturation: An increase in the average antibody affinity acquired during the course of a secondary and following immune responses.

AFP: α-fetoprotein.

Allele: Gene locus variations within a species.

Allergy: An altered response following secondary contact with the same antigen, also defined as type I hypersensitivity.

Allogeneic: Refers to the genetic variety contained within a species.

Allotransplant: Transplanted allogeneic tissue.

Allotype: Different forms of a protein product, usually Ig, recognized as an antigen by another individual of the same species.

Alternative pathway: Activation of the complement system via C3 or other factors, but not via C1q.

ANA (anti-nuclear antibodies): Autoantibody directed against DNA contained within the cell nucleus.

Anaphylatoxins: Complement fragments (C3a and C5a), responsible for mediating mast cell degranulation.

Anaphylaxis: An antigen-specific, primarily systemic IgG- or IgE-mediated-immune response.

Antigens: Molecules which are usually characterized by complex folding, and which can be recognized by antibodies.

Antibody: A molecule which binds to a specific antigen.

APC: Antigen-presenting cell.

Atopic: Increased susceptibility to the clinical manifestations associated with type I hypersensitivity (e.g. eczema, asthma, and rhinitis).

Autologous: Derived from the same individual (or inbred strain).

Autosomes: All chromosomes other than the X or Y sex chromosomes.

Avidity: A measure of the functional binding strength between an antibody and its antigen; dependent on affinity and valences (number of binding sites).

BCA-1: B-cell attractant.

BCG: Bacillus Calmette-Guerin. An attenuated form of *Mycobacterium tuberculosis*.

BCGF: B-cell growth factor.

Bence-Jones proteins: Free light chains of Ig present in the serum and urine of multiple myeloma patients.

Bursa fabricii: Lymphoepithelial organ adjacent to the cloaca of birds, in which B cells mature.

C: Complement (C1–9).

C domain: Constant component of Ig.

C3b inactivator: A component of the complement system, known as factor I.

Capping: Aggregation of surface molecules on the cell membrane.

Carrier: The part of a molecule which is recognized by T cells during an immune response.

CBR: Complement-binding reaction.

CCR: A receptor for those chemokines which contain adjacent cysteine-cysteines (CXC or CXXC, cysteines separated by one or two amino acids).

CD marker: Cluster determinant or cluster of differentiation, characteristic of distinct lymphocyte subpopulations.

CDR: Complementarity determining regions (hypervariable antibody regions).

Chemokines: Chemoattractant cytokines

2

Chimera: A single host bearing cells derived from genetically distinct individuals.

CLIP: A protein which blocks the binding groove of MHC class II prior to its inclusion in the phagolysosome (class II-inhibiting protein).

CMI: Cell-mediated immunity.

Cobra venom factor: A component of cobra venom which exhibits enzymatic activity corresponding to the activity of mammalian C3b.

Combining site: The configuration on an antibody which forms a link with antigen determinants (ABS).

Complement system: A group of serum proteins that are activated in cascades; usually via antibodies, but in some cases directly by infectious agents. Plays an important role during inflammation, chemotaxis, cytolysis, and phagocytosis.

Con A (concanavalin A): A T-cell mitogen.

Cryoglobulin: Antibodies in immune complexes that can be precipitated at 4 °C.

CSF: Colony-stimulating factor (also: cerebrospinal fluid).

CTL: Cytotoxic $CD8^+$ T cell.

CXCR: Receptor for those chemokines which contain a cysteine-x-cysteine motif.

Cyclophosphamide: A toxic substance frequently used to induce immunosuppression.

Cyclosporine A: An immunosuppressant used for the prevention of rejection reactions.

Cytophilic: Exhibiting an affinity towards cells (i.e., binds to cells).

Cytostatic: Exhibiting an inhibitory effect on cell proliferation.

Cytotoxic: Exhibiting a destructive effect towards target cells.

DARC: Duffy antigen receptor for chemokines.

Dendritic cells: Professional APCs derived from the bone marrow. Dendritic cells are mobile and function to transport antigen into lymphoid organs. In the skin they are known as *Langerhans* cells, on the way to the lymph nodes *veiled* cells, and in the lymph nodes *interdigitating* cells.

Desensitization: Repeated exposure to small amounts of an antigen, against which the host shows an allergic reaction; the aim being to downregulate IgE production and upregulate IgG production.

DiGeorge syndrome: Congenital thymic hypoplasia.

DNP: Dinitrophenol, a frequently used small hapten.

Domain: A peptide region with a stable tertiary structure. Immunoglobulins (Ig), MHC class I, and MHC class II molecules all contain comparable Ig domains.

DTH: Delayed type hypersensitivity; A delayed cellular type IV response.

EAE: Experimental allergic encephalitis.

ELISA: Enzyme-linked immunosorbent assay.

ELISPOT: A modified ELISA method used for the detection of specific cell secretion products.

Endotoxins: Bacterial toxins; largely comprised by lipopolysaccharides (LPS) from Gram-negative bacteria.

Eotaxin: A chemokine which regulates eosinophil migration.

Epitope: A special region within an antigen, which is recognized by an antibody binding site.

Epstein-Barr virus: A herpes virus capable of transforming human B cells, and for which B cells possess a special receptor (EBVR). The causative agent of infectious mononucleosis (Pfeiffer disease).

Exon: A protein-coding gene fragment.

Fab: The part of the antibody molecule which contains the antigen-binding site following treatment with papain; comprises a light chain and the first two domains of the heavy chain.

FACS: Fluorescence-activated cell sorter.

Fc: Antibodies use the Fc fragment to bind to cellular receptors (FcR) and C1q complement components.

FcR: Fc receptor.

Fractalkine: A chemokine expressed by endothelial cells; has effects on inflammation and other processe.

Freund's adjuvant (FA): A water-in-oil emulsion. Complete FA contains killed *Mycobacterium tuberculosis*, whilst incomplete FA does not.

GALT: Gut-associated lymphoid tissue.

Gammaglobulins: The serum fraction which migrates most rapidly towards the anode during electrophoresis. Contains all five classes of immunoglobulins.

Gel diffusion test: Immunoprecipitation test; Antigens and antibodies diffuse towards one another, forming a stainable precipitate at the equivalence zone (Ouchterlony test).

Germ line: The genetic material of gametes. Mutations in the germ line, unlike somatic mutations, are inherited by progeny.

GVH: Graft-versus-host reaction; rejection of host tissue by transplanted cells.

H-2: Main histocompatibility complex of mice.

Haplotype: The set of genetic determinants present on one chromosome or chromosome set.

Hapten: A small molecule which can function as an epitope by itself, without being coupled to a carrier, but which alone does not elicit an antibody response.

Helper cells: The CD4+ subclass of T cells which are functionally important for B cells, and which release cytokines; a single helper T-cell clone is specific for one peptide presented by a specific MHC class II molecule.

Hereditary angioedema: Result of congenital C1 inhibitor deficiency.

Heterologous: Belonging to another species.

HEV: High endothelial venules; these are specialized to allow the movement of lymphocytes from the blood into the lymph nodes.

High responder: Individuals (or inbred strains) which exhibit a strong immune response against a defined antigen.

Hinge region: The segment of an immunoglobulin heavy chain which lies between the Fc and Fab regions.

Histocompatibility: Quality which determines rules of acceptance or rejection of a transplant.

HLA: Human leukocyte antigen coded for by the human major histocompatibility gene complex (MHC).

Homologous: Belonging to the same species.

Humoral: Any factor present within extracellular body fluids (e.g. serum, lymph).

HVG: Host-versus-graft reaction. Rejection of transplanted cells by host tissue.

Hybridoma: An antigen-specific B cell that has been successfully fused with a myeloma cell.

Hypervariable region: The three most variable segments present within the V domains of immunoglobulins and T-cell receptors.

Idiotype: The antigenic characteristic of the ABS region of an antibody.

IFN: Interferons; cellular derived substances which contribute to nonspecific cellular resistance, particularly with regard to viral infections.

IL: Interleukins; short-lived substances which mediate the transfer of information between distinct cells (both of the immune system and other tissues).

Immune complex: The product of an antigen-antibody reaction; may also contain components of the complement system.

Immune paralysis: Temporary inability to produce a specific immune response usually resulting from the presence of excessive antigen.

Immunity: Actively or passively acquired immune protection against pathogens and other antigens.

Immunoconglutinins: Auto-antibodies directed against complement components.

Immunofluorescence: Rendering certain antigens visible by binding of a specific fluorescence-labeled antibody.

Immunogen: Any substance which can elicit a specific immune response.

Immunological memory: The ability to produce a faster and stronger immune response following a second, or subsequent, encounter with the same antigen.

Intron: The gene segment present between two exons.

Ir genes: Immune response genes; an early designation used for MHC genes. These code for MHC molecules which control peptide presentation, and thus directly determine the specificity and strength of an immune response.

Isologous: Of identical genetic constitution.

Isotype: The "isotypic" variants of certain proteins coded within the genome, which are identical for all individuals of a species (e.g., immunoglobulin classes).

J genes: Joining genes; a set of gene segments contained within the genetic loci of the heavy and light immunoglobulin chains, or T-cell receptor chains.

K cells: Killer cells; a group of lymphocytes bearing Fc receptors which can destroy their target cells by means of antibody-dependent cell-mediated cytotoxicity (ADCC).

Kupffer cells: Phagocytic cells present in the hepatic sinusoids.

LAK: Lymphokine-activated killer cells (lymphocytes).

LARC: Liver and activation-regulated chemokine.

LCM: Lymphocytic choriomeningitis; an non-bacterial, viral, meningitis.

LGL: Large granular lymphocyte.

Low responder: Individuals (or inbred strains) which exhibit a weak immune response against a given antigen.

LPS: Lipopolysaccharide; a component of the cell wall of certain Gram-negative bacteria, which acts as a B-cell mitogen.

MALT: Mucosa-associated lymphoid tissue.

MBP: Myelin basic protein; functions as an antigen in experimental allergic encephalitis (and probably in multiple sclerosis).

MCP: Monocyte chemoattractant protein.

MDC: Macrophage-derived chemokine.

MHC: Major histocompatibility complex; the main genetic complex responsible for determining histocompatibility. This gene complex codes for the most important transplantation antigens (HLA antigens) in humans. MHC class I molecules are associated with β_2 microglobulin, class II molecules consist of two noncovalently bound transmembrane molecules. The actual function of MHC I, and MHC II, molecules is to present antigenic peptides on the cell surface. Class III molecules comprise complement components, cytokines, and so on.

MHC restriction: Resulting from the interaction of T lymphocytes with other cells, and being controlled by recognition of MHC-presented peptides by the TCR.

MIF: Migration inhibition factors; a group of peptides produced by lymphocytes which inhibit macrophage migration.

MIG: A monokine induced by interferon gamma.

β_2 microglobulin: A protein component of MHC class I molecules.

MIP: Macrophage inflammatory protein.

Mitogen: Any substance which can alone stimulate cells, particularly lymphocytes, to undergo cell division.

MLC: Mixed lymphocyte culture. An in-vitro assay which measures the stimulation response of lymphocytes as alloreactive cytotoxic T-cell reactivity.

MLR: Mixed lymphocyte reaction. An in-vitro assay which measures the stimulation response of lymphocytes as alloreactive proliferation (determined by ^{3}H-thymidine incorporation).

Monoclonal: Any substance derived from a single cell clone, for example monoclonal antibodies.

Myeloma: A B-cell lymphoma, which produces antibodies (plasmocytoma).

NK cells: Natural killer cells. Non-MHC-restricted lymphocytes capable of recognizing and destroying certain cells that are either virally infected or tumorous.

Nude mice: A mouse strain which carries a spontaneous mutation resulting in the animals having no hair, and usually being athymic.

NZB/W: A strain of mouse bred as an animal model for systemic lupus erythematosus.

Opsonization: Depositions of proteins on an infectious pathogen, that facilitate phagocytosis of the pathogen (e.g., antibodies and C3b).

Paratope: The part of an antibody molecule which contacts the antigenic determinant (epitope); the antigen-binding site (ABS) on the antibody.

PC: Phosphorylcholine; a commonly used hapten found on the surface of a number of microorganisms.

PCA: Passive cutaneous anaphylaxis; a classic detection reaction for antigen-specific IgE.

PFC: Plaque forming cell; an antibody-producing cell which can be detected by the hemolysis plaque test.

PHA: Phytohemagglutinin; a mitogen for T cells.

Plasma cell: An antibody-producing B cell which has reached the end of its differentiation pathway.

PMN: Polymorphonuclear neutrophilic granulocytes.

Pokeweed mitogen: A mitogen for B cells.

Polyclonal: A term describing products derived from a number of different cell clones (e.g., polyclonal antibodies).

Primary lymphoid tissues: Thymus, bursa of Fabricius (in birds), bone marrow.

Primary response: The immune response which follows an initial encounter with a particular antigen (see priming, secondary response).

Priming: Following an initial contact with an antigen, an immunocompetent cell becomes sensitized or "primed."

Prozone phenomenon: Lack of a measurable response at high-test substance concentrations.

Pseudoalleles: Tandem variants of a gene, which do not occupy a homologous position on the chromosome.

Pseudogenes: Genes containing structures which are homologous to other genes, but which cannot be expressed.

RANTES: Regulated on activation; this is normally expressed and secreted by T cells.

Reagin: Historical term for IgE.

Rearrangement: For instance the rearrangement of genetic information in somatic B and T cells.

Recombination: A process by which genetic information is rearranged during meiosis.

Reticuloendothelial system (RES): Phagocytic cells distributed within the supportive connective tissue of the liver, spleen, lymph nodes, and other organs (e.g. sinus endothelial cells, Kupffer cells, histiocytes).

Rhesus (Rh) antigens: Antigenic proteins present on the surface of erythrocytes in approximately 85% of all humans.

Rheumatoid factor (RF): Autoantibodies—these are usually IgM but can also be of the IgG and IgA isotypes—which are specifically directed against the body's own IgG molecules.

SCID: Severe combined immunodeficiency disease; a congenital deficiency of the humoral and cellular immune system, resulting from a lack of both T and B cells. The animal model is the SCID mouse and is a spontaneous mutant.

SDF-1alpha: Stromal cell-derived factor.

Secretory piece: An IgA-associated polypeptide produced by epithelial cells, and which facilitates the transmembrane transport of IgA.

Secondary response: The immune response which follows a second encounter with a specific antigen.

Serum sickness: An inflammatory type III reaction, occurring after repeated injection of a foreign protein.

SLC: Secondary lymphoid organ chemokine.

SLE: Systemic lupus erythematosus.

Somatic mutation/recombination: Rearrangements of genes in somatic cells (as opposed to germ line cells), resulting in a newly combined DNA sequence which is not heritable.

Splenomegaly: Splenic enlargement; often observed in cases of hematopoietic cell tumors, vascular circulatory problems, or following various parasitic infections. Can also be used as a measure of GVH reactions.

SRBC: Sheep red blood cells (erythrocytes).

Stripping: The process by which antibodies remove antigen determinants from target cells.

Suppressor cell: A proposed antigen-specific T-cell subpopulation which acts to reduce the immune responses of other T cells or B cells. This suppression can also be of a nonspecific nature.

Syngeneic: Animals produced by repeated inbreeding, or monozygotic twins, which are considered syngeneic when each pair of autosomes within the individuals is identical.

TATA: Tumor-associated transplantation antigens.

Tc: Cytotoxic T cell (CD8+ T cell) or CTL.

TCGF: T-cell growth factor; identical with interleukin 2 (IL-2).

T-dep/T-ind: T cell-dependent/T cell-independent; an antibody response to T-dependent antigens is only possible if (MHC-restricted) T-cell help is also available.

T-DTH: A T cell that contributes to delayed type hypersensitivity reactions.

TECK: Thymus-expressed chemokine.

Tetramer: Biotinylated MHC class I, or class II, molecule complexed to peptide and bound to labeled avidin. Used to determine the presence of peptide-specific T cells.

TGF: Transforming growth factor.

TH: T helper cells (CD4+ T cell; see also Helper cells).

Thy: A cell surface antigen of mouse T cells; there are several allelic variants of this marker.

TNF: Tumor necrosis factor.

Tolerance: A state of specific immunological unresponsiveness.

Transformation (blastic): Morphological changes in a lymphocyte associated with the onset of cell division.

Transplantation antigens: See MHC.

Wiskott-Aldrich syndrome: A sex-linked, inheritable, recessive, combined immune deficiency in which IgM antibody production and cellular immune reactions are impaired.

II
Bacteriology

Escherichia coli

3   General Bacteriology

F. H. Kayser

The Morphology and Fine Structure of Bacteria

■ Bacterial cells are between 0.3 and 5 µm in size. They have three basic forms: cocci, straight rods, and curved or spiral rods. The **nucleoid** consists of a very thin, long, circular DNA molecular double strand that is not surrounded by a membrane. Among the nonessential genetic structures are the **plasmids**. The **cytoplasmic membrane** harbors numerous proteins such as permeases, cell wall synthesis enzymes, sensor proteins, secretion system proteins, and, in aerobic bacteria, respiratory chain enzymes. The membrane is surrounded by the **cell wall**, the most important element of which is the supporting murein skeleton. The cell wall of Gram-negative bacteria features a porous outer membrane into the outer surface of which the lipopolysaccharide responsible for the pathogenesis of Gram-negative infections is integrated. The cell wall of Gram-positive bacteria does not possess such an outer membrane. Its murein layer is thicker and contains teichoic acids and wall-associated proteins that contribute to the pathogenic process in Gram-positive infections. Many bacteria have **capsules** made of polysaccharides that protect them from phagocytosis. Attachment **pili** or **fimbriae** facilitate adhesion to host cells. Motile bacteria possess **flagella**. Foreign body infections are caused by bacteria that form a **biofilm** on inert surfaces. Some bacteria produce **spores**, dormant forms that are highly resistant to chemical and physical noxae. ■

Bacterial Forms

Bacteria differ from other single-cell microorganisms in both their cell structure and size, which varies from 0.3–5 µm. Magnifications of 500–1000×—close to the resolution limits of light microscopy—are required to obtain useful images of bacteria. Another problem is that the structures of objects the size of bacteria offer little visual contrast. Techniques like phase contrast and dark field microscopy, both of which allow for live cell observation, are used to overcome this difficulty. Chemical-staining techniques are also used, but the prepared specimens are dead.

Bacterial Morphology

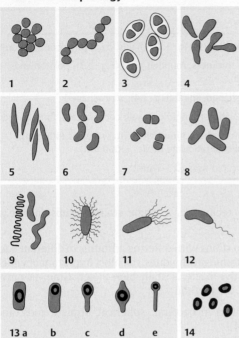

Fig. 3.**1**

1. Gram-positive cocci in grapelike clusters (staphylococci)
2. Gram-positive cocci in chains (streptococci)
3. Gram-positive cocci with capsules (pneumococci)
4. Gram-positive, clubshaped, pleomorphic rods (corynebacteria)
5. Gram-negative rods with pointed ends (fusobacteria)
6. Gram-negative curved rods (here commashaped vibrios)
7. Gram-negative diplococci, adjacent sides flattened (neisseria)
8. Gram-negative straight rods with rounded ends (coli bacteria)
9. Spiral rods (spirilla) and Gram-negative curved rods (*Helicobacter*)
10. Peritrichous flagellation
11. Lophotrichous flagellation
12. Monotrichous flagellation
13. Formation of endospores (sporulation) in cells of the genera *Bacillus* and *Clostridium* (spore stain)
    a) Central spore, vegetative cell shows no swelling
    b) Terminal spore, vegetative cell shows no swelling
    c) Terminal spore ("tennis racquet")
    d) Central spore, vegetative cell shows swelling
    e) Terminal spore ("drumstick")
14. Free spores (spore stain)

Table 3.1 Morphological Characteristics of Bacteria (see Fig. 3.1 for examples)

Bacterial form	Remarks
Cocci	Occur in clusters (Fig. 3.2), chains, pairs (diplococci), packets
Straight rods	Uniform thickness, rounded ends (Fig. 3.3), pointed ends, club form
Curved rods	Commashaped, spiral (Fig. 3.4), screwshaped
Mycoplasmas	Bacteria without a rigid cell wall; coccoid cells, long threads
Chlamydiae	Two forms: spherical/oval elementary bodies (300 nm); spherical/oval reticulate bodies (1000 nm)
Rickettsiae	Short coccoid rods (0.3–1 µm)

■ **Simple staining.** In this technique, a single staining substance, e.g., methylene blue, is used.

■ **Differential staining.** Two stains with differing affinities to different bacteria are used in differential staining techniques, the most important of which is gram staining. Gram-positive bacteria stain blue-violet, Gram-negative bacteria stain red (see p. 211 for method).

Three basic forms are observed in bacteria: spherical, straight rods, and curved rods (see Figs. 3.1–3.4).

Fine Structures of Bacteria

Nucleoid (Nucleus Equivalent) and Plasmids

The "cellular nucleus" in prokaryotes consists of a tangle of double-stranded DNA, not surrounded by a membrane and localized in the cytoplasm (Fig. 3.5). In *E. coli* (and probably in all bacteria), it takes the form of a single circular molecule of DNA. The genome of *E. coli* comprises 4.63×10^6 base pairs (bp) that code for 4288 different proteins. The genomic sequence of many bacteria is known.

The plasmids are nonessential genetic structures. These circular, twisted DNA molecules are $100–1000\times$ smaller than the nucleoid genome structure and reproduce autonomously (Fig. 3.6). The plasmids of human pathogen bacteria often bear important genes determining the phenotype of their cells (resistance genes, virulence genes).

Cocci

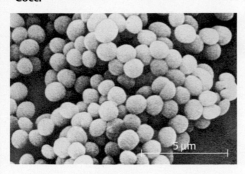

Fig. 3.**2** Cocci are spherical bacteria. Those found in grapelike clusters as in this picture are staphylococci (Scanning electron microscopy (SEM)).

Rod Bacteria

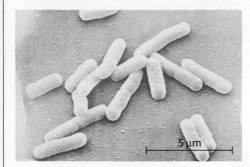

Fig. 3.**3** The straight rod bacteria with rounded ends shown here are coli bacteria (SEM).

Spirilla

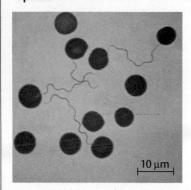

Fig. 3.**4** Spirilla, in this case borrelia are spiral bacteria (light microscopy (LM), Giemsa stain).

Bacteria During Cell Division

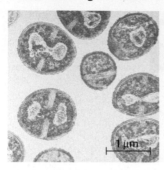

Fig. 3.**5** The nucleoid (nucleus equivalent) of bacteria consists of a tangled circular DNA molecule without a nuclear membrane. Transmission electron microscopy (TEM) image of staphylococci.

DNA Topology in Bacterial Cells

The DNA double helix (one winding/10 base pairs) is also wound counterclockwise about its helical axis (one winding/15 helical windings). This so-called supercoiling is necessary to save space and energy. Only supercoiled DNA can be replicated and transcribed. Topoisomerases steer the supercoiling process. DNA gyrase and topoisomerase IV are topoisomerases that occur only in bacteria. The 4-quinolones, an important group of anti-infection substances, inactivate these enzymes irreversibly.

Plasmids

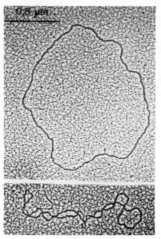

Fig. 3.**6** **a** Open circular form (OC). The result of a rupture in one of the two nucleic acid strands.
b Twisted (CCC = covalently closed circular), native form (TEM image).

Cytoplasm

The cytoplasm contains a large number of solute low- and high-molecular-weight substances, RNA and approximately 20 000 ribosomes per cell. Bacteria have 70S ribosomes comprising 30S and 50S subunits. Bacterial ribosomes function as the organelles for protein synthesis. The cytoplasm is also frequently used to store reserve substances (glycogen depots, polymerized metaphosphates, lipids).

3

■ The Most Important Bacterial Cytoplasmic Membrane Proteins ■

Permeases	Active transport of nutrients from outside to inside against a concentration gradient.
Biosynthesis enzymes	Required for biosynthesis of the cell wall, e.g., its murein (see under "Cell wall" p. 152). The enzymes that contribute to the final murein biosynthesis steps are for the most part identical with the "penicillin-binding proteins" (PBPs).
Secretion system proteins	Four secretion systems differing in structure and mode of action have been described to date. Proteins are moved out of the cell with the help of these systems. A common feature of all four is the formation of protein cylinders that traverse the cytoplasmic membrane and, in Gram-negative bacteria, the outer cell wall membrane as well. See p. 17 on the special relevance of the type III secretion system to virulence.
Sensor proteins (also known as signal proteins)	Transmit information from the cell's environment into its interior. The so-called receiver domain extends outward, the transmitter domain inward. The transmission activity is regulated by the binding of signal molecules to a receiver module. In two-component systems, the transmitter module transfers the information to a regulator protein, activating its functional module. This regulator segment can then bind to specific gene sequences and activate or deactivate one or more genes (see also Fig. 1.**4**, p. 19).
Respiratory chain enzymes	Occur in bacteria with aerobic metabolism. Aerobic respiration functions according to the same principles as cellular respiration in eurkaryotes.

The Cytoplasmic Membrane

This elementary membrane, also known as the plasma membrane, is typical of living cells. It is basically a double layer of phospholipids with numerous proteins integrated into its structure. The most important of these membrane

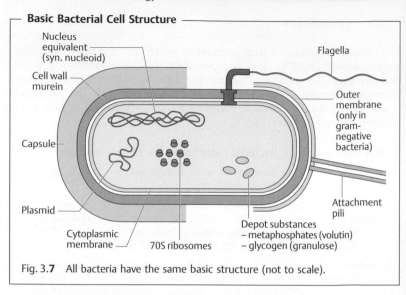

Basic Bacterial Cell Structure

Nucleus equivalent (syn. nucleoid)

Cell wall murein

Capsule

Plasmid

Cytoplasmic membrane

70S ribosomes

Flagella

Outer membrane (only in gram-negative bacteria)

Attachment pili

Depot substances
– metaphosphates (volutin)
– glycogen (granulose)

Fig. 3.7 All bacteria have the same basic structure (not to scale).

proteins are permeases, enzymes for the biosynthesis of the cell wall, transfer proteins for secretion of extracellular proteins, sensor or signal proteins, and respiratory chain enzymes.

In electron microscopic images of Gram-positive bacteria, the mesosomes appear as structures bound to the membrane. How they function and what role they play remain to be clarified. They may be no more than artifacts.

Cell Wall

The tasks of the complex bacterial cell wall are to protect the protoplasts from external noxae, to withstand and maintain the osmotic pressure gradient between the cell interior and the extracellular environment (with internal pressures as high as 500–2000 kPa), to give the cell its outer form and to facilitate communication with its surroundings.

Murein (syn. peptidoglycan). The most important structural element of the wall is murein, a netlike polymer material surrounding the entire cell (sacculus). It is made up of polysaccharide chains crosslinked by peptides (Figs. 3.**8** and 3.**9**).

The cell wall of Gram-positive bacteria (Fig. 3.**10**). The murein sacculus may consist of as many as 40 layers (15–80 nm thick) and account for as much as

The Murein Building Block

CH2OH
CH2OH
O
O
O
OH
O
O
NH–CO–CH3
NH–CO–CH3
O
CH–CH3
CO
(NH)
L-alanine
D-isoglutamine
L-lysine–[glycine]5–
D-alanine
D-alanine (COOH)

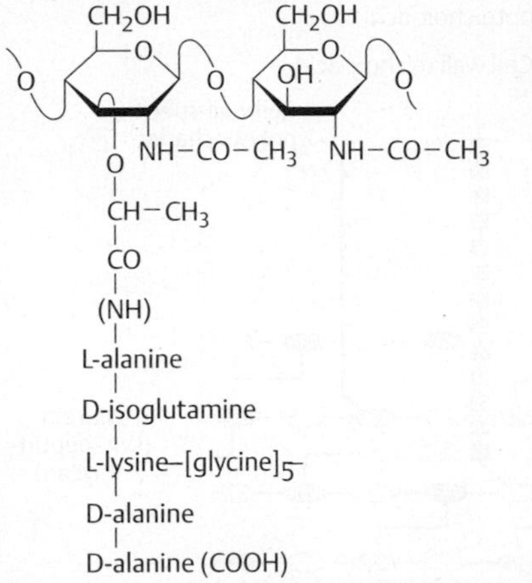

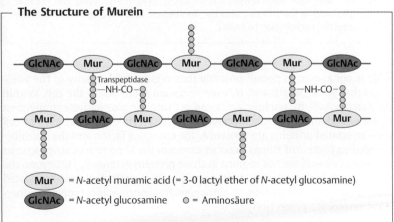

Fig. 3.8 The murein (syn. peptidoglycan) of the cell wall is composed of a series of identical subunits. The terminal D-alanine is split off each time a new crosslink is synthesized. Only in staphylococci is a pentaglycine interpeptide bridge inserted between adjacent peptides.

30% of the dry mass of the cell wall. The membrane lipoteichoic acids are anchored in the cytoplasmic membrane, whereas the cell wall teichoic acids are covalently coupled to the murein. The physiological role of the teichoic

The Structure of Murein

GlcNAc
Mur
GlcNAc
Mur
GlcNAc
Mur
GlcNAc
Transpeptidase
–NH-CO–
–NH-CO–
Mur
GlcNAc
Mur
GlcNAc
Mur
GlcNAc
Mur
Mur = N-acetyl muramic acid (= 3-0 lactyl ether of N-acetyl glucosamine)
GlcNAc = N-acetyl glucosamine
○ = Aminosäure

Fig. 3.9 Soluble murein fragments of Gram-negative and Gram-positive bacteria can stimulate excessive cytokine secretion in macrophages by binding to toll-like receptors and CD14. Cytokines cause the clinical symptoms of sepsis or septic shock syndrome (see under Lipoid A, p. 156).

The Cell Wall of Gram-Positive Bacteria

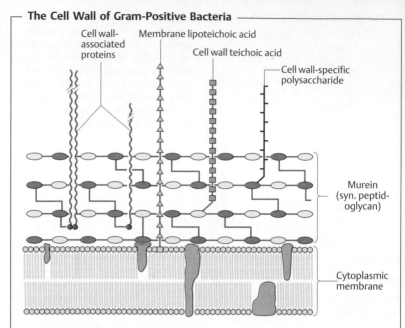

Fig. 3.**10** Note the characteristic thick murein layer, the proteins and teichoic acids anchored in the murein, and the lipoteichoic acid fixed to the membrane by a lipophilic anchor (not to scale).

acids is not known in detail; possibly they regulate the activity of the auto-lysins that steer growth and transverse fission processes in the cell. Within the macroorganism, teichoic acids can activate the alternative complement pathway and stimulate macrophages to secrete cytokines. Examples of cell wall-associated proteins are protein A, the clumping factor, and the fibronec-tin-binding protein of *Staphylococcus aureus* or the M protein of *Streptococcus pyogenes*. Cell wall anchor regions in these proteins extending far beyond the murein are bound covalently to its peptide components. Cell wall-associated proteins frequently function as pathogenicity determinants (specific adher-ence; phagocyte protection).

The cell wall of Gram-negative bacteria. Here, the murein is only about 2 nm thick and contributes up to 10 % of the dry cell wall mass (Fig. 3.**11**). The outer membrane is the salient structural element. It contains numerous proteins (50 % by mass) as well as the medically critical lipopolysaccharide.

The Cell Wall of Gram-Negative Bacteria

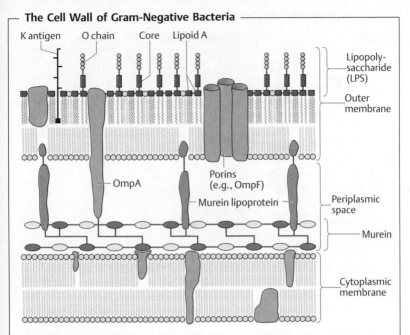

Fig. 3.**11** Note the characteristic thin murein layer and the outer membrane connected to it by proteins (OmpA, murein lipoprotein). Many different proteins are localized in the outer membrane. Its outer layer is made up of closely packed lipopolysaccharide complexes (see Fig. 3.12).

■ **Outer membrane proteins.**
— OmpA (outer membrane protein A) and the murein lipoprotein form a bond between outer membrane and murein.
— Porins, proteins that form pores in the outer membrane, allow passage of hydrophilic, low-molecular-weight substances into the periplasmic space.
— Outer membrane-associated proteins constitute specific structures that enable bacteria to attach to host cell receptors.
— A number of Omps are transport proteins. Examples include the LamB proteins for maltose transport and FepA for transport of the siderophore ferric (Fe^{3+}) enterochelin in *E. coli* (see also p. 13).

■ **Lipopolysaccharide (LPS).** This molecular complex, also known as endotoxin, is comprised of the lipoid A, the core polysaccharide, and the O-specific polysaccharide chain (Fig. 3.**12**).

The Lipopolysaccharide Complex

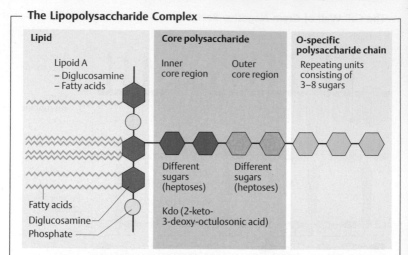

Lipid	Core polysaccharide	O-specific polysaccharide chain
Lipoid A – Diglucosamine – Fatty acids	Inner core region Outer core region	Repeating units consisting of 3–8 sugars
Fatty acids Diglucosamine Phosphate	Different sugars (heptoses) Different sugars (heptoses) Kdo (2-keto-3-deoxy-octulosonic acid)	

Fig. 3.**12** The three-part lipopolysaccharide complex (LPS) of Gram-negative bacteria is anchored in the outer membrane by means of its lipid moiety. LPS is also known as endotoxin.

— **Lipoid A** is responsible for the toxic effect. As a free substance, or bound up in the LPS complex, it stimulates—by binding together with the LPS binding protein (LBP) to the CD14 receptor of macrophages—the formation and secretion of cytokines that determine clinical endotoxin symptomatology. Interleukin 1 (IL-1) and tumor necrosis factor (TNF) induce an increased synthesis of prostaglandin E2 in the hypothalamus, thus setting the "thermostat" in the temperature control center higher, resulting in fever. Other direct and indirect endotoxin effects include granulopoiesis stimulation, aggregation and degeneration of thrombocytes, intravasal coagulation due to factor VII activation, a drop in blood pressure, and cachexia. LPS can also activate the alternative complement pathway. Release of large amounts of endotoxin can lead to septic (endotoxic) shock. Endotoxin is not inactivated by vapor sterilization. Therefore, the parent materials used in production of parenteral pharmaceuticals must be free of endotoxins (pyrogens).
— **The O-specific polysaccharide chain** is the so-called O antigen, the fine chemical structure of which results in a large number of antigenic variants useful in bacterial typing (e.g., detailed differentiation of salmonella types) (see p. 284f.).

L-forms (L = Lister Institute). The L-forms are bacteria with murein defects, e.g., resulting from the effects of betalactam antibiotics. L-forms are highly unstable when subjected to osmotic influences. They are totally resistant to betalactams, which block the biosynthesis of murein. The clinical significance of the L-forms is not clear. They may revert to the normal bacterial form when betalactam therapy is discontinued, resulting in a relapse.

Capsule

Many pathogenic bacteria make use of extracellular enzymes to synthesize a polymer that forms a layer around the cell: the capsule. **The capsule protects bacterial cells from phagocytosis.** The capsule of most bacteria consists of a polysaccharide. The bacteria of a single species can be classified in different capsular serovars (or serotypes) based on the fine chemical structure of this polysaccharide.

Flagella

Flagella give bacteria the ability to move about actively. The flagella (singular flagellum) are made up of a class of linear proteins called flagellins. Flagel-

— **Bacterial flagella** —

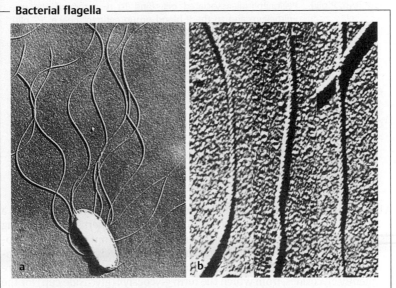

Fig. 3.**13** **a** Flagellated bacterial cell (SEM, 13 000×). **b** Helical structure of bacterial flagella (SEM, 77 000×).

lated bacteria are described as monotrichous, lophotrichous, or peritrichous, depending on how the flagella are arranged (see Fig. 3.**1**, p. 147). The basal body traverses the cell wall and cytoplasmic membrane to anchor the flagellum (see Figs. 3.**7** and 3.**13**) and enables it to whirl about its axis like a propeller. In *Enterobacteriaceae*, the flagellar antigens are called H antigens. Together with the O antigens, they are used to classify bacteria in serovars.

Attachment Pili (Fimbriae), Conjugation Pili

Many Gram-negative bacteria possess thin microfibrils made of proteins (0.1–1.5 nm thick, 4–8 nm long), the attachment pili. They are anchored in the outer membrane of the cell wall and extend radially from the surface. Using these structures, bacteria are capable of specific attachment to host cell receptors (ligand—receptor, key—keyhole).

The conjugation pili (syn. sex pili) in Gram-negative bacteria are required for the process of conjugation and thus for transfer of conjugative plasmids (see p. 175).

Examples of Attachment Pili in Gram-Negative Bacteria

PAP (syn. P pili)	Pyelonephritis-associated pili. Bind to receptors of the uroepithelium and to the P blood group antigen (hence "P" pili). The specific receptors for these pili are plentiful on the uroepithelial surface. PAP are characteristic of the uropathological variety of *Escherichia coli* that causes spontaneous urinary tract infections in patients showing no tract obstruction.
CFA1, CFA2	Colonization factors. Pili responsible for specific binding of enteropathogenic coli bacteria to enterocytes.
Gonococcal attachment pili	Used for specific attachment of gonococci mucosal cells of the urogenital epithelium.

Biofilm

A bacterial biofilm is a structured community of bacterial cells embedded in a self-produced polymer matrix and attached to either an inert surface or living tissue. Such films can develop considerable thickness (mm). The bacteria located deep within such a biofilm structure are effectively isolated from immune system cells, antibodies, and antibiotics. The polymers they secrete are frequently glycosides, from which the term glycocalyx (glycoside cup) for the matrix is derived.

Examples of Medically Important Biofilms

■ Following implantation of endoprostheses, catheters, cardiac pacemakers, shunt valves, etc. these foreign bodies are covered by matrix proteins of the macroorganism such as fibrinogen, fibronectin, vitronectin, or laminin. Staphylococci have proteins on their surfaces with which they can bind specifically to the corresponding proteins, for example the clumping factor that binds to fibrinogen and the fibronectin-binding protein. The adhering bacteria then proliferate and secrete an exopolysaccharide glycocalyx: the biofilm matrix on the foreign body. Such biofilms represent **foreign body-associated infection foci**.

■ Certain oral streptococci (*S. mutans*) bind to the proteins covering tooth enamel, then proceed to build a glucan matrix out of sucrose. Other bacteria then adhere to the matrix to form plaque (Fig. 3.**14**), the precondition for destruction of the enamel and formation of **caries** (see p. 243f.).

■ Oral streptococci and other bacteria attach to the surface of the cardiac valves to form a biofilm. Professional phagocytes are attracted to the site and attempt, unsuccessfully, to phagocytize the bacteria. The frustrated phagocytes then release the tissue-damaging content of their lysosomes (see p. 23), resulting in an inflammatory reaction and the clinical picture of **endocarditis**.

3

Bacterial Spores

Bacterial spores (endospores) are purely dormant life forms. Their development from bacterial cells in a "vegetative" state does not involve assimilation of additional external nutrients. They are spherical to oval in shape and are characterized by a thick spore wall and a high level of resistance to chemical and physical noxae. Among human pathogen bacteria, only the genera *Clostridium* and *Bacillus* produce spores. The heat resistance of these spores is their most important quality from a medical point of view, since heat ster-

--- Dental Plaque ---

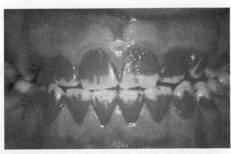

Fig. 3.**14** Dental plaque can be rendered visible with an erythrosin stain.

ilization procedures require very high temperatures to kill them effectively. Potential contributing factors to spore heat resistance include their thick wall structures, the dehydration of the spore, and crosslinking of the proteins by the calcium salt of pyridine-2,6-dicarboxylic acid, both of which render protein denaturing difficult. When a spore's milieu once again provides favorable conditions (nutrient medium, temperature, osmotic pressure, etc.) it returns to the vegetative state in which spore-forming bacteria can reproduce.

3

The Physiology of Metabolism and Growth in Bacteria

■ Human pathogenic bacteria are chemosynthetic and organotrophic (chemo-organotrophic). They derive energy from the breakdown of organic nutrients and use this chemical energy both for resynthesis and secondary activities. Bacteria oxidize nutrient substrates by means of either respiration or fermentation. In respiration, O_2 is the electron and proton acceptor, in fermentation an organic molecule performs this function. Human pathogenic bacteria are classified in terms of their O_2 requirements and tolerance as facultative anaerobes, obligate aerobes, obligate anaerobes, or aerotolerant anaerobes. Nutrient broth or agar is used to cultivate bacteria. Nutrient agar contains the inert substrate agarose, which liquefies at 100 °C and gels at 45 °C. Selective and indicator mediums are used frequently in diagnostic bacteriology.

Bacteria reproduce by means of simple transverse binary fission. The time required for complete cell division is called generation time. The in-vitro generation time of rapidly proliferating species is 15–30 minutes. This time is much longer in vivo. The growth curve for proliferation in nutrient broth is normally characterized by the phases lag, log (or exponential) growth, stationary growth, and death. ■

Bacterial Metabolism

Types of Metabolism

Metabolism is the totality of chemical reactions occurring in bacterial cells. They can be subdivided into anabolic (synthetic) reactions that consume energy and catabolic reactions that supply energy. In the anabolic, endergonic reactions, the energy requirement is consumed in the form of light or chemical energy—by photosynthetic or chemosynthetic bacteria, respectively. Catabolic reactions supply both energy and the basic structural elements for synthesis of specific bacterial molecules. Bacteria that feed on inorganic nutrients are said to be lithotrophic, those that feed on organic nutrients are organotrophic.

Human pathogenic bacteria are always chemosynthetic, organotrophic bacteria (or chemo-organotrophs).

3

Catabolic Reactions

Organic nutrient substrates are catabolized in a wide variety of enzymatic processes that can be schematically divided into four phases:

Digestion. Bacterial exoenzymes split up the nutrient substrates into smaller molecules outside the cell. The exoenzymes represent important pathogenicity factors in some cases.

Uptake. Nutrients can be taken up by means of passive diffusion or, more frequently, specifically by active transport through the membrane(s). Cytoplasmic membrane permeases play an important role in these processes.

Preparation for oxidation. Splitting off of carboxyl and amino groups, phosphorylation, etc.

Oxidation. This process is defined as the removal of electrons and H^+ ions. The substance to which the H_2 atoms are transferred is called the hydrogen acceptor. The two basic forms of oxidation are defined by the final hydrogen acceptor (Fig. 3.**15**).

■ **Respiration.** Here oxygen is the hydrogen acceptor. In anaerobic respiration, the O_2 that serves as the hydrogen acceptor is a component of an inorganic salt.

■ **Fermentation.** Here an organic compound serves as the hydrogen acceptor.

The main difference between fermentation and respiration is the energy yield, which can be greater from respiration than from fermentation for a given nutrient substrate by as much as a factor of 10. Fermentation processes involving microorganisms are designated by the final product, e.g., alcoholic fermentation, butyric acid fermentation, etc.

The energy released by oxidation is stored as chemical energy in the form of a thioester (e.g., acetyl-CoA) or organic phosphates (e.g., ATP).

Bacterial Oxidation Pathways

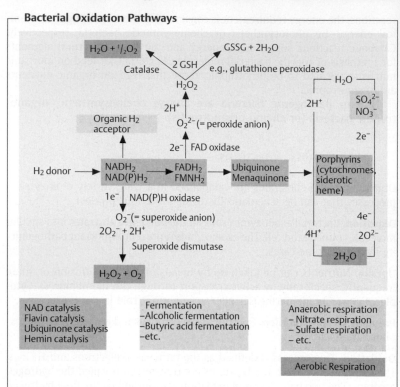

Fig. 3.**15** In oxidation of organic nutrient substrates, protons (H^+) and electrons (e^-) are transferred in more or less long chains. The respiration is aerobic when the final electron acceptor is free oxygen. Anaerobic respiration is when the electrons are transferred to inorganically bound oxygen. Fermentation is the transfer of H^+ and e^- to an organic acceptor.

The role of oxygen. Oxygen is activated in one of three ways:

■ Transfer of $4e^-$ to O_2, resulting in two oxygen ions ($2\ O^{2-}$).

■ Transfer of $2e^-$ to O_2, resulting in one peroxide anion ($1\ O_2^{2-}$).

■ Transfer of $1e^-$ to O_2, resulting in one superoxide anion ($1\ O_2^-$).

Hydrogen peroxide and the highly reactive superoxide anion are toxic and therefore must undergo further conversion immediately (see Fig. 3.**15**).

Bacteria are categorized as the following according to their O_2-related behavior:

■ **Facultative anaerobes.** These bacteria can oxidize nutrient substrates by means of both respiration and fermentation.

■ **Obligate aerobes.** These bacteria can only reproduce in the presence of O_2.

■ **Obligate anaerobes.** These bacteria die in the presence of O_2. Their metabolism is adapted to a low redox potential and vital enzymes are inhibited by O_2.

■ **Aerotolerant anaerobes.** These bacteria oxidize nutrient substrates without using elemental oxygen although, unlike obligate anaerobes, they can tolerate it.

Basic mechanisms of catabolic metabolism. The principle of the biochemical unity of life asserts that all life on earth is, in essence, the same. Thus, the catabolic intermediary metabolism of bacteria is, for the most part, equivalent to what takes place in eukaryotic cells. The reader is referred to textbooks of general microbiology for exhaustive treatment of the pathways of intermediary bacterial metabolism.

Anabolic Reactions

It is not possible to go into all of the biosynthetic feats of bacteria here. Suffice it to say that they are, on the whole, quite astounding. Some bacteria (*E. coli*) are capable of synthesizing all of the complex organic molecules that they are comprised of, from the simplest nutrients in a very short time. These capacities are utilized in the field of microbiological engineering. Antibiotics, amino acids, and vitamins are produced with the help of bacteria. Some bacteria are even capable of using aliphatic hydrocarbon compounds as an energy source. Such bacteria can "feed" on paraffin or even raw petroleum. It is hoped that the metabolic capabilities of these bacteria will help control the effects of oil spills in surface water. Bacteria have also been enlisted in the fight against hunger: certain bacteria and fungi are cultivated on aliphatic hydrocarbon substrates, which supply carbon and energy, then harvested and processed into a protein powder (single cell protein). Culturing of bacteria in nutrient mediums based on methanol is another approach being used to produce biomass.

Metabolic Regulation

Bacteria are highly efficient metabolic regulators, coordinating each individual reaction with other cell activities and with the available nutrients as economically and rationally as possible. One form such control activity takes is regulation of the activities of existing enzymes. Many enzymes are allosteric proteins that can be inhibited or activated by the final products of metabolic pathways. One highly economical type of regulation controls the synthesis of enzymes at the genetic transcription or translation level (see the section on the molecular basis of bacterial genetics (p. 169ff.).

Growth and Culturing of Bacteria

Nutrients

The term bacterial culture refers to proliferation of bacteria with a suitable nutrient substrate. A nutrient medium (Table 3.2) in which chemoorganotrophs are to be cultivated must have organic energy sources (H_2 donors) and H_2 acceptors. Other necessities include sources of carbon and nitrogen for synthesis of specific bacterial compounds as well as minerals such as sulfur, phosphorus, calcium, magnesium, and trace elements as enzyme activators. Some bacteria also require "growth factors," i.e., organic compounds they are unable to synthesize themselves. Depending on the bacterial species involved, the nutrient medium must contain certain amounts of O_2 and CO_2 and have certain pH and osmotic pressure levels.

Table 3.2 Nutrient Mediums for Culturing Bacteria

Nutrient medium	Description
Nutrient broth	Complex liquid nutrient medium.
Nutrient agar	Complex nutrient medium containing the polysaccharide agarose (1.5–2%). Nutrient agar liquefies when heated to 100 °C and does not return to the gel state until cooled to 45 °C. Agarose is not broken down by bacteria.
Selective mediums	Contain inhibitor substances that allow only certain bacteria to proliferate.
Indicator mediums	Indicate certain metabolic processes.
Synthetic mediums	Mediums that are precisely chemically defined.

Growth and Cell Death

Bacteria reproduce asexually by means of simple transverse binary fission. Their numbers (n) increase logarithmically ($n = 2^G$). The time required for a reproduction cycle (G) is called the generation time (g) and can vary greatly from species to species. Fast-growing bacteria cultivated in vitro have a generation time of 15–30 minutes. The same bacteria may take hours to reproduce in vivo. Obligate anaerobes grow much more slowly than aerobes; this is true in vitro as well. Tuberculosis bacteria have an in-vitro generation time of 12–24 hours. Of course the generation time also depends on the nutrient content of the medium.

The so-called **normal growth curve** for bacteria is obtained by inoculating a nutrient broth with bacteria the metabolism of which is initially quiescent, counting them at intervals and entering the results in a semilog coordinate system (Fig. 3.**16**). The lag phase (A) is characterized by an increase in bacterial mass per unit of volume, but no increase in cell count. During this phase, the metabolism of the bacteria adapts to the conditions of the nutrient medium. In the following log (or exponential) phase (C), the cell count increases logarithmically up to about 10^9/ml. This is followed by growth deceleration and transition to the stationary phase (E) due to exhaustion of the nutrients and the increasing concentration of toxic metabolites. Finally, death phase (F) processes begin. The generation time can only be determined during phase C, either graphically or by determining the cell count (n) at two different times and applying the formula:

$$g = \frac{t_2 - t_1}{\log_2 n_2 - \log_2 n_1}.$$

Normal Growth Curve of a Bacterial Culture

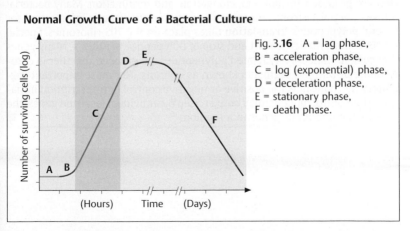

Fig. 3.**16** A = lag phase,
B = acceleration phase,
C = log (exponential) phase,
D = deceleration phase,
E = stationary phase,
F = death phase.

Bacterial Cell Count and Bacterial Mass

The colony counting method. The number of living cells in a given culture or material can be determined by means of the colony counting method. The samples are diluted logarithmically by a dilution factor of 10. Using the pour plate technique, each dilution is mixed with 1 ml of liquid agar and poured out in a plate. In the surface inoculation method, 0.1 ml of each dilution is plated out on a nutrient agar surface. The plates are incubated, resulting in colony growth. The number of colonies counted, multiplied by the dilution factor, results in the original number of viable bacterial cells (CFU = colony forming units).

Bacterial mass. The bacterial mass can be established by weighing (dry or wet weight). The simplest way to determine the mass is by means of photometric adsorption measurement. The increases in mass and cell count run parallel during phase C on the growth curve.

The Molecular Basis of Bacterial Genetics

■ Bacteria possess two genetic structures: the **chromosome** and the **plasmid**. Both of these structures consist of a single circular DNA double helix twisted counterclockwise about its helical axis. **Replication** of this DNA molecule always starts at a certain point (the origin of replication) and is "semiconservative," that is, one strand in each of the two resulting double strands is conserved. Most **bacterial genes** code for proteins (polypeptides). Noncoding interposed sequences (introns), like those seen in eukaryotes, are the exception. Certain bacterial genes have a mosaic structure. The phases of **transcription** are promoter recognition, elongation, and termination. Many bacterial mRNAs are polycistronic, meaning they contain the genetic information for several polypeptides. **Translation** takes place on the 70S ribosomes. Special mRNA codons mark the start and stop of polypeptide synthesis. Many genes that code for functionally related polypeptides are grouped together in chromosome or plasmid segments known as operons. The most important regulatory mechanism is the positive or negative control of transcription initiation. This control function may be exercised by individual localized genes, the genes of an operon or genes in a regulon. ■

The Structure of Bacterial DNA

A bacterium's genetic information is stored in its chromosome and plasmids. Each of these structures is made of a single DNA double helix twisted to the right, then additionally twisted to the left about its helical axis (supercoiled, see p. 148ff. and Fig. 3.**17**). Plasmids consisting of linear DNA also occur, although this is rare. This DNA topology solves spatial problems and enables such functions as replication, transcription, and recombination. Some genes are composed of a mosaic of minicassettes interconnected by conserved DNA sequences between the cassettes (see Fig. 1.**2**, p. 14).

Chromosome. The chromosome corresponds to the nucleoid (p. 148ff.). The *E. coli* chromosome is composed of 4.63×10^6 base pairs (bp). It codes for 4288 proteins. The gene sequence is colinear with the expressed genetic products. The noncoding interposed sequences (introns) normally seen in eukaryotic genes are very rare. The chromosomes of E. coli and numerous other pathogenic bacteria have now been completely sequenced.

Plasmids. The plasmids are autonomous DNA molecules of varying size (3×10^3 to 4.5×10^5 bp) localized in the cytoplasm. Large plasmids are usually present in one to two copies per cell, whereas small ones may be present in 10, 40, or 100 copies. Plasmids are not essential to a cell's survival.

3

Resistance Plasmid in *Escherichia coli*

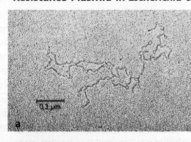

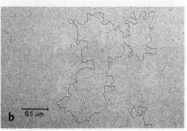

Fig. 3.**17** **a** Covalently closed circle (CCC), also known as a "supercoil" or "supertwist."
b Open circle. This open form is an artifact produced by a nick in one strand of the DNA double helix.

Many of them carry genes that code for certain phenotypic characteristics of the host cell. The following plasmid types are medically relevant:

■ **Virulence plasmids.** Carry determinants of bacterial virulence, e.g., enterotoxin genes or hemolysin genes.

■ **Resistance plasmids.** Carry genetic information bearing on resistance to anti-infective agents. R plasmids may carry several *R* genes at once (see also Fig. 3.**23**, p. 176). Plasmids have also been described that carry both virulence and resistance genes.

DNA Replication

The identical duplication process of DNA is termed semiconservative because the double strand of DNA is opened up during replication, whereupon each strand serves as the matrix for synthesis of a complementary strand. Thus each of the two new double strands "conserves" one old strand. The doubling of each DNA molecule (replicon) begins at a given starting point, the so-called origin of replication. This process continues throughout the entire fission cycle.

Transcription and Translation

■ **Transcription.** Copying of the sense strand of the DNA into mRNA. The continuous genetic nucleotide sequence is transcribed "colinearly" into mRNA. This principle of colinearity applies with very few exceptions. The transcription process can be broken down into the three phases *promoter recognition*, *elongation*, and *termination*. The promoter region is the site where the RNA polymerase begins reading the DNA sequence. A sigma factor is required for binding to the promoter. Sigma factors are proteins that associate temporarily with the RNA polymerase (core enzyme) to form a holoenzyme, then dissociate themselves once the transcription process has begun, making them available to associate once again. Specific sigma factors recognize the standard promoters of most genes. Additional sigma factors, the expression of which depends on the physiological status of the cell, facilitate the transcription of special determinants. Genes that code for functionally related proteins, for example proteins that act together to catalyze a certain metabolic step, are often arranged sequentially at specific locations on the chromosome or plasmid. Such DNA sequences are known as operons (Fig. 3.**18**). The mRNA synthesized by the transcription of an operon is polycistronic, i.e., it contains the information sequences of several genes. The information sequences are

Bacterial Operon and Regulator Gene

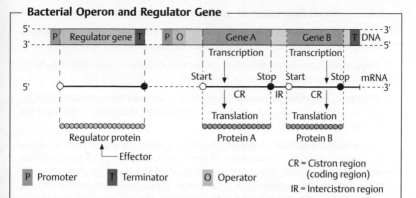

Fig. 3.**18** An operon is a DNA sequence that usually includes several structural genes. These genes code for proteins that are functionally related. Transcription of an operon is often activated or repressed by the product of a regulator gene located elsewhere on the chromosome.

3

separated by intercistronic regions. Each cistron has its own start and stop codon in the mRNA.

■ **Translation.** Transformation of the nucleotide sequence carried by the mRNA into the polypeptide amino acid sequence at the 70S ribosomes. In principle, bacterial and eukaryotic translation is the same. The enzymes and other factors involved do, however, differ structurally and can therefore be selectively blocked by antibiotics (p. 198ff.).

Regulation of Gene Expression

Bacteria demonstrate a truly impressive capacity for adapting to their environment. A number of regulatory bacterial mechanisms are known, for example posttranslational regulation, translational regulation, transcription termination, and quorum sensing (see Fig. 1.**5**, p. 20). The details of all these mechanisms would exceed the scope of this book. The most important is regulation of the initiation of transcription by means of activation or repression, a process not observed in this form in eukaryotes: a single gene, or several genes in an operon at one DNA location, may be affected (see Fig. 3.**18**). The mechanism that has been investigated most thoroughly is transcriptional regulation of catabolic and anabolic operons by a repressor or activator.

3

Transcriptional Regulation of an Operon:

■ **Catabolic operons** have genes that code for enzymes of catabolic metabolism. Anabolic operons code for enzymes of anabolic metabolism.

■ **Regulators.** Code for proteins that can repress or activate transcription by binding to the operator or promoter of an operon.

■ **Effectors.** Low-molecular-weight signal molecules from the immediate environment of the bacterial cell. Can activate (= corepressor) or inactivate (= inducer) the repressor by means of an allosteric effect.

■ **Induction of a catabolic operon.** The effector molecule is a nutrient substrate that is broken down by the products of the operon genes (e.g., lactose). Lactose inactivates the repressor, initializing transcription of the genes for *β-galactosidase* and *β-galactoside permease* in the lactose operon. These genes are normally not read off because the repressor is bound to the operator. The cell is not induced to produce the necessary catabolic enzymes until the nutrient substrate is present.

■ **Repression of an anabolic operon.** The signal molecule is the final product of an anabolic process, for instance an amino acid. If this acid is present in the medium, it can be obtained from there and the cell need not synthesize the anabolic enzymes it would require to produce it. In such a case, binding to the effector is what turns the regulator protein into an active repressor.

A single regulator protein can also activate or repress several genes not integrated in an operon, i.e., at various locations on the DNA. Such functional gene groups are called **regulons**. Alternative **sigma factors** (see p. 168) may be involved in the transcriptional activation of special genes with special promoters. Physiological cell status determines whether or not these alternative factors are produced.

The Genetic Variability of Bacteria

■ Changes in bacterial DNA are the result of spontaneous **mutations** in individual genes as well as recombination processes resulting in new genes or genetic combinations. Based on the molecular mechanisms involved, bacterial **recombinations** are classified as homologous, site-specific, and transpositional. The latter two in particular reflect the high level of mobility of many genes and have made essential contributions to the evolution of bacteria.

Although sexual heredity is unknown in bacteria, they do make use of the mechanisms of intercellular transfer of genomic material known as parasexual processes. **Transformation** designates transfer of DNA that is essentially chemically pure from a donor into a receptor cell. In **transduction**, bacteriophages serve as the vehicles for DNA transport. **Conjugation** is the transfer of DNA by means of cell-to-cell contact. This process, made possible by conjugative plasmids and transposons, can be a high-frequency one and may even occur between partners of different species, genera, or families. The transfer primarily involves the conjugative elements themselves. Conjugative structures carrying resistance or virulence genes are of considerable medical significance.

The processes of **restriction** and **modification** are important factors limiting genetic exchange among different taxa. Restriction is based on the effects of restriction endonucleases capable of specific excision of foreign DNA sequences. These enzymes have become invaluable tools in the field of genetic engineering.   ∎

Molecular Mechanisms of Genetic Variability

Spontaneous Mutation

In the year 1943, Luria and Delbrück used the so-called fluctuation test to demonstrate that changes in the characteristics of bacterial populations were the results of rare, random mutations in the genes of individual cells, which then were selected. Such mutations may involve substitution of a single nucleotide, frame-shifts, deletions, inversions, or insertions. The frequency of mutations is expressed as the **mutation rate**, which is defined as the probability of mutation per gene per cell division. The rate varies depending on the gene involved and is approximately 10^{-6} to 10^{-10}. Mutation rates may increase drastically due to mutagenic factors such as radioactivity, UV radiation, alkylating chemicals, etc.

Recombination

The term recombination designates processes that lead to the restructuring of DNA, formation of new genes or genetic combinations.

Homologous (generalized) recombination. A precise exchange of DNA between corresponding sequences. Several enzymes contribute to the complex breakage and reunion process involved, the most important being the RecA enzyme and another the RecBC nuclease. Fig. 1.2 (p. 14) shows an example of homologous recombination resulting in the exchange of minicassettes between two genes.

Site-specific recombination. Integration or excision of a sequence in or from target DNA. Only a single sequence of a few nucleotides of the integrated DNA needs to be homologous with the recombination site on the target DNA. The integration of bacteriophage genomes is an example of what this process facilitates (p. 184f.) Integration of several determinants of antibiotic resistance in one integron can also utilize this process (Fig. 3.**19**). Resistance integrons may be integrated in transposable DNA.

Transposition. The transposition process does not require the donor and target DNA to be homologous. DNA sequences can either be transposed to a different locus on the same molecule or to a different replicon. Just as in site-specific recombination, transposition has always played a major role in the evolution of multi-resistance plasmids (see Fig. 3.**23**, p. 176).

Site-Specific Recombination (Integron)

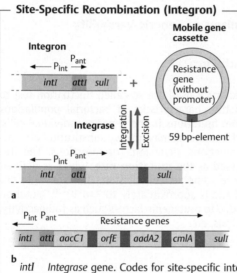

Fig. 3.**19 a** Integration or excision of a circular gene cassette into or out of an integron. An integron is a genetic structure containing the determinants of a site-specific recombination system. This structure is capable of capturing or mobilizing mobile gene cassettes. It also provides the promoter for transcription of the cassette genes, which themselves have no promoter. The cassettes occur in both free circularized and integrated forms.

intI Integrase gene. Codes for site-specific integrase (int = integrase).
attI Attachment sequence for the integrase. Site of recombination (att = attachment).
P_{ant} Promoter for the integrated gene cassette (P = promoter).
P_{int} Promoter for the *integrase* gene.
sulI Gene for sulfonamide resistance (sul = sulfonamide).
59bp Integrase-specific recombination site in cassette.
b Model of integron 4 (In4), which contains three resistance genes and an open reading frame (*orfE*), the function of which is unknown. In4 is the result of successive integration of several resistance genes at the *att1* site.

Transposable DNA Elements

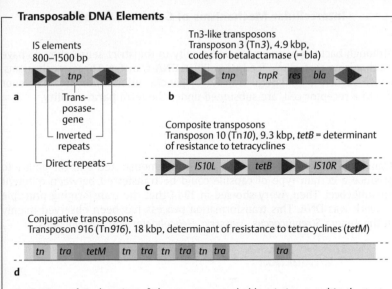

IS elements
800–1500 bp

Tn3-like transposons
Transposon 3 (Tn3), 4.9 kbp,
codes for betalactamase (= bla)

a Trans-
posase-
gene
Inverted
repeats
Direct repeats

b

Composite transposons
Transposon 10 (Tn10), 9.3 kbp, *tetB* = determinant
of resistance to tetracyclines

c

Conjugative transposons
Transposon 916 (Tn916), 18 kbp, determinant of resistance to tetracyclines (*tetM*)

d

Fig. 3.**20**   **a–d** Explanation of the structures and abbreviations used in the text box "Details of Transposable DNA elements" below.

▪ Details of Transposable DNA Elements

▪ **Insertion sequences (IS elements**, Fig. 3.**20**). These are the simplest transposable DNA sequences. They are terminated by identical, but reversed, sequences of 10–40 nucleotides known as inverted repeats (IR). They frame the segment that codes for the enzyme transposase. The target structures for this enzyme are the so-called *direct repeats*, nucleotide sequences comprising 5–9 bp that are duplicated in the integration process.

▪ **Tn3 transposons** (Fig. 3.**20b**). In addition to the transposase gene *tnpA*, they contain the regulator sequence *tnpR* and the *res* site to which resolvase must bind. Tn3-like transposons are duplicated in the transposition process, so that one copy remains at the original location and the other is integrated at the new location.

▪ **Composite transposons** (Fig. 3.**20c**). They consist of two IS elements framing a sequence of variable size that is not required for transposition, e.g., a resistance gene.

▪ **Conjugative transposons** (Fig. 3.**20d**). These genetic elements code in certain regions for factors that control the transfer (Tra) and transposition (Tn) processes. Conjugative transposons have been discovered mainly in Gram-positive cocci and Gram-negative anaerobes (*Bacteroides*).

Intercellular Mechanisms of Genetic Variability

Although bacteria have no sexual heredity in the strict sense, they do have mechanisms that allow for intercellular DNA transfer. These mechanisms, which involve a unilateral transfer of genetic information from a donor cell to a receptor cell, are subsumed under the term **parasexuality**.

Transformation

Transfer of "naked" DNA. In 1928, Griffith demonstrated that the ability to produce a certain type of capsule could be transferred between different pneumococci. Then Avery showed in 1944 that the transforming principle at work was DNA. This transformation process has been observed mainly in the genera *Streptococcus*, *Neisseria*, *Helicobacter* and *Haemophilus*.

Transduction

Transfer of DNA from a donor to a receptor with the help of transport bacteriophages (Fig. 3.**21**).

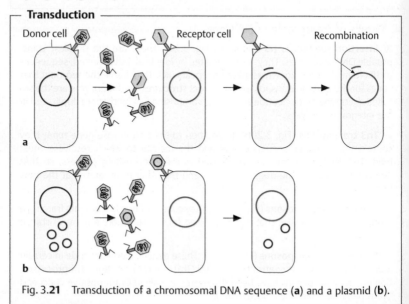

Transduction

Fig. 3.**21** Transduction of a chromosomal DNA sequence (**a**) and a plasmid (**b**).

Bacteriophages are viruses that infect bacteria (p. 182ff.). During their replication process, DNA sequences from the host bacterial cell may replace all or part of the genome in the phage head. Such phage particles are then defective. They can still dock on receptor cells and inject their DNA, but the infected bacterial cell will then neither produce new phages nor be destroyed.

Conjugation

Conjugation is the transfer of DNA from a donor to a receptor in a conjugal process involving cell-to-cell contact. Conjugation is made possible by two genetic elements: the conjugative plasmids and the conjugative transposons.

Conjugation

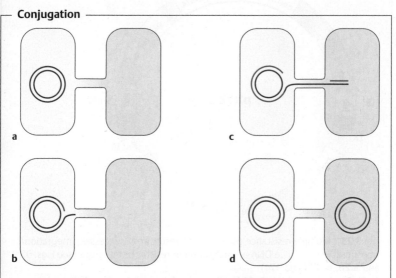

Fig. 3.**22**   Transfer/replication process of a conjugative plasmid.
a Conjugation: connection between two bacterial cells by means of sex pili. This initial step alone does not necessarily always lead to effective conjugation.
b Effective conjugation: formation of a specific conjugal bridge between donor cell and receptor cell.
c Plasmid mobilization and transfer: an endonuclease cleaves one strand of the circular DNA double helix at a specific point (**b**). The single strand with the "leader region" enters the receptor cell.
d Synthesis: the double-stranded structure of both the transferred single strand and the remaining DNA strand is restored by means of complementary DNA synthesis. The receptor cell, now plasmid-positive, is called a transconjugant.

In the conjugation process, the conjugative elements themselves are what are primarily transferred. However, these elements can also mobilize chromosomal genes or otherwise nontransferable plasmids. Conjugation is seen frequently in Gram-negative rods (*Enterobacteriaceae*), in which the phenomenon has been most thoroughly researched, and enterococci.

The F-factor in *Escherichia coli*. This is the prototype of a conjugative plasmid. This factor contains the so-called *tra* (transfer) genes responsible both for

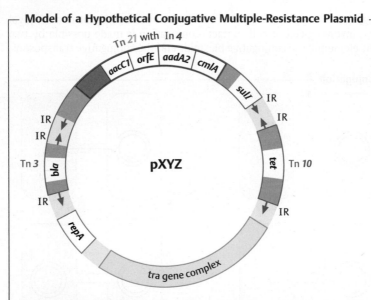

Model of a Hypothetical Conjugative Multiple-Resistance Plasmid

Fig. 3.**23**   Multiple resistance plasmids can result from successive integration of transposable resistance DNA or integration of resistance integrons (see Figs. 3.**19** and 3.**20**, p. 173 and 174)

Tn*21*   Transposon of the Tn*21* family, codes for resistance to sulfonamides (*sulI*) and contains an R integron (In*4*).

In*4*   Codes for chloramphenicol acetyltransferase (= *cmlA*), an aminoglycoside acetyltransferase (= *aacC1*) and an aminoglycoside adenylyltransferase (= *aadA2*); also contains an open reading frame (*orfE*) of unknown function.

Tn*3*   Transposon 3; codes for a betalactamase (= *bla*).

Tn*10*   Transposon 10; codes for resistance to tetracyclines (= *tet*).

repA   Codes for the replication enzyme of the plasmid.

tra   Plasmid DNA region containing 25 *tra* genes; *tra* genes are responsible for the transfer and replication process (see Fig. 3.**22**).

the formation of conjugal pili on the surface of F cells and for the transfer process. The transfer of the conjugative plasmid takes place as shown here in schematic steps (Fig. 3.**22**).

Occasional integration of the F factor into the chromosome gives it the conjugative properties of the F factor. Such an integration produces a sort of giant conjugative element, so that chromosomal genes can also be transferred by the same mechanism. Cells with an integrated F factor are therefore called Hfr ("high frequency of recombination") cells.

Conjugative resistance and virulence plasmids. Conjugative plasmids that carry determinants coding for antibiotic resistance and/or virulence in addition to the *tra* genes and *repA* are of considerable medical importance. Three characteristics of conjugative plasmids promote a highly efficient horizontal spread of these determinant factors among different bacteria:

■ **High frequency of transfer.** Due to the "transfer replication" mechanism, each receptor cell that has received a conjugative plasmid automatically becomes a donor cell. Each plasmid-positive cell is also capable of multiple plasmid transfers to receptor cells.

■ **Wide range of hosts.** Many conjugative plasmids can be transferred between different taxonomic species, genera, or even families.

■ **Multiple determinants.** Many conjugative plasmids carry several genes determining the phenotype of the carrier cell. The evolution of a hypothetical conjugative plasmid carrying several resistance determinants is shown schematically in Fig. 3.**23**.

Conjugative transposons. These are DNA elements (p. 173) that are usually integrated into the bacterial chromosome. They occur mainly in Gram-positive cocci, but have also been found in Gram-negative bacteria (*Bacteroides*). Conjugative transposons may carry determinants for antibiotic resistance and thus contribute to horizontal resistance transfer. In the transfer process, the transposon is first excised from the chromosome and circularized. Then a single strand of the double helix is cut and the linearized single strand—analogous to the F factor—is transferred into the receptor cell. Conjugative transposons are also capable of mobilizing nonconjugative plasmids.

Restriction, Modification, and Gene Cloning

The above descriptions of the mechanisms of genetic variability might make the impression that genes pass freely back and forth among the different bacterial species, rendering the species definitions irrelevant. This is not the case. A number of control mechanisms limit these genetic exchange processes. Among the most important are **restriction** and **modification**. Re-

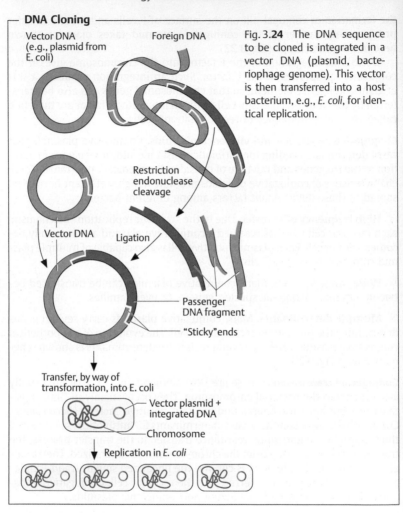

DNA Cloning

Vector DNA (e.g., plasmid from E. coli)

Foreign DNA

Fig. 3.**24** The DNA sequence to be cloned is integrated in a vector DNA (plasmid, bacteriophage genome). This vector is then transferred into a host bacterium, e.g., E. coli, for identical replication.

Restriction endonuclease cleavage

Vector DNA

Ligation

Passenger DNA fragment

"Sticky" ends

Transfer, by way of transformation, into E. coli

Vector plasmid + integrated DNA

Chromosome

Replication in E. coli

striction endonucleases can destroy foreign DNA that bears no "fingerprint" (modification) signifying "self." These modifications take the form of methylation of the DNA bases by modification enzymes.

Bacterial restriction endonucleases are invaluable tools in modern **gene cloning** techniques. The process is termed gene "cloning" because it involves replication of DNA that has been manipulated in vitro in a suitable host cell so as to produce identical copies of this DNA: molecular clones or gene clones.

The technique simplifies the replication of DNA, making experimental manipulations easier. On the other hand, the bacteria can also be used to synthesize gene products of the foreign genes. Such foreign proteins are called recombinant proteins. Bacterial plasmids often function in the role of vectors into which the sequences to be cloned are inserted. Fig. 3.**24** illustrates the principle of gene cloning in simplified form.

Table 3.**3** lists the most important terms used in the field of bacterial genetics.

3

Table 3.**3**   Glossary of Important Terminology in Bacterial Genetics

Anticodon	Triplet sequences of transfer RNA complementary to the codons of mRNA
Chromosome	See nucleoid
Cistron	Genetic unit, identical to "gene"
Code	Key relating the DNA nucleotide (n = 3) sequence to the polypeptide amino acid sequence
Codon	Sequence of three nucleotides, triplet
Corepressor	See effector molecules
Deletion	Loss of a DNA sequence in a replicon
Effector molecules	Small molecules that inactivate (= inductor) or activate (= corepressor) a regulator protein by means of an allosteric effect
Episome	Historical term; characterizes a replicon (e.g., F plasmid) occurring either in the cytoplasm or integrated in the bacterial chromosome
F factor	Prototype of a conjugative plasmid (fertility factor)
Gene	DNA segment containing the information used in synthesis of a polypeptide or RNA
Genome	All of the genetic information contained in a cell
Genotype	The totality of genetically determined characteristics
Hfr cells	Coli bacteria with F factor integrated into their chromosomes, therefore capable of transferring chromosomal genes at a high frequency by means of conjugation (Hfr = high frequency of recombination)
Inductor	See effector molecules
Integron	Genetic structure containing the determinants for a site-specific recombination system; responsible for integration or excision of mobile gene cassettes

Table 3.3 *Continued: Glossary of Important Terminology...*

Inverted repeats	Nucleotide sequences repeated in reverse order at the ends of transposable DNA
IS	Insertion sequences; transposable DNA elements
Cassette	Sequence in a gene that can be transferred to other genes by homologous recombination
Clone	Population of identical cells or DNA molecules
Conjugation	Transfer of hereditary material in a pairing process
Lysogenic bacteria	Cells with a phage genome (prophage) integrated into their chromosomes
Lysogenic conversion	Change in cell phenotype brought about by prophage genes
Messenger RNA	Synthesized at the DNA by transcription; carries genetic information to the ribosomes
Modification enzymes	Methylases that label DNA as "self" by methylation
Mutation	A permanent alteration of the genome
Nucleoid	Nuclear region, nucleus equivalent
Operator	DNA sequence of an operon; regulator binding site
Operon	Regulatory unit comprising the promoter, operator, structural genes, and terminator
Parasexuality	Unilateral gene transfer from a donor to a receptor
Phenotype	The totality of characteristics expressed in a bacterial cell
Plasmid	Extrachromosomal, autonomous, in most cases circular DNA molecule
Promoter	Recognition and binding site for RNA polymerase
Prophage	Phage genome integrated into the chromosome
Regulator	Regulatory protein that controls gene transcription; repressor or activator
Regulon	Functional unit of genes at different loci controlled by the same regulator
Recombination, Legitimate or homologous recombination	Replacement of a DNA sequence by a homologous sequence from a different genome; breakage and reunion model

Table 3.**3**   *Continued: Glossary of Important Terminology...*

Recombination,	
Illegitimate recombination	Insertion of transposable DNA
Site-specific recombination	Integration or excision of a DNA sequence by means of homologous recombination in a specific DNA segment comprising only a small number of nucleotides
Replication	Reproduction, duplication of DNA
Replicon	DNA molecule that replicates autonomously
Restriction endonucleases	Enzymes that recognize and cleave specific DNA nucleotide sequences
Semiconservative replication	DNA duplication mechanism in which one old strand is conserved in each of the two new double strands
Conjugal (or sex) pili	Surface structures essential to conjugation in Gram-negative rod bacteria
Sigma factors	Proteins that temporarily associate with prokaryotic RNA polymerase for specific promoter binding
Supercoil	Circular DNA molecule additionally twisted about the helical axis in the opposite direction
Terminator	Sequence marking the end of a transcription process
Transduction	Gene transfer using bacteriophages as vehicles
Transfer RNA	Specifically binds an amino acid (aminoacyl tRNA) and transfers it to the ribosome
Transformation	Transfer of genes from a donor in the form of "naked" DNA
Transcription	RNA synthesis at DNA
Translation	Ribosomal synthesis of polypeptides
Transposase	Transposition enzyme; facilitates illegitimate recombination
Transposition	Translocation of a mobile DNA element within a replicon or between different replicons
Transposon	Transposable DNA; frequently contains—in addition to the genes for transposition—determinants that change the phenotype of a bacterial cell
Triplet code	Three nucleotides coding for one amino acid
Vector	Vehicle for foreign (passenger) DNA; usually a plasmid or phage genome

3

Bacteriophages

■ Bacteriophages, or simply phages, are viruses that infect bacteria. They possess a protein shell surrounding the phage genome, which with few exceptions is composed of DNA. A bacteriophage attaches to specific receptors on its host bacteria and injects its genome through the cell wall. This forces the host cells to synthesize more bacteriophages. The host cell lyses at the end of this reproductive phase. So-called temperate bacteriophages lysogenize the host cells, whereby their genomes are integrated into the host cell chromosomes as the so-called prophage. The phage genes are inactive in this stage, although the prophage is duplicated synchronously with host cell proliferation. The transition from prophage status to the lytic cycle is termed spontaneous or artificial induction. Some genomes of temperate phages may carry genes which have the capacity to change the phenotype of the host cell. Integration of such a prophage into the chromosome is known as lysogenic conversion. ■

Definition

Bacteriophages are viruses the host cells of which are bacteria. Bacteriophages are therefore obligate cell parasites. They possess only one type of nucleic acid, either DNA or RNA, have no enzymatic systems for energy supply and are unable to synthesize proteins on their own.

Morphology

Similarly to the viruses that infect animals, bacteriophages vary widely in appearance. Fig. 3.**25a** shows a schematic view of a T series coli phage. Research on these phages has been particularly thorough. Fig. 3.**25b** shows an intact T phage next to a phage that has injected its genome.

T Phages

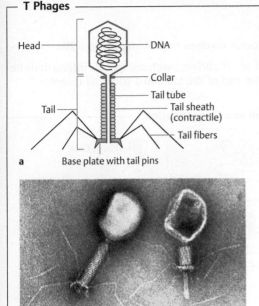

Head — Head

DNA — DNA

Collar

Tail tube

Tail — Tail

Tail sheath (contractile)

Tail fibers

a — Base plate with tail pins

Fig. 3.**25** **a** Morphology of a T series phage (complex structure).

b Electron microscopic image of T bacteriophages. Left: intact, infectious phage. Right: phage shell after injection of the genome with phage head empty and tail sheath contracted.

3

100 nm

b

Composition

Phages are made up of protein and nucleic acid. The proteins form the head, tail, and other morphological elements, the function of which is to protect the phage genome. This element bears the genetic information, the structural genes for the structural proteins as well as for other proteins (enzymes) required to produce new phage particles. The nucleic acid in most phages is DNA, which occurs as a single DNA double strand in, for example, T series phages. These phages are quite complex and have up to 100 different genes. In spherical and filamentous phages, the genome consists of single-stranded DNA (example: ΦX174). RNA phages are less common.

Reproduction

The phage reproduction process involves several steps (Fig. 3.**26**).

■ **Adsorption.** Attachment to cell surface involving specific interactions between a phage protein at the end of the tail and a bacterial receptor.

3

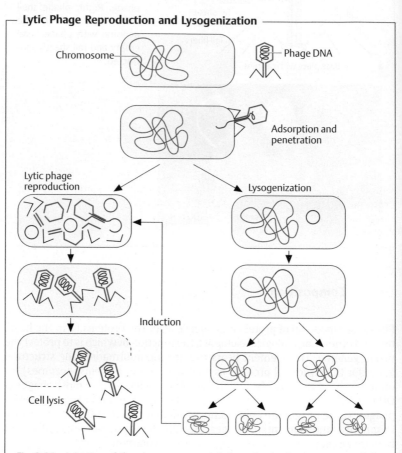

Lytic Phage Reproduction and Lysogenization

Chromosome

Phage DNA

Adsorption and penetration

Lytic phage reproduction

Lysogenization

Induction

Cell lysis

Fig. 3.**26** Injection of the phage genome is followed either by direct intracellular (lytic) phage reproduction or lysogenization of the host cell. In the lysogenization process, the phage DNA is integrated into the host cell chromosome and replicated together with it in the process of cell fission.

Release of Phages from the Host Cell

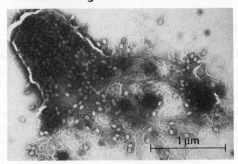

Fig. 3.**27** At the end of the phage maturation process, the host cell is lysed to release the new phages. Lysis occurs by a phage-encoded murein hydrolase, which gains access to the murein through membrane channels formed by the phage-encoded protein holin.

3

■ **Penetration.** Injection of the phage genome. Enzymatic penetration of the wall by the tail tube tip and injection of the nucleic acid through the tail tube.

■ **Reproduction.** Beginning with synthesis of early proteins (zero to two minutes after injection), e.g., the phage-specific replicase that initiates replication of the phage genome. Then follows transcription of the late genes that code for the structural proteins of the head and tail. The new phage particles are assembled in a maturation process toward the end of the reproduction cycle.

■ **Release.** This step usually follows the lysis of the host cell with the help of murein hydrolase coded by a phage gene that destroys the cell wall (Fig. 3.**27**).

Depending on the phage species and milieu conditions, a phage reproduction cycle takes from 20 to 60 minutes. This is called the **latency period**, and can be considered as analogous to the generation time of bacteria. Depending on the phage species, an infected cell releases from 20 to several hundred new phages, which number defines the **burst size**. Thus phages reproduce more rapidly than bacteria. In view of this fact, one might wonder how any bacteria have survived in nature at all. It is important not to forget that cell population density is a major factor determining the probability of finding a host cell in the first place and that such densities are relatively small in nature. Another aspect is that only a small proportion of phages reproduce solely by means of these lytic or vegetative processes. Most are temperate phages that lysogenize the infected host cells.

Lysogeny

Fig. 3.**26** illustrates the **lysogeny** of a host cell. Following injection of the phage genome, it is integrated into the chromosome by means of region-specific recombination employing an integrase. The phage genome thus integrated is called a **prophage**. The prophage is capable of changing to the vegetative state, either spontaneously or in response to induction by physical or chemical noxae (UV light, mitomycin). The process begins with excision of the phage genome out of the DNA of the host cell, continues with replication of the phage DNA and synthesis of phage structure proteins, and finally ends with host cell lysis. Cells carrying a prophage are called **lysogenic** because they contain the genetic information for lysis. Lysogeny has advantages for both sides. It prevents immediate host cell lysis, but also ensures that the phage genome replicates concurrently with host cell reproduction.

Lysogenic conversion is when the phage genome lysogenizing a cell bears a gene (or several genes) that codes for bacterial rather than viral processes. Genes localized on phage genomes include the gene for diphtheria toxin, the gene for the pyrogenic toxins of group A streptococci and the *cholera toxin* gene.

The Importance of the Bacteriophages

Biological research	Bacteriophages are often used as models in studies of fundamental biological processes: DNA replication, gene expression, gene regulation, viral morphogenesis, studies of the details, and function of supramolecular structures
Genetic engineering	Vectors for gene cloning, adjuvants in sequencing
Therapy and prevention	An older concept now receiving increased attention. Administration of suitable phage mixtures in therapy and prevention of gastrointestinal infections. In animal husbandry, a number of phages that attack only EHEC (enterohemorrhagic *E. coli*) are used against EHEC infections
Epidemiology	Bacterial typing. Strains of a bacterial species are classified in phagovars (syn. lysotypes) based on their sensitivity to typing bacteriophages. Recognition of the bacterial strain responsible for an epidemic, making it possible to follow up the chain of infection and identify the infection sources. This typing method has been established for *Salmonella typhi*, *Salmonella paratyphi B*, *Staphylococcus aureus*, *Pseudomonas aeruginosa*, and other bacteria, although it is now increasingly being replaced by new molecular methods, in particular DNA typing

The Principles of Antibiotic Therapy

■ Specific antibacterial therapy refers to treatment of infections with anti-infective agents directed against the infecting pathogen. The most important group of anti-infective agents are the antibiotics, which are products of fungi and bacteria (*Streptomycetes*). Anti-infective agents are categorized as having a broad, narrow, or medium spectrum of action. The efficacy, or effectiveness, of a substance refers to its bactericidal or bacteriostatic effect. Anti-infective agents have many different mechanisms of action. Under the influence of sulfonamides and trimethoprim, bacteria do not synthesize sufficient amounts of tetrahydrofolic acid. All betalactam antibiotics irreversibly block the biosynthesis of murein. Rifamycin inhibits the DNA-dependent RNA polymerase (transcription). Aminoglycosides, tetracyclines, and macrolides block translation. All 4-quinolones damage cellular DNA topology by inhibiting bacterial topoisomerases. Due to their genetic variability, bacteria may develop resistance to specific anti-infective agents. The most important resistance mechanisms are: inactivating enzymes, resistant target molecules, reduced influx, increased efflux. Resistant strains (problematic bacteria) occur frequently among hospital flora, mainly *Enterobacteriaceae*, pseudomonads, staphylococci, and enterococci. Laboratory resistance testing is required for specific antibiotic therapy. Dilutions series tests are quantitative resistance tests used to determine the minimum inhibitory concentration (MIC). The disk test is a semiquantitative test used to classify the test bacteria as resistant or susceptible. In combination therapies it must be remembered that the interactions of two or more antibiotics can give rise to an antagonistic effect. Surgical chemoprophylaxis must be administered as a short-term antimicrobial treatment only. ■

Definitions

Specific **antibacterial therapy** designates treatment of infections with **anti-infective agents** directed against the infecting pathogen (syn. **antibacterial chemotherapeutics, antibiotics**). One feature of these pharmaceuticals is "selective toxicity," that is, they act upon bacteria at very low concentration levels without causing damage to the macroorganism. The most important group of anti-infective agents is the **antibiotics**. These natural substances are produced by fungi or bacteria (usually *Streptomycetes*). *The term "antibiotic" is often used in medical contexts to refer to all antibacterial pharmaceuticals, not just to antibiotics in this narrower sense.* Fig. 3.**28** illustrates

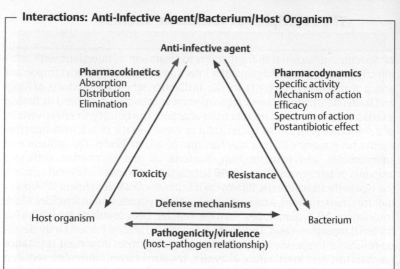

Fig. 3.**28** Interactions between the anti-infective agent and host organism are characterized by the terms pharmacokinetics and toxicity; interactions between the anti-infective agent and the bacterial pathogen are characterized in terms of pharmacodynamics and resistance.

the relations between an anti-infective agent, the host organism, and a bacterial pathogen. Table 3.**4** lists frequently used anti-infective agents. The most important groups (cephalosporins, penicillins, 4-quinolones, macrolides, tetracyclines) are in bold print. Fig. 3.**29** presents the basic chemical structures of the most important anti-infective agents.

Table 3.**4**   Frequently Used Anti-Infective Agents

Class/active substance	Remarks
Aminoglycoside/aminocyclitol antibiotics	
(dihydro)streptomycin	For treatment of tuberculosis
neomycin, paramomycin	Only for oral or topical application
kanamycin	Parenteral administration; resistance frequent
gentamicin, tobramycin, amikacin, netilmicin, sisomicin	Newer aminoglycosides; broad spectrum; no effect on streptococci and enterococci; ototoxicity and nephrotoxicity; control of serum levels during therapy
spectinomycin	Against penicillinase-positive gonococci, in urogenital gonorrhea
Carbacephems	Betalactams structured like cephalosporins, but with a C atom instead of sulfur in the second ring system (see fig. 3.**29**, p. 195)
loracarbef	Oral carbacephem; stable in the presence of penicillinases from *Haemophilus* and *Moraxella*
4-Quinolones	
norfloxacin, pefloxacin	Oral quinolones; only in urinary tract infections
ciprofloxacin, ofloxacin, fleroxacin, enoxacin	Oral and systemic quinolones with broad spectrum of indications
levofloxacin, sparfloxacin	Quinolones with enhanced activity against Gram-positive and "atypical" pathogens (chlamydias, mycoplasmas); caution—sparfloxacin is phototoxic
gatifloxacin, moxifloxacin	Quinolones with enhanced activity against Gram-positive and "atypical" pathogens (chlamydias, mycoplasmas) and Gram-negative anaerobes
Cephalosporins	
Group 1 cefazolin, cephalothin	Effective against Gram-positive and some Gram-negative bacteria; stable in the presence of staphylococci penicillinases; unstable in the presence of betalactamases of Gram-negative bacteria

Table 3.**4** *Continued: Frequently Used Anti-Infective Agents*

Class/active substance	Remarks
Group 2 cefuroxime, cefotiam, cefamandole	Effective against Gram-positive bacteria; more effective against Gram-negative bacteria than Group 1; stable in the presence of staphylococci penicillinases; stable in the presence of some betalactamases of Gram-negative bacteria
Group 3a cefotaxime, ceftriaxone, ceftizoxime, cefmenoxime, cefodizime	Much more effective than Group 1 against Gram-negative bacteria; stable in the presence of numerous betalactamases of Gram-negative bacteria; show weak activity against staphylococci
Group 3b Ceftazidime, cefepime, cefpirome, cefoperazone	Spectrum of action as in Group 3a; also effective against *Pseudomonas aeruginosa*
Further cephalosporins cefsulodin	Narrow spectrum of action; the only therapeutically relevant activity is that against *Pseudomonas aeruginosa*
cefoxitin	Effective against the anaerobic *Bacteroidaceae*; activity against Gram-negative bacteria as in Group 2; insufficient activity against staphylococci
Oral cephalosporins ceflaclor, cefadroxil, cephalexin, cefradine	Spectrum of action similar as cephalothin
cefpodoxime, cefuroxime (axetil), cefixime, cefprozil, cefdinir, cefetamet, ceftibuten	Newer oral cephalosporins with broad spectra of action
Chloramphenicol	Broad spectrum, mainly bacteriostatic effect; risk of aplastic anemia
Diaminobenzyl pyrimidine trimethoprim	Broad spectrum; inhibition of dihydrofolic acid reductase; frequent bactericidal synergism with sulfonamides (e.g., cotrimoxazole)

Table 3.**4** *Continued: Frequently Used Anti-Infective Agents*

Class/active substance	Remarks
Ethambutol	Only against tuberculosis bacteria
Fosfomycin	Broad spectrum, bactericidal effect in bacterial cell division phase; blocks murein biosynthesis; rapid development of resistance; use in combination therapy
Fusidic acid	Steroid antibiotic; only against Gram-positive bacteria; bacteriostatic; blocks protein biosynthesis (translation); development of resistance is frequent
Glycopeptides vancomycin teicoplanin	Narrow spectrum including only Gram-positive bacteria; moderate bactericidal efficacy during bacterial cell division phase; blocks murein biosynthesis; nephrotoxicity, allergy, thrombophlebitis
Isonicotinamides isoniazid (INH)	Only against tuberculosis bacteria, inhibition of enzymes requiring pyridoxal or pyridoxamine as a coenzyme
Lincosamides lincomycin, clindamycin	Effective against Gram-positive bacteria and Gram-negative anaerobes; good penetration into bone tissue
Macrolides/ketolides	
erythromycin, roxithromycin, clarithromycin, azithromycin	Against Gram-positive and Gram-negative cocci, chlamydias, and mycoplasmas
telithromycin	Ketolide; effective against many macrolide-resistant strains

Table 3.**4** *Continued: Frequently Used Anti-Infective Agents*

Class/active substance	Remarks
Monobactams	Betalactam antibiotics with only the betalactam ring (see fig. 3.**29**, p. 195)
aztreonam, carumonam	Good activity against *Enterobacteriaceae*; moderate efficacy against *Pseudomonas*; very high level of betalactamase stability; no effect against Gram-positive bacteria
Nitrofurans nitrofurantoin, furazolidone, nitrofural, etc.	Against Gram-positive and Gram-negative bacteria; use only in urinary tract infections
Nitroimidazoles metronidazole, tinidazole, omidazole	Active against various protozoans and obligate anaerobic bacteria; bactericidal effect
Oxalactams	Betalactam antibiotics with oxygen instead of sulfur in the second ring system (see Fig. 3.**29**, p. 195)
lamoxactam	Broad spectrum; moderate efficacy against *Pseudomonas*; poor efficacy against Gram-positive cocci; highly stable in the presence of beta-lactamases; also effective against Gram-negative anaerobes
flomoxef	No activity against *Pseudomonas*; good activity against staphylococci; otherwise like lamoxactam
clavulanic acid	Only minimum antibacterial activity; inhibits beta-lactamases; used in combination with amoxicillin (Augmentin)
Oxazolidinones linezolid	Only against Gram-positive bacteria; inhibits bacterial translation; no crossresistance with other translation inhibitors
Para-aminosalicylic acid (PAS)	Only against tuberculosis bacteria; affects folic acid biosynthesis

Table **3.4**   *Continued: Frequently Used Anti-Infective Agents*

Class/active substance	Remarks
Penicillins	

Classic penicillins
penicillin G (benzyl penicillin), penicillin V (oral penicillin), pheneticillin, propicillin — Effective against Gram-positive bacteria and Gram-negative cocci; bactericidal effect during bacterial cell division phase; inactivated by penicillinase of staphylococci, gonococci, *Haemophilus influenzae*, *Moraxella catarrhalis*

Penicillinase-resistant penicillins
methicillin, oxacillin, cloxacillin, flucloxacillin — Stable in the presence of penicillinase of staphylococci; agent of choice in staphylococci infections (flucloxacillin)

Aminopenicillins
ampicillin, amoxicillin, epicillin, hetacillin, etc. — Also effective against *Enterobacteriaceae*; labile against Gram-positive and Gram-negative penicillinases

Carboxyl penicillins
carbenicillin, ticarcillin, carfecillin, etc. — Effective against *Enterobacteriaceae* and *Pseudomonas*; labile against Gram-positive and Gram-negative penicillinases

temocillin (6-α-methoxy ticarcillin) — No effect against *Pseudomonas*; highly stable in the presence of betalactamases

Acylureidopenicillins
azlocillin, mezlocillin, piperacillin, apalcillin — Effective against *Enterobacteriaceae* and *Pseudomonas*; despite lability against beta-lactamases active against many enzyme-producing strains due to good penetration and high levels of sensitivity of the target molecules

Penems — Penicillins with a double bond in the second ring system

N-formimidoyl thienamycin (imipenem = N-F-thienamycin + cilastatin) — A carbapenem (C atom instead of sulfur in second ring); very broad spectrum and high level of activity against Gram-positive and Gram-negative bacteria, including anaerobes; frequently effective against *Enterobacteriaceae* and *Pseudomonas* with resistance to the cephalosporins of Group 3b; inactivated by renal enzymes; is therefore administered in combination with the enzyme inhibitor cilastatin

3

Table 3.**4**   *Continued: Frequently Used Anti-Infective Agents*

Class/active substance	Remarks
meropenem	Like imipenem, but stable against renal dehydropeptidase
Polypeptides bacitracin	Only against Gram-positive bacteria; is only used topically
Polymyxin B, colistin	Only against Gram-negative rod bacteria; neuro-toxicity, nephrotoxicity
Rifamycins rifampicin	Against Gram-positive bacteria and tuberculosis bacteria; mainly bacteriostatic; rapid development of resistance, for which reason combination therapy is recommended
Streptogramins quinopristin/dalfopristin	Fixed combination preparation of two streptogramins; effective mainly against Gram-positive bacteria
Sulfamethoxazole/trimethoprim (cotrimoxazole)	Fixed combination; five parts sulfamethoxazole and one part trimethoprim
Sulfonamides sulfanilamide, sulfamethoxazole, sulfafurazole, etc.	Broad spectrum; bacteriostatic effect only; resistance frequent
Sulfones dapsone	diaminodiphenylsulfone; for therapy of leprosy
Tetracyclines **doxycycline** tetracycline, oxytetracycline, rolitetracycline, minocycline	Broad spectrum including all bacteria, chlamydias, and rickettsias; resistance frequent; dental deposits in small children

Basic Chemical Structures of the Most Important Anti-infectives

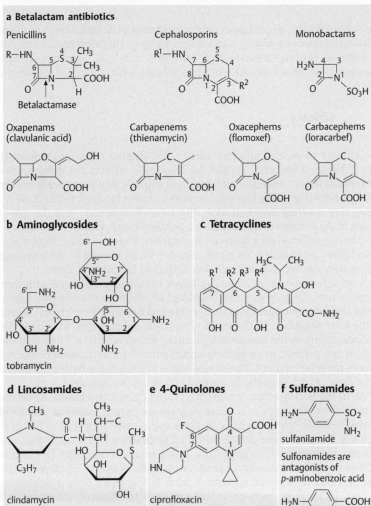

a Betalactam antibiotics

Penicillins

Cephalosporins

Monobactams

Betalactamase

Oxapenams
(clavulanic acid)

Carbapenems
(thienamycin)

Oxacephems
(flomoxef)

Carbacephems
(loracarbef)

b Aminoglycosides

tobramycin

c Tetracyclines

d Lincosamides

clindamycin

e 4-Quinolones

ciprofloxacin

f Sulfonamides

sulfanilamide

Sulfonamides are
antagonists of
p-aminobenzoic acid

Fig. 3.**29**   Antibiotic groups often include many drug substances with different substituents.

Spectrum of Action

Each anti-infective agent has a certain **spectrum of action**, which is a range of bacterial species showing natural sensitivity to the substance. Some anti-infective agents have a narrow spectrum of action (e.g., vancomycin). Most, however, have broad spectra like tetracyclines, which affect all eubacteria.

Efficacy

The efficacy of an anti-infective agent (syn. kinetics of action) defines the way it affects a bacterial population. Two basic effects are differentiated: **bacteriostasis**, i.e., reversible inhibition of growth, and irreversible **bactericidal activity** (Fig. 3.**30**). Many substances can develop both forms of efficacy depending on their concentration, the type of organism, and the growth phase. Many of these drugs also have a **postantibiotic effect (PAE)** reflecting the damage inflicted on a bacterial population. After the anti-infective agent is no longer present, the bacterial cells not killed require a recovery phase before they can reproduce again. The PAE may last several hours.

A bacteriostatic agent alone can never completely eliminate pathogenic bacteria from the body's tissues. "Healing" results from the combined effects of the anti-infective agent and the specific and nonspecific immune defenses of the host organism. In tissues in which this defense system is inefficient (endocardium), in the middle of a purulent lesion where no functional phagocytes are present, or in immunocompromised patients, bactericidal substances must be required. The clinical value of knowing whether an antibacterial drug is bacteriostatic or bactericidal is readily apparent.

All of the bacteria from an infection focus cannot be eliminated without support from the body's immune defense system. A bacterial population always includes several cells with phenotypic resistance that is not genotypically founded. These are the so-called **persisters**, which occur in in-vitro cultures at frequencies ranging from $1:10^6$ to $1:10^8$ (Fig. 3.**30**). The cause of such persistence is usually a specific metabolic property of these bacteria that prevents bactericidal substances from killing them. Following discontinuation of therapy, such persisters can lead to relapses. Infections with **L-forms** show a special type of persistence when treated with antibiotics that block murein synthesis (p. 156).

Efficacy of Selected Anti-Infective Agents

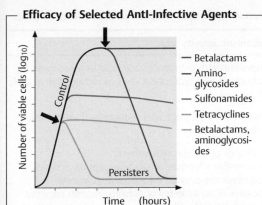

— Betalactams
— Amino-
  glycosides
— Sulfonamides
— Tetracyclines
— Betalactams,
  aminoglycosi-
  des

Fig. 3.**30**   The arrows indicate addition of substances in the different phases of the normal growth curve (see Fig. 3.**16**). Betalactams are bactericidal only during the bacterial cell division phase, whereas aminoglycosides show this activity in all growth phases. Sulfonamides are always bacteriostatic, tetracyclines are mainly bacteriostatic. Some cells in every culture (so-called persisters) are phenotypically (but not genotypically) resistant to the bactericidal effects of anti-infective agents.

Mechanisms of Action

Table 3.**5** provides a concise summary of the molecular mechanisms of action of the most important groups of anti-infective agents.

Table 3.5 Mechanisms of Action of the Most Important Anti-Infective Agents

Substance group	Mechanism, activity site
Sulfonamides	Competition with p-aminobenzoic acid as a substrate for dihydropteric acid synthetase, thus too little tetrahydrofolic acid
Trimethoprim	Inhibition of dihydrofolic acid reductase, thus too little tetrahydrofolic acid
Betalactam antibiotics	Disturbance of murein biosynthesis: — Irreversible inhibition of DD-transpeptidase, which catalyzes the peptide crosslinkage in murein — Release of an inhibitor of autolytic murein enzymes — Enzymatic destruction of murein architecture with autolysins: "wrong place at the wrong time" — Lysis due to high internal osmotic pressure
Vancomycin Teicoplanin Fosfomycin Bacitracin	Disturbance of murein biosynthesis at various different molecular stages
Rifamycin	Transcription: Blockage of DNA-dependent RNA polymerase
Aminoglycosides	Translation: — Genetic code is not read correctly (miscoding) — Blockage of e-type (elongation ribosome) A-position occupancy by AA-tRNA
Tetracyclines	Translation: — Blockage of e-type (elongation ribosome) and i-type (initiation ribosome) A-position occupancy by AA-tRNA
Chloramphenicol	Translation: Inhibition of peptidyl transferase activity
Macrolides, ketolides	Translation: Inhibition of elongation of the polypeptide chain
4-Quinolones	Inhibition of the DNA gyrase and topoisomerase IV resulting in the inhibition of DNA replication
Polymyxins	Cytoplasmic membrane: Structural disruption

Details of the Mechanisms of Action of Anti-Infective Agents

Sulfonamides and trimethoprim   Tetrahydrofolic acid (THFA) acts as a coenzyme to regulate the C1 metabolism for transfer of the hydroxymethyl and formyl groups. Too little THFA results in the cessation of growth. The combination of sulfamethoxazole and trimethoprim (cotrimoxazole) results in a potentiated efficacy.

Betalactam antibiotics   The mechanisms described in Table 3.**5** refer to penicillin and pneumococci. They probably hold in similar form for other betalactams and other bacteria as well. All bacteria with cell walls containing murein possess autolysins. These enzymes create gaps in the murein sacculus while the bacterium is growing, these gaps are then filled in with new murein material. Bacteria the growth of which is inhibited, but which are not lysed, show betalactam **tolerance** (bacteriostatic, but not bactericidal effects).

Protein synthesis inhibitors   The biosynthesis of bacterial proteins differs in detail from that observed in eukaryotes, permitting a selective inhibition by antibiotics. The principle of selective toxicity still applies.

4-Quinolones   DNA gyrase, which only occurs in bacteria, catalyzes the counterclockwise supercoiling of the double helix, which is, in itself, wound to the right, about its helical axis (see Fig. 3.**17**, p. 167). Only in supercoiled form can the DNA fit economically into the cell. DNA replication depends on this supercoiled topology. 4-Quinolones also inhibit bacterial topoisomerase IV of Gram-positive bacteria.

Pharmacokinetics

Pharmacokinetics covers the principles of absorption, distribution, and elimination of pharmacons by the macroorganism. The reader is referred to standard textbooks of pharmacology for details. The dosage and dosage interval recommendations for antibacterial therapy take into account the widely differing pharmacokinetic parameters of the different anti-infective agents, among them:

- Absorption rate and specific absorption time
- Volume of distribution
- Protein binding
- Serum (blood) concentration
- Tissue concentration
- Metabolization
- Elimination

Side Effects

Treatment with anti-infective agents can cause side effects, resulting either from noncompliance with important therapeutic principles or specific patient reactivity. On the whole, such side effects are of minor significance.

■ **Toxic effects.** These effects arise from direct cell and tissue damage in the macroorganism. Blood concentrations of some substances must therefore be monitored during therapy if there is a risk of cumulation due to inefficient elimination (examples: aminoglycosides, vancomycin).

■ **Allergic reactions.** See p. 108 for possible mechanisms (example: penicillin allergy).

■ **Biological side effects.** Example: change in or elimination of normal flora, interfering with its function as a beneficial colonizer (see p. 25).

The Problem of Resistance

Definitions

Clinical resistance. Resistance of bacteria to the concentration of anti-infective agents maintained at the infection site in the macroorganism.

Natural resistance. Resistance characteristic of a bacterial species, genus, or family.

Acquired resistance. Strains of sensitive taxa can acquire resistance by way of changes in their genetic material.

Biochemical resistance. A biochemically detectable resistance observed in strains of sensitive taxa. The biochemical resistance often corresponds to the clinically relevant resistance. Biochemically resistant strains sometimes show low levels of resistance below the clinically defined boundary separating resistant and sensitive strains. Such strains may be medically susceptible.

Incidence, Significance

Problematic bacteria. Strains with acquired resistance are encountered frequently among *Enterobacteriaceae*, pseudomonads, staphylococci, and enterococci. Specific infection therapy directed at these pathogens is often fraught with difficulties, which explains the label problematic bacteria. They are responsible for most nosocomial infections (p. 342f.). Usually harmless in otherwise healthy persons, they may cause life-threatening infections in highly susceptible, so-called **problematic patients**. Problematic bacteria are often characterized by **multiple resistance**. Resistance to anti-infective agents is observed less frequently in nonhospital bacteria.

Genetic variability. The basic cause of the high incidence of antibiotic resistance experienced with problematic bacteria is the pronounced genetic variability of these organisms, the mechanisms of which are described in the section "Genetic variability" (p. 171 and p. 174). Most important are the mechanisms of horizontal transfer of resistance determinants responsible for the efficient distribution of resistance markers among these bacteria.

Selection. The origin and distribution of resistant strains is based to a significant extent on selection of resistance variants. The more often anti-infective substances are administered therapeutically, the greater the number of strains that will develop acquired resistance. Each hospital has a characteristic flora reflecting its prescription practice. A physician must be familiar with the resistance characteristics of this hospital flora so that the right anti-infective agents for a **"calculated antibiotic therapy"** can be selected even before the resistance test results are in. Such therapies take into account the frequency of infections by certain bacterial species (pathogen epidemiology) as well as current resistance levels among these bacteria (resistance epidemiology).

Resistance Mechanisms

Inactivating enzymes. Hydrolysis or modification of anti-infective agents.

■ **Betalactamases.** Hydrolyze the betalactam ring of betalactam antibiotics (see Fig. 3.**29**). Over 200 different betalactamases are known. A course classification system is based on the substrate profile in penicillinases and cephalosporinases. Production of some betalactamases is induced by betalactams (see p. 169), others are produced constitutively (unregulated).

■ **Aminoglycosidases.** Modify aminoglycosides by means of phosphorylation and nucleotidylation of free hydroxyl groups (phosphotransferases and nucleotidyl transferases) or acetylation of free amino groups (acetyltransferases).

■ **Chloramphenicol acetyltransferases.** Modification, by acetylation, of chloramphenicol.

Resistant target molecules.

■ Gene products with a low affinity to anti-infective agents are produced based on mutations in natural genes. Example: DNA gyrase subunit A, resistant to 4-quinolones.

■ Acquisition of a gene that codes for a target molecule with low affinity to anti-infective agents. The resistance protein assumes the function of the sensitive target molecule. Example: methicillin resistance in staphylococci; acquisition of the penicillin-binding protein 2a, which is resistant to betalactam antibiotics and assumes the function of the naturally sensitive penicillin-binding proteins.

■ Acquisition of the gene for an enzyme that alters the target structure of an anti-infective agent to render it resistant. Example: 23S rRNA methylases; modification of ribosomal RNA to prevent binding of macrolide antibiotics to the ribosome.

Permeability mechanisms.

■ **Reduced influx.** Reduction of transport of anti-infective agents from outside to inside through membranes; rare.

■ **Increased efflux.** Active transport of anti-infective agents from inside to outside by means of efflux pumps in the cytoplasmic membrane, making efflux greater than influx; frequent.

Evolution of Resistance to Anti-Infective Agents

Resistance to anti-infective agents is genetically determined by resistance genes. Many resistance determinants are not new developments in response to the use of medical antibiotics, but developed millions of years ago in bacteria with no human associations. The evolutionary process is therefore a **"nonanthropogenic"** one. The determinants that code for resistance to anti-infective agents that are not antibiotics did develop after the substances began to be used in therapy, hence this is **"anthropogenic"** evolution. Factors contributing to the resistance problem have included the molecular mechanisms of genetic variability (mutation, homologous recombination, site-specific integration, transposition) and the mechanisms of intercellular gene transfer in bacteria (transformation, transduction, conjugation).

Nonanthropogenic and Anthropogenic Evolution

Nonanthropogenic evolution. The need for resistance developed parallel to the ability to produce antibiotics. The producing organisms protect themselves from their own products by means of such R mechanisms. Resistance genes also evolved in bacteria that shared the natural habitat of the antibiotic producers. They secured their own ecological niche in the presence of the producers by means of the characteristic of resistance. The genetic sequences from which the resistance genes evolved were those that coded for the anabolic or catabolic metabolism genes. At a later point in evolutionary history, such "nonanthropogenic" genes have accidentally, and rarely, found their way into the genetic material of human pathogen bacteria. Therefore, when new antibiotic substances come to be used for therapeutic purposes, there are always a small number of bacteria that already show resistance to them.

Anthropogenic evolution. This term refers to the evolution of resistance genes in bacteria associated with humans based on mutations in native genes. An example is the mutation that brings about resistance to 4-quinolones in gene *gyrA*, which codes for subunit A of the DNA gyrase. A special case of anthropogenic evolution is the development of new resistance genes resulting from mutations in "nonanthropogenic" resistance genes already established in human pathogen bacteria.

The best-known example of this is provided by mutations in TEM and SHV *betalactamase* genes that code for betalactamases with a very broad substrate profile (ESBL = extended spectrum betalactamases).

Resistance Tests

Two standard test systems are used to determine the in-vitro resistance levels of bacteria.

In **dilution series tests**, the minimum inhibitory concentration (MIC) of an anti-infective agent required to inhibit proliferation of a bacterial population is determined. A factor 2 geometrical dilution series of the agent is prepared in a nutrient medium, inoculated with the test organism and incubated, whereupon the lowest growth-inhibiting concentration level (mg/l) is determined. Three standardized dilution methods are available. In the agar dilution test, nutrient agar plates containing antibiotic are inoculated ("spotted") with the test organisms. In the microbroth dilution test, the final volume is usually 100 µl per microplate well. This test type can also be automated. The final volume in a macrobroth dilution test is 2 ml per tube.

Due to the complexity and time-consuming nature of the above test types, routine laboratories often use the **agar diffusion test**. This involves diffuse inoculation of the nutrient agar plate with the test strain. Then disks of filter paper containing the anti-infective agents are placed on the agar. After the plates thus prepared are incubated, the inhibition zones around the disks (i.e., whether or not they develop and their size) provide information on the resistance of the microorganisms tested (Fig. 3.**31**). This is possible because of the linear relation between the $\log_2$ MIC and the diameter of the inhibition zones (Fig. 3.**32**).

To **interpret the results**, the MICs or inhibition zones are brought into relation with the substance concentrations present at a site of infection at standard dosage levels. This calculation is based on known averages for various pharmacokinetic parameters (serum concentration, half-life) and pharmacodynamic parameters (bactericidal activity or not, postantibiotic effect,

---

Agar Diffusion Test

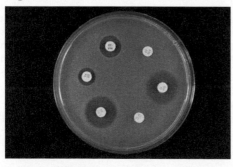

Fig. 3.**31**   This method, also known as the "disk test," is used to test the resistance of a bacterial culture to various anti-infective agents. The method provides a basis for classification of a bacterial strain as "susceptible," "resistant," or "intermediate" according to the dimension of the inhibition zone.

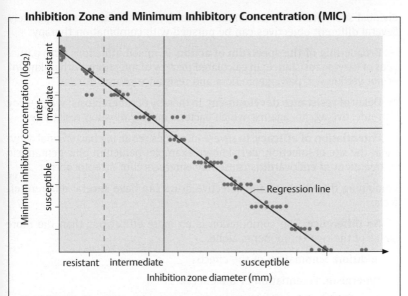

Fig. 3.32 Each point represents a bacterial strain. The size of the inhibition zone is determined in the agar diffusion test (disk test) and the minimum inhibitory concentration (MIC) in the dilution test. The MIC corresponds logarithmically ($\log_2$) with the diameter of the inhibition zone.

etc.). The interpretation also takes into account clinical experience gained from therapy of infections with pathogens of given suceptibility. Such data are used to establish general guideline values defining the boundary between susceptible and resistant bacteria.

The **minimum bactericidal concentration** (MBC) is the smallest concentration of a substance required to kill 99.9% of the cells in an inoculum.

The MBC is determined using quantitative subcultures from the macroscopically unclouded tubes or (microplate) wells of an MIC dilution series.

Combination Therapy

Combination therapy is the term for concurrent administration of two or more anti-infective agents. Some galenic preparations combine two components in a fixed ratio (example: cotrimoxazole). Normally, however, the individual substances in a combination therapy are administered separately. Several different objectives can be pursued with combination therapy:

■ **Broadening of the spectrum of action.** In mixed infections with pathogens of varying resistance; in calculated therapy of infections with unknown, or not yet known, pathogenic flora and resistance characteristics.

■ **Delay of resistance development.** In therapy of tuberculosis; when using anti-infective agents against which bacteria quickly develop resistance.

■ **Potentiation of efficacy.** In severe infections requiring bactericidal activity at the site of infection. Best-known example: penicillin plus gentamicin in treatment of endocarditis caused by enterococci or streptococci.

Combining the effects of anti-infective drugs can have several different effects:

■ **No difference.** The combination is no more efficacious than the more active of the two components alone.

■ **Addition.** Summation of the effects.

■ **Synergism.** Potentiation of the effects.

■ **Antagonism.** The combination is less efficacious than one of the two components alone.

Rule of thumb: combinations of bacteriostatics with substances that are bactericidal in the cell division phase only often result in antagonism, e.g., penicillin plus tetracycline in therapy of pneumococcal pneumonia.

In-vitro investigations of the mechanism of action of a combination when used against a pathogen usually employ the so-called "checkerboard titration" technique, in which the combinatory effects of substances A and B are compared using a checkerboard-like pattern.

Chemoprophylaxis

One of the most controversial antibiotic uses is prophylactic antibiosis. There are no clear-cut solutions here. There are certain situations in which chemoprophylaxis is clearly indicated and others in which it is clearly contraindicated. The matter must be decided on a case-by-case basis by weighing potential benefits against potential harm (side effects, superinfections with highly virulent and resistant pathogens, selection of resistant bacteria).

Chemoprophylaxis is considered useful in malaria, rheumatic fever, pulmonary cystic fibrosis, recurring pyelonephritis, following intensive contact with meningococci carriers, before surgery involving massive bacterial contamination, in heavily immunocompromised patients, in cardiac surgery or in femoral amputations due to circulatory problems. Chemoprophylaxis aimed at preventing a postsurgical infection should begin a few hours before the operation and never be continued for longer than 24–72 hours.

Immunomodulators

Despite the generally good efficacy of anti-infective agents, therapeutic success cannot be guaranteed. Complete elimination of bacterial pathogens also requires a functioning immune defense system. In view of the fact that the number of patients with severe immunodeficiencies is on the rise, immunomodulators are used as a supportive adjunct to specific antibiotic therapy in such patients. Many of these "cytokines" (see p. 77ff.) produced by the cells of the immune system can now be produced as "recombinant proteins." Myelopoietic growth factors have now been successfully used in patients suffering from neutropenia. Additional immunomodulators are also available, e.g., interferon gamma (IFNγ) and interleukin 2 (IL-2).

Laboratory Diagnosis

■ Infections can be diagnosed either directly by detection of the pathogen or components thereof or indirectly by antibody detection methods. The reliability of laboratory results is characterized by the terms sensitivity and specificity, their value is measured in terms of positive to negative predictive value. These predictive values depend to a great extent on prevalence. In direct laboratory diagnosis, correct material sampling and adequate transport precautions are an absolute necessity. The classic methods of direct laboratory diagnosis include microscopy and culturing. Identification of pathogens is based on morphological, physiological, and chemical characteristics. Among the latter, **the importance of detection of pathogen-specific nucleotide sequences is constantly increasing**. Development of sensitive test systems has made direct detection of pathogen components in test materials possible in some cases. The molecular biological methods used are applied with or without amplification of the sequence sought as the case warrants. Direct detection can also employ polyclonal or monoclonal antibodies to detect and identify antigens. ■

Preconditions, General Methods, Evaluation

Preconditions

The field of medical microbiology dealing with laboratory diagnosis of infectious diseases is known as diagnostic or clinical microbiology. Modern medical practice, and in particular hospital-based practice, is inconceivable without the cooperation of a special microbiological laboratory.

To ensure optimum patient benefit, the physician in charge of treatment and the laboratory staff must cooperate closely and efficiently. The preconditions include a basic knowledge of pathophysiology and clinical infectiology on the part of the laboratory staff and familiarity with the laboratory work on the part of the treating physician. The following sections provide a brief rundown on what physicians need to know about laboratory procedures.

General Methods and Evaluation

An infectious disease can be diagnosed **directly** by finding the causal pathogen or its components or products. It can also be diagnosed **indirectly** by means of antibody detection (Chapter 2, p. 121ff.). The accuracy and value of each of the available diagnostic methods are characterized in terms of sensitivity, specificity, and positive or negative predictive value. These parameters are best understood by reference to a 2 × 2 table (Table 3.**6**).

By inserting fictitious numbers into the 2 × 2 table, it readily becomes apparent that a positive predictive value will fall rapidly, despite high levels of specificity and sensitivity, if the prevalence level is low (Baye's theorem).

Sampling and Transport of Test Material

It is very important that the material to be tested be correctly obtained (sampled) and transported. In general, material from which the pathogen is to be isolated should be sampled as early as possible before chemotherapy is begun. Transport to the laboratory must be carried out in special containers provided by the institutes involved, usually containing transport mediums—either enrichment mediums (e.g., blood culture bottle), selective growth mediums or simple transport mediums without nutrients. An invoice must be attached to the material containing the information required for processing (using the form provided).

Table 3.6 2 × 2 Table: Explanation and Calculation of Sensitivity, Specificity, and Predictive Value (Positive–Negative)

Collective	Test positive	Test negative
Infected	Correct positive cp	False negative fn
Noninfected	False positive fp	Correct negative cn

■ Sensitivity (%) measures the frequency of correct positive results in the **infected** collective (horizontal addition).

■ Specificity (%) measures the frequency of correct negative results in the **noninfected** collective (horizontal addition).

$$\text{Sensitivity (\%)} = \frac{cp}{cp + fn} \times 100; \quad \text{Specificity (\%)} = \frac{cn}{fp + cn} \times 100$$

■ The predictive value of the positive result expresses the probability that a positive result indicates an infection. It analyzes the positive test results both in the infected collective and in the noninfected collective (vertical addition).

■ The predictive value of the negative result expresses the probability that a negative result indicates noninfection.

$$\text{Pos. pred. value (\%)} = \frac{cp}{cp + fp} \times 100; \quad \text{Neg. pred. value (\%)} = \frac{cn}{cn + fn} \times 100$$

Material from the respiratory tract:
— Swab smear from tonsils.
— Sinus flushing fluid.
— Pulmonary secretion. Expectorated sputum is usually contaminated with saliva and the flora of the oropharynx. Since these contaminations include pathogens that may cause infections of the lower respiratory tract organs, the value of positive findings would be limited. The material can be considered unsuitable for diagnostic testing if more than 25 oral epithelia are present per viewing frame at 100× magnification. Morning sputum from flushing the mouth or after induction will result in suitable samples. Sputum is not analyzed for anaerobes.
— Useful alternatives to expectorated sputum include bronchoscopically sampled bronchial secretion, flushing fluid from bronchoalveolar lavage (BAL), transtracheal aspirate or a pulmonary puncture biopsy. These types of material are required if an anaerobe infection is suspected. The material must then be transported in special anaerobe transport containers.

3

Material from the urogenital tract:

— Urine. Midstream urine is in most cases contaminated with the flora of the anterior urethra, which often corresponds to the pathogen spectrum of urinary tract infections. Bacterial counts must be determined if "contamination" is to be effectively differentiated from "infection." At counts in morning urine of $\geq 10^5$/ml an infection is highly probable, at counts of $\leq 10^3$ rather improbable. At counts of around 10^4/ml the test should be repeated. Lower counts may also be diagnostically significant in urethrocystitis. The dipstick method, which can be used in any medical practice, is a simple way of estimating the bacterial count: a stick coated with nutrient medium is immersed in the midstream urine, then incubated. The colony count is then estimated by comparing the result with standardized images.

— Catheterizing the urinary bladder solely for diagnostic purposes is inadvisable due to the potential for iatrogenic infection. Uncontaminated bladder urine is obtainable only by means of a suprapubic bladder puncture.

— Genital secretions are sampled with smear swabs and must be transported in special transport mediums.

Blood:

— For a blood culture, at least 10–20 ml of venous blood should be drawn sterilely into one aerobic and one anaerobic blood culture bottle. Sample three times a day at intervals of several hours (minimum interval one hour).

— For serology, (2–)5 ml of native blood will usually suffice. Take the initial sample as early as possible and a second one 1–3 weeks later to register any change in the antibody titer.

Pus and wound secretions:

— For surface wounds sample material with smear swabs and transport in preservative transport mediums. Such material is only analyzed for aerobic bacteria.

— For deep and closed wounds, liquid material (e.g., pus) should be sampled, if possible, with a syringe. Use special transport mediums for anaerobes.

Material from the gastrointestinal tract:

— Use a small spatula to place a portion of stool about the size of a cherry in liquid transport medium for shipment.

— Transport duodenal juice and bile in sterile tubes. Use special containers if anaerobes are suspected.

Cerebrospinal fluid, puncture biopsies, exudates, transudates:

— Ensure sampling sterility. Use special containers if anaerobes are suspected.

3

Microscopy

Bacteria are so small that a magnification of $1000\times$ is required to view them properly, which is at the limit of light microscope capability. At this magnification, bacteria can only be discerned in a preparation in which their density is at least 10^4–10^5 bacteria per ml.

Microscopic examination of such material requires a slide preparation:

■ **Native preparations**, with or without vital staining, are used to observe living bacteria. The poor contrast of such preparations makes it necessary to amplify this aspect (dark field and phase contrast microscopy). Native preparations include the coverslip and suspended drop types.

■ **Stained preparations** are richer in contrast so that bacteria are readily recognized in an illuminated field at $1000\times$. The staining procedure kills the bacteria. The material is first applied to a slide in a thin layer, dried in the air, and fixed with heat or methyl alcohol. **Simple** and **differential staining techniques** are used. The best-known simple staining technique employs methylene blue. **Gram staining** is the most important differential technique (Table 3.**7**): Gram-positive bacteria stain blue-violet, Gram-negative bacteria stain red. The Gram-positive cell wall prevents alcohol elution of the stain-

Table 3.**7** Procedure for the Three Most Important Types of Staining

Methylene blue	Gram staining	Ziehl–Neelsen staining
Methylene blue 1–5 minutes	Gentian violet or crystal violet, 1 minute	Concentrated carbolfuchsin; heat three times until vapor is observed
Rinse off with water	Pour off stain, rinse off with Lugol's solution, then cover with Lugol's solution for 2–3 minutes	Rinse off with water Destain with HCl (3%)/alcohol mixture
	Pour off Lugol's solution	Counterstain with methylene blue, 1–5 minutes
	Destain with acetone/ethyl alcohol (1:4)	Rinse off with water
	Rinse off with water	
	Counterstain with dilute carbolfuchsin, 1 minute	
	Rinse off with water	

iodine complex. In old cultures in which autolytic enzymes have begun to break down the cell walls, Gram-positive cells may test Gram-negative ("Gram-labile" bacteria).

Another differential stain is the **Ziehl-Neelsen** technique. It is used to stain mycobacteria, which do not "take" gram or methylene blue stains due to the amounts of lipids in their cell walls. Since mycobacteria cannot be destained with HCl-alcohol, they are called acid-resistant rods. The mycobacteria are stained red and everything else blue.

■ **Fluorescence microscopy** is another special technique. A fluorochrome absorbs shortwave light and emits light with a longer wavelength. Preparations stained with fluorochromes are exposed to light at the required wavelength. The stained particles appear clearly against a dark background in the color of the emitted light. This technique requires special equipment. Its practical application is in the observation of mycobacteria. In **immunofluorescence** detection, a fluorochrome (e.g., fluorescein isothiocyanate) is coupled to an antibody to reveal the presence of antigens on particle surfaces.

Culturing Methods

Types of nutrient mediums. Culturing is required in most cases to detect and identify bacteria. Almost all human pathogen bacteria can be cultivated on nutrient mediums. Nutrient mediums are either liquid (nutrient broth) or gelatinous (nutrient agar, containing 1.5–2% of the polysaccharide agarose). Enrichment mediums are complex mediums that encourage the proliferation of many different bacterial species. The most frequently used enrichment medium is the blood agar plate containing 5% whole blood. Selective mediums allow only certain bacteria to grow and suppress the reproduction of others. Indicator mediums are used to register metabolic processes.

Proliferation forms. Most bacteria show diffuse proliferation in **liquid mediums**. Some proliferate in "crumbs," other form a grainy bottom sediment, yet others a biofilm skin at the surface (pseudomonads). Isolated colonies are observed to form on, or in, **nutrient agar** if the cell density is not too high. These are pure cultures, since each colony arises from a single bacterium or colony-forming unit (CFU). The pure culture technique is the basis of bacteriological culturing methods. The procedure most frequently used to **obtain isolated colonies** is fractionated inoculation of a nutrient agar plate (Figs. 3.**33**–3.**35**).

Use of this technique ensures that isolated colonies will be present in one of the three sectors. Besides obtaining pure cultures, the isolated colony technique has the further advantage of showing the form, appearance, and

Fractionated Inoculation of Nutrient Agar

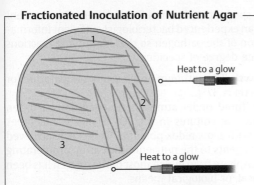

Fig. 3.**33** Isolated colonies are obtained by means of fractionated inoculation of nutrient agar. The wire loop must be sterilized between inoculations.

Heat to a glow

Heat to a glow

Blood Agar Plate Following Fractionated Inoculation and Incubation

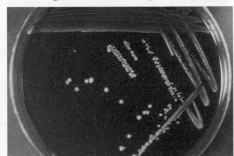

Fig. 3.**34** Blood agar is frequently used as a universal enrichment medium. Most human bacterial pathogens grow on it. Here is a pure culture of *Staphylococcus aureus*.

Endo Agar Following Fractionated Inoculation with a Mixed Culture

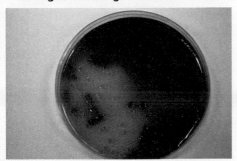

Fig. 3.**35** Endo agar is a combined selective/indicator medium. It allows growth of *Enterobacteriaceae*, *Pseudomonadaceae*, and other Gram-negative rod bacteria but inhibits the growth of Gram-positive bacteria and Gram-negative cocci. The red color of the colonies and agar is characteristic of lactose breakdown (= *Escherichia coli*); the light-colored colonies are lactose-negative (= *Salmonella enterica*).

color of single colonies. The special proliferation forms observed in nutrient broth and nutrient agar give an experienced bacteriologist sufficient information for an initial classification of the pathogen so that identifying reactions can then be tested with some degree of specificity.

Conditions required for growth. The optimum proliferation temperature for most human pathogen bacteria is 37 °C.

Bacteria are generally cultured under atmospheric conditions. It often proves necessary to incubate the cultures in 5% CO_2. Obligate anaerobes must be cultured in a milieu with a low redox potential. This can be achieved by adding suitable reduction agents to the nutrient broth or by proliferating the cultures under a gas atmosphere from which most of the oxygen has been removed by physical, chemical, or biological means.

Identification of Bacteria

The essential principle of bacterial identification is to assign an unknown culture to its place within the taxonomic classification system based on as few characteristics as possible and as many as necessary (Table 3.**8**).

■ **Morphological characteristics**, including staining, are determined under the microscope.

■ **Physiological characteristics** are determined with indicator mediums. Commercially available miniaturized systems are now frequently used for this purpose (Fig. 3.**36**).

Determination of Metabolic Characteristics with Indicator Mediums

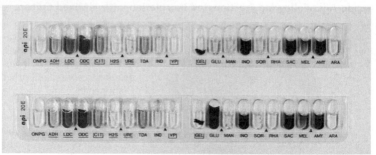

Fig. 3.**36** Identification of *Enterobacteriaceae* using API 20E, a standardized microplate method. Positive and negative reactions are shown by color reactions.

Table 3.8   Characteristics Useful in Identification of Bacteria

Morphological characteristics

Form (sphere, rod, spiral)

Size; pseudogroupings (clusters, chains, diplococci)

Staining (Gram-positive, Gram-negative); flagella (presence, arrangement); capsule (yes, no); spores (form, within cell formation)

Physiological characteristics

Respiratory chain enzymes (oxidases, catalases)

Enzymes that break down carbohydrates, alcohols, glycosides (e.g., betagalactosidase)

Protein metabolism enzymes (e.g., gelatinase, collagenase)

Amino acid metabolism enzymes (e.g., decarboxylases, deaminases, urease)

Other enzymes: hemolysins, lipases, lecithinases, DNases, etc.

End products of metabolism (e.g., organic acids detected by gas chromatography)

Resistance/sensitivity to chemical noxae

Characteristics of anabolic metabolism (e.g., citrate as sole source of C)

Chemical characteristics

DNA structure (base sequences)

Structure of cell wall murein

Antigen structure: fine structures detectable with antibodies (e.g., flagellar protein or polysaccharides of the cell wall or capsule)

Fatty acids in membranes and cell wall; analysis using different chromatographic methods

■ **Chemical characteristics** have long been in use to identify bacteria, e.g., in detection of antigen structures. Molecular genetic methods (see below) will play an increasing role in the future.

Molecular Methods

The main objective of the molecular methods of bacterial identification is direct recognition of pathogen-specific nucleotide sequences in the test material. These methods are used in particular in the search for bacteria that are not culturable, are very difficult to culture, or proliferate very slowly. Of course, they can also be used to identify pure bacterial cultures (see above). In principle, any species-specific sequence can be used for identification, but the specific regions of genes coding for 16S rRNA and 23S rRNA are particularly useful in this respect. The following methods are used:

■ **DNA probes.** Since DNA is made up of two complementary strands of nucleic acids, it is possible to detect single-strand sequences with the hybridization technique using complementary marking of single strands. The probes can be marked with radioactivity (^{32}P, ^{35}S) or nonradioactive reporter molecules (biotin, dioxigenin):

— *Solid phase hybridization.* The reporter molecule or probe is fixed to a nylon or nitrocellulose membrane (colony blot technique, dot blot technique).
— *Liquid phase hybridization.* The reporter molecule and probe are in a solute state.
— *In-situ hybridization.* Detection of bacterial DNA in infected tissue.

■ **Amplification.** The main objective here is to increase the sensitivity level so as to find the "needle in a haystack." A number of techniques have been developed to date, which can be classified in three groups:

— *Amplification of the target sequence.* The oldest and most important among the techniques in this group is the polymerase chain reaction (PCR), which is described on p. 409f.). With "real time PCR," a variant of PCR, the analysis can be completed in 10 minutes.
— *Probe amplification.*
— *Signal amplification.*

Identification by Means of Amplification and Sequencing

The target sequence for identification of bacteria that have not yet been cultured (e.g., *Tropheryma whipplei*, the causal pathogen in Whipple's disease) or of pathogens very difficult to identify with classic methods, is often a certain region of the 16S rRNA, some sections of which are identical in all bacteria. Between these highly conservative segments are other sections that are specific for a species or genus. Using primers that can recognize the conserved regions of 16S rDNA to the right and left of the specific regions, the specific sequence is amplified, then sequenced. The base sequence thus obtained is then identified by comparison with a reference data library.

Identification by Means of Amplification and Gene Chips

In this technique, thousands of oligonucleotides specific for human pathogen bacteria are deposited on the surface of a chip about $2\,cm^2$ in size. This chip is then charged with amplified and marked single-strand DNA from the test material (containing, for example, species-specific sequences of the 16S rDNA or other species-specific sequences). Then the level of binding to complementary nucleotide sequences is measured as fluorescence using confocal laser scanning microscopy. The occurrence of antibiotic resistance genes can also be measured by this method.

3

Direct Detection of Bacterial Antigens

Antigens specific for particular species or genera can be detected directly by means of polyclonal or (better yet) monoclonal antibodies present in the test material. This allows for rapid diagnosis. Examples include the detection of bacterial antigens in cerebrospinal fluid in cases of acute purulent meningitis, detection of gonococcal antigens in secretion from the urogenital tract, and detection of group A streptococcal antigen in throat smear material. These direct methods are not, however, as sensitive as the classic culturing methods. Adsorbance, coagglutination, and latex agglutination tests are frequently used in direct detection. In the agglutination methods, the antibodies with the Fc components are fixed either to killed staphylococcal protein A or to latex particles.

Diagnostic Animal Tests

Animal testing is practically a thing of the past in diagnostic bacteriology. Until a few years ago, bacterial toxins (e.g., diphtheria toxin, tetanus toxin, botulinus toxin) were confirmed in animal tests. Today, molecular genetic methods are used to detect the presence of the toxin gene, which process usually involves an amplification step.

Bacteriological Laboratory Safety

Microbiologists doing diagnostic work will of course have to handle potentially pathogenic microorganisms and must observe stringent regulations to avoid risks to themselves and others. Laboratory safety begins with suitable room designs and equipment (negative-pressure lab rooms, safety hoods) and goes on to include compliance with the basic rules of work in a microbiological laboratory: protective clothing, no eating, drinking, or smoking, mechanical pipetting aids, hand and working surface disinfection (immediately in case of contamination, otherwise following each procedure), proper disposal of contaminated materials, staff health checks, and proper staff training.

Taxonomy and Overview of Human Pathogenic Bacteria

■ Taxonomy includes the two disciplines of classification and nomenclature. The bacteria are classified in a hierarchic system based on phenotypic characteristics (morphological, physiological, and chemical characteristics). The basic unit is the species. Similar and related species are classified in a single genus and related genera are placed in a single family. Classification in yet higher taxa often takes practical considerations into account, e.g., division into "descriptive sections." A species is designated by two Latin names, the first of which denotes the genus, both together characterizing the species. Family names end in -aceae. Table 3.**9** provides an overview of human pathogenic bacteria. ■

Classification

Bacteria are grouped in the domain bacteria to separate them from the domains archaea and eucarya (see p. 5). Within their domain, bacteria are further broken down into taxonomic groups (taxa) based on relationships best elucidated by knowledge of the evolutionary facts. However, little is known about the phylogenetic relationships of bacteria, so their classification is often based on similarities among phenotypic characteristics (phenetic relationships). These characteristics are **morphological**, **physiological** (metabolic), or **chemical** (see Table 3.**8**, p. 215) in nature. The role of chemical characteristics in classification is growing in importance, for instance, murein composition or the presence of certain fatty acids in the cell wall. DNA and RNA structure is highly important in classification. DNA composition can be roughly estimated by determining the proportions of the bases: mol/l of guanine + cytosine (GC). The GC content (in mol%) of human pathogenic bacteria ranges from 25% to 70%. Measurement of how much heterologous duplex DNA is formed, or of RNA-DNA hybrids, provides information on the similarity of different bacteria and thus about their degree of relationship. Another highly useful factor in determining phylogenetic relationship is the sequence analysis of the (16S/23S) rRNA or (16S/23S) rDNA. This genetic material contains highly conserved sequences found in all bacteria alongside sequences characteristic of the different taxa.

In formal terms, the prokaryotes are classified in phyla, classes, orders, families, genera, and species, plus subtaxa if any:

Family (familia)	*Enterobacteriaceae*
Genus	*Escherichia*
Species	*E. coli*
Var(iety) or type	Serovar O157:H7
Strain	xyz

Taxonomic classification is based on the concept of the species. Especially in an epidemiological setting, we often need to subclassify a species in **vars** or (syn.) **types**, in which cultures of a species that share certain characteristics are grouped together. Examples: biovar, phagovar, pathovar, morphovar, serovar (also biotype, phagotype, etc.). Use of the term **strain** varies somewhat: in clinical bacteriology it often designates the first culture of a species isolated from an infected patient. In an epidemiological context, isolates of the same species obtained from different patients are considered to belong to the same epidemic strain.

There is no official, internationally recognized classification of bacteria. The higher taxa therefore often reflect practical considerations.

Table 3.**9** Overview of the Medically Most Important Bacteria[1]

Family Genus, species	Characteristics	Clinical manifestations
Section 1. Gram-positive cocci		
Staphylococcaceae	Cluster-forming cocci, nonmotile; catalase-positive	
Staphylococcus aureus	Coagulase-positive, yellow-pigmented colonies	Pyogenic infections, toxicoses
S. epidermidis	Coagulase-negative, whitish colonies, normal flora	Foreign body infections
S. saprophyticus	Coagulase-negative	Urinary tract infections in young women
Streptococcaceae	Chain-forming cocci and diplococci, nonmotile, catalase-negative	
Streptococcus pyogenes	Chain-forming cocci, Lancefield group A, β-hemolysis	Tonsillitis, scarlet fever, skin infections
S. pneumoniae	Diplococci, no group antigen present, α-hemolysis	Pneumonia, otitis media, sinusitis
S. agalactiae	Chain-forming cocci, group antigen B, β-hemolysis	Meningitis/sepsis in neonates
"*Enterococcaceae*"	Chain-forming cocci and diplococci, α, β, or γ-hemolysis, group antigen D, catalase-negative	Part of the flora of intestines of humans and animals
Enterococcus faecalis *Enterococcus faecium*	Aesculin-positive, growth in 6.5% NaCl, pH 9.6	Opportunistic infections
Section 2. Endospore-forming Gram-positive rods		
Bacillaceae	Aerobic soil bacteria	
Bacillus anthracis	Nonmotile, ubiquitous	Anthrax
Clostridiaceae	Anaerobic soil bacteria	
Clostridium tetani	Motile, anaerobic, tetanus toxin (tetanospasmin)	Tetanus

[1] (Nomenclature according to Bergey's *Manual of Systematic Bacteriology*, 2001, Vol. 1, pp. 155–166. Names in quotation marks not yet validated).

Table **3.9**   *Continued: Overview of the Medically Most Important Bacteria*

Family Genus, species	Characteristics	Clinical manifestations
Continued: Section 2.		
Clostridium botulinum	Motile, neurotoxins A, B, and G	Botulism, usually ingestion of toxin with food
Clostridium perfringens and further clostridiae	Nonmotile, exotoxins, and exoenzymes	1. Anaerobic cellulitis 2. Gas gangrene (myonecrosis)
Clostridium difficile	Motile, enterotoxin (toxin A), cytotoxin (toxin B)	Pseudomembranous colitis (often antibotic associated)

Section 3. Regular, nonsporing, Gram-positive rods

Family Genus, species	Characteristics	Clinical manifestations
Listeria monocytogenes	Slender rods, weak β-hemolysis on blood agar, motile at 20 °C, ubiquitous (soil)	Meningitis, sepsis (neonates, immunocompromised persons), epidemic gastroenteritis
Erysipelothrix rhusiopathiae	Transmitted from diseased pigs	Erysipeloid (today rare)
Gardnerella vaginalis	Flora of the normal genital mucosa	Contributes to vaginosis

Section 4. Irregular, nonsporing, Gram-positive rods

Family Genus, species	Characteristics	Clinical manifestations
Corynebacteriaceae	Mostly normal bacterial flora of the skin and mucosa, aerobic	Only few species cause disease
Corynebacterium diphtheriae	Club shape, pleomorphic, diphtheria exotoxin (A + B)	Diphtheria (throat, nose, wounds)
Actinomycetaceae	Normal bacterial flora of the mucosa, anaerobic or micro-aerophilic	
Actinomyces israelii and further *Actinomyces* spp.	Filaments (also branched)	Actinomycosis (cervicofacial, thoracic, abdominal, pelvic)
Nocardiaceae	Nonmotile, obligately aerobic, filaments, partially acid-fast	Habitat: soil and aquatic biotopes

3

Table **3.9** *Continued: Overview of the Medically Most Important Bacteria*

Family Genus, species	Characteristics	Clinical manifestations
Continued: Section 4.		
Nocardia asteroides *Nocardia brasiliensis* and further species	Infections in patients with impaired cell-mediated immunity	Pulmonary, systemic, and dermal nocardioses

Section 5. Mycobacteria (acid-fast rods)

Mycobacteriaceae	Slender rods, Ziehl-Neelsen staining (Gram-positive cell wall), aerobic, nonmotile	
Mycobacterium tuberculosis	Slow proliferation (culturing 3–6–8 weeks)	Tuberculosis (pulmonary and extrapulmonary)
Mycobacterium leprae	In-vitro culture not possible	Leprosy (lepromatous, tuberculoid)
Nontuberculous mycobacteria (NTM) (e.g., *Mycobacterium avium/intracellulare* complex, and numerous other species)	Ubiquitous. Low level of pathogenicity, opportunists	Pulmonary disease, lymphadenitis, infections of skin, soft tissue, bones, joints, tendons. Disseminated disease in immunosuppressed patients (AIDS)

Section 6. Gram-negative aerobic cocci and coccobacilli

Neisseriaceae	Coffee bean-shaped diplococci, nonmotile, oxidase (+), catalase (+)	
Neisseria gonorrheae	Cocci often in phagocytes, acid from fermentation of glucose	Gonorrhea
Neisseria meningitidis	Acid from fermentation of glucose and maltose	Meningitis/sepsis
Eikenella corrodens	HACEK-group. Low pathogenicity	Nosocomial infections
Kingella kingae	HACEK-group. Low pathogenicity	Nosocomial infections

Table 3.9 *Continued: Overview of the Medically Most Important Bacteria*

Family Genus, species	Characteristics	Clinical manifestations
Continued: Section 6.		
Moraxellaceae	Cocci and short rods	
Moraxella catarrhalis	Normal respiratory tract flora	Sinusitis, otitis media in children
Acinetobacter baumannii *Acinetobacter calcoaceticus*	Ubiquitous, coccobacillary rods	Nosocomial infections, often multiple resistance against anti-infective agents
Section 7. Gram-negative facultatively anaerobic rods		
Enterobacteriaceae	Inhabitat intestine of man and animals. Genera (41) and species (hundreds) identified biochemically	
Escherichia coli	Lactose-positive, most frequent human pathogen, various pathovars.	Nosocomial infections, Gut disease caused by pathovars EPEC, ETEC, EIEC, EHEC, and EAggEC
Salmonella enterica	Lactose-negative, motile, over 2000 serovars	Typhoid/paratypoid fever, gastroenteritis
Shigella dysenteriae, S. flexneri, S. boydii, S. sonnei	Lactose-negative (in most cases), nonmotile, O-serovars	Bacterial dysentery
Klebsiella, Enterobacter, Citrobacter, Proteus, Serratia, Morganella, Providencia, and other genera	Opportunists, frequently resistant to antibiotics	Nosocomial infections
Yersinia pestis	Bipolar staining, motile, no acid from lactose. Rodent pathogen	Bubonic plague, pulmonary plague
Yersinia enterocolitica	Reservoir: wild animals, domestic animals, pets	Enteritis, lymphadenitis
Calymmatobacterium granulomatis	Encapsulated, nonmotile	Granuloma inguinale (venereal disease)

3

Table 3.**9** *Continued: Overview of the Medically Most Important Bacteria*

Family Genus, species	Characteristics	Clinical manifestations
Continued: Section 7.		
Vibrionaceae	Comma-shaped, polar flagella, oxidase-positive	
Vibrio cholerae	Alkaline tolerance, exotoxin, no invasion of the small intestine's mucosa	Cholera, massive watery diarrhea
Aeromonadaceae		
Aeromonas spp.	Aquatic biotopes, fish infections	Occasionally the cause of enteritis in man
Pasteurellaceae	Small straight rods, nonmotile	
Pasteurella multocida	Pathogen of various animals (sepsis)	Infections via dermal injuries (rare)
Haemophilus influenzae	X and V factors for culturing, capsule serovar "b" (Hib)	Meningitis, respiratory tract infections
Cardiobacteriaceae *Cardiobacterium hominis*	HACEK group. Normal mucosal flora of humans, nonmotile	Endocarditis (rare). Opportunistic infections

Section 8. Gram-negative aerobic rods

Pseudomonadaceae	Straight or curved rods, motile, oxidase-positive. Ubiquitous bacteria	Nosocomial infections
Pseudomonas aeruginosa and many further species	Fluorescent pigments produced. Other properties as above	Nosocomial infections, frequent multiple antibiotic resistance
"Burkholderiaceae" *Burkholderia cepacia*	Ubiquitous	Nosocomial infections. Often resistance to multiple antibiotics
B. mallei	Malleus of horses	Skin abscesses. Very rare
B. pseudomallei	Habitat: soil	Melioidosis (Asia)

Table 3.**9** *Continued: Overview of the Medically Most Important Bacteria*

Family Genus, species	Characteristics	Clinical manifestations
Continued: Section 8.		
"Xanthomonadaceae"		
Stenotrophomonas maltophilia	Low pathogenicity	Nosocomial infections. Often resistance to multiple antibiotics
Legionellaceae	Motile, difficult to stain, requires special culturing mediums	
Legionella pneumophila	Most frequent species, aquatic biotopes	Legionnaire's pneumonia, Pontiac fever
Brucellaceae	Short rods, nonmotile, facultative intracellular parasite, fastidious growth	Zoonoses
Brucella abortus *Brucella melitensis* *Brucella suis* *Brucella canis*	Transmission via direct contact or foods (milk and milk products)	Brucellosis (Bang disease, Malta fever)
Alcaligenaceae *Bordetella pertussis*	Short rods, nonmotile, only in humans	Pertussis (whooping cough)
"Francisellaceae" *Francisella tularensis*	Minute pleomorphic rods. Requires enriched media for culturing	Tularemia, zoonosis (rodents)

Section 9. Gram-negative rods, straight, curved, and helical, strictly anaerobic

Bacteroidaceae "*Fusobacteriaceae*" "*Porphyromonadaceae*" "*Prevotellaceae*"	Pleomorphic rods, major component of normal mucosal flora	Subacute necrotic infections, mostly together with other bacteria
Bacteroides spp. *Porphyromonas* spp. *Prevotella* spp. *Fusobacterium* spp.		Necrotic abscesses in CNS, head region, lungs, abdomen, female genital tract

3

Table 3.9 *Continued: Overview of the Medically Most Important Bacteria*

Family Genus, species	Characteristics	Clinical manifestations
Continued: Section 9.		
Streptobacillus monili-formis (belongs new to *Fusobacteriaceae*)	Normal flora in rats, mice, and cats	Rat-bite fever (also caused by *Spirillum minus* (= Sodoku)

Section 10. Aerobic/microaerophilic, motile, helical/vibrioid Gram-negative rod bacteria

Campylobacteriaceae	Thin, helical, and vibrioid, culturable	
Campylobacter jejuni	Animal pathogen	Enteritis
Campylobacter fetus		Opportunistic infections: sepsis, endocarditis
"Helicobacteriaceae" *Helicobacter pylori*	Helical, culturing difficult, produces large amounts of urease	Type B gastritis, peptic ulcers of stomach and duodenum

Section 11. The Spirochetes. Gram-negative, helical bacteria

Spirochaetaceae	Helical, motile, thin	
Treponema pallidum	Only in humans, not culturable	Syphilis, three stages
Borrelia burgdorferi *B. afzelii* *B. garinii*	Tickborne, culturable	Lyme disease, three stages
Borrelia duttonii *Borrelia hermsii* and further species	Tickborne, antigen variability	Endemic relapsing fever
Borrelia recurrentis	Transmitted by body lice	Epidemic relapsing fever
Leptospiraceae	Helical, motile, culturable	
Leptospira interrogans	Serogroups and serovars (e.g., icterohemorrhagiae, pomona, grippotyphosa, etc.)	Leptospirosis, morbus Weil

Table 3.**9** *Continued: Overview of the Medically Most Important Bacteria*

Family Genus, species	Characteristics	Clinical manifestations
Section 12. Rickettsiae, Coxiellae, Ehrlichiae, Bartonellae, and Chlamydiae		
Rickettsiaceae	Small short rods, usually intracellular bacteria transmitted by arthropods	Rickettsioses
Rickettsia prowazekii	Transmitted by body lice	Typhus
Rickettsia rickettsii	Transmitted by ticks	Rocky Mountains Spotted Fever (RMSF)
"Coxelliaceae" *Coxiella burnetii*	Reservoir: sheep, cattle, rodents; infection by inhalation	Q fever (pneumonia)
Ehrlichiaceae	Coccobacillary. Culture possible	Zoonoses
Ehrlichia chaffeensis	Transmission by ticks	Human monocytrophic ehrlichiosis (HME)
Ehrlichia ewingii and *Anaplasma* (formerly *Ehrlichia*) *phagocytophilum*	Transmission by ticks	Human granulocytotrophic ehrlichiosis (HEG)
Bartonellaceae	Short pleomorphic rods	
Bartonella bacilliformis	Tropism for erythrocytes/endothelia. Transmitted by sand flea	Oroya fever and verruga peruana
Bartonella henselae and *Bartonella claridgeia*	Animal reservoir: cats	Sepsis, bacillary angiomatosis in immunosuppressed patients (AIDS). Cat scratch disease in immunocompetent persons
Bartonella quintana	Transmission by body lice	Five-day fever
Chlamydiaceae	Obligate intracellular pathogen, reproductive cycle	
Chlamydia trachomatis	Biovar trachoma	Trachoma, inclusion conjunctivitis, urethritis (nonspecific)
	Biovar lymphogranuloma venerum	Lymphogranuloma venereum

3

Table 3.**9** *Continued: Overview of the Medically Most Important Bacteria*

Family Genus, species	Characteristics	Clinical manifestations
Continued: Section 12.		
Chlamydia psittaci	Reservoir: infected birds. Infection by inhalation of pathogen-containing dust	Ornithosis (pneumonia)
Chlamydia pneumoniae	Only in humans, aerogenic transmission	Infections of the respiratory tract, often subacute. Role in atherosclerosis of coronary arteries still unclear

Section 13. Mycoplasmas (bacteria without cell walls)

Family Genus, species	Characteristics	Clinical manifestations
Mycoplasmataceae	Pleomorphic; no murein, therefore resistant to antibiotics that attack the cell wall	
Mycoplasma pneumoniae	Reservoir human, aerogenic infection	Pneumonia (frequently atypical)
Ureaplasma urealyticum	Component of the normal flora of the urogenital tract	Urethritis (nonspecific)

Nomenclature

The rules of bacterial nomenclature are set out in the *International Code for the Nomenclature of Bacteria.* A species is designated with two latinized names, the first of which characterizes the genus and the second the species. Family names always end in *-aceae*. Taxonomic names approved by the "International Committee of Systematic Bacteriology" are considered official and binding. In medical practice, short handles have become popular in many cases, for instance gonococci instead of *Neisseria gonorrheae* or pneumococci (or even "strep pneumos") instead of *Streptococcus pneumoniae*.

4 Bacteria as Human Pathogens

F. H. Kayser

Staphylococcus

■ Staphylococci are Gram-positive cocci occurring in clusters. They can be cultured on normal nutrient mediums both aerobically and anaerobically. The most important species from the viewpoint of human medicine is *S. aureus*. A number of extracellular enzymes and exotoxins such as coagulase, alphatoxin, leukocidin, exfoliatins, enterotoxins, and toxic shock toxin are responsible for the clinical symptoms of infections by this pathogen, which are observed in the three types invasive infections, pure toxicoses, and mixed forms. The antibiotics of choice for therapy of these infections are penicillinase-resistant penicillins. Laboratory diagnosis involves identification of the pathogen by means of microscopy and culturing. *S. aureus* is a frequent pathogen in nosocomial infections and limited outbreaks in hospitals. Hand washing by medical staff is the most important prophylactic measure in hospitals.

Coagulase-negative staphylococci are classic opportunists. *S. epidermidis* and other species are frequent agents in foreign body infections due to their ability to form biofilms on the surfaces of inert objects. *S. saprophyticus* is responsible for between 10 and 20 % of acute urinary tract infections in young women. ■

Staphylococci are small spherical cells (1 μm) found in grapelike clusters. Staphylococci are nonmotile, catalase-producing bacteria. The genus *Staphylococcus* includes over 30 species and subspecies. Table 4.1 briefly summarizes the characteristics of those most important in the medical context. *S. aureus* (and *E. coli*) are among the most frequent causal organisms in human bacterial infections.

Table **4.1** Overview of the *Staphylococcus* Species That Affect Humans Most
Frequently

Species	Parameter
S. aureus	Coagulase-positive; colonies golden yellow. Local purulent infections: furuncles, carbuncles, bullous impetigo, wound infections, sinusitis, otitis media, mastitis puerperalis, ostitis, postinfluenza pneumonia, sepsis. Toxin-caused illnesses: food poisoning, dermatitis exfoliativa, toxic shock syndrome
S. epidermidis	Coagulase-negative; sensitive to novobiocin; most frequent CNS* pathogen; opportunist; infection requires host predisposition; foreign body infections with discrete clinical symptoms
S. saprophyticus	Coagulase-negative; resistant to novobiocin. Urinary tract infections in young women (10–20%); occasional nonspecific urethritis in men

* CNS: coagulase-negative staphylococci

Staphylococcus Aureus

Morphology and culturing. Fig. **4.1a** shows the appearance of Gram-stained *S. aureus*. This is a facultative anaerobe that is readily cultured on normal nutrient mediums at $37\,°C$. Colonies as in Fig. **4.1b** develop after 24 hours of incubation. Hemolytic zones are frequently observed around the colonies.

Fine structure. The cell wall consists of a thick layer of murein. Linear teichoic acids and polysaccharides are covalently coupled to the murein polysaccharide (Fig. 3.**10**, p. 154). The lipoteichoic acids permeating the entire murein layer are anchored in the cell membrane. Teichoic and lipoteichoic acids can trigger activation of complement by the alternative pathway and stimulate macrophages to secrete cytokines. Cell wall-associated proteins are bound to the peptide components of the murein. Clumping factor, fibronectin-binding protein, and collagen-binding protein bind specifically to fibrinogen, fibronectin, and collagen, respectively, and are instrumental in adhesion to tissues and foreign bodies covered with the appropriate matrix protein. Protein A binds to the Fc portion of immunoglobulins (IgG). It is assumed that "false" binding of immunoglobulins by protein A prevents "correct" binding of opsonizing antibodies, thus hindering phagocytosis.

Staphylococcus aureus

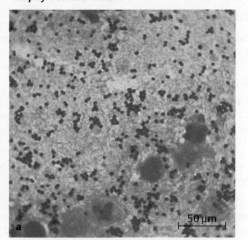

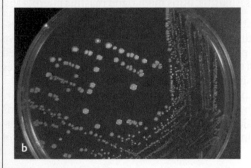

Fig. 4.**1 a** Gram staining of a pus preparation: Gram-positive cocci, some in grapelike clusters. Clinical diagnosis: furunculosis. **b** Culture on blood agar: convex colonies with yellowish pigment and porcelainlike surface.

50 µm

4

Extracellular toxins and enzymes. *S. aureus* secretes numerous enzymes and toxins that determine, together with the fine structures described above, the pathogenesis of the attendant infections. The most important are:

■ **Plasma coagulase** is an enzyme that functions like thrombin to convert fibrinogen into fibrin. Tissue microcolonies surrounded by fibrin walls are difficult to phagocytose.

■ **α-toxin** can have lethal CNS effects, damages membranes (resulting in, among other things, hemolysis), and is responsible for a form of dermonecrosis.

■ **Leukocidin** damages microphages and macrophages by degranulation.

■ **Exfoliatins** are responsible for a form of epidermolysis.

■ Food poisoning symptoms can be caused by eight serologically differentiated **enterotoxins** (A-E, H, G, and I). These proteins (MW: 35 kDa) are not inactivated by heating to 100 °C for 15–30 minutes. *Staphylococcus* enterotoxins are superantigens (see p. 72).

■ **Toxic shock syndrome toxin-1** (TSST-1) is produced by about 1% of *Staphylococcus* strains. TSST-1 is a superantigen that induces clonal expansion of many T lymphocyte types (about 10%), leading to massive production of cytokines, which then give rise to the clinical symptoms of toxic shock.

Pathogenesis and clinical pictures. The pathogenesis and symptoms of *S. aureus* infections take one of three distinct courses:

■ **Invasive infections.** In this type of infection, the pathogens tend to remain in situ after penetrating through the derma or mucosa and to cause local infections characterized by purulence. Examples include furuncles (Fig. 4.**2**), carbuncles, wound infections, sinusitis, otitis media, and mastitis puerperalis.

Other kinds of invasive infection include postoperative or posttraumatic ostitis/osteomyelitis, endocarditis following heart surgery (especially valve replacement), postinfluenza pneumonia, and sepsis in immunocompromised patients. *S. aureus* and *E. coli* are responsible for approximately equal shares of nearly half of all cases of inpatient sepsis.

Inert foreign bodies (see p. 158 for examples) can be colonized by *S. aureus*. Colonization begins with specific binding of the staphylococci, by means of cell wall-associated adhesion proteins, to fibrinogen or fibronectin covering the foreign body, resulting in a biofilm that may function as a focus of infection.

Multiple Furuncles

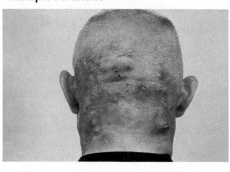

Fig. 4.**2** Furuncles in a patient with type 2 diabetes mellitus.

■ **Toxicoses.** Food poisoning results from ingestion of food contaminated with enterotoxins. The onset a few hours after ingestion takes the form of nausea, vomiting, and massive diarrhea.

■ **Mixed forms.** Dermatitis exfoliativa (staphylococcal scalded skin syndrome, Ritter disease), pemphigus neonatorum, and bullous impetigo are caused by exfoliatin-producing strains that infect the skin surface. Toxic shock syndrome (TSS) is caused by strains that produce TSST-1. These strains can cause invasive infections, but may also only colonize mucosa. The main symptoms are hypotension, fever, and a scarlatiniform rash.

Diagnosis. This requires microscopic and culture-based pathogen identification. Differentiating *S. aureus* from the coagulase-negative species is achieved by detection of the plasma coagulase and/or the clumping factor. The enterotoxins and TSST-1 can be detected by means of immunological and molecular biological methods (special laboratories).

Plasma Coagulase and Clumping Factor Test

■ To detect plasma coagulase, suspend several colonies in 0.5 ml of rabbit plasma, incubate the inoculated plasma for one, four, and 24 hours and record the levels of coagulation.

■ For the clumping factor test, suspend colony material in a drop of rabbit plasma on a slide. Macroscopically visible clumping confirms the presence of the factor.

Therapy. Aside from surgical measures, therapy is based on administration of antibiotics. The agents of choice for severe infections are penicillinase-resistant penicillins, since 70–80% of all strains produce penicillinase. These penicillins are, however, ineffective against methicillin-resistant strains, and this resistance applies to all betalactams.

Epidemiology and prevention. *S. aureus* is a frequent colonizer of skin and mucosa. High carrier rates (up to 80%) are the rules among hospital patients and staff. The principle localization of colonization in these persons is the anterior nasal mucosa area, from where the bacteria can spread to hands or with dust into the air and be transmitted to susceptible persons.

S. aureus is frequently the causal pathogen in nosocomial infections (see p. 343f.). Certain strains are known to cause hospital epidemics. Identification of the epidemic strain requires differentiation of relevant infection isolates from other ubiquitous strains. Lysotyping (see p. 186) can be used for this purpose, although use of molecular methods to identify genomic DNA "fingerprints" is now becoming more common.

The most important preventive measure in hospitals is washing the hands thoroughly before medical and nursing procedures. Intranasal application of antibiotics (mupirocin) is a method of reducing bacterial counts in carriers.

Coagulase-Negative Staphylococci (CNS)

CNS are an element in the normal flora of human skin and mucosa. They are classic opportunists that only cause infections given a certain host disposition.

■ **S. epidermidis.** This is the pathogen most frequently encountered in CNS infections (70–80% of cases). CNS cause mainly foreign body infections. Examples of the foreign bodies involved are intravasal catheters, continuous ambulant peritoneal dialysis (CAPD) catheters, endoprostheses, metal plates and screws in osteosynthesis, cardiac pacemakers, artificial heart valves, and shunt valves. These infections frequently develop when foreign bodies in the macroorganism are covered by matrix proteins (e.g., fibrinogen, fibronectin) to which the staphylococci can bind using specific cell wall proteins. They then proliferate on the surface and produce a polymeric substance—the basis of the developing biofilm. The staphylococci within the biofilm are protected from antibiotics and the immune system to a great extent. Such biofilms can become infection foci from which the CNS enter the bloodstream and cause sepsislike illnesses. Removal of the foreign body is often necessary.

■ **S. saprophyticus** is responsible for 10–20% of acute urinary tract infections, in particular dysuria in young women, and for a small proportion of cases of nonspecific urethritis in sexually active men.

Antibiotic treatment of CNS infections is often problematic due to the multiple resistance often encountered in these staphylococci, especially *S. hemolyticus*.

Streptococcus and Enterococcus

■ **Streptococci** are Gram-positive, **nonmotile**, catalase-negative, facultatively anaerobic cocci that occur in chains or pairs. They are classified based on their hemolytic capacity (α-, β-, γ-hemolysis) and the antigenicity of a carbohydrate occurring in their cell walls (Lancefield antigen).

β-hemolytic group A streptococci (*S. pyogenes*) cause infections of the upper respiratory tract and invasive infections of the skin and subcutaneous connective tissue. Depending on the status of the immune defenses and the genetic disposition, this may lead to scarlet fever and severe infections such as necrotizing fasciitis, sepsis, or septic shock. Sequelae such as acute rheumatic fever and glomerulonephritis have an autoimmune pathogenesis. The α-hemolytic pneumococci (*S. pneumoniae*) cause infections of the respiratory tract. Penicillins are the antibiotics of choice. Resistance to penicillins is known among pneumococci, and is increasing. Laboratory diagnosis involves pathogen detection in the appropriate material. Persons at high risk can be protected from pneumococcal infections with an active prophylactic vaccine containing purified capsular polysaccharides. Certain oral streptococci are responsible for dental caries. Oral streptococci also cause half of all cases of endocarditis.

Although **enterococci** show only low levels of pathogenicity, they frequently cause nosocomial infections in immunocompromised patients (usually as elements of a mixed flora). ■

Streptococci are round to oval, Gram-positive, nonmotile, nonsporing bacteria that form winding chains (streptos [greek] = twisted) or diplococci. They do not produce catalase. Most are components of the normal flora of the mucosa. Some can cause infections in humans and animals.

Classification. The genera *Streptococcus* and *Enterococcus* comprise a large number of species. Table 4.**2** lists the most important.

■ **α-, β-, γ-hemolysis.**

α-hemolysis. Colonies on blood agar are surrounded by a green zone. This "greening" is caused by H_2O_2, which converts hemoglobin into methemoglobin.

β-hemolysis. Colonies on blood agar are surrounded by a large, yellowish hemolytic zone in which no more intact erythrocytes are present and the hemoglobin is decomposed.

γ-hemolysis. This (illogical) term indicates the absence of macroscopically visible hemolytic zones.

■ **Lancefield groups.** Many streptococci and enterococci have a polymeric carbohydrate (C substance) in their cell walls called the Lancefield antigen. They are classified in Lancefield groups A–V based on variations in the antigenicity of this antigen.

Specific characteristics of enterococci that differentiate them from streptococci include their ability to proliferate in the presence of 6.5% NaCl, at 45 °C and at a pH level of 9.6.

Table **4.2** The Most Important Human Pathogen Streptococci and Enterococci

Species	Hemolysis	Group antigen	Remarks
Pyogenic, hemolytic streptococci			
Streptococcus pyogenes (A streptococci)	β	A	Frequent pathogen in humans; invasive infections, sequelae
S. agalactiae (B streptococci)	β	B	Meningitis/sepsis in neonates; invasive infections in predisposed persons
C streptococci	β(α; γ)	C	Rare; purulent infections (similar to *S. pyogenes* infections)
G streptococci	β	G	Rare; purulent infections (similar to *S. pyogenes* infections)
S. pneumoniae	α	–	Pneumococci; respiratory tract infections; sepsis; meningitis
S. bovis	α; γ	D	Not enterococci, although in group D; rare sepsis pathogen; if isolated from blood work up for pathological colon processes
Oral streptococci (selection)			
S. salivarius *S. sanguis* *S. mutans* *S. mitis* *S. anginosus* *S. constellatus* *S. intermedius* etc.	α; γ	A, C, E, F, G, H, K occasionally detectable *S. milleri* group	Greening (viridans) streptococci; occur in oral cavity; endocarditis; caries (*S. mutans*, *S. sanguis*, *S. mitis*) Purulent abscesses
Enterococci (Enterococcus)			
E. faecalis *E. faecium*	α; γ; β α	D D	Occur in human and animal intestines; low-level pathogenicity; endocarditis; nosocomial infections. Often component of mixed florae.

Streptococcus pyogenes (A Streptococci)

Morphology and culturing. Gram-positive cocci with a diameter of 1 μm that form chains (Fig. 4.**3a**). Colonies on blood agar (Fig. 4.**3b**) show β-hemolysis caused by streptolysins (see below).

Fine structure. The murein layer of the cell wall is followed by the serogroup A carbohydrate layer, which consists of C substance and is covalently bound to the murein. Long, twisted protein threads that extend outward are anchored in the cell wall murein: the M protein. A streptococci are classified in serovars with characteristic M protein chemistry. Like the hyaluronic acid capsules seen in some strains, the M protein has an antiphagocytic effect.

4

--- *Streptococcus Pyogenes* ---

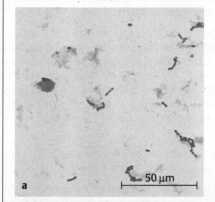

50 μm

a

Fig. 4.**3** **a** Gram staining of pleural puncture biopsy material: gram-positive cocci in twisted chains. **b** Culture on blood agar: small, whitish-gray colonies surrounded by large β-hemolysis zones; a 5% CO_2 atmosphere provides optimum conditions for β-hemolysis.

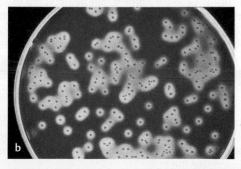

b

Extracellular toxins and enzymes. The most important in the context of pathogenicity are:

■ **Streptolysin O, streptolysin S.** Destroy the membranes of erythrocytes and other cells. Streptolysin O acts as an antigen. Past infections can be detected by measuring the antibodies to this toxin (antistreptolysin titer).

■ **Pyrogenic streptococcal exotoxins** (PSE) A, B, C. Responsible for fever, scarlet fever exanthem and enanthem, sepsis, and septic shock. The pyrogenic exotoxins are superantigens and therefore induce production of large amounts of cytokines (p. 77).

■ **Streptokinase.** Dissolves fibrin; facilitates spread of streptococci in tissues.

■ **Hyaluronidase.** Breaks down a substance that cements tissues together.

■ **DNases.** Breakdown of DNA, producing runny pus.

Pathogenesis and clinical pictures. Streptococcal diseases can be classified as either acute, invasive infections or sequelae to them.

■ **Invasive infections.** The pathogens enter through traumas or microtraumas in the skin or mucosa and cause invasive local or generalized infections (Fig. 4.**4**). The rare cases of severe septic infection and necrotizing fasciitis occur in persons with a high-risk MHC II allotype. In these patients, the PSE superantigens (especially PSEA) induce large amounts of cytokine by binding at the same time to the MHC II complex and the β chain of the T cell receptor. The excess cytokines thus produced are the cause of the symptoms.

■ **Sequelae.** Glomerulonephritis is an immune complex disease (p. 113) and acute rheumatic fever may be a type II immune disease (p. 109).

Diagnosis. What is involved in diagnosis is detection of the pathogen by means of microscopy and culturing. Group A antigen can be detected using particles coated with antibodies that precipitate agglutination (latex agglutination, coagglutination). Using these methods, direct detection of A streptococci in tonsillitis is feasible in the medical practice. However, this direct detection method is not as sensitive as the culture. Differentiation of A streptococci from other β-hemolytic streptococci can be realized in the laboratory with the bacitracin disk test, because A streptococci are more sensitive to bacitracin than the other types.

Therapy. The agents of choice are penicillin G or V. Resistance is unknown. Alternatives are oral cephalosporins or macrolide antibiotics, although resistance to the latter can be expected. In treatment of septic shock, a polyvalent immunoglobulin is used to inactivate the PSE.

Streptococcus pyogenes Infections

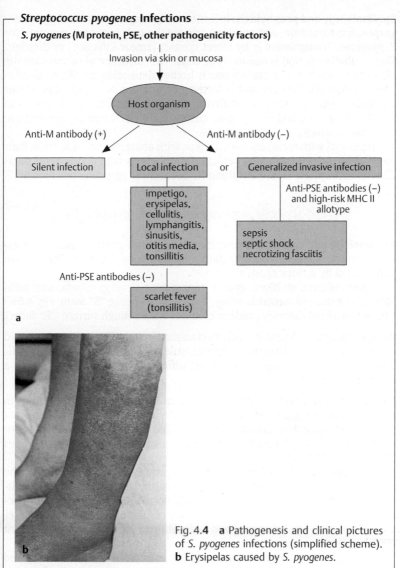

Fig. 4.4 **a** Pathogenesis and clinical pictures of *S. pyogenes* infections (simplified scheme). **b** Erysipelas caused by *S. pyogenes*.

Epidemiology and prophylaxis. Infection frequency varies according to geographical area, season, and age. Humans are the only pathogen reservoir for *S. pyogenes*. Transmission is by direct contact (smear infection) or droplets. The incubation period is one to three days. The incidence of carriers among children is 10–20%, but can be much higher depending on the epidemiological situation. Carriers and infected persons are no longer contagious 24 hours after the start of antibiotic therapy. Microbiological follow-up checks of patients and first-degree contacts are not necessary (exception: rheumatic history).

In persons with recurring infections or with acute rheumatic fever in their medical histories, continuous penicillin prophylaxis with a long-term penicillin is appropriate (e.g., 1.2 million IU benzathine penicillin per month).

Streptococcus pneumoniae (Pneumococci)

Morphology and culturing. Pneumococci are Gram-positive, oval to lancet-shaped cocci that usually occur in pairs or short chains (Fig. **4.5a**). The cells are surrounded by a thick capsule.

When cultured on blood agar, *S. pneumoniae* develop α-hemolytic colonies with a mucoid (smooth, shiny) appearance (hence "S" form, Fig. **4.5b**). Mutants without capsules produce colonies with a rough surface ("R" form).

Antigen structure. Pneumococci are classified in 90 different serovars based on the fine chemical structure of the capsule polysaccharides acting as antigens. This capsule antigen can be identified using specific antisera in a reaction known as capsular swelling.

Pathogenesis and clinical pictures. The capsule protects the pathogens from phagocytosis and is the most important determinant of pneumococcal virulence. Unencapsulated variants are not capable of causing disease. Other potential virulence factors include pneumolysin with its effects on membranes and an IgA_1 protease.

The natural habitat of pneumococci is provided by the mucosa of the upper respiratory tract. About 40–70% of healthy adults are carriers. Pneumococcal infections usually arise from this normal flora (endogenous infections). Predisposing factors include primary cardiopulmonary diseases, previous infections (e.g., influenza), and extirpation of the spleen or complement system defects.

The most important pneumococcal infections are **lobar pneumonia** and **bronchopneumonia**. Other infections include acute exacerbation of chronic bronchitis, otitis media, sinusitis, meningitis, and corneal ulcer. Severe pneumococcal infections frequently involve sepsis.

Streptococcus pneumoniae

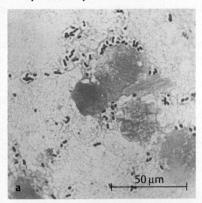

Fig. 4.5 **a** Gram staining of a preparation of middle ear secretion: gram-positive, round-oval, encapsulated cocci; clinical diagnosis: otitis media.

b Culture on blood agar: gray colonies showing little intrinsic color, often mucoid (due to capsules); a zone of greening is often observed around the colonies, caused by α-hemolysis; the shiny appearance of the colonies is caused by light reflections from their mucoid surface.

50 μm

4

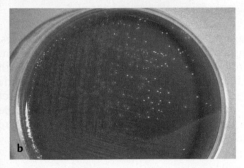

Diagnosis. The laboratory diagnosis includes detection of the pathogen in appropriate test samples by means of microscopy and culturing. Pneumococci can be differentiated from other α-hemolytic streptococci based on their greater sensitivity to optochin (ethyl hydrocuprein hydrochloride) in the disk test or their bile solubility. Bile salts increase autolysis in pneumococci.

Therapy. Penicillin is still the antibiotic of choice. There have been reports of high-frequency occurrence of strains resistant to penicillin (South Africa, Spain, Hungary, USA). These strains are still relatively rare in Germany, Switzerland, and Austria (5–10%). Macrolide antibiotics are an alternative to penicillins, but resistance to them is also possible.

Penicillin resistance is not due to penicillinase, but rather to modified penicillin-binding proteins (PBPs) to which penicillins have a lower level of affinity. PBPs are required for murein biosynthesis. Biochemically, penicillin resistance extends to cephalosporins as well. However, certain cephalosporins (e.g., ceftriaxone) can be used against penicillin-resistant pneumococci due to their higher levels of activity.

Epidemiology and prophylaxis. Pneumococcal infections are endemic and occur in all seasons, more frequently in the elderly. Humans are the natural pathogen reservoir.

The vaccine product Pneumovax® is available for immunization purposes. It contains 25 mg of the purified capsule polysaccharides of each of 23 of the most frequent serovars. Eighty to ninety percent of all isolated pneumococci have antigens contained in this vaccine, which is primarily indicated in persons with predisposing primary diseases. There is also a seven-valent conjugate vaccine that is effective in children under two years of age (p. 33). Exposure prophylaxis is not necessary.

Streptococcus agalactiae (B Streptococci)

B streptococci occasionally cause infections of the skin and connective tissues, sepsis, urinary tract infections, pneumonia, and peritonitis in immunocompromised individuals. About one in 1000 neonates suffers from a sepsis with or without meningitis. These infections manifest in the first days of life (early onset type) or in the first weeks of life (late onset type). In the early onset form, the infection is caused intra partum by B streptococci colonizing the vagina. Potential predisposing factors include birth complications, premature birth, and a lack of antibodies to the capsule in mother and neonate.

Oral Streptococci

Most of the oral streptococci of the type often known as the viridans group have no group antigen. They usually cause α-hemolysis, some γ-hemolysis as well.

Oral streptococci are responsible for 50–70% of all cases of bacterial **endocarditis**, overall incidence of which is one to two cases per 100 000 annually. The origins of endocarditis lie in invasion of the vascular system through lesions in the oral mucosa. A transitory bacteremia results. The heart valves are colonized and a biofilm is formed by the organism. Predisposing factors include congenital heart defects, acute rheumatic fever, cardiac surgery, and scarred heart valves. Laboratory diagnosis of endocarditis involves isolation of the pathogen from blood cultures. Drug therapy of endocarditis is carried out with either penicillin G alone or combined with an aminoglycoside (mostly gentamicin). Bactericidal activity is the decisive parameter.

Pronounced Dental Caries

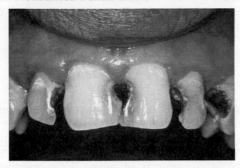

Fig. 4.**6** Certain oral streptococci (*S. mutans*) are the main culprits in tooth decay.

4

S. mutans, *S. sanguis*, and *S. mitis* are, besides *Actinomyces viscosus* and *A. naeslundii*, responsible for **dental caries** (Fig. 4.**6**). These streptococci can attach to the proteins covering the tooth enamel, where they then convert sucrose into extracellular polysaccharides (mutan, dextran, levan). These sticky substances, in which the original bacterial layer along with secondary bacterial colonizers are embedded, form dental plaque. The final metabolites of the numerous plaque bacteria are organic acids that breach the enamel, allowing the different caries bacteria to begin destroying the dentin.

Enterococcus (Enterococci)

Enterococci are a widespread bacterial genus (p. 220) normally found in the intestines of humans and other animals. They are nonmotile, catalase-negative, and characterized by group antigen D. They are able to proliferate at 45 °C, in the presence of 6.5% NaCl and at pH 9, qualities that differentiate them from streptococci. As classic opportunists, enterococci show only low levels of pathogenicity. However, they are frequently isolated as components of a mixed flora in nosocomial infections (p. 343). Ninety percent of such isolates are identified as *E. faecalis*, 5–10% as *E. faecium*. Among the most dangerous enterococcal infections is endocarditis, which must be treated with a combination of an aminopenicillin and streptomycin or gentamicin. Therapeutic success depends on the bactericidal efficacy of the combination used. The efficacy level will be insufficient in the presence of high levels of resistance to either streptomycin (MIC >1000 mg/l) or gentamicin (MIC >500 mg/l) or resistance to the aminopenicillin. Enterococci frequently develop resistance to antibiotics. Strains manifesting multiple resistance are found mainly in hospitals, in keeping with the classic opportunistic character of these pathogens. Recently observed epidemics on intensive care wards involved strains that were resistant to all standard anti-infective agents including the glycopeptides vancomycin and teicoplanin.

Gram-Positive, Anaerobic Cocci

Gram-positive, strictly anaerobic cocci are included in the genera *Peptococcus* and *Peptostreptococcus*. The only species in the first genus is *Peptococcus niger*, whereas the latter comprises a number of species. The anaerobic cocci are commonly observed in normal human flora. In a pathogenic context they are usually only encountered as components of mixed florae together with other anaerobes or facultative anaerobes. These bacteria invade tissues through dermal or mucosal injuries and cause subacute purulent infections. Such infections are either localized in the head area (cerebral abscess, otitis media, mastoiditis, sinusitis) or lower respiratory tract (necrotizing pneumonia, pulmonary abscess, empyema). They are also known to occur in the abdomen (appendicitis, peritonitis, hepatic abscess) and female genitals (salpingitis, endometriosis, tubo-ovarian abscess). Gram-positive anaerobic cocci may also contribute to soft-tissue infections and postoperative wound infections. See p. 317ff. for clinical details of anaerobe infections.

Bacillus

■ The natural habitat of *Bacillus anthracis*, a Gram-positive, sporing, obligate aerobic rod bacterium, is the soil. The organism causes **anthrax** infections in animals. Human infections result from contact with sick animals or animal products contaminated with the spores. Infections are classified according to the portal of entry as dermal anthrax (95% of cases), primary inhalational anthrax, and intestinal anthrax. Sepsis can develop from the primary infection focus. Laboratory diagnosis includes microscopic and cultural detection of the pathogen in relevant materials and blood cultures. The therapeutic agent of choice is penicillin G. ■

The genera *Bacillus* and *Clostridium* belong to the *Bacillaceae* family of sporing bacteria. There are numerous species in the genus *Bacillus* (e.g., *B. cereus*, *B. subtilis*, etc.) that normally live in the soil. The organism in the group that is of veterinary and human medical interest is *Bacillus anthracis*.

Bacillus anthracis (Anthrax)

Occurrence. Anthrax occurs primarily in animals, especially herbivores. The pathogens are ingested with feed and cause a severe clinical sepsis that is often lethal.

Morphology and culturing. The rods are 1 µm wide and 2–4 µm long, non-flagellated, with a capsule made of a glutamic acid polypeptide. The bacterium is readily grown in an aerobic milieu.

Pathogenesis and clinical picture. The pathogenicity of *B. anthracis* results from its antiphagocytic capsule as well as from a toxin that causes edemas and tissue necrosis. Human infections are contracted from diseased animals or contaminated animal products. Anthrax is recognized as an occupational disease.

4

Dermal, primary inhalational, and intestinal anthrax are differentiated based on the pathogen's portal of entry. In dermal anthrax, which accounts for 90–95 % of human *B. anthracis* infections) the pathogens enter through injuries in the skin. A local infection focus similar to a carbuncle develops within two to three days. A sepsis with a foudroyant (highly acute) course may then develop from this primary focus. Inhalational anthrax (bioterrorist anthrax), with its unfavorable prognosis, results from inhalation of dust containing the pathogen. Ingestion of contaminated foods can result in intestinal anthrax with vomiting and bloody diarrheas.

Diagnosis. The diagnostic procedure involves detection of the pathogen in dermal lesions, sputum, and/or blood cultures using microscopic and culturing methods.

Therapy. The antimicrobial agent of choice is penicillin G. Doxycycline (a tetracycline) or ciprofloxacin (a fluoroquinolone) are possible alternatives. Surgery is contraindicated in cases of dermal anthrax.

Epidemiology and prophylaxis. Anthrax occurs mainly in southern Europe and South America, where economic damage due to farm animal infections is considerable. Humans catch the disease from infected animals or contaminated animal products. Anthrax is a classic zoonosis.

Prophylaxis involves mainly exposure prevention measures such as avoiding contact with diseased animals and disinfection of contaminated products. A cell-free vaccine obtained from a culture filtrate can be used for vaccine prophylaxis in high-risk persons.

Clostridium

■ Clostridia are 3–8 μm long, thick, Gram-positive, sporing rod bacteria that can only be cultured anaerobically. Their natural habitat is the soil. The pathogenicity of the disease-causing species in this genus is due to production of exotoxins and/or exoenzymes. The most frequent causative organism in **anaerobic cellulitis** and **gas gangrene** (clostridial myonecrosis) is *C. perfringens*. **Tetanus** is caused by *C. tetani*. This pathogen produces the exotoxin tetanospasmin, which blocks transmission of inhibitory CNS impulses to motor neurons. **Botulism** is a type of food poisoning caused by the neurotoxins of *C. botulinum*. These substances inhibit stimulus transmission to the motor end plates. **Pseudomembranous colitis** is caused by *C. difficile*, which produces an enterotoxin (A) and a cytotoxin (B). Diagnosis of clostridial infections requires identification of the pathogen (gas gangrene) and/or the toxins (tetanus, botulism, colitis). All clostridia are readily sensitive to penicillin G. Antitoxins are used in therapy of tetanus and botulism and hyperbaric O_2 is used to treat gas gangrene. The most important preventive measure against tetanus is active vaccination with tetanus toxoid. ■

Occurrence. Clostridia are sporing bacteria that naturally inhabit the soil and the intestinal tracts of humans and animals. Many species are apathogenic saprophytes. Under certain conditions, several species cause gas gangrene, tetanus, botulism, and pseudomembranous colitis.

Morphology and culturing. All clostridia are large, Gram-positive rod bacteria about 1 μm thick and 3–8 μm in length (Fig. 4.**7**). Many cells in older cultures show a Gram-negative reaction. With the exception of *C. perfringens*, clostridia are flagellated. Clostridia sporulate. They are best cultured in an anaerobic atmosphere at 37 °C. *C. perfringens* colonies are convex, smooth, and surrounded by a hemolytic zone. Colonies of motile clostridia have an irregular, ragged edge.

The Pathogens That Cause Gas Gangrene (Clostridial Myonecrosis) and Anaerobic Cellulitis

Pathogen spectrum. The pathogens that cause these clinical pictures include *Clostridium perfringens*, *C. novyi*, *C. septicum*, and *C. histolyticum*. Species observed less frequently include *C. sporogenes*, *C. sordellii*, and *C. bifermentans*. The most frequent causative pathogen in gas gangrene is *C. perfringens*.

Toxins, enzymes. The toxins produced by invasive clostridia show necrotizing, hemolytic, and/or lethal activity. They also produce collagenases,

Clostridium perfringens and sporogenes

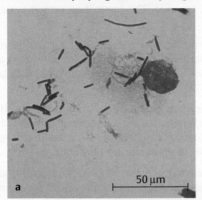

Fig. 4.**7** **a** *C. perfringens*: gram staining of a preparation of wound pus. Large, thick, gram-positive rods. Clinical diagnosis: gas gangrene in a gunshot wound.

b *C. sporogenes*: Spore staining of a preparation from an aged broth culture. Thick-walled spores stained red. Occasionally "tennis racquet" forms.

4

a   50 μm

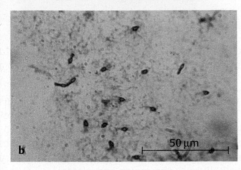

b   50 μm

proteinases, DNases, lecithinases, and hyaluronidase, all of which destroy tissue structures, resulting in accumulations of toxic metabolites.

Pathogenesis and clinical picture. Due to the ubiquitous presence of clostridia, they frequently contaminate open wounds, often together with other microorganisms. Detection of clostridia in a wound is therefore no indication of a clostridial infection. These infections develop when a low tissue redox potential makes anaerobe reproduction possible, resulting in tissue necrosis. Two such infections of differing severity are described below:

■ **Anaerobic cellulitis.** Infection restricted to the fascial spaces that does not affect musculature. Gas formation in tissues causes a cracking, popping sensation under the skin known as crepitus. There is no toxemia.

■ **Gas gangrene (clostridial myonecrosis).** An aggressive infection of the musculature with myonecrosis and toxemia. The incubation period varies from hours to a few days.

Diagnosis. The diagnostic procedure includes identification of the pathogens in relevant materials by means of microscopy and culturing. Identification of anaerobically grown cultures is based on morphological and physiological characteristics.

Therapy. Primary treatment is surgical, accompanied by antibiosis (penicillins, cephalosporins). Treatment with hyperbaric O_2 in special centers has proved effective: patients breathe pure O_2 through a tube or mask in a pressure chamber (3 atm = 303 kPa) several times during two-hour periods.

Epidemiology and prevention. True gas gangrene is now a rare condition. Timely operation of contaminated wounds is the main preventive measure.

Clostridium tetani (Tetanus)

Tetanus (lockjaw) is an acute clostridial disease, its clinical manifestations do not result directly from the invasive infection, but are rather caused by a strong neurotoxin.

Toxin. Tetanospasmin (an AB toxin, p. 16) consists of two polypeptide chains linked by a disulfide bridge. The heavy chain binds specifically to neuron receptors. The light chain is a zinc-metalloprotease that is responsible for proteolysis of components of the neuroexocytosis apparatus in the synapses of the anterior horns of the spinal cord. This stops transmission of inhibitory efferent impulses from the cerebellum to the motor end plates.

Pathogenesis and clinical picture. These ubiquitous pathogens invade tissues following injuries (Fig. 4.**8a**). Given anaerobic conditions, they proliferate and produce the toxin (see above), which reaches the anterior horns of the spinal cord or brain stem via retrograde axonal transport. The clinical picture resulting from the effects of the toxin is characterized by increased muscle tone and spasms induced by visual or acoustic stimuli. The cramps often begin in the facial musculature (risus sardonicus, Fig. 4.**8b**), then spread to neck and back muscles (opisthotonus). The patient remains lucid.

Diagnosis. The preferred method is toxin detection in wound material in an animal test (mouse) based either on neutralization or detection of the toxin gene with PCR. The pathogen is difficult to culture.

Therapy. Antitoxic therapy with immune sera is applied following a meticulous wound cleaning. The patient's musculature must also be relaxed with curare or similar agents.

— Tetanus

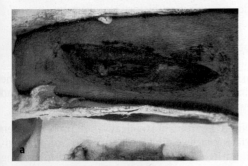

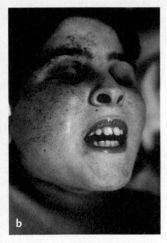

Fig. 4.**8** **a** Open lower-leg fracture following a traffic accident; the portal of entry of *C. tetani*.
b Risus sardonicus: fully manifest case of tetanus in a patient with lower-leg fracture. Patient was not vaccinated.

4

Epidemiology and prophylaxis. Tetanus is now rare in developed countries due to widespread vaccination practice with incidence rates of approximately one case per million inhabitants per year. The frequency of occurrence is much higher in developing or underdeveloped countries. Worldwide, about 300 000 persons contract tetanus every year, with a lethality rate of approximately 50%. Thus, the importance of the active vaccination as a protective measure can hardly be overstated (see p. 33 for vaccination schedule). A dose of Td should be administered once every 10 years to sustain protection (p. 33). A booster shot is also required in case of severe injury if the patient's last inoculation was administered longer than five years before, and in case of minor injury longer than 10 years. Human tetanus immunoglobulin (250 IU) must be administered to severely injured persons with insufficient vaccination protection or if the basic immunization history is uncertain.

Clostridium botulinum (Botulism)

Foodborne botulism is not an infection, but rather an intoxication, that is, the toxin is ingested with food. Infant botulism involves ingestion of spores and wound botulism results from infection of a wound.

Toxin. The very strong botulinum neurotoxin is a heat-labile protein. Seven toxigenic types are differentiated, each of which produces an immunologically distinct form of botulinum toxin. Types A, B, and E cause poisoning in humans. The toxin is a metalloprotease that catalyzes the proteolysis of components of the neuroexocytosis apparatus in the motor end plates, resulting in flaccid paralysis of the musculature.

Pathogenesis and clinical picture. Classic botulism results from eating spoiled foods in which the toxin has been produced under anaerobic conditions by *C. botulinum*. The toxin is absorbed in the gastrointestinal tract, and then transported to the peripheral nervous system in the bloodstream.

   Within a matter of hours or days paralysis symptoms occur, especially in the nerves of the head. Frequent symptoms include seeing double, difficulty swallowing and speaking, constipation, and dry mucosa. Lethality rates range from 25–70%, depending on the amount of toxin ingested. Death usually results from respiratory paralysis. **Wound botulism** results from wound infection by *C. botulinum* and is very rare. **Infant botulism**, first described in 1976, results from ingestion of spores with food (e.g., honey). Probably due to the conditions prevailing in the intestines of infants up to the age of six months, the spores are able to proliferate there and produce the toxin. The lethality of infant botulism is low (<1%).

Diagnosis. Based on toxin detection by means of the mouse neutralization test.

Therapy. Urgent administration of a polyvalent antitoxin.

Epidemiology and prevention. Botulism is a rare disease. Exposure to the toxin is a food hygiene problem that can be avoided by taking appropriate precautions during food production. Aerosolized botulinum toxin has been used experimentally as a bioweapon.

Clostridium difficile (Pseudomembranous Colitis)

C. difficile occurs in the fecal flora of 1–4% of healthy adults and in 30–50% of children during the first year of life. The factors that lead to development of the disease are not known with certainty. Cases of pseudomembranous colitis are observed frequently under treatment with clindamycin, aminopenicillins, and cephalosporins (hence the designation **antibiotic-associated colitis**), but also occur in persons not taking antibiotics. Occasional outbreaks are seen in hospitals. The **pathological mechanism** is based on formation of two toxins. Toxin A is an enterotoxin that causes a dysfunction characterized by increased secretion of electrolytes and fluids. Toxin B is a cytotoxin that damages the mucosa of the colon.

The **clinical course** includes fever, diarrhea, and spasmodic abdominal pains. Coloscopy reveals edematous changes in the colon mucosa, which is also covered with yellowish-whitish matter. **Laboratory diagnosis** involves culturing the pathogen from patient stool and detection of the cytotoxin in bacteria-free stool filtrates on the basis of a cytopathic effect (CPE) observed in cell cultures, which CPE is then no longer observed after neutralization with an antiserum. Toxins A and B can also be detected with immunological test kits (ELISA tests, see p. 127f.). A specific **therapy** is not required in many cases. Antibiotic treatment is indicated in severe cases. The agent of choice is currently metronidazole.

Listeria, Erysipelothrix, and Gardnerella

■ *Listeria monocytogenes* are diminutive Gram-positive rods with peritrichous flagellation that are quite motile at 20 °C and can be cultured aerobically on blood agar. They occur ubiquitously in nature. Human infections may result if 10^6–10^9 pathogens enter the gastrointestinal tract with food. Listeriae are classic opportunists. In immunocompetent persons, an infection will either be clinically silent or present the picture of a mild flu. In immunocompromised patients, the disease manifests as a primary sepsis and/or meningoencephalitis. More rarely, listeriae cause endocarditis. Listeriosis during pregnancy may result in spontaneous abortion or connatal listeriosis (granulomatosis infantiseptica). Penicillins (amoxicillin) and cotrimoxazole, sometimes in combination with aminoglycosides, are used in therapy. Listeriosis is a rare infection characterized by sporadic occurrence. Occasional gastrointestinal epidemics due to contaminated food may result from the coincidence of unfortunate circumstances.

Erysipelothrix rhusiopathiae, the pathogen that causes the zoonosis swine erysipelas, is the causative organism in the human infection erysipeloid, now a rare occupational disease.

Gardnerella vaginalis is usually responsible, in combination with other bacteria, for nonspecific vaginitis (vaginosis). ■

Listeria monocytogenes

The only listeriae that cause human disease are *L. monocytogenes* and the rare species *L. ivanovii*. The designation *L. monocytogenes* results from the observation that infections of rodents, which are much more susceptible than humans, are accompanied by a monocytosis.

Morphology and culturing. The small Gram-positive rods feature peritrichous flagellation. They show greater motility at 20 °C than at 37 °C. Culturing is most successful under aerobic conditions on blood agar. Following incubation for 18 hours, small gray colonies surrounded by inconspicuous hemolytic zones appear. The zones are caused by listeriolysin O. Listeriae can also reproduce at 5–10 °C, which fact can be used in their selective enrichment ("cold enrichment").

Pathogenesis. Studies of the molecular processes involved have used mainly systemically infected mice.

■ **Adherence.** To phagocytic cells (e.g., macrophages) and nonphagocytic cells (e.g., enterocytes).

■ **Invasion.** Endocytosis, induced by the protein internalin on the surface of the listeriae. Formation of the endosome.

■ **Destruction of the endosome.** The virulence factor listeriolysin forms pores in the endosomal membrane, releasing the listeriae into the cytoplasm.

■ **Replication** of the listeriae in the cytoplasm of infected cells.

■ **Local intercellular dissemination.** Polymerization of the actin of infected cells at one pole of the listeriae to form so-called actin tails that move the listeriae toward the membrane. Formation of long membrane protuberances (known as listeriopods) containing listeriae. Neighboring cells engulf the listeriopods, whereupon the process of listeria release by means of endosome destruction is repeated.

■ **Dissemination is generally** by means of hematogenous spread.

Clinical characteristics. Listeriae are classic opportunists. The course of most infections is clinically silent. Symptoms resembling a mild flu do not occur in immunocompetent persons until large numbers of pathogens (10^6–10^9) enter the gastrointestinal tract with food. Massive infections frequently cause symptoms of gastroenteritis.

Listeriosis can take on the form of a **sepsis** and/or **meningoencephalitis** in persons with T cell defects or malignancies, in alcoholics, during cortisone therapy, during pregnancy, in elderly persons and in infants.

Connatal listeriosis is characterized by sepsis with multiple abscesses and granulomas in many different organs of the infant (**granulomatosis infantiseptica**).

The lethality rate in severe cases of listeriosis varies between 10% and 40%. The incubation period can vary from one to three days to weeks.

4

Diagnosis requires pathogen identification by means of microscopy and culturing.

Therapy. Amoxicillin, penicillin G, or cotrimoxazole.

Epidemiology and prevention. Listeriae occur ubiquitously in soil, surface water, plants, and animals and are also found with some frequency (10%) in the intestines of healthy humans. Despite the fact that contact with listeriae is, therefore, quite normal and even frequent, listeriosis is not at all common. The incidence of severe infections is estimated at six cases per 10^6 inhabitants per year. Occurrence is generally sporadic. Small-scale epidemics caused by food products—such as milk, milk products (cheese), meat products, and other foods (e.g., coleslaw)—contaminated with very high numbers of listeriae have been described. Preventive measures include proper processing and storage of food products in keeping with relevant hygienic principles.

Erysipelothrix rhusiopathiae

This bacterium is a slender, nonmotile, Gram-positive rod. *E. rhusiopathiae* causes a septic disease in pigs, swine erysipelas. The correlate in humans is now quite rare and is a recognized occupational disease. Following contact with infectious animal material, the pathogens enter body tissues through dermal injuries. After an incubation period of one to three days, the so-called **erysipeloid**—a hivelike, bluish-red swelling—develops at the site of entry. The lymph nodes are also affected. These benign infections often heal spontaneously and disappear rapidly under treatment with penicillin G. Laboratory diagnostic procedures involve identification of the pathogen in wound secretion using the methods of microscopy and culturing.

Gardnerella vaginalis

G. vaginalis is a Gram-variable, nonmotile, nonencapsulated rod bacterium. Its taxonomy has changed repeatedly in recent decades. It has thus also been designated as *Corynebacterium vaginalis* and *Haemophilus vaginalis*. Based on DNA hybridization, the pathogen is now classified with the regularly shaped, Gram-positive, nonsporing rod bacteria. The natural habitat of this organism is the vagina of sexually mature women. It can also cause vulvovaginitis (vaginosis). *G. vaginalis* is found in over 90% of women showing the symptoms of this infection, usually together with other bacteria including in particular obligate anaerobes (*Mobiluncus*, *Bacteroides*, *Peptostreptococcus*). The organism can be detected in vaginal discharge by means of microscopy and culturing. In the microscopic analysis, so-called clue cells (vaginal epithelia densely covered with Gram-labile rods) provide evidence of the role played by *G. vaginalis*. This bacterium can be cultured on blood-enriched agar incubated in an atmosphere containing 5% CO_2. The therapeutic agent of choice is metronidazole.

Corynebacterium, Actinomyces, Other Gram-Positive Rod Bacteria

■ **Diphtheria bacteria** are pleomorphic, club-shaped rod bacteria that often have polar bodies and group in V, Y, or palisade forms. They can be grown on enriched nutrient media. Their pathogenicity derives from diphtheria toxin, which binds to receptors of sensitive cells with the B fragment. Once the binding process is completed, the active A fragment invades the cell. This substance irreversibly blocks translation in the protein biosynthesis chain. The toxin gene is a component of the β prophage. Local and systemic intoxications are differentiated when evaluating the clinical picture. Local infection usually affects the tonsils, on which the diphtherial pseudomembrane develops. Systemic intoxications affect mainly the liver, kidneys, adrenal glands, cardiac muscle, and cranial nerves. Laboratory diagnosis is based on pathogen identification. The most important treatment is antitoxin therapy. Diphtheria occurs only in humans. Thanks to extensive diphtheria toxoid vaccination programs, it is now rare.

Actinomycetes are part of the normal mucosal flora. These are Gram-positive rods that often occur in the form of branched filaments in young cultures. Conglomerates of microcolonies in pus form so-called sulfur granules. Actinomycetes are obligate anaerobes. The pathogens enter body tissues through mucosa defects. Monoinfections are rare, the most frequent case being actinomycetes-dominated endogenous polyinfections. Cervicofacial actinomycosis, caused by oral cavity colonizer *A. israelii*, is the most frequent form of actinomycosis. Treatment includes surgical procedures and antibiosis with aminopenicillins. ■

The group of Gram-positive, irregular (pleomorphic), nonsporing rod bacteria includes many different genera that are normal components of the skin and mucosal flora (Table 4.**3**, p. 261). Pathogens in this group cause two characteristic diseases: diphtheria, caused by *Corynebacterium diphtheriae* and actinomycosis, caused mainly by *Actinomyces israelii*.

Corynebacterium diphtheriae (Diphtheria)

4

Morphology and culturing. Diphtheria bacteria are Gram-positive, pleomorphic, often club-shaped rods. The individual cells tend to group in V, Y, or palisade arrangements (Fig. 4.**9**). Neisser staining reveals the polar bodies (polyphosphates stored at one end of the rod).

Löffler nutrient medium, which consists of coagulated serum and nutrient broth, is still used for the primary cultures. Selective indicator mediums containing tellurite are used in selective culturing. K tellurite is used to inhibit the accompanying flora. The K tellurite is also reduced to tellurium, coloring the colonies a brownish black.

Extracellular toxin. Diphtheria toxin consists of two functionally distinct fragments, A and B, whereby **B** stands for **binding** to receptors of target cells and **A** stands for toxic **activity**. Fragment A irreversibly blocks protein synthesis translation in the target cells, which then die. The toxin gene is always a prophage genome component (see lysogenic conversion, p. 186).

Corynebacterium diphtheriae

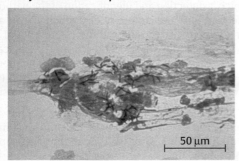

Fig. 4.**9** Gram staining of a wound secretion preparation in wound diphtheria: typical configuration of Gram-positive rods of irregular thickness, often with a clublike enlargement at one end.

50 μm

■ **Diphtheria toxin**

Fragment A is an ADP ribosyl transferase. The enzyme transfers adenosine diphosphate ribose from NAD to the elongation factor eEF2, thereby inactivating it:

$$NAD + eEF2 \rightarrow ADP\ ribosyl\ eEF2 + nicotinamide + H^+$$

eEF2 "translocates" the peptidyl tRNA from the amino acid position A to the peptide position P on the eukaryotic ribosome. Although the toxin gene is integrated in a phage genome, its activity is regulated by the gene product DtxR of the *dtxR* gene of the bacterial cell's genome. DtxR combines with Fe^{2+} to become an active repressor that switches off the transcription of the toxin gene.

Pathogenesis and Clinical Picture

■ **Local infection.** Infection of the mucosa of tonsils, pharynx, nose, and conjunctiva (Fig. 4.**10**). Wounds and skin lesions can also be infected. The pathogens invade the host through these portals, reproduce, and produce toxin, resulting in local cell damage. The inflammatory reaction leads to collection of a grayish-white exudate, the matrix of the "diphtherial pseudomembrane" consisting of fibrin, dead granulocytes, and necrotic epithelial cells. This coating adheres quite strongly to the mucosa. It may extend into the larynx, thus eventually hindering respiration. Regional lymph nodes are highly swollen.

■ **Systemic intoxication.** Parenchymal degeneration in the cardiac muscle, liver, kidneys, and adrenal glands. Motor cranial nerve paralysis. Late sequel damage due to the intoxication is frequently seen after the acute infection has subsided.

Toxin-negative strains of *C. diphtheriae* are occasionally observed as pathogens in endocarditis or dermal infections. The pathogenicity of such strains corresponds to that of commensal corynebacteria (see Table 4.**3**, p. 261).

Diagnosis. The method of choice is detection and identification of the pathogen in cultures from local infection foci. The culture smear, which arrives at the laboratory in transport medium, is plated out on Löffler medium and a selective indicator medium. Identification is based on both morphological and physiological characteristics. The toxin is detected by the Elek-Ouchterlony immunodiffusion test. A molecular method is now also being used to identify the toxin gene. Toxin detection is necessary for a laboratory diagnosis of diphtheria because of the occurrence of toxin-negative strains.

Therapy. Antitoxic serum therapy is the primary treatment and it must commence as soon as possible if diphtheria is suspected. This treatment is supplemented by administration of penicillin or erythromycin.

Nose and Throat (Nasopharyngeal) Diphtheria

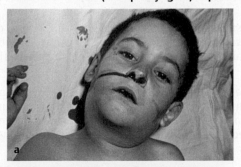

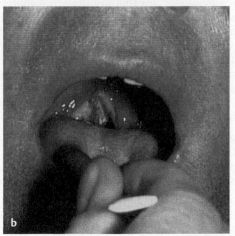

Fig. 4.**10** **a** Hemorrhaging of the nasal mucosa (endothelial damage). Pronounced cervical adenopathy and swelling, creating a bull neck appearance.
b Thick coating (membrane) on highly swollen tonsils (so-called diphtherial pseudomembrane), causing respiratory stridor.

Epidemiology and prevention. Humans are the sole *pathogen reservoir* for diphtheria. *Infection sources* include infected persons and carriers (rare). The disease is usually *transmitted* by droplet infection, or less frequently indirectly via contaminated objects. The *incubation period* is two to five days. Incidence levels in central Europe are low. From 1975 to 1984, only 113 cases were reported in Germany. Incidence levels are higher in other countries (Russia). *Protective immunization* with diphtheria toxoid is the most important preventive measure (see Table 1.**13**, p. 33). *Exposure prophylaxis* involves isolation of infected persons until two cultures from specimens taken at least 24 hours apart are negative.

Actinomyces

Actinomycetes are Gram-positive bacteria that tend to grow in the form of branched filaments. The resulting mycelial masses are, however, not observed in older cultures, which strongly resemble those of corynebacteria in their morphology.

Occurrence. Actinomycetes are part of the normal mucosal flora in humans and animals. They colonize mainly the oral cavity, and an actinomycosis infection is therefore always endogenous. Ninety percent of actinomycetes infections in humans are caused by *A. israelii*, with far fewer cases caused by *A. naeslundii* and other species.

Morphology and culture. Actinomycetes are Gram-positive, pleomorphic rod bacteria that sometimes also show genuine branching (Fig. 4.11). The yellowish **sulfur granules**, measuring 1–2 mm, can be observed macroscopically in actinomycetes pus. These particles are conglomerates of small *Actinomyces* colonies surrounded by a wall of leukocytes. Mycelial filaments extend radially from the colonies (actinium = Greek for raylike). Culturing the organism requires enriched mediums and an anaerobic milieu containing 5–10% CO_2. Mycelial microcolonies form only during the first days. Whitish macrocolonies, often with a rough surface, begin to appear after two weeks.

Pathogenesis and clinical picture. The pathogens breach mucosa (perhaps normal dermis as well) and are able to establish themselves in tissue in the presence of a low redox potential. The factors responsible for these conditions include poor blood perfusion and, above all, contributing bacterial

---

Actinomyces israelii

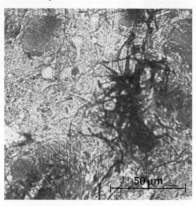

Fig. 4.**11** Gram staining of a pus preparation in cervicofacial actinomycosis: mass of Gram-positive, branched rods; next to them mixed Gram-negative flora. Tentative clinical diagnosis: actinomycosis.

50 μm

pathogens. Genuine actinomycoses are actually always polymicrobial. The mixed flora found includes mainly the anaerobes of the oral cavity. *Actinobacillus actinomycetemcomitans* is frequently isolated along with various species of *Bacteroidaceae*. Facultative anaerobes such as staphylococci, streptococci, and *Enterobacteriaceae* are, however, also found among the contributing flora.

■ **Cervicofacial actinomycosis.** This is the most frequent form of actinomycetes infection (>90%). The abscesses are hard and tumorlike at first, then they necrotize. They may also break through to the dermal surface to create fistulae.

■ **Thoracic actinomycosis.** This rare form results from aspiration of saliva; sometimes this type also develops from an actinomycosis in the throat or hematogenous spread.

■ **Abdominal actinomycosis.** This type results from injuries to the intestine or female genitals.

■ **Genital actinomycosis.** May result from use of intrauterine contraceptive devices.

■ **Canaliculitis.** An inflammation of the lacrimal canaliculi caused by any of several *Actinomyces* species.

■ **Caries.** The *Actinomyces* species involved in caries development are *A. viscosus*, *A. naeslundii*, and *A. odontolyticus* (p. 243f.). A possible contribution to periodontitis is also under discussion.

Diagnosis involves identification of the pathogen by microscopy and culturing in pus, fistula secretion, granulation tissue, or bronchial secretion. The samples must not be contaminated with other patient flora, in particular from the oral cavity and must be transported to the laboratory in special anaerobe containers. Microscopic detection of branched rods suffices for a tentative diagnosis. Detection of mycelial microcolonies on enriched nutrient mediums after one to two weeks further consolidates this diagnosis. Final identification by means of direct immunofluorescence, cell wall analysis, and metabolic analysis requires several weeks.

Therapy. Treatment includes both surgical and antibiotic measures. The antibiotic of choice is an aminopenicillin. Antibiosis that also covers the contributing bacterial pathogens is important.

Epidemiology and prevention. Actinomycoses occur sporadically worldwide. Average morbidity (incidence) levels are between 2.5 and five cases per 100 000 inhabitants per year. Men are infected twice as often as women. Prophylactic considerations are irrelevant due to the endogenous nature of actinomycetes infections.

Other Gram-Positive Rod Bacteria

Table 4.3 lists bacteria that are rarely involved in infections and normally infect only persons with defective immune defenses. Recent years have seen considerable changes in their classification and nomenclature—still an ongoing process. Many of these bacteria are part of the normal dermal and mucosal flora. They are frequently found in sampled materials as contaminants, but also occasionally cause infections. Some of these bacteria are designated by collective terms such as "diphtheroid rods" or "coryneform bacteria."

Table 4.**3**   Gram-Positive Rods with (Generally) Low-Level Pathogenicity

Actinomyces pyogenes	Cutaneous and subcutaneous purulent infections.
Arcanobacterium hemolyticum	Purulent dermal infections; pharyngitis?
Corynebacterium ulcerans	Can produce diphtheria toxin and therefore cause diphtherialike clinical symptoms
C. jeikeium	Dermal pathogen. Occasionally isolated from blood, wounds, or intravasal catheters. Often shows multiple antibiotic resistance.
C. xerosis *C. pseudodiphtheriticum*	Rare endocarditis pathogens.
Gordona bronchialis	Colonizes and infects the respiratory tract.
Rhodococcus equi	Infections of the respiratory tract in immunosuppressed persons.
Tsukamurella sp.	Infections of the respiratory tract in immunosuppressed persons; meningitis.
Turicella otitidis	Infections of the ear in predisposed persons.
Propionibacterium acnes *P. granulosum* *P. avidum*	Anaerobic or microaerophilic. Rarely involved in endocarditis. *P. acnes* is thought to be involved in the development of acne.
Eubacterium sp.	Obligate anaerobe. Normal flora of the intestinal tract. Sometimes component of an anaerobic mixed flora.
Tropheryma whipplei (nov. gen.; nov. spec.; formerly *T. whippelii*)	Causal pathogen in Whipple's disease. Culture growth of this organism has not been possible to date. Probable taxonomic classification in proximity to actinomycetes. Little is known about this organism. Rare, chronic systemic disease. Dystrophy of small intestine mucosa (100%). Also involvement of cardiovascular system (55%), respiratory tract (50%), central nervous system (25%), and eyes (10%). Primary clinical symptoms are weight loss, arthralgias, diarrhea, abdominal pain. Microscopic detection and identification in small intestine biopsies, other biopsies or cerebrospinal fluid (PAS staining) or by molecular methods (see p. 216). Cotrimoxazole is the antibiotic agent of choice.
Mobiluncus mulieri *M. curtisii*	Obligate anaerobic. Colonize the vagina; frequently isolated in cases of bacterial vaginosis together with *Gardnerella vaginalis* and other bacteria.

4

Mycobacterium

■ Mycobacteria are slender rod bacteria that are stained with special differential stains (Ziehl-Neelsen). Once the staining has taken, they cannot be destained with dilute acids, hence the designation acid-fast. In terms of human disease, the most important mycobacteria are the tuberculosis bacteria (TB) *M. tuberculosis* and *M. bovis* and the leprosy pathogen (LB) *M. leprae*.

TB can be grown on lipid-rich culture mediums. Their generation time is 12–18 hours. Initial droplet infection results in **primary tuberculosis**, localized mainly in the apices of the lungs. The primary disease develops with the Ghon focus (Ghon's complex), whereby the hilar lymph nodes are involved as well. Ninety percent of primary infection foci remain clinically silent. In 10% of persons infected, primary tuberculosis progresses to the **secondary** stage (reactivation or organ tuberculosis) after a few months or even years, which is characterized by extensive tissue necrosis, for example pulmonary caverns. The specific immunity and allergy that develop in the course of an infection reflect T lymphocyte functions. The allergy is measured in terms of the tuberculin reaction to check for clinically inapparent infections with TB. Diagnosis of tuberculosis requires identification of the pathogen by means of microscopy and culturing. Modern molecular methods are now coming to the fore in TB detection. Manifest tuberculosis is treated with two to four antitubercule chemotherapeutics in either a short regimen lasting six months or a standard regimen lasting nine months.

In contrast to TB, the LB pathogens do not lend themselves to culturing on artificial nutrient mediums. **Leprosy** is manifested mainly in skin, mucosa, and nerves. In clinical terms, there is a (malignant) lepromatous type leprosy and a (benign) tuberculoid type. Nondifferential forms are also frequent. Humans are the sole infection reservoir. Transmission of the disease is by close contact with skin or mucosa. ■

The genus *Mycobacterium* belongs to the *Mycobacteriaceae* family. This genus includes saprophytic species that are widespread in nature as well as the causative pathogens of the major human disease complexes tuberculosis and leprosy. Mycobacteria are Gram-positive, although they do not take gram staining well. The explanation for this is a cell wall structure rich in lipids that does not allow the alkaline stains to penetrate well. At any rate, once mycobacteria have been stained (using radical methods), they resist destaining, even with HCl-alcohol. This property is known as **acid fastness**.

Tuberculosis Bacteria (TB)

History. The tuberculosis bacteria complex includes the species *Mycobacterium tuberculosis*, *M. bovis*, and the rare species *M. africanum*. The clinical etiology of tuberculosis, a disease long known to man, was worked out in 1982 by R. Koch based on regular isolation of pathogens from lesions. Tuberculosis is unquestionably among the most intensively studied of all human diseases. In view of the fact that tuberculosis can infect practically any organ in the body, it is understandable why a number of other clinical disciplines profit from these studies in addition to microbiology and pathology.

Morphology and culturing. TB are slender, acid-fast rods, 0.4 µm wide, and 3–4 µm long, nonsporing and nonmotile. They can be stained with special agents (Ziehl-Neelsen, Kinyoun, fluorescence, p. 212f.) (Fig. 4.**12a**).

4

--- *Mycobacterium Tuberculosis* ---

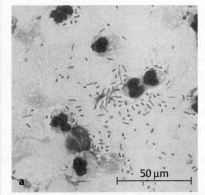

Fig. 4.**12** **a** Ziehl-Neelsen staining of a urine preparation: Fine, red, acid-fast rods, which tend to stick together. Clinical diagnosis: renal tuberculosis.
b Culture of *M. tuberculosis* on egg nutrient substrate according to Löwenstein-Jensen: after four weeks of incubation rough, yellowish, cauliflowerlike colonies.

50 µm

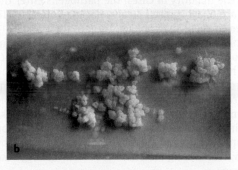

TB are obligate anaerobes. Their reproduction is enhanced by the presence of 5–10% CO_2 in the atmosphere. They are grown on culture mediums with a high lipid content, e.g., egg-enriched glycerol mediums according to Löwenstein-Jensen (Fig. **4.12b**). The generation time of TB is approximately 12–18 hours, so that cultures must be incubated for three to six or eight weeks at 37 °C until proliferation becomes macroscopically visible.

Cell wall. Many of the special characteristics of TB are ascribed to the chemistry of their cell wall, which features a murein layer as well as numerous lipids, the most important being the glycolipids (e.g., lipoarabinogalactan), the mycolic acids, mycosides, and wax D.

Glycolipids and wax D.
- Responsible for **resistance** to chemical and physical noxae.
- **Adjuvant effect** (wax D), i.e., enhancement of antigen immunogenicity.
- **Intracellular persistence** in nonactivated macrophages by means of inhibition of phagosome-lysosome fusion.
- **Complement resistance**.
- **Virulence.** Cord factor (trehalose 6,6-dimycolate).

Tuberculoproteins.
- **Immunogens.** The most important of these is the 65 kDa protein.
- **Tuberculin.** Partially purified tuberculin contains a mixture of small proteins (10 kDa). Tuberculin is used to test for TB exposure. Delayed allergic reaction.

Polysaccharides. Of unknown biological significance.

Pathogenesis and clinical picture. It is necessary to differentiate between primary and secondary tuberculosis (reactivation or postprimary tuberculosis) (Fig. **4.13**). The clinical symptoms are based on reactions of the cellular immune system with TB antigens.

■ **Primary tuberculosis.** In the majority of cases, the pathogens enter the lung in droplets, where they are phagocytosed by alveolar macrophages. TB bacteria are able to reproduce in these macrophages due to their ability to inhibit formation of the phagolysosome. Within 10–14 days a reactive inflammatory focus develops, the so-called primary focus from which the TB bacteria move into the regional hilar lymph nodes, where they reproduce and stimulate a cellular immune response, which in turn results in clonal expansion of specific T lymphocytes and attendant lymph node swelling. The Ghon's complex (primary complex, PC) develops between six and 14 weeks after infection. At the same time, granulomas form at the primary infection site and in the affected lymph nodes, and macrophages are activated by the cytokine MAF (macrophage activating factor). A tuberculin allergy also develops in the macroorganism.

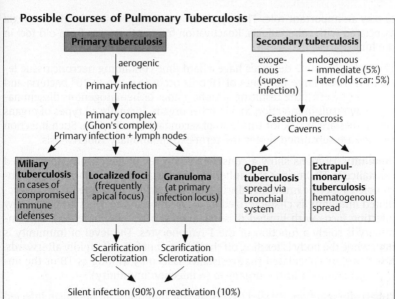

Possible Courses of Pulmonary Tuberculosis

Primary tuberculosis

aerogenic

Primary infection

↓

Primary complex
(Ghon's complex)
Primary infection + lymph nodes

Miliary tuberculosis in cases of compromised immune defenses

Localized foci (frequently apical focus)

Granuloma (at primary infection locus)

Secondary tuberculosis

| exoge-nous (super-infection) | endogenous – immediate (5%) – later (old scar: 5%) |

Caseation necrosis
Caverns

Open tuberculosis spread via bronchial system

Extrapul-monary tuberculosis hematogenous spread

Scarification Sclerotization

Scarification Sclerotization

Silent infection (90%) or reactivation (10%)

Fig. 4.**13** The primary tuberculosis that develops immediately post infection is clinically silent in most cases thanks to an effective immune response. However, in 10% of cases a so-called secondary tuberculosis develops, either immediately or years later, and may spread to the entire bronchial system or other organ systems.

The further course of the disease depends on the outcome of the battle between the TB and the specific cellular immune defenses. Postprimary dissemination foci are sometimes observed as well, i.e., development of local tissue defect foci at other localizations, typically the apices of the lungs. Mycobacteria may also be transported to other organs via the lymph vessels or bloodstream and produce dissemination foci there. The host eventually prevails in over 90% of cases: the granulomas and foci fibrose, scar, and calcify, and the infection remains clinically silent.

■ **Secondary tuberculosis.** In about 10% of infected persons the primary tuberculosis reactivates to become an organ tuberculosis, either within months (5%) or after a number of years (5%). Exogenous reinfection is rare in the populations of developed countries. Reactivation begins with a caseation necrosis in the center of the granulomas (also called tubercles) that may progress to cavitation (formation of caverns). Tissue destruction is caused by cytokines, among which tumor necrosis factor α (TNFα) appears to play an important role. This cytokine is also responsible for the cachexia associated with tuberculosis. Reactivation frequently stems from old foci in the lung apices.

The body's immune defenses have a hard time containing necrotic tissue lesions in which large numbers of TB cells occur (e.g., up to 10^9 bacteria and more per cavern); the resulting lymphogenous or hematogenous dissemination may result in infection foci in other organs. Virtually all types of organs and tissues are at risk for this kind of secondary TB infection. Such infection courses are subsumed under the term extrapulmonary tuberculosis.

Immunity. Humans show a considerable degree of genetically determined resistance to TB. Besides this inherited faculty, an organism acquires an (incomplete) specific immunity during initial exposure (first infection). This acquired immunity is characterized by localization of the TB at an old or new infection focus with limited dissemination (Koch's phenomenon). This immunity is solely a function of the T lymphocytes. The level of immunity is high while the body is fending off the disease, but falls off rapidly afterwards. It is therefore speculated that resistance lasts only as long as TB or the immunogens remain in the organism (= infection immunity).

Tuberculin reaction. Parallel to this specific immunity, an organism infected with TB shows an altered reaction mechanism, the tuberculin allergy, which also develops in the cellular immune system only. The tuberculin reaction, positive six to 14 weeks after infection, confirms the allergy. The tuberculin proteins are isolated as purified tuberculin (PPD = purified protein derivative). Five tuberculin units (TU) are applied intracutaneously in the tuberculin test (Mantoux tuberculin skin test, the "gold standard"). If the reaction is negative, the dose is sequentially increased to 250 TU. A positive reaction appears within 48 to 72 hours as an inflammatory reaction (induration) at least 10 mm in diameter at the site of antigen application. A positive reaction means that the person has either been infected with TB or vaccinated with BCG. It is important to understand that a positive test is not an indicator for an active infection or immune status. While a positive test person can be assumed to have a certain level of specific immunity, it will by no means be complete. One-half of the clinically manifest cases of tuberculosis in the population are secondary reactivation tuberculoses that develop in tuberculin-positive persons.

Diagnosis requires microscopic and cultural identification of the pathogen or pathogen-specific DNA.

Traditional method

■ **Workup of test material**, for example with *N*-acetyl-L-cysteine-NaOH (NALC-NaOH method) to liquefy viscous mucus and eliminate rapidly proliferating accompanying flora, followed by centrifugation to enrich the concentration.

■ **Microscopy.** Ziehl-Neelsen and/or auramine fluorescent staining (p. 212). This method produces rapid results but has a low level of sensitivity ($>10^4$–10^5/ml) and specificity (acid-fast rods only).

■ **Culture** on special solid and in special liquid mediums. Time requirement: four to eight weeks.

■ **Identification.** Biochemical tests with pure culture if necessary. Time requirement: one to three weeks.

■ **Resistance test** with pure culture. Time requirement: three weeks.

Rapid methods. A number of different rapid TB diagnostic methods have been introduced in recent years that require less time than the traditional methods.

■ **Culture.** Early-stage growth detection in liquid mediums involving identification of TB metabolic products with highly sensitive, semi-automated equipment. Time requirement: one to three weeks. Tentative diagnosis.

■ **Identification.** Analysis of cellular fatty acids by means of gas chromatography and of mycolic acids by means of HPLC. Time requirement: 12 days with a pure culture.

■ **DNA probes.** Used to identify *M. tuberculosis* complex and other mycobacteria. Time requirement: several hours with a pure culture.

■ **Resistance test.** Use of semi-automated equipment (see above). Proliferation/nonproliferation determination in liquid mediums containing standard antituberculotic agents (Table 4.**4**). Time requirement: 7–10 days.

Table 4.**4**   Scheme for Chemotherapy of Tuberculosis

	Standard scheme	Months	Short scheme *	Months
Initial phase	isoniazid (INH) rifampicin (RMP) ethambutol (EMB)	2	isoniazid rifampicin ethambutol pyrazinamide (PZA)	2
Continuation phase	isoniazid rifampicin	7	isoniazid rifampicin	4

* Alternative in cases of confirmed INH sensitivity or mild clinical picture: initial treatment with a combination of fixed INH + RMP + PZA for two months

Direct identification in patient material. Molecular methods used for direct detection of the *M. tuberculosis* complex in (uncultured) test material. These methods involve amplification of the search sequence.

Therapy. The previous method of long-term therapy in sanatoriums has been replaced by a standardized chemotherapy (see Table 4.4 for examples), often on an outpatient basis.

Epidemiology and prevention. Tuberculosis is endemic worldwide. The disease has become much less frequent in developed countries in recent decades, where its **incidence** is now about five to 15 new infections per 100 000 inhabitants per year and **mortality** rates are usually below one per 100 000 inhabitants per year. Seen from a worldwide perspective, however, tuberculosis is still a major medical problem. It is estimated that every year approximately 15 million persons contract tuberculosis and that three million die of the disease. The main **source of infection** is the human carrier. There are no healthy carriers. Diseased cattle are not a significant source of infection in the developed world. **Transmission** of the disease is generally direct, in most cases by droplet infection. Indirect transmission via dust or milk (udder tuberculosis in cattle) is the exception rather than the rule. The **incubation period** is four to 12 weeks.

■ **Exposure prophylaxis.** Patients with open tuberculosis must be isolated during the secretory phase. Secretions containing TB must be disinfected. Tuberculous cattle must be eliminated.

■ **Disposition prophylaxis.** An active vaccine is available that reduces the risk of contracting the disease by about one-half. It contains the live vaccine BCG (lyophilized bovine TB of the Calmette-Guérin type). Vaccination of tuberculin-negative persons induces allergy and (incomplete) immunity that persist for about five to 10 years. In countries with low levels of tuberculosis prevalence, the advisory committees on immunization practices no longer recommend vaccination with BCG, either in tuberculin-negative children at high risk or in adults who have been exposed to TB. Preventive chemotherapy of clinically inapparent infections (latent tuberculosis bacteria infection, LTBI) with INH (300 mg/d) over a period of six months has proved effective in high-risk persons, e.g., contact persons who therefore became tuberculin-positive, in tuberculin-positive persons with increased susceptibility (immunosuppressive therapy, therapy with corticosteroids, diabetes, alcoholism) and in persons with radiologically confirmed residual tuberculosis. Compliance with the therapeutic regimen is a problem in preventive chemotherapy.

Leprosy Bacteria (LB)

Morphology and culture. *Mycobacterium leprae* (Hansen, 1873) is the causative pathogen of leprosy. In morphological terms, these acid-fast rods are identical to tuberculosis bacteria. They differ, however, in that they cannot be grown on nutrient mediums or in cell cultures.

Pathogenesis. The pathomechanisms of LB are identical to those of TB. The host organism attempts to localize and isolate infection foci by forming granulomas. Leprous granulomas are histopathologically identical to tuberculous granulomas. High counts of leprosy bacteria are often found in the macrophages of the granulomas.

Immunity. The immune defenses mobilized against a leprosy infection are strictly of the cellular type. The lepromin skin test can detect a postinfection allergy. This test is not, however, very specific (i.e., positive reactions in cases in

4

Tuberculoid Leprosy

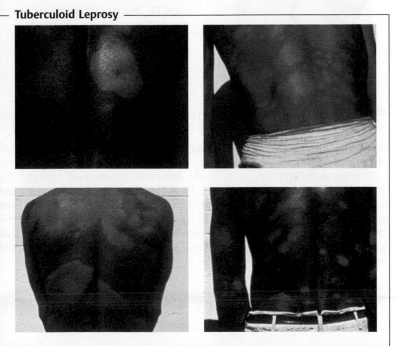

Fig. 4.**14** Tuberculoid leprosy is the benign, nonprogressive form of the disease, characterized by spotty dermal depigmentations.

Lepromatous Leprosy

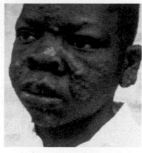

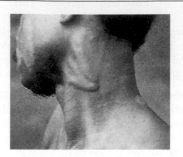

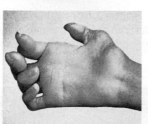

Fig. 4.**15** In lepromatous leprosy, nodular dermal and mucosal lesions develop. Nerve inflammation and neuroparalysis follow, eventually resulting in mutilations.

which no leprosy infection is present). The clinically differentiated infection course forms observed are probably due to individual immune response variants.

Clinical picture. Leprosy is manifested mainly on the skin, mucosa, and peripheral nerves.

A clinical differentiation is made between tuberculoid leprosy (TL, Fig. 4.**14**) and lepromatous leprosy (LL, Fig. 4.**15**). There are many intermediate forms. TL is the benign, nonprogressive form characterized by spotty dermal lesions. The LL form, on the other hand, is characterized by a malignant, progressive course with nodular skin lesions and cordlike nerve thickenings that finally lead to neuroparalysis. The inflammatory foci contain large numbers of leprosy bacteria.

Diagnosis. Detection of the pathogens in skin or nasal mucosa scrapings under the microscope using Ziehl-Neelsen staining (p. 212). Molecular confirmation of DNA sequences specific to leprosy bacteria in a polymerase chain reaction is possible.

Therapy. Paucibacillary forms are treated with dapson plus rifampicin for six months. Multibacillary forms require treatment with dapson, rifampicin, and clofazimine over a period of at least two years.

Epidemiology and prevention. Leprosy is now rare in socially developed countries, although still frequent in developing countries. There are an estimated 11 million victims worldwide. Infected humans are the only source of infection. The details of the transmission pathways are unknown. Discussion of the topic is considering transmission by direct contact with skin or mucosa injuries and aerogenic transmission. The incubation period is 2–5–20 years. Isolation of patients under treatment is no longer required. An effective epidemiological reaction requires early recognition of the disease in contact persons by means of periodical examinations every six to 12 months up to five years following contact.

Nontuberculous Mycobacteria (NTM)

4

Mycobacteria that are neither tuberculosis nor leprosy bacteria are categorized as atypical mycobacteria (old designation), nontuberculous mycobacteria (NTM) or MOTT (mycobacteria other than tubercle bacilli).

Morphology and culture. In their morphology and staining behavior, NTM are generally indistinguishable from tuberculosis bacteria. With the exception of the rapidly growing NTM, their culturing characteristics are also similar to TB. Some species proliferate only at 30 °C. NTM are frequent inhabitants of the natural environment (water, soil) and also contribute to human and animal mucosal flora. Most of these species show resistance to the antituberculoid agents in common use.

Clinical pictures and diagnosis. Some NTM species are apathogenic, others can cause mycobacterioses in humans that usually follow a chronic course (Table 4.**5**). NTM infections are generally rare. Their occurrence is encouraged by compromised cellular immunity. Frequent occurrence is observed together with certain malignancies, in immunosuppressed patients and in AIDS patients, whereby the NTM isolated in 80% of cases are *M. avium* or *M. intercellulare*. As a rule, NTM infections are indistinguishable from tuberculous lesions in clinical, radiological, and histological terms. Diagnosis therefore requires culturing and positive identification. The clinical significance of a positive result is difficult to determine due to the ubiquitous occurrence of these pathogens. They are frequent culture contaminants. Only about 10% of all persons in whom NTM are detected actually turn out to have a mycobacteriosis.

Therapy. Surgical removal of the infection focus is often indicated. Chemotherapy depends on the pathogen species, for instance a triple combination (e.g., INH, ethambutol, rifampicin) or, for resistant strains, a combination of four or five antituberculoid agents.

Table 4.5 Infections Caused by Nontuberculous Mycobacteria

Disease	Frequent species	Rare species
Chronic pulmonary disease (adults)	M. kansasii M. avium/M. intracellulare (M. avium complex) M. abscessus	M. malmoense M. xenopi M. scrofulaceum M. fortuitum M. chelonae and others
Local lymphadenitis (children, adolescents)	M. avium complex	M. kansasii, M. malmoense M. fortuitum
Skin and soft tissue infections	M. marinum M. fortuitum M. chelonae M. ulcerans	M. haemophilum M. smegmatis M. hansasii
Bone, joint, tendon infections	M. kansasii M. avium complex M. fortuitum M. abscessus	M. smegmatis M. chelonae M. marinum M. malmoense
Disseminated diseases in immunocompromised patients	M. kansasii M. avium complex	M. fortuitum M. chelonae M. genavense M. xenopi and others

Nocardia

Occurrence. The genus *Nocardia* includes species with morphology similar to that of the actinomycetes, differing from them in that the natural habitat of these obligate aerobes is the soil and damp biotopes. The pathogens known for involvement in nocardioses, a generally very rare type of infection, include *N. asteroides, N. brasiliensis, N. farcinia, N. nova,* and *N. otitidiscaviarum.*

Morphology and culture. Nocardia are Gram-positive, fine, pleomorphic rods that sometimes show branching. They can be cultured on standard nutrient mediums and proliferate particularly well at 30 °C. Nocardia are obligate aerobes.

Pathogenesis and clinical picture. Nocardia penetrate from the environment into the macroorganism via the respiratory tract or dermal wounds. An infection develops only in patients with predisposing primary diseases directly affecting the immune defenses. Monoinfections are the rule. There are no typical clinical symptoms. Most cases of infection involve pyogenic inflammations with central necroses. The following types have been described: **pulmonary nocardioses** (bronchial pneumonia, pulmonary abscess), **systemic nocardioses** (sepsis, cerebral abscess, abscesses in the kidneys and musculature), and **surface nocardioses** (cutaneous and subcutaneous abscesses, lymphocutaneous syndrome).

Actinomycetomas are tumorlike processes affecting the extremities, including bone. An example of such an infection is Madura foot, caused by *Nocardia* species, the related species *Actinomadura madurae*, and *Streptomyces somaliensis*. Fungi (p. 355) can also be a causal factor in this clinical picture.

Diagnosis. Detection of the pathogen by means of microscopy and culturing techniques is required in materials varying with the specific disease. Due to the long generation time of these species, cultures have to be incubated for at least one week. Precise identification to differentiate pathogenic and apathogenic species is desirable, but difficult.

4

Therapy. The anti-infective agents of choice are sulfonamides and cotrimoxazole. Surgery may be required.

Epidemiology and prevention. Nocardioses are rare infections. Annual incidence levels range from about 0.5 to 1 case per 1 000 000 inhabitants. The pathogens, which are present in the natural environment, are carried by dust to susceptible patients. There are no practicable prophylactic measures.

Neisseria, Moraxella, and Acinetobacter

■ Neisseria are Gram-negative, aerobic cocci that are often arranged in pairs. They are typical mucosal parasites that die rapidly outside the human organism. Culturing on enriched nutrient mediums is readily feasible.

Neisseria gonorrheae is the pathogen responsible for gonorrhea ("clap"). Infection results from sexual intercourse. The organisms adhere to cells of the urogenital tract by means of attachment pili and the protein Opa, penetrate into the organism using parasite-directed endocytosis and cause a pyogenic infection, mainly of the urogenital epithelium. An infection is diagnosed mainly by means of microscopy and culturing of purulent secretions. The therapeutic of choice is penicillin G. Alternatives for use against penicillinase-positive gonococci include third-generation cephalosporins and 4-quinolones.

N. meningitidis is a parasite of the nasopharyngeal mucosa. These meningococci cause meningitis and sepsis. Diagnosis involves detection of the pathogens in cerebrospinal fluid and blood. The disease occurs sporadically or in the form of minor epidemics in children, youths, and young adults. The antibiotics of choice are penicillin G and third-generation cephalosporins.

■

The family *Neisseriaceae* includes aerobic, Gram-negative cocci and rods (see Table 3.**9**, p. 222), the most important of which are the human pathogens *N. gonorrheae* and *N. meningitidis*. Other species in the genus *Neisseria* are elements of the normal mucosal flora.

Neisseria gonorrheae (Gonorrhea)

Morphology and culture. Gonococci are Gram-negative, coffee-bean-shaped cocci that are usually paired and have a diameter of approximately 1 μm (Fig. 4.**16**). Attachment pili on the bacterial cell surface are responsible for their adhesion to mucosal cells.

Gonococci can be grown on moist culture mediums enriched with protein (blood). The atmosphere for primary culturing must contain 5–10 % CO_2.

Pathogenesis and clinical picture. Gonorrhea is a sexually transmitted disease. The pathogens penetrate into the urogenital mucosa, causing a local purulent infection. In men, the prostate and epididymis can also become infected. In women, the gonococci can also cause salpingitis, oophoritis, or even peritonitis. Gonococci reaching the conjunctival membrane may cause a purulent conjunctivitis, seen mainly in newborn children. Gonococci can also infect the rectal or pharyngeal mucosa. Hematogenously disseminated gonococci may also cause arthritis or even endocarditis.

Determinants of the Pathogenicity of Gonococci

Attachment pili on the surface and the outer membrane protein Opa are responsible for adhesion to cells of the urogenital tract. Opa also directs the invasion process by means of endocytosis. Immune defenses against granulocytes are based on the outer membrane porin Por that prevents the phagosome from fusing with lysosomes, resulting in the survival—and proliferation—of phagocytosed gonococci in granulocytes. The lipo-oligosaccharide (LOS) in the outer membrane is responsible for resistance to complement (serum resistance) as well as for the inflammatory tissue reaction in a manner analogous to the more complexly structured LPS of enterobacteria. Gonococci can capture iron from the siderophilic proteins lactoferrin and transferrin, accumulating it inside the bacterial cells to facilitate their rapid proliferation. An IgA_1 protease produced by the gonococci hydrolyzes secretory antibodies in the mucosal secretions. The pronounced antigen variability of the attachment pili (p. 14) and the Opa protein make it possible for gonococci to thwart specific immune defense mechanisms repeatedly.

Neisseria gonorrhoeae and *Neisseria meningitidis*

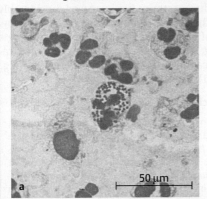

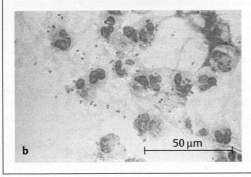

Fig. 4.**16 a** *N. gonorrheae*: gram staining of a preparation of urethral secretion: coffee-bean-shaped diplococci, grouped within a granulocyte. Clinical diagnosis: gonorrhea. **b** *N. meningitidis*: gram staining of a preparation of cerebrospinal fluid sediment. Clinical diagnosis: acute purulent meningitis.

4

Diagnosis. The method of choice is detection of the pathogens by means of methylene blue and gram staining and culturing. Gonococci are sensitive in cultures and the material must be used immediately after they are obtained to inoculate Thayer-Martin blood agar with antibiotics added to eliminate accompanying flora, on which medium the cultures are then transported to the laboratory. The identification procedure involves both morphology and biochemical characteristics. Techniques developed recently utilize immunofluorescence or coagglutination methods (p. 217) utilizing monoclonal antibodies to the main protein of the outer membrane, Por.

Direct detection in pus and secretion samples is possible using an enzymatic immunosorbence test or detection of gonococcus-specific DNA sequences coding for rRNA using a gene probe.

Therapy. The agent of choice used to be penicillin G. In recent years, however, the percentage of penicillinase-producing strains has increased considerably all over the world. For this reason, third-generation cephalosporins are now used to treat uncomplicated cases of gonorrhea. They are applied in a single dose (e.g., ceftriaxone, 250–500 mg i.m.). Good results have also been reported with single-dose oral application of fluorinated 4-quinolones (e.g., 0.5 g ciprofloxacin or 0.4 g ofloxacin).

Penicillin Resistance in Gonococci

The determinants of high-level penicillin resistance in gonococci are small, nonconjugative plasmids, which are mobilized by a conjugative helper plasmid for transmission from one gonococcal cell to another. The penicillin resistance plasmids code for the TEM betalactamase that occurs frequently in *Enterobacteriaceae*. It is therefore assumed that the *penicillinase* gene in gonococci derived from the *Enterobacteriaceae* gene pool. Low-level, inherent resistance to penicillin is based on chromosomal genes (*penA*, *penB*) that code for penicillin-binding proteins with reduced affinity to penicillin. These genes are products of mutations.

Epidemiology and prevention. Gonorrhea is a worldwide sexually transmitted disease that occurs only in humans. Its level of annual incidence in developed countries is estimated at 12 cases per 1000 inhabitants. The actual figures are likely to be much higher due to large numbers of unreported cases. A reduction in incidence seen in recent years may be due to AIDS prophylaxis. Protective immunization for high-risk persons is not feasible due to the antigen variability of the organism as described above. Stopping the spread of gonorrhea involves mainly rapid recognition of infections and treatment accordingly.

One hundred percent prevention of ophthalmia neonatorum is possible with a single parenteral dose of 125 mg ceftriaxone. Local prophylaxis is also practiced using a 1% solution of silver nitrate or eye ointments containing 1% tetracycline or 0.5% erythromycin.

Neisseria meningitidis (Meningitis, Sepsis)

Morphology and culture. Meningococci are Gram-negative, coffee-bean-shaped cocci that are frequently pleomorphic and have a diameter of 1 μm (Fig. 4.**16b**). They are nonmotile and feature a polysaccharide capsule.

Growing meningococci in cultures requires mediums containing blood. A concentration of 5–10% CO_2 encourages proliferation.

Antigen structure. Serogroups A, B, C, D, etc. (a total of 12) are differentiated based on the capsule chemistry. Epidemics are caused mainly by strains of serogroup A, sometimes by B strains as well and, more rarely, by group C strains. Serogroups are divided into serovars based on differences in the outer membrane protein antigens.

Pathogenesis and clinical picture. Meningococci are parasites of the nasopharynx. These microorganisms are carried by 5–10% of the population. If virulent meningococci colonize the nasopharyngeal mucosa of a host lacking the antibodies, pathogen invasion of the mucosa by means of "parasite-directed endocytosis" becomes possible (see p. 12). The CNS is doubtless the preferred compartment for secondary infections, although hematogenously disseminated pathogens can also infect the lungs, the endocardium, or major joints.

Onset of the meningitis is usually sudden, after an incubation period of two to three days, with severe headache, fever, neck stiffness, and severe malaise. Severe hemorrhagic sepsis sometimes develops (Waterhouse-Friedrichsen syndrome).

Diagnosis requires detection of the pathogen in cerebrospinal fluid or blood by means of microscopy and culturing techniques. For success in culturing, the material must be used to inoculate blood agar without delay. Identification of the pathogen is based on identification of metabolic properties. The slide agglutination test is used to determine the serogroup.

Latex agglutination or coagglutination (p. 217) can be used for direct antigen detection in cerebrospinal fluid.

Therapy. The antibiotic of choice is penicillin G. Very good results have also been obtained with third-generation cephalosporins, e.g., cefotaxime or ceftriaxone. It is important to start treatment as quickly as possible to prevent delayed damage.

The advantage of cephalosporins is that they are also effective against other meningitis pathogens due to their broad spectrum of action (with the exception of *Listeria monocytogenes*).

Epidemiology and prevention. Meningococcal infections are more frequent in the winter and spring months. **Transmission** of meningococci is by droplet infection. Humans are the only pathogen reservoir. **Sources of infection** include both carriers and infected persons with manifest disease. In developed countries, meningitis occurs sporadically or in the form of minor epidemics in more or less isolated collectives (work camps, recruiting camps, school camping facilities). The **incidence** level is approximately 12 cases per 100 000 inhabitants per year. In parts of the developing world (African meningitis belt) the level is higher. Lethality runs to 85% if the disease is left untreated, but is reduced to less than 1% if treatment is begun early enough. **Prophylactic antibiosis** is indicated for those in close contact with diseased persons (e.g., in the same family). Prophylactic measures also include treatment of carriers to eliminate this reservoir, whereby minocylin or rifampicin must be used instead of penicillin G. **Prophylactic immunization** can be achieved with a vaccine made from the purified capsule polysaccharides A, C, Y, and W-135. There is no serogroup B vaccine, since the capsule in serogroup B consists of polyneuraminic acid, which the immune system does not recognize as a foreign substance.

Moraxella and Acinetobacter

The taxonomic definitions of these genera are still inconclusive. Bergey's *Manual of Systematic Bacteriology* groups both under the family *Moraxella-ceae*. These bacteria are short, rounded rods, often coccoid, sometimes also diplococcoid. Their natural habitat is either human mucosa (*Moraxella*) or the natural environment (*Acinetobacter*).

■ *Moraxella.* The genus comprises two medically important species:
— *Moraxella catarrhalis.* Component of the normal flora of the upper respiratory tract. May be responsible for: pneumonia, acute exacerbation of chronic bronchitis, otitis media (up to 20% in children), and sinusitis. About 90% of all strains produce one of the so-called BRO penicillinases, so that therapy with a penicillinase-stable betalactam antibiotic is indicated.
— *Moraxella lacunata.* Formerly *Diplobacterium Morax-Axenfeld*. Can cause conjunctivitis and keratitis. The reason why this organism is now rarely found as a pathogen in these eye infections is unknown.

■ *Acinetobacter.* In immunodeficient persons, *A. baumannii*, *A. calcoaceti-cus*, and other species can cause nosocomial infections (urinary tract infections, pneumonias, wound infections, sepsis). Clinical strains of these species often show multiresistance to antibiotics, so that treatment of these infections may prove difficult.

Enterobacteriaceae, Overview

■ The most important bacterial family in human medicine is the *Enterobac-teriaceae*. This family includes genera and species that cause well-defined diseases with typical clinical symptoms (typhoid fever, dysentery, plague) as well as many opportunists that cause mainly nosocomial infections (urinary tract infections, pneumonias, wound infections, sepsis). *Enterobacteria-ceae* are Gram-negative, usually motile, facultatively anaerobic rod bacteria. The high levels of metabolic activity observed in them are made use of in identification procedures. The species are subdivided into epidemiologically significant serovars based on O, H, and K antigens. The most important pathogenicity factors of *Enterobacteriaceae* are colonizing factors, invasins, endotoxin, and various exotoxins. *Enterobacteriaceae* are the most significant contributors to intestinal infections, which are among the most frequent diseases of all among the developing world populace.

Definition and significance. Together with the families *Vibrionaceae* and others (p. 224), the *Enterobacteriaceae* form the group of Gram-negative, facultatively anaerobic rod bacteria. Their natural habitat is the intestinal tract of humans and animals. Some species cause characteristic diseases. While others are facultatively pathogenic, they are still among the bacteria most frequently isolated as pathogens (e.g., *E. coli*). They are often responsible for nosocomial diseases (see p. 343ff.).

4

Taxonomy. The taxonomy of the *Enterobacteriaceae* has seen repeated changes in recent decades and has doubtless not yet assumed its final form. The family includes 41 genera with hundreds of species. Table 4.**6** provides an overview of the most important *Enterobacteriaceae* in the field of human medicine.

The taxonomic system applied to *Enterobacteriaceae* is based on varying patterns of metabolic processes (Fig. 3.**36**, p. 214). One of the important characteristics of this bacterial family is lactose breakdown (presence of the lac operon). The lac operon includes the genes *lacZ* (codes for β-galactosidase), *lacY* (codes for β-galactoside permease), and *lacA* (codes for transacetylase). Lactose-positive *Enterobacteriaceae* are grouped together as coliform *Enterobacteriaceae*. Salmonellae and most of the shigellae are lactose-negative.

Morphology and culture. *Enterobacteriaceae* are short Gram-negative rods with rounded ends, 0.5–1.5 μm thick, and 24 μm long (Fig. 4.**17a**). Many have peritrichous flagellation. Species with many flagella (e.g., *Proteus* species) show motility on the agar surface, which phenomenon is known as "swarming." Some *Enterobacteriaceae* possess a capsule.

All bacteria in this family can readily be cultured on simple nutrient mediums. They are rapidly growing facultative anaerobes. Their mean generation time in vitro is 20–30 minutes. They show resistance to various chemicals (bile salts, crystal violet), which fact is made use of in selective culturing. Endo agar is an important selective indicator medium; it allows only Gram-negative rod bacteria to grow and indicates lactose breakdown (Fig. 4.**17b**).

Table 4.**6** The Most Important Genera/Species/Vars of *Enterobacteriaceae* and the Corresponding Clinical Pictures

Genera/species/var	Disease	Remarks
Salmonella enterica		
S. Typhi	Typhus abdominalis (syn. typhoid fever)	Generalized septic infection
S. Typhimurium S. Enteritidis and others	Gastroenteritis (diarrhea)	Profuse watery diarrhea
Shigella	Bacterial dysentery	Diarrhea, abdominal cramping, tenesmus, stool frequently contains blood and mucus
Klebsiella pneumoniae	Pneumonia (Friedländer's)	Severe pneumonia in predisposed persons
Escherichia coli *Citrobacter* *Klebsiella* *Enterobacter* *Serratia* *Proteus* *Providencia* *Morganella* and others	Sepsis, wound infections, infections of the urinary tract and respiratory tract	Facultatively pathogenic bacteria; disease only manifests if host organism immune defenses are weakened; often cause nosocomial infections; frequently resistant to antibiotics
Yersinia		
Y. pestis	Plague	Generalized systemic infection; rare
Y. enterocolitica Y. pseudotuberculosis	Enterocolitis, lymphadenitis of the mesenteric lymph nodes	Pseudoappendicitis, reactive arthritis, erythema nodosum
Escherichia coli	Intestinal infections	
Enteropathogenic E. coli (EPEC)	Classic infant diarrhea	Epidemics in hospitals, children's homes
Enterotoxic E. coli (ETEC)	Diarrhea, choleralike	Cause of travelers' diarrhea (50%)
Enteroinvasive E. coli (EIEC)	Dysenterylike	Invasion and verocytotoxins
Enterohemorrhagic E. coli (EHEC)	Hemorrhagic colitis	Hemolytic–uremic syndrome (HUS) in 5% of EHEC cases
Enteroaggregative E. coli (EAggEC)	Watery diarrhea, mainly in infants	Adhesion to small intestine mucosa; production of a toxin

Escherichia coli

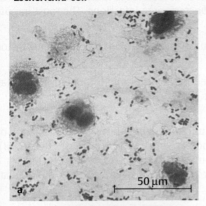

Fig. 4.**17** **a** Gram staining of a urine sediment preparation: rounded gram-negative rods, some coccoid. Clinical diagnosis: acute cystitis.
b Culture on endo agar, a combined selective/indicator medium. The red color of the colony and agar indicates the lactose breakdown process.

4

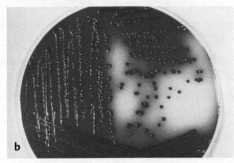

Antigen structure. The most important antigens of the *Enterobacteriaceae* are:

■ **O antigens.** Specific polysaccharide chains in the lipopolysaccharide complex of the outer membrane (p. 156).

■ **H antigens.** Flagellar antigens consisting of protein.

■ **K antigens.** Linear polymers of the outer membrane built up of a repeated series of carbohydrate units (sometimes proteins as well). They can cover the cell densely and render them O inagglutinable (p. 155).

■ **F antigens.** Antigens of protein attachment fimbriae.

Pathogenicity determinants. A number of factors are known to play a role in the pathogenicity of various *Enterobacteriaceae* infections. The most important are:

■ **Adhesion factors.** Attachment fimbriae, attachment pili, colonizing factor antigens (CFAs).

■ **Invasive factors.** Proteins localized in the outer membrane (invasins) that facilitate the invasion of target cells.

■ **Exotoxins.**
— *Enterotoxins* disturb the normal functioning of enterocytes. Stimulation of adenylate or guanylate cyclase; increased production of cAMP (see p. 298). This results in the loss of large amounts of electrolytes and water.
— *Cytotoxins* exert a direct toxic effect on cells (enterocytes, endothelial cells).

■ **Endotoxin.** Toxic effect of lipoid A as a component of LPS (p. 156).

■ **Serum resistance.** Resistance to the membrane attack complex C5b6789 of the complement system (p. 86ff.).

■ **Phagocyte resistance.** Makes survival in phagocytes possible. Resistance against defensins and/or oxygen radicals (p. 23).

■ **Cumulation of Fe^{2+}.** Active transport of Fe^{2+} by siderophores in the bacterial cell (p. 13).

Salmonella (Gastroenteritis, Typhoid Fever, Paratyphoid Fever)

■ All salmonellae are classified in the species *Salmonella enterica* with seven subspecies. Nearly all human pathogen salmonellae are grouped under *S. enterica*, subsp. *enterica*. Salmonellae are further subclassified in over 2000 serovars based on their O and H antigens, which used to be (incorrectly) designated as species.

Typhoid salmonelloses are caused by the serovars *typhi* and *paratyphi A, B*, and *C*. The salmonellae are taken up orally and the invasion pathway is through the intestinal tract, from where they enter lymphatic tissue, first spreading lymphogenously, then hematogenously. A generalized septic clinical picture results. Human carriers are the only source of infection. Transmission is either direct by smear infection or indirect via food and drinking water. Anti-infective agents are required for therapy (ampicillin, cotrimoxazole, 4-quinolones). An active vaccine is available to protect against typhoid fever.

Enteric salmonelloses develop when pathogens are taken up with food. The primary infection source is usually livestock. These relatively frequent infections remain restricted to the gastrointestinal tract. Treatment with anti-infective agents is necessary in exceptional cases only. ∎

Taxonomy. The salmonellae that cause significant human disease are classified in most countries under the taxon *Salmonella enterica,* subsp. *enterica* (synonymous with *S. choleraesuis,* subsp. *choleraesuis*). However, this nomenclature has still not been officially adopted by the *Enterobacteriaceae* Subcommittee. *Salmonella enterica,* spp. *enterica* includes over 2000 serovars, which were formerly (incorrectly) designated with species names. The serovars are capitalized to differentiate them from species.

4

Taxonomy of the Salmonellae

The problems involved in the taxonomy and nomenclature of this group of bacteria can only be understood in the historical perspective. At first, the genus *Salmonella* appeared to comprise species that differed only in their antigen structures. Species names were therefore used for what turned out to be serovars. More recent molecular studies have demonstrated that the genus *Salmonella* contains only a single species that can be subdivided into seven subspecies. All of the important human pathogen salmonellae belong to the subspecies *enterica*. The (false) species names for the serovars had, however, already become normal usage. In view of the fact that the causative pathogens in typhoid salmonelloses, a clinical picture clearly differentiated from *Salmonella* gastroenteritis, are only serovars of the same species/subspecies, the official committee has, however, not adopted the new nomenclature as yet.

The serovars are determined by O and H antigens. The Kauffman–White scheme is used to arrange them (see Table 4.**7** for an excerpt).

This taxonomic arrangement classifies the serovars in groups characterized by certain O antigens (semibold). This results in a clinically and epidemiologically useful grouping, since certain serovars are responsible for typhoid salmonelloses and others for enteric salmonelloses. The serovars are determined by means of antisera in the slide agglutination test.

Phase Variations of the H Antigens

H antigens occur with two different antigen structures. The primary structure of flagellin is determined by two genes on the chromosome, only one of which is read off. Whether a gene is read off or not is determined by spontaneous inversion of a DNA sequence before the *H2* gene, which inversion occurs with a frequency of approximately 10^{-4} per cell division (Fig. 4.**18**).

Table **4.7** Excerpt from the Kauffmann–White Scheme which Covers Over 2000 Serovars

Group	Serovar	O antigens	H antigens Phase 1	Phase 2
A	*Paratyphi A*	1, **2**, 12	a	–
B	*Schottmuelleri* (syn. *Paratyphi B*)	1, **4**, (5), 12	b	1, 2
	Typhimurium	1, **4**, (5), 12	i	1, 2
C1	*Hirschfeldii* (syn. *Paratyphi C*)	**6**, 7, (Vi)	c	1, 5
	Choleraesuis	**6**, 7	(c)	1, 5
C2	*Newport*	**6**, 8	e, h	1, 2
D1	*Typhi*	**9**, 12, (Vi)	d	–
	Enteritidis	1, **9**, 12, (Vi)	g, m	(1, 7)
	Dublin	1, **9**, 12, (Vi)	g, p	–
	Gallinarum	1, **9**, 12	–	–
	Panama	1, **9**, 12	l, v	1, 5
E1	*Oxford*	**3**, 10	a	1, 7

Parentheses indicate that the antigen is often not present. The Vi antigen is, strictly speaking, actually a K antigen. The numbers in bold type indicate the antigen that characterizes the O group.

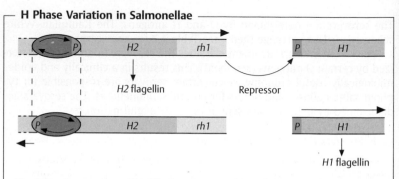

H Phase Variation in Salmonellae

Fig. 4.**18** *P* = promoter, *H2* = H2 phase gene, *H1* = H1 phase gene, *rh1* = regulator gene for *H1*, *hin* = gene coding for the DNA invertase. The horizontal arrows show the direction in which the genetic information is read off.

Pathogenesis and clinical pictures. Salmonellae are classified as either typhoid or enteric regarding the relevant clinical pictures and epidemiologies. It is not known why typhoid salmonellae only cause systemic disease in humans, whereas enteric salmonella infections occur in animals as well and are usually restricted to the intestinal tract.

■ **Typhoid salmonelloses.** Attachment of typhoid salmonellae to cells of the jejunum (M cells). Invasion by means of endocytosis, transfer, and exocytosis. Phagocytosis in the subserosa by macrophages and translocation into the mesenteric lymph nodes. Proliferation occurs. Lymphogenous and hematogenous dissemination. Secondary foci in the spleen, liver, bone marrow, bile ducts, skin (roseola), Peyer's patches.

Manifest illness begins with fever, rising in stages throughout the first week to 39/40/41 °C. Further symptoms: stupor (typhos [greek] = fog), leukopenia, bradycardia, splenic swelling, abdominal roseola, beginning in the third week diarrhea, sometimes with intestinal bleeding due to ulceration of the Peyer's patches.

■ **Enteric salmonelloses.** Attachment to enterocytes of the ileum and colon. Invasion of mucosa induced by invasin proteins on the surface of the salmonella cells. Persistence in epithelial cells, possibly in macrophages as well. Production of *Salmonella* enterotoxin. Local inflammation. Manifest illness usually begins suddenly with diarrhea and vomiting, accompanied in some cases by high fever. The symptoms abate after several days without specific therapy. In cases of massive diarrhea, symptoms may be observed that result from the loss of water and electrolytes (Table 4.**8**).

Diagnosis. The method of choice is detection of the pathogens in cultures. Selective indicator mediums are used to isolate salmonellae in stool. Identification is done using metabolic patterns (see Fig. 3.**36**, p. 214). Serovar classification is determined with specific antisera in the slide agglutination test. Culturing requires at least two days. Typhoid salmonelloses can be diagnosed indirectly by measuring the titer of agglutinating antibodies to O and H antigens (according to Gruber-Widal). To provide conclusive proof the titer must rise by at least fourfold from blood sampled at disease onset to a sample taken at least one week later.

Therapy. Typhoid salmonelloses must be treated with anti-infective agents, whereas symptomatic treatment will suffice for enteric infections. Symptomatic treatment encompasses slowing down intestinal activity (e.g., with loperamide) and replacing fluid and electrolyte losses orally as required (WHO formula: 3.5 g NaCl, 2.5 g $NaHCO_3$, 1.5 g KCl, 20 g glucose per liter of water).

Table 4.8   Overview of the Most Important Differences between Typhoid and Enteric Salmonellae and Salmonelloses

Parameter	Typhoid salmonellae/salmonelloses	Enteric salmonellae/salmonelloses
Serovars	*Typhi*; *Paratyphi A, B, C* (see Table 4.**7**)	Often *Enteritidis* and *Typhimurium*; more rarely: numerous other serovars
Infection spectrum	Humans	Animals and humans
Source of infection	Humans: infected persons, chronic carriers	Mainly livestock; possibly humans as well
Mode of infection	Oral	Oral
Transmission	Indirect: water, contaminated food Direct: smear infection	Indirect: contaminated food
Infective dose	Small: 10^2–10^3 bacteria	Large: $>10^6$ bacteria; in most cases proliferation in food
Incubation time	1–3 weeks	1–2 days
Clinical picture	**Generalized infection.** Sepsis	**Acute diarrhea with vomiting.** Fever. Self-limiting infection in most cases
Diagnosis	Identification of pathogen in blood, stool, urine. Antibody detection using Gruber-Widal quantitative agglutination reaction	Identification of pathogen in stool
Therapy	Antibiotics: aminopenicillins, 4-quinolones	Symptomatic therapy: loperamide, replacement of water and electrolyte losses as required (WHO formula)
Occurrence	Sporadic; usually imported from countries with endemic typhoid fever	Endemic, epidemics in small groups (family, cafeteria, etc.) or as mass infection
Prevention	**Exposure prophylaxis:** Drinking water and food hygiene; elimination of pathogen in chronic carriers. **Immunization prophylaxis:** Active immunization possible (travelers) (see p. 287f.)	**Exposure prophylaxis:** Food hygiene

Eliminating the infection in chronic stool carriers of typhoid salmonellae, 2–5% of cases, presents a problem. Chronic carriers are defined as convalescents who are still eliminating pathogens three months after the end of the manifest illness. The organisms usually persist in the scarified wall of the gallbladder. Success is sometimes achieved with high-dose administration of anti-infective agents, e.g., 4-quinolones or aminopenicillins. A cholecystectomy is required in refractory cases.

Epidemiology. The cases of typhoid salmonellosis seen in northern and central Europe are imported by travelers. Cases arise only sporadically or in form of an epidemic because of a chain of unfortunate circumstances. Humans are the only primary source of infection.

By contrast, enteric salmonelloses occur in this population both endemically and epidemically. Case counts are steadily increasing. Exact morbidity data are hard to come by due to the large numbers of unreported cases. Livestock represents the most important source of infection. The pathogens are transmitted to humans in food.

Prevention. The main method of effective prevention is to avoid exposure: this means clean drinking water, prevention of food contamination, avoidance of uncooked foods in countries where salmonellae occur frequently, disinfection of excreta containing salmonellae or from chronic carriers, etc. It is also important to report all cases to health authorities so that appropriate measures can be taken.

Typhoid fever vaccinations for travelers to endemic areas can best be done with the oral attenuated vaccine Virotif Ty 21a.

Shigella (Bacterial Dysentery)

■ Shigella is the causative pathogen in bacterial dysentery. The genus comprises the species *S. dysenteriae*, *S. flexneri*, *S. boydii*, and *S. sonnei*. Shigellae are nonmotile. The three primary species can be classified in serovars based on the fine structure of their O antigens. Shigellae are characterized by invasive properties. They can penetrate the colonic mucosa to cause local necrotic infections. Humans are the sole source of infection since shigellae are pathologically active in humans only. The pathogens are transmitted directly, more frequently indirectly, via food and drinking water. Antibiotics can be used therapeutically. ■

Classification. The genus *Shigella* includes four species: *S. dysenteriae*, *S. flexneri*, *S. boydii*, and *S. sonnei*. The first three are subdivided into 10, six, and

15 servars, respectively, based on their antigen structures. Shigellae are non-motile and therefore have no flagellar (H) antigens.

Pathogenesis. Shigellae are only pathogenic in humans. The pathogens are ingested orally. Only a few hundred bacteria suffice for an infective dose. Shigellae enter the terminal ileum and colon, where they are taken up by the M cells in the intestinal mucosa, which in turn are in close vicinity to the macrophages. Following phagocytosis by the macrophages, the shigellae lyse the phagosome and actively induce macrophage apoptosis. The shigellae released from the dead macrophages are then taken up by enterocytes via the basolateral side of the mucosa (i.e., retrograde transport). The invasion is facilitated by outer membrane polypeptides, the invasins, which are coded by *inv* genes localized on 180–240 kb plasmids. Adjacent enterocytes are invaded by means of lateral transfer from infected cells. In the enterocytes, the shigellae reproduce, finally destroying the cells. *Shigella dysenteriae* produces **shigatoxin**, the prototype for the family of **shigalike toxins** (or **verocytotoxins**), which also occur in several other *Enterobacteriaceae*. The toxin inhibits protein synthesis in eukaryotic cells by splitting the 23S rRNA at a certain locus. Shigatoxin contributes to the colonic epithelial damage, the small intestine diarrhea with watery stools at the onset of shigellosis and (less frequent) the hemolytic-uremic syndrome (HUS).

Clinical picture. Following an incubation period of two to five days, the disease manifests with profuse watery diarrhea (= small intestine diarrhea). Later, stools may contain mucus, pus, and blood. Intestinal cramps, painful stool elimination (tenesmus), and fever are observed in the further course of the infection. Complications include massive intestinal bleeding and perforation peritonitis. These severe effects are caused mainly by *S. dysenteriae*, whereas *S. sonnei* infections usually involve only diarrhea.

Diagnosis requires identification of the pathogen in a culture. Combined selective/indicator mediums must be used for the primary culture. Suspected colonies are identified by using indicator media to detect certain metabolic characteristics (p. 214). The serovar is determined with specific antisera in the slide agglutination test.

Therapy. Anti-infective agents are the first line of treatment (aminopenicillins, 4-quinolones, cephalosporins). Losses of water and electrolytes may have to be replaced.

Epidemiology and prevention. Bacterial dysentery occurs worldwide, although it is usually seen only sporadically in developed countries. In developing countries, its occurrence is more likely to be endemic and even epidemic. The source of infection is always humans, in most cases infected persons whose stools contain pathogens for up to six weeks after the disease has abated. Transmission is by direct contact (smear infection) or indirect uptake via food, surface water, or flies. Control of dysentery includes exposure prophylaxis measures geared to prevent susceptible persons from coming into contact with the pathogen.

Yersinia (Plague, Enteritis)

■ *Y. pestis* is the causative pathogen of plague (black death, bubonic plague). Plague is a classic rodent zoonosis. It occurred in epidemic proportions in the Middle Ages, but is seen today only sporadically in persons who have had direct contact with diseased wild rodents. The pathogens penetrate into the skin through microtraumata, from where they reach regional lymph nodes in which they proliferate, resulting in the characteristic buboes. In the next stage, the pathogens may enter the bloodstream or the infection may generalize to affect other organs. Laboratory diagnosis involves isolation and identification of the organism in pus, blood, or other material. Therapy requires use of antibiotics.

Y. enterocolitica and *Y. pseudotuberculosis* cause generalized zoonoses in wild animals and livestock. Diseased animals contaminate their surroundings. Humans then take up the pathogens orally in water or food. The organisms penetrate the mucosa of the lower intestinal tract, causing enteritis accompanied by mesenteric lymphadenitis.

Extramesenteric forms are observed in 20% of infected persons (sepsis, lymphadenopathies, various focal infections). Secondary immunopathological complications include arthritis and erythema nodosum. Diagnosis involves identification of the pathogen by means of selective culturing. ■

To date, 10 different species have been classified in the genus *Yersinia*. The species most frequently isolated is *Y. enterocolitica*. *Y. pestis*, the "black death" pathogen responsible for epidemics in the Middle Ages, today no longer presents a significant threat.

Yersinia pestis

Morphology and culture. *Y. pestis* is a nonflagellated, short, encapsulated, Gram-negative rod bacteria that often shows bipolar staining. This bacterium is readily cultured on standard nutrient mediums at 30 °C.

Pathogenesis and clinical picture. The plague is primarily a disease of rodents (rats). It spreads among them by direct contact or via the rat flea. Earlier plague epidemics in humans resulted from these same transmission pathways. The rare human infections seen today result from contact with rodents that are infected with or have died of plague. The pathogen breaches the skin through dermal injuries. From such a location, the bacteria reach regional lymph nodes in which they proliferate. Two to five days after infection, hemorrhagically altered, blue, and swollen lymph nodes (buboes) are observed. Over 90% of *pestis* infections show the "bubonic plague" course. In 50–90% of untreated cases, the organisms break out into the bloodstream to cause a clinical sepsis, in the course of which they may invade many different organs. Dissemination into the pulmonary circulation results in secondary pulmonary plague with bloody, bacteria-rich, highly infectious sputum. Contact with such patients can result in primary pulmonary plague infections due to direct, aerogenic transmission. Left untreated, this form of plague is lethal in nearly 100% of cases.

Diagnosis. The pathogen must be identified in bubo punctate, sputum, or blood by means of microscopy and culturing.

Therapy. In addition to symptomatic treatment, antibiotics are the primary method (streptomycin, tetracyclines, in the case of meningitis, chloramphenicol). Incision of the buboes is contraindicated.

Epidemiology and prevention. Plague still occurs **endemically** in wild rodents over large areas of Asia, Africa, South America, and North America. Human plague infections have been reduced to sporadic instances. The **sources of infection** are mainly diseased rodents. **Transmission** of the disease is mainly via **direct contact** with such animals.

Prevention involves **exposure prophylactic** measures. Persons with manifest disease, in particular the pulmonary form, must be isolated. Contact persons must be quarantined for six days (= incubation period). Cases of plague infection must be reported to health authorities.

Yersinia enterocolitica and Yersinia pseudotuberculosis

Occurrence and significance. *Y. enterocolitica* and *Y. pseudotuberculosis* cause generalized infections in domestic and wild animals, especially rodents. The pathogens can be transmitted from animals to humans. *Y. enterocolitica* is responsible for about 1% of acute enteritis cases in Europe. *Y. pseudotuberculosis* is insignificant in terms of human pathology.

Morphology, culture, and antigen structure. These are pleomorphic, short rods with peritrichous flagellation. They can be cultured on all standard mediums. These *Yersinia* bacteria grow better at 20–30 °C than at 37 °C.

Pathogenesis and clinical pictures. All of the strains isolated as human pathogens bear a 70 kb virulence plasmid with several vir determinants. They code for polypeptides that direct the functions cell adhesion, phagocytosis resistance, serum resistance, and cytotoxicity. Yersiniae also have chromosomal virulence genes, for example markers for invasins, enterotoxins, and an iron capturing system. Exactly how these virulence factors interact to produce the disease is too complex to be described in detail here.

Yersiniae are usually ingested indirectly with food. Although much less frequent, infections can also occur by way of direct contact with diseased animals or animal carriers. The bacteria enter the lower intestinal tract, penetrate the mucosa and are transported with the macrophages into the mesenteric lymph nodes. A simplified overview of the resulting clinical pictures follows:

4

■ **Intestinal yersinioses.** The clinically dominant symptom is enteritis together with mesenteric lymphadenitis. This form is frequently observed in youths and children. Other enteric forms include pseudoappendicitis in youths and children, ileitis (pseudo Crohn disease), and colitis in adults.

■ **Extraintestinal yersinioses.** These infections account for about 20% of cases, usually adults. Notable features of the clinical picture include sepsis, lymphadenopathy, rarely hepatitis, and various local infections (pleuritis, endocarditis, osteomyelitis, cholecystitis, localized abscesses).

■ **Other sequelae.** The immunopathological complications observed in about 20% of acutely infected patients one to six weeks after onset of the intestinal symptoms include reactive arthritis and erythema nodosum.

Diagnosis. A confirmed diagnosis is only possible with identification of the pathogen in a culture based on physiological characteristics. Special mediums are used to isolate the pathogen from stool. The agglutination reaction, an ELISA or immunoblot assay can be used to detect the antibodies.

Therapy. Generally, favorable courses require no chemotherapy. Clinically difficult cases can be treated with cotrimoxazole, second- or third-generation cephalosporins, or fluorinated 4-quinolones.

Epidemiology and prevention. Prevalence of *Y. enterocolitica* and *Y. pseudotuberculosis* in animals is widespread. The most important reservoirs in epidemiological terms are mammals that are diseased or carry latent infections. From these sources, vegetation, soil, and surface water are contaminated. Transmission is by the oral pathway in food. Contact zoonosis is possible, but rare. There are no specific prophylactic measures.

Escherichia coli

■ The natural habitat of *E. coli* is the intestinal tract of humans and animals. It is therefore considered an indicator organism for fecal contamination of water and foods. *E. coli* is the most frequent causative pathogen in human bacterial infections. **Extraintestinal infections** include urinary tract infections, which occur when the tract is obstructed or spontaneously caused by the pathovar UPEC. The most important other coli infections are cholecystitis, appendicitis, peritonitis, postoperative wound infections, and sepsis. **Intestinal infections** are caused by the pathovars EPEC, ETEC, EIEC, EHEC, and EAggEC. EPEC and EAggEC frequently cause diarrhea in infants. ETEC produce enterotoxins that cause a choleralike clinical picture. EIEC cause a dysenterylike infection of the large intestine. EHEC produce verocytotoxins and cause a hemorrhagic colitis as well as the rare hemolytic-uremic syndrome. *E. coli* bacteria infections are diagnosed by means of pathogen identification.   ■

General characteristics. The natural habitat of *E. coli* is the intestines of animals and humans. This bacterium is therefore used as an indicator for fecal contamination of drinking water, bathing water, and foods. Guideline regulations: 100 ml of drinking water must not contain any *E. coli*. Surface water approved for bathing should not contain more than 100 (guideline value) to 2000 (absolute cutoff value) *E. coli* bacteria per 100 ml.

E. coli is also an important human pathogen. It is the bacterial species most frequently isolated from pathological materials.

Morphology, culture, and antigen structure. The Gram-negative, straight rods are peritrichously flagellated. Lactose is broken down rapidly. The complex antigen structure of these bacteria is based on O, K, and H antigens. Fimbrial antigens have also been described. Specific numbers have been assigned to the antigens, e.g., serovar O18:K1:H7.

Pathogenesis and clinical picture of extraintestinal infections. Extraintestinal infections result from relocation of *E. coli* bacteria from one's own flora to places on or in the macroorganism where they are not supposed to be but where conditions for their proliferation are favorable.

■ **Urinary tract infection.** Such an infection manifests either solely in the lower urinary tract (**urethritis, cystitis, urethrocystitis**) or affects the renal pelvis and kidneys (**cystopyelitis, pyelonephritis**). In acute urinary tract infections, *E. coli* is the causative organism in 70–80% of cases and in chronic, persistent infections in 40–50% of cases.

Urinary tract infections result from ascension of the pathogen from the ostium urethrae. Development of such an infection is also furthered by obstructive anomalies, a neurogenic bladder or a vesicoureteral reflux. Urinary tract infections that occur in the absence of any physical anomalies are often caused by the pathovar UPEC (uropathogenic *E. coli*). UPEC strains can attach specifically to receptors of the renal pelvis mucosa with pyelonephritis-associated pili (PAP, P fimbriae, p. 158) or nonfimbrial adhesins (NFA). They produce the hemolysin HlyA.

■ **Sepsis.** *E. coli* causes about 15% of all cases of nosocomial sepsis (*S. aureus* 20%). An *E. coli* sepsis is frequently caused by the pathovar SEPEC, which shows serum resistance (p. 13).

■ **Other *E. coli* infections.** Wound infections, infections of the gallbladder and bile ducts, appendicitis, peritonitis, meningitis in premature infants, neonates, and very elderly patients.

Pathogenesis and clinical pictures of intestinal infections. *E. coli* that cause intestinal infections are now classified in five pathovars with differing pathogenicity and clinical pictures:

■ **Enteropathogenic *E. coli* (EPEC).** These bacteria cause epidemic or sporadic infant diarrheas, now rare in industrialized countries but still a main contributor to infant mortality in developing countries. EPEC attach themselves to the epithelial cells of the small intestine by means of the EPEC adhesion factor (EAF), then inject toxic molecules into the enterocytes by means of a type III secretion system (see p. 17).

■ **Enterotoxic *E. coli* (ETEC).** The pathogenicity of these bacteria is due to the heat-labile enterotoxin LT (inactivation at 60 °C for 30 minutes) and the heat-stable toxins STa and STb (can tolerate temperatures up to 100 °C). Some strains produce all of these toxins, some only one. LT is very similar to cholera toxin. It stimulates the activity of adenylate cyclase (see p. 298). STa stimulates the activity of guanylate cyclase. (cGMP mediates the inhibition of Na^+ absorption and stimulates Cl^- secretion by enterocytes.) ETEC pathogenicity also derives from specific fimbriae, so-called colonizing factors (CFA) that allow these bacteria to attach themselves to small intestine epithelial cells, thus preventing their rapid removal by intestinal peristalsis. The enterotoxins and CFA are determined by plasmid genes. The clinical picture of an ETEC infection is characterized by massive watery diarrhea. The disease can occur at any age. Once the illness has abated, a local immunity is conferred lasting several months.

■ **Enteroinvasive *E. coli* (EIEC).** These bacteria can penetrate into the colonic mucosa, where they cause ulcerous, inflammatory lesions. The pathogenesis and clinical picture of EIEC infections are the same as in bacterial dysentery (p. 288). EIEC strains are often lac-negative.

■ **Enterohemorrhagic *E. coli* (EHEC).** These bacteria are the causative pathogens in the hemorrhagic colitis and hemolytic-uremic syndrome (HUS) that occur in about 5% of EHEC infections, accompanied by acute renal failure, thrombocytopenia, and anemia. EHEC possess specific, plasmid-coded fimbriae for adhesion to enterocytes. They can also produce pro-phage-determined cytotoxins (shigalike toxins or verocytotoxins). Some authors therefore designate them as VTEC (verotoxin-producing *E. coli*). EHEC strains have been found in the O serogroups O157, O26, O111, O145, and others. The serovar most frequently responsible for HUS is O157:H7.

■ **Enteroaggregative *E. coli* (EAggEC).** These bacteria cause watery, and sometimes hemorrhagic, diarrhea in infants and small children. Adhesion to enterocytes with specific attachment fimbriae. Production of a toxin identical to STa in ETEC.

Diagnosis. Extraintestinal infections are diagnosed by identifying the pathogen in relevant materials. Diagnosis of a urinary tract infection with midstream urine requires determination of the bacterial count to ensure that an infection can be distinguished from a contamination. Counts $\geq 10^5$/ml tend to indicate an infection, $\leq 10^3$/ml a contamination, 10^4/ml could go either way. Specific gene probes are now being used to make identification of intestinal pathogen *E. coli* bacteria less difficult.

Therapy. Antibiotic therapy must take into consideration the resistance pattern of the pathogen. Aminopenicillins, ureidopenicillins, cephalosporins, 4-quinolones, or cotrimoxazole are useful agents. Severe diarrhea necessitates oral replacement of fluid and electrolyte losses according to the WHO formula: 3.5 g NaCl, 2.5 g $NaHCO_3$, 1.5 g KCl, 20 g glucose per liter of water. When required, intestinal activity is slowed down with loperamide.

Epidemiology and prevention. Transmission of intestinal infections is usually indirect via food, drinking water, or surface water. Fifty percent of travelers' diarrhea cases are caused by *E. coli*, in most cases ETEC.

The most effective preventive measures against intestinal infections, e.g., when travelling in countries with warm climates, is to eat only thoroughly cooked foods and drink only disinfected water. Studies have demonstrated the efficacy of chemoprophylaxis with anti-infective agents in preventing traveler's diarrhea, whereby the agents used must not reduce the normal aerobic intestinal flora (4-quinolones and cotrimoxazole are suitable). This method is hardly practicable, however, in view of the large numbers of travelers.

Opportunistic Enterobacteriaceae

Many *Enterobacteriaceae* with minimum pathogenicity are classic opportunists. The most frequent opportunistic infections caused by them are: **urinary tract infections, respiratory tract infections, wound infections,**

Table 4.**9** Overview of the Most Important *Enterobacteriaceae* That Cause Opportunistic Infections

Bacterial species	Properties
Escherichia coli	See p. 280ff., p. 292ff.
Citrobacter freundii; C. divs.; C. amalonaticus	Can use citrate as its sole source of C; delayed breakdown of lactose; nonmotile
Klebsiella pneumoniae; K. oxytoca and others	Lactose-positive; nonmotile; many strains have a polysaccharide capsule. Cause approx. 10% of nosocomial infections. Causative organism in so-called Friedländer's pneumonia in predisposed persons, especially in the presence of chronic pulmonary diseases.
Klebsiella ozaenae	Causative pathogen in ozena; atrophy of nasal mucosa
Klebsiella rhinoscleromatis	Causative pathogen in rhinoscleroma; granuloma in the nose and pharynx
Enterobacter cloace; E. aerogenes; E. agglomerans; E. sakazakii, and others	Lactose-positive; motile; frequent multiple resistance to antibiotics
Serratia marcescens and others	Lactose-positive; motile; frequent multiple resistance to antibiotics, some strains produce red pigment at 20 °C
Proteus mirabilis *Proteus vulgaris*	Lactose-negative; highly motile; wanders on surface of nutrient agar (swarming). O antigens OX-2, OX-19, and OX-K from *P. vulgaris* are identical to rickettsiae antigens. For this reason, antibodies to rickettsiae were formerly identified using these strains (Weil-Felix agglutination test)
Morganella morganii	Lactose-negative; frequent multiple resistance to antibiotics
Providencia rettgeri; P. stuartii	Lactose-negative; frequent multiple resistance to antibiotics

4

dermal and subcutaneous infections, and sepsis. Such infections only occur in predisposed hosts, they are frequently seen in patients with severe primary diseases. Another reason why opportunistic *Enterobacteriaceae* have become so important in hospital medicine is the frequent development of resistance to anti-infective agents, which ability enables them to persist at locations where use of such agents is particularly intensive, i.e., in hospitals. Occurrence of multiple resistance in *Enterobacteriaceae* is due to the impressive genetic variability of these organisms (p. 170). Table 4.**9** provides an overview of the most important opportunistic *Enterobacteriaceae*.

Vibrio, Aeromonas, and Plesiomonas

■ *Vibrio cholerae* is the most important species in this group from a medical point of view. Cholera vibrios are Gram-negative, comma-shaped, monotrichously flagellated rods. They show alkali tolerance (pH 9), which is useful for selective culturing of *V. cholerae* in alkaline peptone water. The primary cholera pathogen is serovar O:1. NonO:1 strains (e.g., O:139) cause the typical clinical picture in rare cases. O:1 vibrios are further subdivided into the biovars *cholerae* and *eltor*. The disease develops when the pathogens enter the intestinal tract with food or drinking water in large numbers ($\geq 10^8$). The vibrios multiply in the proximal small intestine and produce an enterotoxin. This toxin stimulates a series of reactions in enterocytes, the end result of which is increased transport of electrolytes out of the enterocytes, whereby water is also lost passively. Massive watery diarrhea (up to 20 l/day) results in exsiccosis. The initial therapeutic focus is thus on replacement of lost electrolytes and water. Cholera occurs only in humans. Preventive measures concentrate on protection from exposure to the organism. A killed whole cell vaccine and an attenuated live vaccine are available. They provide only a moderate degree of protection over a period of only six months. International healthcare sources report an incubation period of five days.　■

The bacteria in these groups are Gram-negative rods with a comma or spiral shape. Their natural habitat is in most cases damp biotopes including the ocean. Some of them cause infections in fish (e.g., *Aeromonas salmonicida*). By far the most important species in terms of human medicine is *Vibrio cholerae*.

Vibrio cholerae (Cholera)

Morphology and culture. Cholera vibrios are Gram-negative rod bacteria, usually slightly bent (comma-shaped), 1.5–2 μm in length, and 0.3–0.5 μm wide, with monotrichous flagellation (Fig. 4.**19**).

Culturing of *V. cholerae* is possible on simple nutrient mediums at 37 °C in a normal atmosphere. Owing to its pronounced alkali stability, *V. cholerae* can be selectively cultured out of bacterial mixtures at pH 9.

Antigens and classification. *V. cholerae* bacteria are subdivided into serovars based on their O antigens (lipopolysaccharide antigens). The serovar pathogen is usually serovar O:1. Strains that do not react to an O:1 antiserum are grouped together as nonO:1 vibrios. NonO:1 strains were recently described in India (O:139) as also causing the classic clinical picture of cholera. O:1 vibrios are further subclassified in the biovars *cholerae* and *eltor* based on physiological characteristics. The var *eltor* has a very low level of virulence.

Cholera toxin. Cholera toxin is the sole cause of the clinical disease. This substance induces the enterocytes to increase secretion of electrolytes, above all Cl⁻ ions, whereby passive water loss also occurs. The toxin belongs to the group of AB toxins (see p. 16). Subunit **B** of the toxin **b**inds to enterocyte receptors, the **a**ctive toxin subunit **A** causes the adenylate cyclase in the enterocytes to produce cAMP continuously and in large amounts (Fig. 4.**20**). cAMP in turn acts as a second messenger to activate protein kinase A, which then activates the specific cell proteins that control secretion of electrolytes. The toxin genes *ctxA* and *ctxB* are components of the so-called CTX element, which is integrated in the nucleoid of toxic cholera vibrios (see lysogenic conversion, p. 186) as part of the genome of the filamentous prophage CTXφ. The CTX element also includes several regulator genes that regulate both produc-

Vibrio cholerae

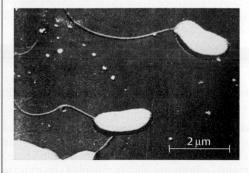

Fig. 4.**19** Comma-shaped rod bacteria with monotrichous flagellation (SEM image).

2 μm

Mechanism of Action of Cholera Toxin

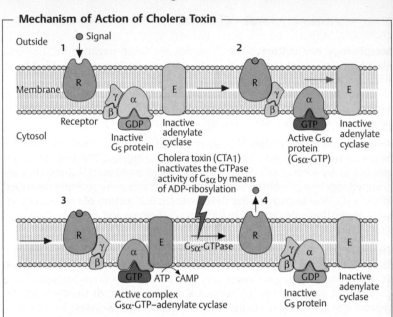

Fig. 4.**20** Cholera toxin disrupts the G_s protein-mediated signal cascade.

1 The G_s proteins in the membrane comprise the three subunits α, β, and γ. GDP is bound to subunit α. G_s is inactive in this configuration.

2 After a signal molecule is bound to the membrane receptor R, the subunits dissociate from G_s; also, the GDP on the $G_{s\alpha}$ is phosphorylated to GTP.

3 $G_{s\alpha}$–GTP then combines with adenylate cyclase to form the active enzyme that transforms ATP into the second messenger cAMP.

4 When the signal molecule once again dissociates from the receptor, the GTP bound to the $G_{s\alpha}$ is dephosphorylated to GDP, i.e., inactive status is restored. This is the step that cholera toxin prevents: the A_1 subunit of the cholera toxin (CTA_1) catalyzes ADP-ribosylation of $G_{s\alpha}$, which thus loses its GTPase activity so that the adenylate cyclase is not "switched off" and synthesis of cAMP continues unchecked.

tion of the toxin and formation of the so-called toxin-coregulated pili (TCP) on the surface of the *Vibrio* cells.

Pathogenesis and clinical picture. Infection results from oral ingestion of the pathogen. The infective dose must be large ($\geq 10^8$), since many vibrios are killed by the hydrochloric acid in gastric juice. Based on their pronounced stability in alkaline environments, vibrios are able to colonize the mucosa of the proximal small intestine with the help of TCP (see above) and secrete cholera toxin (see Fig. 4.**20**). The pathogen does not invade the mucosa.

The incubation period of cholera is two to five days. The clinical picture is characterized by voluminous, watery diarrhea and vomiting. The amount of fluids lost per day can be as high as 20 l. Further symptoms derive from the resulting exsiccosis: hypotension, tachycardia, anuria, and hypothermia. Lethality can be as high as 50% in untreated cases.

Diagnosis requires identification of the pathogen in stool or vomit. Sometimes a rapid microscopical diagnosis succeeds in finding numerous Gram-negative, bent rods in swarm patterns. Culturing is done on liquid or solid selective mediums, e.g., alkaline peptone water or taurocholate gelatin agar. Suspected colonies are identified by biochemical means or by detection of the O:1 antigen in an agglutination reaction.

Therapy. The most important measure is restoration of the disturbed water and electrolyte balance in the body. Secondly, tetracyclines and cotrimoxazole can be used, above all to reduce fecal elimination levels and shorten the period of pathogen secretion.

Epidemiology and prevention. Nineteenth-century Europe experienced several cholera pandemics, all of which were caused by the classic *cholerae* biovar. An increasing number of cases caused by the biovar *eltor*, which is characterized by a lower level of virulence, have been observed since 1961. With the exception of minor epidemics in Italy and Spain, Europe, and the USA have been spared major outbreaks of cholera in more recent times. South America has for a number of years been the venue of epidemics of the disease.

Humans are the only **source of infection**. Infected persons in particular eliminate large numbers of pathogens. Convalescents may also shed *V. cholerae* for weeks or even months after the infection has abated. Chronic carriers as with typhoid fever are very rare. **Transmission** of the disease is usually via foods, and in particular drinking water. This explains why cholera can readily spread to epidemic proportions in countries with poor hygiene standards.

Protection from exposure to the pathogen is the main thrust of the relevant **preventive measures**. In general, control of cholera means ensuring adequate food and water hygiene and proper elimination of sewage. In case of an outbreak, infected persons must be isolated. Infectious excreta and contaminated objects must be disinfected. Even suspected cases of cholera must be reported to health authorities without delay. The incubation period of the cholera *vibrio* is reported in international health regulations to be five days. A vaccine containing killed cells as well an attenuated live vaccine are available. The level of immunization protection is, however, incomplete and lasts for only six months.

Other Vibrio Bacteria

Vibrio parahemolyticus is a halophilic (salt-friendly) species found in warm ocean shallows and brackish water. These bacteria can cause gastroenteritis epidemics. The pathogen is transmitted to humans with food (seafood, raw fish). The illness is transient in most cases and symptomatic therapy is sufficient.

Vibrio vulnificus is another aquatic organism that produces a very small number of septic infections, mainly in immunosuppressed patients.

Aeromonas and Plesiomonas

The bacteria of these two genera live in freshwater biotopes. Some are capable of causing infection in fish (*A. salmonicida*). They are occasionally observed as contaminants of moist parts of medical apparatus such as dialysis equipment, vaporizers, and respirators. They can cause nosocomial infections in hospitalized patients with weakened immune systems. Cases of gastroenteritis may result from eating foods contaminated with large numbers of these bacteria.

Haemophilus and Pasteurella

■ The most important species of *Pasteurellaceae* from the medical point of view is *Haemophilus influenzae*. This is a nonmotile, Gram-negative rod that is often encapsulated. Capsule serovar b is the main pathogenic form. *H. influenzae* is a facultative anaerobe that requires growth factors X (hemin) and V (NAD, NADP) in its culture medium. *H. influenzae* is a typical parasite of the respiratory tract mucosa. It occurs only in humans. It causes infections of the upper and lower respiratory tract in individuals with weakened immune defenses and in children under the age of four or five. Invasive infections—meningitis and sepsis—are also observed in small children. A betalactamase-stable betalactam antibiotic is required for treatment since the number of betalactamase-producing strains observed is increasing. Conjugate vaccines in which the capsule polysaccharide is coupled with proteins are available for prophylactic immunization. These vaccines can be administered beginning in the third month of life. ■

Haemophilus influenzae

Hemophilic bacteria are so designated because they require growth factors contained in blood. The most important human pathogen in this genus is *H. influenzae*. Other *Haemophilus* species either infect only animals or are found in the normal human mucosal flora. These latter include *H. parainfluenzae*, *H. hemolyticus*, *H. segnis*, *H. aphrophilus*, and *H. paraphrophilus*. These species can cause infections on occasion.

Morphology and culture. *Haemophilus* are small (length: 1.0–1.5 μm, width: 0.3 μm), often encapsulated, nonmotile, Gram-negative rods (Fig. 4.**21a**). The encapsulated strains are subclassified in serovars a-f based on the fine structure of their capsule polysaccharides. Serovar b (Hib) causes most *Haemophilus* infections in humans.

4

Haemophilus influenzae

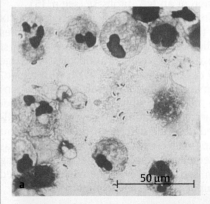

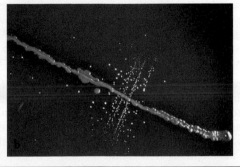

Fig. 4.**21 a** Gram-stained cerebrospinal fluid sediment preparation. Fine, Gram-negative rods surrounded by a capsule (serovar b). Clinical diagnosis: purulent meningitis.

b Satellite colonies of *Haemophilus influenzae* surrounding the *Staphylococcus aureus* streak. *S. aureus* provides small amounts of V factor. The blood agar contains free X factor.

H. influenzae is a facultative anaerobe requiring growth factors X and V in its culture medium. The X factor is hemin, required by the bacteria to synthesize enzymes containing heme (cytochromes, catalase, oxidases). The X factor requirement is greatly reduced in anaerobic culturing. The V factor was identified as NAD or NADP. A standard blood agar plate does not contain sufficient free V factor. Some bacteria, in particular *Staphylococcus aureus*, produce excess NAD and even secrete this coenzyme into the medium. That is why *H. influenzae* can proliferate in the immediate vicinity of *S. aureus* colonies. This is known as the **satellite phenomenon** (Fig. 4.**21b**). The medium normally used to culture *H. influenzae* is chocolate agar containing sufficient amounts of the X and V factors.

Pathogenesis and clinical pictures. *H. influenzae* is a mucosal parasite of the upper respiratory tract present in 30–50% of healthy persons. The strains usually found are nonencapsulated and therefore hardly virulent. The capsule protects the cells from phagocytosis and is thus the primary determinant of pathogenicity. Others include the affinity of *H. influenzae* to respiratory tract mucosa and meninges and production of an IgA_1 protease (see p. 15).

H. influenzae infections are seen frequently in children aged from six months to four years of age due to the low levels of anticapsule antibodies in this age group. Maternal antibodies still protect children during the first months of life. The body has built up a sufficient store of antibodies by the age of four. Any list of potential clinical developments must begin with meningitis, followed by epiglottitis, pneumonia, empyema, septic arthritis, osteomyelitis, pericarditis, cellulitis, otitis media, and sinusitis. *Haemophilus* infections in adults are usually secondary complications of severe primary illnesses or the result of compromised immune defenses. The most frequent complication is an acute exacerbation of chronic bronchitis. Pneumonias caused by *H. influenzae* are also observed, often as superinfections following viral influenza. In immunocompromised adults, even the nonencapsulated strains can cause infections of the upper and lower respiratory tract.

Diagnosis. The method of choice is identification of the pathogen in cerebrospinal fluid, blood, pus, or purulent sputum using microscopy and culture assays. Satelliting on blood agar is an indication of a V factor requirement. An X factor requirement is confirmed most readily by the porphyrin test, with a negative result in the presence of *H. influenzae*.

Therapy. In view of the increasing number of betalactamase-producing *H. influenzae* strains observed in recent years, penicillinase-stable betalactam antibiotics should be used to treat these infections. The likelihood that a strain produces betalactamase is 5–30% in most countries. 4-quinolones are an alternative to betalactams that should not, however, be used in children. The agent of choice in meningitis is ceftriaxone.

Epidemiology and prevention. *H. influenzae* is found only in humans. The incidence of severe invasive infections (meningitis, sepsis, epiglottitis) in children has been reduced drastically—to about one in 10 of the numbers seen previously—since a vaccination program was started, and will continue to fall assuming the vaccinations are continued (see vaccination schedule, p. 33).

Immunization is achieved with the conjugate vaccine Hib in which the capsule polysaccharide epitope "b" conferring immunity is conjugated to protein. Such a conjugate vaccine can be administered as early as the first month of life. The immune system does not respond to pure polysaccharide vaccines until about the age of two, since polysaccharides are T-independent antigens against which hardly any antibodies are produced in the first two years of life. There is also no booster response. A four-day regimen of rifampicin has proved to be an effective chemoprophylactic treatment for nonvaccinated small children who have been exposed to the organism.

4

Haemophilus ducreyi and Haemophilus aegyptius

H. ducreyi are short, Gram-negative, nonmotile rods that are difficult to culture and require special mediums. This bacterium causes ulcus molle (soft chancre) a tropical venereal disease seen rarely in central Europe. The infection locus presents as a painful, readily bleeding ulcer occurring mainly in the genital area. Regional lymph nodes are quite swollen. Identification of the pathogen by means of microscopy and culturing are needed to confirm the diagnosis. Therapeutic alternatives include sulfonamides, streptomycin, and tetracyclines.

H. aegyptius (possibly identical with biovar III of **Haemophilus influenzae**) causes a purulent conjunctivitis occurring mainly in northern Africa, in particular Egypt. A raised incidence of Brazilian purpuric fever, a systemic infection with this organism, has been observed in Brazil in recent years.

Pasteurella

Various different species belonging to the genus *Pasteurella* occur in the normal mucosal flora of animals and humans; some are pathogenic in animals. Their significance as human pathogens is minor. Infections by **Pasteurella multocida** are described here as examples of human pasteurelloses. The bacteria invade the organism through bite or scratch injuries or in droplets during contact with infected animals. Weakened immune defenses may then result in either local wound infections with lymphadenitis, subacute to chronic infections of the lower respiratory tract, or CNS infections (after cerebral trauma or brain surgery). Diagnosis is based on pathogen identification.

A penicillin or cephalosporin is recommended for therapy. Sources of infection include domestic animals (dogs, cats, birds, guinea pigs) and livestock (cattle, sheep, goats, pigs).

Gram-Negative Rod Bacteria with Low Pathogenic Potential

The bacterial species listed in Table 4.**10** are typical opportunists that occasionally cause infections in persons with defective specific or nonspecific immune defenses. When they are isolated from infective material, their pathological significance is in most cases difficult to interpret.

Table 4.**10** Overview of Gram-Negative Rod Bacteria with Low Pathogenic Potential

Bacterial species	Most important characteristics
HACEK group	
– Hemophilus aphrophilus	Endocarditis, cerebral abscesses
– Actinobacillus actinomycetemcomitans	Part of normal oral cavity flora. Nonmotile, slender rods; microaerophilic; colonies on blood agar with "starfish" appearance. Accompanying bacterium in approx. 25% of oral-cervicofacial **actinomycoses**. Penicillin G resistance. Also a pathogen in endocarditis.
– Cardiobacterium hominis	Nonmotile; pleomorphic. Normal flora of the respiratory tract. Culturing on blood agar in 5% CO_2 at 35 °C for 4 days. **Endocarditis**. Occasionally observed as component of mixed flora in facial purulent infections.
– Eikenella corrodens	Nonmotile, coccoid. Normal flora of respiratory and intestinal tracts. Cultures, on blood agar, show corrosion of the agar surface. **Abscesses, wound infections, peritonitis, empyemas, septic arthritis**, often as part of a mixed flora. Also reports of **endocarditis** and **meningitis**.
– Kingella kingae	Normal flora of the upper respiratory tract. Rare cases of endocarditis, arthritis, osteomyelitis.

Table 4.**10**   *Continued: Overview of Other Gram-Negative Rod Bacteria*

Bacterial species	Most important characteristics
Calymmatobacterium granulomatis (syn. *Donovania granulomatis*)	Nonmotile, capsule, culturing on mediums containing egg yolk; facultative anaerobe. **Granuloma inguinale**. Venereal disease; indolent, ulcerogranulomatous lesions on skin and mucosa. Sporadic occurrence in Europe. Diagnosis involves identification of bacteria in vacuoles of large mononuclear cells using Giemsa staining (Donovan bodies). Antibiotics: aminoglycosides, tetracyclines
Streptobacillus moniliformis	Pronounced pleomorphism; frequent production of filaments because of defective cell walls. Culturing in enriched mediums at 35 °C, 5% CO_2, 3 days. Component of oral cavity flora in rats, mice, cats **Rat bite fever**. Incubation period 1–22 days. Fever, arthralgias, myalgias, exanthema. Possible inflammation at site of bite. Polyarthritis in 50% of patients. Therapy with penicillin G.
Chryseobacterium (formerly *Flavobacterium*) *meningosepticum* (and other flavobacteria)	Strictly aerobic; often with yellow pigment; nonfermenter. Natural habitat soil and natural bodies of water. **Meningitis.** In neonates. Poor prognosis. **Sepsis, pneumonia** in immunocompromised patients. All infections rare.
Alcaligenes faecalis (and other species of the genus *Alcaligenes*)	Strictly aerobic; nonfermenter. Natural habitat soil and surface water. Various **opportunistic infections** in patients with severe primary illnesses; usually isolated as a component in mixed flora; data difficult to interpret.
Capnocytophaga spp.	Component of normal oral cavity flora in humans and dogs. Long, thin, fusiform rods. Proliferation on blood agar in presence of 5–10% CO_2. Can contribute to pathogenesis of **periodontitis**. **Sepsis** in agranulocytosis, leukemias, malignancys. Wide variety of purulent processes. Often component of mixed flora.

4

Campylobacter, Helicobacter, Spirillum

■ *Campylobacter*, *Helicobacter*, and *Spirillum* belong to the group of spiral, motile, Gram-negative, microaerophilic bacteria. *C. jejuni* causes a form of enteritis. The sources of infection are diseased animals. The pathogens are transmitted to humans in food. The diseases are sometimes also communicable among humans. The pathogens are identified for diagnostic purposes in stool cultures using special selective mediums. *Helicobacter pylori* contribute to the pathogenesis of type B gastritis and peptic ulcers. *Spirillum minus* causes rat bite fever, known as sodoku in Japan where it is frequent. ■

4

The genera *Campylobacter*, *Helicobacter*, and *Spirillum* belong to the group of aerobic, microaerophilic, motile, Gram-negative rod bacteria with a helical/vibrioid form (p. 220). Human pathogens are found in all three genera.

Campylobacter

Classification. For several years now, *Campylobacter* bacteria have been classified together with *Arcobacter* (medically insignificant) in the new family *Campylobacteriaceae* (fam. nov.). The genus *Campylobacter* comprises numerous species, among which *C. jejuni* (more rarely *C. coli*, *C. lari*) as well as *C. fetus* have been observed as causative pathogens in human infections.

Morphology and culture. *Campylobacter* are slender, spirally shaped rods 0.2–0.5 μm thick and 0.5–5 μm long. Individual cells may have one spiral winding or several. A single flagellum is attached to either one or both poles.

Campylobacter can, under microaerophilic conditions, and in an atmosphere containing 5% O_2 and 10% CO_2, be cultured on blood agar plates. The optimum proliferation temperature for *C. fetus* is 25 °C and for *C. jejuni* 42 °C.

Pathogenesis and clinical pictures. The details of the pathogenic mechanisms of these pathogens are largely unknown. *C. jejuni* produces an enterotoxin similar to the STa produced by *E. coli* as well as a number of cytotoxins. *C. jejuni* causes a form of enterocolitis with watery, sometimes bloody diarrhea and fever. The incubation period is two to five days. The manifest illness lasts less than one week.

C. fetus has been identified in isolated cases as a pathogen in endocarditis, meningitis, peritonitis, arthritis, cholecystitis, salpingitis, and sepsis in immunocompromised patients.

Diagnosis. To isolate *C. jejuni* in stool cultures, mediums are used containing selective supplements (e.g., various anti-infective agents). The cultures are incubated for 48 hours at 42 °C in a microaerophilic atmosphere. Identification is based on growth requirements as well as detection of catalase and oxidase.

C. fetus is readily isolated in most cases, since it is usually the only organism found in the material (e.g., blood, cerebrospinal fluid, joint punctate, pus, etc.).

Therapy. Severe *Campylobacter* infections are treated with macrolides or 4-quinolones. Resistance is known to occur.

Epidemiology and prevention. *Campylobacter jejuni* is among the most frequent enteritis pathogens worldwide. The bacteria are transmitted from animals to humans via food and drinking water. Direct smear infection transmission among humans is possible, especially in kindergarten or family groups. There are no specific preventive measures.

Helicobacter pylori

Morphology and culture. *H. pylori* are spirally shaped, Gram-negative rods with lophotrichous flagellation. Cultures from stomach biopsies are grown on enriched mediums and selective mediums under microaerobic conditions (90% N_2, 5% CO_2, and 5% O_2) for three to four days. Identification is based on detection of oxidase, catalase, and urease.

Pathogenesis and clinical pictures. *H. pylori* occurs only in humans and is transmitted by the fecal-oral pathway. The pathogen colonizes and infects the stomach mucosa. The pathogenicity factors include pronounced motility for efficient target cell searching, adhesion to the surface epithelial cells of the stomach, urease that releases ammonia from urea to facilitate survival of the cells in a highly acidic environment and a vacuolizing cytotoxin (VacA) that destroys epithelial cells.

Once the pathogen has infected the stomach tissues an acute gastritis results, the course of which may or may not involve overt symptoms. Potential sequelae include:

1. Mild chronic gastritis type B that may persist for years or even decades and is often asymptomatic.
2. Duodenal ulceration, sometimes gastric ulceration as well.
3. Chronic atrophic gastritis from which a gastric adenocarcinoma sometimes develops.
4. Rarely B cell lymphomas of the gastric mucosa (MALTomas).

Diagnosis. Histopathological, cultural and, molecular identification of the bacteria in stomach lining biopsies. A noninvasive breath test involving ingestion of ^{13}C-labeled urea and measurement of $^{13}CO_2$ in the expelled air. Antigen detection in stool. Antibodies can be identified with an ELISA or Western blotting.

Therapy. In patients with ulcers and/or gastritis symptoms, a triple combination therapy with omeprazole (proton pump blocker), metronidazole, and clarithromycin lasting seven days is successful in 90% of cases.

Epidemiology. Based on seroepidemiological studies we know that *H. pylori* occur worldwide. Generalized contamination of the population begins in childhood and may reach 100% in adults in areas with poor hygiene. The contamination level is about 50% among older adults in industrialized countries. Transmission is by the fecal-oral route.

Spirillum minus

This species is a motile bacterium only 0.2 μm thick and 3–5 μm long with two to three spiral windings. It cannot be grown on culture mediums. *S. minus* causes spirillary rat bite fever, also known as sodoku. This disease occurs worldwide, with a high level of incidence in Japan. The organism is transmitted to humans by the bites of rats, mice, squirrels, and domestic animals that eat rodents. Following an incubation period of seven to 21 days a febrile condition develops with lymphangitis and lymphadenitis. Ulcerous lesions develop at the portal of entry. Diagnosis can be done by using dark field or phase contrast microscopy to detect the spirilla in blood or ulcerous material. Penicillin G is used to treat the infection.

Pseudomonas, Stenotrophomonas, Burkholderia

■ Pseudomonads are Gram-negative, aerobic, rod-shaped bacteria with widespread occurrence in nature, especially in damp biotopes. The most important species from a medical point of view is *Pseudomonas aeruginosa*. Free O_2 is required as a terminal electron acceptor to grow the organism in cultures. The pathogenesis of *Pseudomonas* infections is complex. The organism can use its attachment pili to adhere to host cells. The relevant virulence factors are: exotoxin A, exoenzyme S, cytotoxin, various metal proteases, and two types of phospholipase C. Of course, the lipopolysaccharide of the outer membrane also plays an important role in the pathogenesis. *Pseudomonas* infections occur only in patients with weakened immune defense systems, notably pneumonias in cystic fibrosis, colonization of burn wounds, endocarditis in drug addicts, postoperative wound infection, urinary tract infection, sepsis. *P. aeruginosa* frequently contributes to nosocomial infections. Diagnosis requires identification of the pathogen in cultures. Multiple resistance to anti-infective agents presents a therapeutic problem.

Numerous other *Pseudomonas* species and the species of the genera *Burkholderia* and *Stenotrophomonas* are occasionally found in pathogenic roles in immunosuppressed patients. *B. mallei* causes malleus (glanders) and *B. pseudomallei* causes melioidosis. ∎

Pseudomonas aeruginosa

4

Occurrence, significance. All pseudomonads are widespread in nature. They are regularly found in soils, surface water, including the ocean, on plants and, in small numbers, in human and animal intestines. They can proliferate in a moist milieu containing only traces of nutrient substances. The most important species in this group from a medical point of view is *P. aeruginosa*, which causes infections in person with immune defects.

Morphology and culture. *P. aeruginosa* are plump, 2–4 µm long rods with one to several polar flagella. Some strains can produce a viscous extracellular slime layer. These mucoid strains are frequently isolated in material from cystic fibrosis patients. *P. aeruginosa* possesses an outer membrane as part of its cell wall. The architecture of this membrane is responsible for the natural resistance of this bacterium to many antibiotics.

P. aeruginosa can only be grown in culture mediums containing free O_2 as a terminal electron acceptor. In nutrient broth, the organism therefore grows at the surface to form a so-called pellicle. Colonies on nutrient agar often have a metallic sheen (*P. aeruginosa*; Latin: aes = metal ore). Given suitable conditions, *P. aeruginosa* can produce two pigments, i.e., both yellow-green fluorescein and blue-green pyocyanin.

Pathogenesis and clinical pictures. The pathomechanisms involved are highly complex. *P. aeruginosa* usually enters body tissues through injuries. It attaches to tissue cells using specific attachment fimbriae. The most important virulence factor is exotoxin A (ADP ribosyl transferase), which blocks translation in protein synthesis by inactivating the elongation factor eEF2. The exoenzyme S (also an ADP ribosyl transferase) inactivates cytoskeletal proteins and GTP-binding proteins in eukaryotic cells. The so-called cytotoxin damages cells by creating transmembrane pores. Various different metalloproteases hydrolyze elastin, collagen, or laminin. Two type C phospholipases show membrane activity. Despite these pathogenic determinants, infections are rare in immunocompetent individuals. Defective nonspecific and specific immune defenses are preconditions for clinically manifest infections. Patients suffering from a neutropenia are at high risk. The main infections are pneumonias in cystic fibrosis or in patients on respiratory equipment, infections of burn wounds, postoperative wound infections, chronic pyelonephritis, endocarditis in drug addicts, sepsis, and malignant otitis externa. *P. aeruginosa* frequently causes nosocomial infections (see p. 343).

Diagnosis. Laboratory diagnosis includes isolation of the pathogen from relevant materials and its identification based on a specific pattern of metabolic properties.

Therapy. The antibiotics that can be used to treat *P. aeruginosa* infections are aminoglycosides, acylureidopenicillins, carboxylpenicillins, group 3b cephalosporins (see p. 190), and carbapenems. Combination of an aminoglycoside with a betalactam is indicated in severe infections. Susceptibility tests are necessary due to frequent resistance.

Epidemiology and prevention. Except in cystic fibrosis, *P. aeruginosa* is mainly a hospital problem. Since this ubiquitous organism can proliferate under the sparest of conditions in a moist milieu, a number of sources of infection are possible: sinks, toilets, cosmetics, vaporizers, inhalers, respirators, anesthesiology equipment, dialysis equipment, etc. Infected patients and staff carrying the organism are also potential primary sources of infection. Neutropenic patients are particularly susceptible. Preventive measures i.e., above all disinfection and clinical hygiene, concentrate on avoiding exposure.

Other Pseudomonas species, Stenotrophomonas and Burkholderia

Opportunistic pseudomonads. Other *Pseudomonas* species besides *P. aeruginosa* are capable of causing infections in immunosuppressed patients. These nosocomial infections are, however, infrequent. It would therefore not be particularly useful here to list all of the species that occasionally come to the attention of physicians. Classic opportunists also include *Stenotrophomonas maltophilia* (formerly *Xanthomonas maltophilia*) and *Burkholderia cepacia* (formerly *Pseudomonas cepacia*). These species all occur in hospitals and frequently show resistance to anti-infective agents. Antibiotic therapy must therefore always be based on a resistance test.

Burkholderia mallei. This species is the causative organism in malleus or glanders, a disease of solipeds. The bacteria invade the human organism through microtraumata, e.g., in the skin or mucosa, and form local ulcers. Starting from these primary infection foci they can move to other organs, either lymphogenously or hematogenously, and cause secondary abscesses there. Malleus no longer occurs in Europe.

Burkholderia pseudomallei. This species is the causative organism in melioidosis, a disease of animals and humans resembling malleus. The natural reservoirs of *B. pseudomallei* are soil and surface water. The pathogen invades the body through injuries of the skin or mucosa and causes multiple subcutaneous and subserous abscesses and granulomas. Starting from primary foci, the infection can disseminate and cause abscesses in a number of different organs. This disease is observed mainly in Asia.

Legionella (Legionnaire's Disease)

■ *Legionella* is the only genus in the family *Legionellaceae*. The species *Legionella pneumophila* is responsible for most legionelloses in humans. Legionellae are difficult to stain. They are Gram-negative, aerobic rod bacteria. Special mediums must be used to grow them in cultures. Infections with *Legionella* occur when droplets containing the pathogens are inhaled. Two clinically distinct forms are on record: legionnaire's disease leading to a multifocal pneumonia and nonpneumonic legionellosis or Pontiac fever. The persons most likely to contract legionnaire's disease are those with a primary cardiopulmonary disease and generally weakened immune defenses. Laboratory diagnostic methods include microscopy with direct immunofluorescence, culturing on special mediums and antibody assays. The antibiotics of choice are the macrolides. The natural habitat of legionellae is damp biotopes. The sources of infection listed in the literature include hot and cold water supply systems, cooling towers, moisturizing units in air conditioners, and whirlpool baths. Legionelloses can occur both sporadically and in epidemics. ■

Classification. *Legionella* bacteria were discovered in 1976, occasioned by an epidemic among those attending a conference of American Legionnaires (former professional soldiers). They are now classified in the family *Legionellaceae*, which to date comprises only the genus *Legionella*. This genus contains numerous species not listed here. Most human infections are caused by *L. pneumophila*, which species is subdivided into 12 serogroups. Human infections are caused mainly by serogroup 1.

Morphology and culture. *L. pneumophila* is a rod bacterium 0.3–1 µm wide and 2–20 µm long. Its cell wall structure is of the Gram-negative type, but gram staining hardly "takes" with these bacteria at all. They can be rendered visible by means of direct immunofluorescence.

Legionella grow only on special mediums in an atmosphere containing 5% CO_2.

Pathogenesis and clinical picture. The pathomechanisms employed by legionellae are not yet fully clarified. These organisms are facultative intracellular bacteria that can survive in professional phagocytes and in alveolar macrophages. They are capable of preventing the phagosome from fusing with lysosomes. They also produce a toxin that blocks the oxidative burst.

Two clinical forms of legionellosis have been described:

■ **Legionnaire's disease.** Infection results from inhalation of droplets containing the pathogens. The incubation period is two to 10 days. The clinical picture is characterized by a multifocal, sometimes necrotizing pneumonia. Occurrence is more likely in patients with cardiopulmonary primary diseases or other immunocompromising conditions. Lethality >20%.

■ **Pontiac fever.** Named after an epidemic in Michigan. Incubation period one to two days. Nonpneumonic, febrile infection. Self-limiting. Rare.

Diagnosis. Specific antibodies marked with fluorescein are used to detect the pathogens in material from the lower respiratory tract. For cultures, special culture mediums must be used containing selective supplements to exclude contaminants. The mediums must be incubated for three to five days. *Legionella* antigen can be identified in urine with an EIA. A gene probe can also be used for direct detection of the nucleic acid (rDNA) specific to the genus *Legionella* in the material. Antibodies can be assessed using the indirect immunofluorescence technique.

Therapy. Macrolide antibiotics are now the agent of choice, having demonstrated clinical efficacy. Alternatively, 4-quinolones can be used.

Epidemiology and prevention. Legionellosis can occur in epidemic form or in sporadic infections. It is estimated that one third of all pneumonias requiring hospitalization are legionelloses. Soil and damp biotopes are the natural habitat of *Legionella*. Sources of infection include hot and cold water supply systems, cooling towers, air moisturizing units in air conditioners, and whirlpool baths. Human-to-human transmission has not been confirmed. *Legionella* bacteria tolerate water temperatures as high as 50 °C and are not killed until the water is briefly heated to 70 °C.

Brucella, Bordetella, Francisella

■ The genera *Brucella*, *Bordetella*, and *Francisella* are small, coccoid, Gram-negative rods. They can be cultured under strict aerobic conditions on enriched nutrient mediums.

Brucella abortus, *B. melitensis*, and *B. suis* cause **brucellosis**, a classic zoonosis that affects cattle, goats, and pigs. The pathogens can be transmitted to humans directly from diseased animals or indirectly in food. They cause characteristic granulomas in the organs of the RES. The primary clinical symptom is the undulant fever. Diagnosis is by means of pathogen identification or antibody assay using a standardized agglutination reaction.

Bordetella pertussis is the causative organism of **whooping cough**, which affects only humans. The pathogens are transmitted by aerosol droplets. The organism is not characterized by specific invasive properties, although it is able to cause epithelial and subepithelial necroses in the mucosa of the lower respiratory tract. The catarrhal phase, paroxysmal phase, and convalescent phase characterize the clinical picture of whooping cough (pertussis), which is usually diagnosed clinically. During the catarrhal and early paroxysmal phases, the pathogens can be cultured from nasopharyngeal secretions. The most important prophylactic measure is the vaccination in the first year of life.

Francisella tularensis causes **tularemia**. This disease, rare in Europe, affects wild rodents and can be transmitted to humans by direct contact, by arthropod vectors, and by dust particles. ■

Brucella (Brucellosis, Bang's Disease)

Occurrence and classification. The genus *Brucella* includes three medically relevant species—*B. abortus*, *B. melitensis*, and *B. suis*—besides a number of others. These three species are the causative organisms of classic zoonoses in livestock and wild animals, specifically in cattle (*B. abortus*), goats (*B. melitensis*), and pigs (*B. suis*). These bacteria can also be transmitted from diseased animals to humans, causing a uniform clinical picture, so-called undulant fever or Bang's disease.

Morphology and culture. Brucellae are slight, coccoid, Gram-negative rods with no flagella.

They only reproduce aerobically. In the initial isolation the atmosphere must contain 5–10% CO_2. Enriched mediums such as blood agar are required to grow them in cultures.

Pathogenesis and clinical picture. Human brucellosis infections result from direct contact with diseased animals or indirectly by way of contaminated foods, in particular unpasteurized milk and dairy products. The bacteria invade the body either through the mucosa of the upper intestinal and respiratory tracts or through lesions in the skin, then enter the subserosa or subcutis. From there they are transported by microphages or macrophages, in which they can survive, to the lymph nodes, where a lymphadenitis develops. The pathogens then disseminate from the affected lymph nodes, at first lymphogenously and then hematogenously, finally reaching the liver, spleen, bone marrow, and other RES tissues, in the cells of which they can survive and even multiply. The granulomas typical of intracellular bacteria develop. From these inflammatory foci, the brucellae can enter the bloodstream intermittently, each time causing one of the typical febrile episodes, which usually occur in the evening and are accompanied by chills. The incubation period is one to four weeks. *B. melitensis* infections are characterized by more severe clinical symptoms than the other brucelloses.

Diagnosis. This is best achieved by isolating the pathogen from blood or biopsies in cultures, which must be incubated for up to four weeks. The laboratory must therefore be informed of the tentative diagnosis. Brucellae are identified based on various metabolic properties and the presence of surface antigens, which are detected using a polyvalent *Brucella*-antiserum in a slide agglutination reaction. Special laboratories are also equipped to differentiate the three *Brucella* species.

Antibody detection is done using the agglutination reaction according to Gruber-Widal in a standardized method. In doubtful cases, the complement-binding reaction and direct Coombs test can be applied to obtain a serological diagnosis.

Therapy. Doxycycline is administered in the acute phase, often in combination with gentamicin. A therapeutic alternative is cotrimoxazole. The antibiotic regimen must be continued for three to four weeks.

Epidemiology and prevention. Brucellosis is a zoonosis that affects animals all over the world. Infections with *B. melitensis* occur most frequently in Mediterranean countries, in Latin America, and in Asia. The *melitensis* brucelloses seen in Europe are either caused by milk products imported from these countries or occur in travelers. *B. abortus* infections used to be frequent in central Europe, but the disease has now practically disappeared there thanks to the elimination of *Brucella*-infested cattle herds. Although control of brucellosis infections focuses on prevention of exposure to the pathogen, it is not necessary to isolate infected persons since the infection is not communicable between humans. There is no vaccine.

Bordetella (Whooping Cough, Pertussis)

The genus *Bordetella*, among others, includes the species *B. pertussis, B. parapertussis,* and *B. bronchiseptica.* Of the three, the pathogen responsible for whooping cough, *B. pertussis,* is of greatest concern for humans. The other two species are occasionally observed as human pathogens in lower respiratory tract infections.

Morphology and culture. *B. pertussis* bacteria are small, coccoid, nonmotile, Gram-negative rods that can be grown aerobically on special culture mediums at 37 °C for three to four days.

Pathogenesis. Pertussis bacteria are transmitted by aerosol droplets. They are able to attach themselves to the cells of the ciliated epithelium in the bronchi. They rarely invade the epithelium. The infection results in (sub-) epithelial inflammations and necroses.

4

Pathogenicity Factors of *Bordetella pertussis*

■ **Adhesion factors.** The two most important factors are filamentous hemagglutin (FHA) and pertussis toxin (Ptx). The latter can function both as an exotoxin and as an adhesin. The pathogenic cells attach themselves to the epithelial cilia.

■ **Exotoxins.** Pertussis toxin: AB toxin (see p. 16); the A component is an ADP-ribosyl transferase; mechanism of action via G_s proteins (as with cholera toxin A1); increased amount of cAMP in target cells, with a variety of effects depending on the type of cell affected by the toxin.

Invasive adenylate cyclase: AB toxin; A enters cells, acts in addition to pertussis toxin to increase levels of cAMP.

■ **Endotoxins.** Tracheal cytotoxin: murein fragment; kills ciliated epithelial cells. Lipopolysaccharide: stimulates cytokine production; activates complement by the alternative pathway.

Clinical picture. The onset of whooping cough (pertussis) develops after an incubation period of about 10–14 days with an uncharacteristic catarrhal phase lasting 1–2 weeks, followed by the two to three week-long paroxysmal phase with typical convulsive coughing spells. Then comes the convalescent phase, which can last for several weeks. Frequent complications, especially in infants, include secondary pneumonias caused by pneumococci or *Haemophilus,* which are able to penetrate readily through the damaged mucosa, and otitis media. Encephalopathy develops as a delayed complication in a small number of cases (0.4%), whereby the pathomechanism has not yet been clarified. The lethality level for pertussis during the first year of life is approximately 1–2%. The infection confers a stable immunity. Adults who were vaccinated as children have little or no residual immunity and often present atypical pertussis.

Diagnosis. The pathogen can only be isolated and identified during the catarrhal and early paroxysmal phases. Specimen material is taken from the nasopharynx through the nose using a special swabbing technique. A special medium is then carefully inoculated or the specimen is transported to the laboratory using a suitable transport medium. *B. pertussis* can also be identified in nasopharyngeal secretion using the direct immunofluorescence technique. Cultures must be aerobically incubated for three to four days. Antibodies cannot be detected by EIA until two weeks after onset at the earliest. Only a seroconversion is conclusive.

Therapy. Antibiotic treatment can only be expected to be effective during the catarrhal and early paroxysmal phases before the virulence factors are bound to the corresponding cell receptors. Macrolides are the agents of choice.

Epidemiology and prevention. Pertussis occurs worldwide. Humans are the only hosts. Sources of infection are infected persons during the catarrhal phase, who cough out the pathogens in droplets. There are no healthy carriers.

The most important preventive measure is the active vaccination (see vaccination schedule, p. 33). Although a whole-cell vaccine is available, various acellular vaccines are now preferred.

Francisella tularensis (Tularemia)

F. tularensis bacteria are coccoid, nonmotile, Gram-negative, aerobic rods. They cause a disease similar to plague in numerous animal species, above all in rodents. Humans are infected by contact with diseased animals or ectoparasites or dust. The pathogens invade the host either through microtraumata in the skin or through the mucosa. An ulcerous lesion develops at the portal of entry that also affects the local lymph nodes (ulceroglandular, glandular, or oculoglandular form). Via lymphogenous and hematogenous dissemination the pathogens then spread to parenchymatous organs, in particular RES organs such as the spleen and liver. Small granulomas develop, which develop central caseation or purulent abscesses. In pneumonic tularemia, as few as 50 CFU cause disease. The incubation period is three to four days. Diagnostic procedures aim to isolate and identify the pathogen in cultures and under the microscope. Agglutinating antibodies can be detected beginning with the second week. A seroconversion is the confirming factor. Antibiosis is carried out with streptomycin or gentamicin.

Gram-Negative Anaerobes

■ The obligate anaerobic, Gram-negative, pleomorphic rods are components of the normal mucosal flora of the respiratory, intestinal, and genital tracts. Among the many genera, *Bacteroides*, *Prevotella*, *Porphyromonas*, and *Fusobacterium*, each of which comprises numerous species, are of medical significance. They cause endogenous necrotic infections with subacute to chronic courses in the CNS, head, lungs, abdomen, and female genitals. A typical characteristic of such infections is that a mixed flora including anaerobes as well as aerobes is almost always found to be causative. Laboratory diagnostic procedures seek to identify the pathogens. Special transport vessels are required to transport specimens to the laboratory. Identification is based on morphological and physiological characteristics. A special technique is GC organic acid assay. Potentially effective antibiotics include certain penicillins and cephalosporins, clindamycin, and metronidazole.   ■

4

Occurrence. These bacteria include a large and heterogeneous group of Gram-negative, nonsporing, obligate anaerobe rods, many of which are components of the normal human mucosal flora.

Their numbers are particularly large in the intestinal tract, where they are found $1000\times$ as frequently as *Enterobacteriaceae*. They also occur regularly in the oral cavity, upper respiratory tract, and female genitals.

Classification. The taxonomy and nomenclature has changed considerably in recent years. The families *Bacteroidaceae*, *Prevotellaceae* (nov. fam.), *Porphyromonadaceae* (nov. fam.), and *Fusobacteriaceae* (nov. fam.) include significant human pathogens (Table 4.**11**).

Morphology and culture. The Gram-negative anaerobes show a pronounced pleomorphy; they are straight or curved, in most cases nonmotile, Gram-negative rods. Fusobacteria often take on gram staining irregularly and frequently feature pointed poles (Fig. 4.**22**).

Culture growth is only achieved under stringent anaerobic conditions. Some species are so sensitive to oxygen that the entire culturing procedure must be carried out in an anaerobic chamber (controlled atmosphere glove box). Anaerobes proliferate more slowly than aerobes, so the cultures must be incubated for two days or more.

Pathogenesis and clinical pictures. Infections with Gram-negative anaerobes participation are almost exclusively endogenous infections. The organisms show low levels of pathogenicity. They therefore are not found to feature any spectacular pathogenicity factors like clostridial toxins. Some have a capsule to protect them from phagocytosis. Some produce various enzymes that

4

Mixed Anaerobic Flora

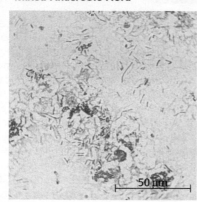

Fig. 4.**22**   Gram staining of a pleural punctate preparation: Gram-negative, fusiform, pleomorphic, and coccoid rods. Clinical diagnosis: pleural empyema.

destroy tissues (hyaluronidase, collagenase, neuraminidase). Gram-negative anaerobes are almost never the sole pathogens in an infection focus, but are rather found there together with other anaerobes and aerobes.

The clinical course of infections is subacute to chronic. Necrotic abscesses are seen frequently. The compartments infected are the CNS, the oral cavity, the upper and lower respiratory tract, the abdominal cavity, and the urogenital tract (Table 4.**11**). These pathogens can infect wounds following bite injuries or surgery in areas colonized by them (intestine, oral cavity, genital tract).

Diagnosis requires isolation and identity of the bacteria involved. Since these anaerobes are components of normal flora, correct sampling techniques are very important. The material must be transported in special anaerobe containers. Cultures should always be grown under both anaerobic and aerobic conditions. Selective culture mediums are available. Identification is based on morphological and physiological characteristics. Gas chromatography can be used for organic acid assays (butyric acid, acetic acid, propionic acid, etc.). These acids are produced as final products of certain bacterial metabolic steps.

Therapy. Penicillin, usually in combination with a betalactamase inhibitor, clindamycin, cefoxitin, imipenem, and nitroimidazoles are potentially effective antibiotics. Resistance testing is only necessary in certain cases.

Table 4.**11**   Overview of Medically Significant Genera and Species of
Gram-Negative Anaerobes

Taxonomy	Remarks and clinical pictures

Bacteroides
  B. fragilis
  B. distasonis
  B. thetaiotaomicron
  B. merdae
  B. caccae
  B. vulgatus and others
	Bacteria of the normal intestinal flora; in large intestine $> 10^{11}$/g of stool. These species are also classified under the designation *Bacteroides fragilis* group.
	
	Mainly peritonitis, intraabdominal abscesses, hepatic abscesses.

Prevotella
  P. bivia
  P. disiens
  P. buccae
  P. oralis
  P. buccalis and others
	Normal flora of the urogenital tract and/or oropharynx. Also known as the *Prevotella oralis* group (formerly *Bacteroides oralis* group).
	
	Chronic otitis media and sinusitis, dental abscesses, ulcerating gingivostomatitis, infections of the female genital tract, cerebral abscesses.

Prevotella
  P. melaninogenica
  P. intermedia and others
	Normal oral flora; blackish-brown hematin pigment. Also known as the *Prevotella melaninogenica* group.
	
	Aspiration pneumonia, pulmonary abscesses, pleural empyema, cerebral abscesses.

Porphyromonas
  P. asaccharolytica
  P. endodontalis
  P. gingivalis, and others
	Normal oral flora.
	
	Dental abscesses, gingivostomatitis, periodontitis; also contribute to infections of the lower respiratory tract (see above); cerebral abscesses.

Fusobacterium
  F. nucleatum
  F. necropherum
  F. periodonticum
  F. sulci (nov. sp.)
  F. ulcerans (nov. sp.), and others
	Rods with pointed ends. Spindle forms. Normal oral and intestinal flora.
	
	Infections in the orofacial area, lower respiratory tract, and abdomen; Plaut-Vincent angina

4

Epidemiology and prevention. Most infections arise from the patient's own flora. Exogenous infections can be contracted from animal bites. Following intestinal surgery, suitable anti-infective agents (see above) are administered for one to two days to prevent infections.

Treponema (Syphilis, Yaws, Pinta)

■ *Treponema pallidum*, subsp. *pallidum* is the causative pathogen of syphilis. Treponemes feature 10–20 primary spiral windings and can be viewed using dark field microscopy. They cannot be grown on artificial nutrient culture mediums. Syphilis affects only humans. The pathogens are transmitted by direct contact, in most cases during sexual intercourse. They invade the sub-cutaneous and subserous connective tissues through microtraumata in skin or mucosa. The disease progresses in stages designated as primary, second-ary, and tertiary syphilis or stages I, II, and III. **Stage I** is characterized by the painless primary affect and local lymphadenitis. Dissemination leads to **stage II**, characterized by polylymphadenopathy as well as generalized exanthem and enanthem. **Stage III** is subdivided into neurosyphilis, cardiovascular sy-philis, and gummatous syphilis. In stages I and II the lesion pathogens can be viewed under a dark field microscope. Antibody assays include the VDRL floc-culation reaction, TP-PA particle agglutination, and the indirect immuno-fluorescence test FTA-ABS. The therapeutic of choice is penicillin G. This dis-ease is known in all parts of the world. Preventive measures concentrate on protection from exposure. Other *Treponema*-caused diseases that do not oc-cur in Europe include nonvenereal syphilis, caused by *T. pallidum*, subsp. *en-demicum*, yaws, caused by *T. pallidum*, subsp. *pertenue*, and pinta, caused by *Treponema carateum*. ■

The genus *Treponema* belongs to the family of *Spirochaetaceae* and includes several significant human pathogen species and subspecies. *T. pallidum*, subsp. *pallidum* is the syphilis pathogen. *T. pallidum*, subsp. *endemicum* is the pathogen that causes a syphilislike disease that is transmitted by direct, but not sexual contact. *T. pallidum*, subsp. *pertenue* is the pathogen that causes yaws, and *T. carateum* causes pinta, two nonvenereal infections that occur in the tropics and subtropics.

Treponema pallidum, subsp. pallidum (Syphilis)

Morphology and culture. These organisms are slender bacteria, 0.2 μm wide and 5–15 μm long; they feature 10–20 primary windings and move by rotat-ing around their lengthwise axis. Their small width makes it difficult to ren-der them visible by staining. They can be observed in vivo using dark field microscopy. In-vitro culturing has not yet been achieved.

Pathogenesis and clinical picture. Syphilis affects only humans. The disease is normally transmitted by sexual intercourse. Infection comes about because of direct contact with lesions containing the pathogens, which then invade the host through microtraumata in the skin or mucosa. The incubation period is two to four weeks. Left untreated, the disease manifests in several stages:

■ **Stage I (primary syphilis).** Hard, indolent (painless) lesion, later infiltration and ulcerous disintegration, called hard chancre. Accompanied by regional lymphadenitis, also painless. Treponemes can be detected in the ulcer.

■ **Stage II (secondary syphilis).** Generalization of the disease occurs four to eight weeks after primary syphilis. Frequent clinical symptoms include micropolylymphadenopathy and macular or papulosquamous exanthem, broad condylomas, and enanthem. Numerous organisms can be detected in seeping surface efflorescences.

■ **Latent syphilis.** Stage of the disease in which no clinical symptoms are manifested, but the pathogens are present in the body and serum antibody tests are positive. Divided into early latency (less than four years) and late latency (more than four years).

■ **Stage III (tertiary or late syphilis).** Late gummatous syphilis: manifestations in skin, mucosa, and various organs. Tissue disintegration is frequent. Lesions are hardly infectious or not at all. Cardiovascular syphilis: endarteritis obliterans, syphilitic aortitis. Neurosyphilis: two major clinical categories are observed: meningovascular syphilis, i.e., endarteritis obliterans of small blood vessels of the meninges, brain, and spinal cord; parenchymatous syphilis, i.e., destruction of nerve cells in the cerebral cortex (paresis) and spinal cord (tabes dorsalis). A great deal of overlap occurs.

■ **Syphilis connata.** Transmission of the pathogen from mother to fetus after the fourth month of pregnancy. Leads to miscarriage or birth of severely diseased infant with numerous treponemes in its organs.

Diagnosis. Laboratory diagnosis includes both isolation and identification of the pathogen and antibody assays.

Pathogen identification. Only detectable in fluid pressed out of primary chancre, in the secretions of seeping stage II efflorescences or in lymph node biopsies. Methods: dark field microscopy, direct immunofluorescence (Fig. 4.**23**).

Antibody assays. Two antibody groups can be identified:

■ **Antilipoidal antibodies (reaginic antibodies).** Probably produced in response to the phospholipids from the mitochondria of disintegrating somatic cells. The antigen used is **cardiolipin**, a lipid extract from the heart muscle of cattle. This serological test is performed according to the standards

Treponema pallidum

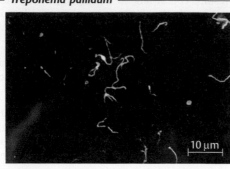

Fig. 4.**23** Serous transudate from moist mucocutaneous primary chancre. Direct immunofluorescence.

10 µm

4

of the Venereal Disease Research Laboratory (USA) and is known as the VDRL flocculation reaction.

- ■ **Antitreponema antibodies.** Probably directed at *T. pallidum*.
- — *Treponema pallidum* **particle agglutination (TP-PA).** This test format has widely replaced the *Treponema pallidum* hemagglutination assay (TPHA). The antigens (ultrasonically-treated suspension of *Treponema pallidum*, Nichols strain, cultured in rabbit testicles) are coupled to particles or erythrocytes.
- — **Immunofluorescence test (FTA-ABS).** In this **f**luorescence **t**reponemal **a**ntibody **abs**orption test the antigen consists of killed Nichols strain treponemes mounted on slides and coated with patient serum. Bound antibodies are detected by means of fluorescein-marked antihuman IgG antibodies. Selective antitreponeme IgM antibodies can be assayed (= 19S-FTA-ABS) using antihuman IgM antibodies (µ capture test).
- — *Treponema pallidum* **immobilization test (TPI test).** Living treponemes (Nichols strain) are immobilized by antibodies in the patient serum. This test is no longer used in routine diagnostics. It is considered the gold standard for evaluation of antitreponeme antibody tests.

The antibody tests are used as follows:
- — **Screening:** TP-PA or TPHA (qualitative).
- — **Primary diagnostics:** TP-PA or TPHA, VDRL, FTA-ABS (all qualitative).
- — **Special diagnostics:** VDRL (quantitative); 19S-FTA-ABS.

Therapeutic success can be determined by the quantitative VDRL test. A rapid drop in reagins indicates an efficacious therapy. The 19S-FTA-ABS can be used to find answers to specialized questions. Example: does a positive result in primary diagnostic testing indicate a serological scar or a fresh infection?

Therapy. Penicillin G is the antibiotic agent of choice. Dosage and duration of therapy depend on the stage of the disease and the galenic formulation of the penicillin used.

Epidemiology and prevention. Syphilis is known all over the world. Annual prevalence levels in Europe and the US are 10–30 cases per 100 000 inhabitants. The primary preventive measure is to avoid any contact with syphilitic efflorescences. When diagnosing a case, the physician must try to determine the first-degree contact person, who must then be examined immediately and provided with penicillin therapy as required. National laws governing venereal disease management in individual countries regulate the measures taken to diagnose, prevent, and heal this disease. There is no vaccine.

4

Treponema pallidum, subsp. endemicum (Nonvenereal Syphilis)

This subspecies is responsible for nonvenereal syphilis, which occurs endemically in certain circumscribed areas in the Balkans, the eastern Mediterranean, Asia, and Africa. The disease manifests with maculous to papulous, often hypertrophic lesions of the skin and mucosa. These lesions resemble the venereal efflorescences. The pathogens are transmitted by direct contact or indirectly on everyday objects such as clothes, tableware, etc. The incubation period is three weeks to three months. Penicillin is the therapy of choice. Serological syphilis tests are positive.

Treponema pallidum, subsp. pertenue (Yaws)

This species causes yaws (German "Frambösie," French "pian"), a chronic disease endemic in moist, warm climates characterized by epidermal proliferation and ulceration. Transmission is by direct contact. The incubation period is three to four weeks. Treponemes must be found in the early lesions to confirm diagnosis. Serological syphilis reactions are positive. Penicillin G is the antibiotic of choice.

Treponema carateum (Pinta)

This species causes pinta, an endemic treponematosis that occurs in parts of Central and South America, characterized by marked dermal depigmentations. The pathogens are transmitted by direct contact. The incubation period is one to three weeks. The disease often has a chronic course and can persist for years. Diagnosis is confirmed by identification of treponemes from the skin lesions. Penicillin G is used in therapy.

Borrelia (Relapsing Fever, Lyme Disease)

■ *Borrelia recurrentis* is the pathogen of an epidemic relapsing fever transmitted by body lice that no longer occurs in the population of developed countries. *B. duttonii, B. hermsii,* and other borreliae are the causative pathogens of the endemic, tickborne relapsing fever, so called for the periodic relapses of fever characterizing the infection. The relapses are caused by borreliae that have changed the structure of the variable major protein in their outer membranes so that the antibodies produced by the host in the previous episode are no longer effective against them. Laboratory diagnostic confirmation requires identification of the borreliae in the blood. Penicillin G is the antibiotic of choice.

B. burgdorferi is the causative pathogen in Lyme disease, a tickborne infection. Left untreated, the disease has three stages. The primary clinical symptom of stage I is the erythema chronicum migrans. Stage II in the European variety is clinically defined by chronic lymphocytic meningitis Bannwarth. Meningitis is frequent in children. The primary symptoms of stage III are acrodermatitis chronica atrophicans Herxheimer and Lyme arthritis. Laboratory diagnostics comprises detection of specific antibodies by means of immunofluorescent or EIA methods. Betalactam antibiotics are used to treat the infection. Lyme disease is the most frequent tickborne disease in central Europe.   ■

Borrelia that Cause Relapsing Fevers

Taxonomy and significance. The genus *Borrelia* belongs to the family *Spirochaetaceae*. The body louseborne epidemic form of relapsing fever is caused by the species *B. recurrentis*. The endemic form, transmitted by various tick species, can be caused by any of a number of species (at least 15), the most important being *B. duttonii* and *B. hermsii*.

Morphology and culture. Borreliae are highly motile spirochetes with three to eight windings, 0.3–0.6 µm wide, and 8–18 µm in length. They propel themselves forward by rotating about their lengthwise axis. They can be rendered visible with Giemsa stain (Fig. 4.**24**). It is possible to observe live borreliae using dark field or phase contrast microscopy.

Borrelia duttonii

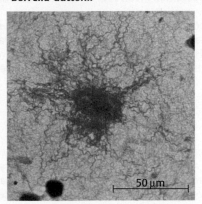

Fig. 4.**24** Preparation from the blood of an experimentally infected mouse. Giemsa staining.

50 µm

4

Borreliae can be cultured using special nutrient mediums, although it must be added that negative results are not reliable.

Pathogenesis and clinical picture. _B. recurrentis_ is pathogenic only in humans. The pathogens are transmitted by body lice. _B. duttonii_, _B. hermsii_, and other species are transmitted by ticks.

Following an incubation period of five to eight days, the disease manifests with fever that lasts three to seven days, then suddenly falls. A number of feverfree intervals, each longer than the last, are interrupted by relapses that are less and less severe. The borreliae can be detected in the patient's blood during the febrile episodes. The disease got its name from these recurring febrile attacks. The relapses are caused by borreliae that have changed their antigen structure in such a way that the antibodies produced in response to the last proliferative episode cannot attack them effectively. Borreliae possess a highly variable gene coding for the adhesion protein VMP (variable major protein) in the outer membrane of the cell wall.

Diagnosis. Borreliae can be detected in patients' blood when the fever rises. They cannot be reliably cultured. One method is to inject patient blood i.p. into mice. After two to three days, the mouse develops a bacteremia that can be verified by finding the pathogens in its blood under a microscope.

Therapy. The antibiotic of choice is penicillin G. Alternatives include other betalactam antibiotics and doxycycline.

Epidemiology and prevention. _B. recurrentis_ causes the **epidemic form of relapsing fever**, which still occurred worldwide at the beginning of the 20th century but has disappeared for the most part today. The pathogens are transmitted by the body louse. Prevention involves eradication of the lice with insecticides.

B. duttonii, *B. hermsii*, and other borreliae cause **endemic relapsing fever**, which is still observed today in Africa, the Near and Middle East, and Central America. This is a tickborne disease. Here again, the main preventive measure is elimination of the insect vectors (ticks) with insecticides, especially in residential areas.

Borrelia burgdorferi (Lyme Disease)

Classification. The etiology of an increase in the incidence of acute cases of arthritis among youths in the Lyme area of Connecticut in 1977 was at first unclear. The illness was termed Lyme arthritis. It was not until 1981 that hitherto unknown borreliae were found to be responsible for the disease. They were classified as *B. burgdorferi* in 1984 after their discoverer. Analysis of the genome of various isolates has recently resulted in a proposal to subclassify *B. burgdorferi* sensu lato in three species: *B. burgdorferi* sensu stricto, *B. garinii*, *B. afzelii*.

Morphology and culture. These are thin, flexible, helically wound, highly motile spirochetes. They can be rendered visible with Giemsa staining or by means of dark field or phase contrast microscopy methods.

These borreliae can be grown in special culture mediums at 35 °C for five to 10 days, although culturing these organisms is difficult and often unsuccessful.

Pathogenesis and clinical picture. The pathogens are transmitted by the bite of various tick species (see p. 607). The incubation period varies from three to 30 days. Left untreated, the disease goes through three stages (Table 4.12), though individual courses often deviate from the classic

— **Lyme Disease** —

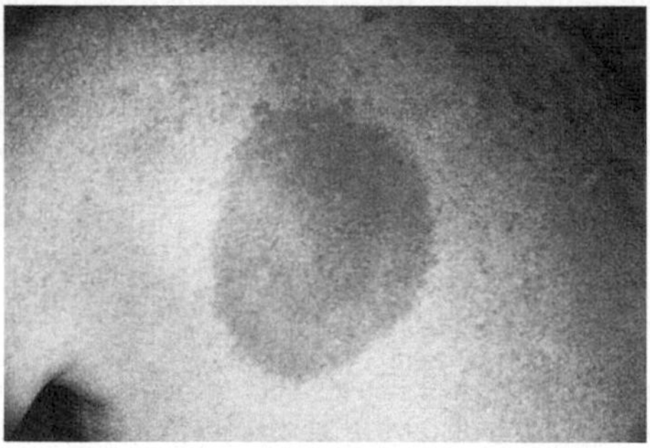

Fig. 4.25 Erythema chronicum migrans.

Table **4.12**   Clinical Manifestations of Lyme Disease

Organ/organ system	Stage I	Stage II	Stage III
Skin	**Erythema migrans**	Diffuse erythema Lymphadenosis benigna cutis (Lymphocytoma)	**Acrodermatitis chronica atrophicans**
Lymphatic system	Local lymphadenopathy	Regional lympha-denopathy	
Nervous system		**Lymphocytic meningoradiculitis Bannwarth**, facialis paresis, aseptic meningitis	Chronic encephalo-myelitis (rare delayed complication)
Joints		Brief attacks of arthritis	**Arthritis**
Heart		Carditis, atrioventricular block	

The clinical pictures in bold type represent the primary disease manifestations of the three stages.

pattern. The presenting symptom in stage I is the erythema chronicum migrans (Fig. 4.**25**).

Diagnosis. Direct detection and identification of the pathogen by means of microscopy and culturing techniques is possible, but laden with uncertainties. In a recent development, the polymerase chain reaction (PCR) is used for direct detection of pathogen-specific DNA. However, the method of choice is still the antibody test (EIA or indirect immunofluorescence, Western blotting if the result is positive).

Therapy. Stages I and II: amoxicillin, cefuroxime, doxycycline, or a macrolide. Stage III: ceftriaxone.

Epidemiology and prevention. Lyme disease occurs throughout the northern hemisphere. There are some endemic foci where the infection is more frequent. The disease is transmitted by various species of ticks, in Europe mostly by *Ixodes ricinus* (sheep tick). In endemic areas of Germany, approximately 3–7% of the larvae and 10–34% of nymphs and adult ticks are infected with *B. burgdorferi* sensu lato. The annual incidence of acute Lyme disease (stage I) in central Europe is 20–50 cases per 100 000 inhabitants. Wild animals from rodents on up to deer are the natural reservoir of the Lyme disease *Borrelia*, although these species seldom come down with the disease. The ticks obtain their blood meals from these animals.

Leptospira (Leptospirosis, Weil Disease)

■ The pathogenic species *Leptospira interrogans* is subclassified in over 100 serovars reflecting different surface antigens. The serovars are divided into 19 serogroups (*icterohemorrhagiae, canicola, pomona*, etc.). These organisms are in the form of spiral rods and can be grown in in-vitro cultures. Leptospirosis is a zoonosis that occurs worldwide. The sole sources of infection are diseased rodents and domestic animals (pigs), which excrete the pathogen in their urine. Upon contact, leptospirae penetrate skin or mucosa, are disseminated hematogenously and cause a generalized vasculitis in various organs. The incubation period is seven to 12 days. The disease at first presents as a sepsis, followed after three to seven days by the so-called immune stage. In the milder form, anicteric leptospirosis, the most frequent manifestation in stage two is an aseptic meningitis. The icteric form of leptospirosis (Weil disease) can cause dysfunction of liver and kidneys, cardiovascular disruptions, and hemorrhages. The method of choice in laboratory diagnostics is antibody identification in a lysis-agglutination reaction. The therapeutic agent of choice is penicillin G.   ■

Classification. Leptospirae belong to the family *Leptospiraceae*. The genus *Leptospira* comprises two species. *L. biflexa* includes all apathogenic leptospirae and *L. interrogans* represents the pathogenic species. Based on its specific surface antigen variety, *L. interrogans* is subclassified in over 100 serovars in 19 serogroups. Some of the most important serogroups are: *icterohemorrhagiae, canicola, pomona, australis, grippotyphosa, hyos*, and *sejroe*.

Morphology and culture. Leptospirae are fine spirochetes, 10–20 μm long, and 0.1–0.2 μm thick (Fig. 4.**26**). They possess no flagella, but rather derive their motility from rotating motions of the cell corpus. Visualization of leptospirae is best done using dark field or phase contrast microscopy. Leptospirae can be grown in special culture mediums under aerobic conditions at temperatures between 27–30 °C

Pathogenesis and clinical picture. Leptospirae invade the human organism through microinjuries in the skin or the intact conjunctival mucosa. There are no signs of inflammation in evidence at the portal of entry. The organisms spread to all parts of the body, including the central nervous system, hematogenously. Leptospirosis is actually a generalized vasculitis. The pathogens

Leptospira interrogans

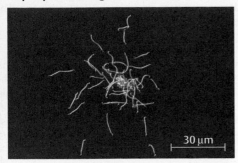

Fig. 4.**26** Serogroup *icterohemorrhagiae*. Culture preparation. Dark field microscopy.

4

damage mainly the endothelial cells of the capillaries, leading to greater permeability and hemorrhage and interrupting the O_2 supply to the tissues. Jaundice is caused by a nonnecrotic hepatocellular dysfunction. Disturbances of renal function result from hypoxic tubular damage. A clinical distinction is drawn between **anicteric leptospirosis**, which has a milder course, and the severe clinical picture of **icteric leptospirosis (Weil disease)**. In principle, any of the serovars could potentially cause either of these two clinical courses. In practice, however, the serogroup *icterohemorrhagiae* is isolated more frequently in Weil disease.

Both types of leptospirosis are characterized by fever with chills, headache, and myalgias that set in after an incubation period of seven to 12 days. This initial **septic** stage of the disease lasts three to seven days and is then followed by the second, so-called **immune stage**, which lasts from four to 30 days. The most important clinical manifestation of stage two anicteric leptospirosis is a mild, aseptic meningitis. The second stage of Weil disease is characterized by hepatic and renal dysfunctions, extensive hemorrhaging, cardiovascular symptoms, and clouding of the state of consciousness. The immunity conferred by survival of the infection is reliable, but only protects against the one specific serovar.

Diagnosis. Detection and identification of leptospirae are accomplished by growing the organisms in **cultures**. Blood, cerebrospinal fluid, urine, or organ biopsies, which must not be contaminated with other bacteria, are incubated in special mediums at 27–30 °C for three to four weeks. A microscope check (dark field) is carried out every week to see if any leptospirae are proliferating. The *Leptospirae* are typed serologically in a lysis-agglutination reaction with specific test sera.

The method of choice for a laboratory diagnosis is an **antibody assay**. The antibodies produced after the first week of the infection are detected in patient serum using a quantitative lysis-agglutination test. Viable culture strains of the regionally endemic serovars provide the test antigens. The reaction is read off under the microscope.

Therapy. The agent of choice is penicillin G.

Epidemiology and prevention. Leptospiroses are typical zoonotic infections. They are reported from every continent in both humans and animals. The most important sources of infection are rodents and domestic animals, mainly pigs. The animals excrete the pathogen with urine. Leptospirae show little resistance to drying out so that infections only occur because of contact with a moist milieu contaminated with urine. The persons most at risk are farmers, butchers, sewage treatment workers, and zoo staff.

Prevention of these infections involves mainly avoiding contact with material containing the pathogens, control of *Muridae* rodents and successful treatment of domestic livestock. It is not necessary to isolate infected persons or their contacts. There is no commercially available vaccine.

Rickettsia, Coxiella, Orientia, and Ehrlichia (Typhus, Spotted Fever, Q Fever, Ehrlichioses)

■ The genera of the *Rickettsiaceae* and *Coxelliaceae* contain short, coccoid, small rods that can only reproduce in host cells. With the exception of *Coxiella* (aerogenic transmission), they are transmitted to humans via the vectors lice, ticks, fleas, or mites. *R. prowazekii* and *R. typhi* cause typhus, a disease characterized by high fever and a spotty exanthem. Several rickettsiae species cause spotted fever, a milder typhuslike disease. *Orientia tsutsugamushi* is transmitted by mite larvae to cause tsutsugamushi fever. This disease occurs only in Asia. *Coxiella burnetii* is responsible for Q fever, an infection characterized by a pneumonia with an atypical clinical course.

Several species of *Ehrlichiaceae* cause ehrlichiosis in animals and humans. The method of choice for laboratory diagnosis of the various rickettsioses and ehrlichioses is antibody assay by any of several methods, in most cases indirect immunofluorescence. Tetracyclines represent the antibiotic of choice for all of these infections. Typhus and spotted fever no longer occur in Europe. Q fever infections are reported from all over the world. Sources of infection include diseased sheep, goats, and cattle. The prognosis for the rare chronic form of Q fever (syn. Q fever endocarditis) is poor. Ehrlichiosis infects mainly animals, but in rare cases humans as well. ■

Classification. The bacteria of this group belong to the families *Rickettsiaceae* (*Rickettsia* and *Orientia*), *Coxelliaceae* (*Coxiella*), and *Ehrlichiaceae* (*Ehrlichia*, *Anaplasma*, *Neorickettsia*). Some of these organisms can cause mild, self-limiting infections in humans, others severe disease. Arthropods are the transmitting vectors in many cases.

Morphology and culture. These obligate cell parasites are coccoid, short rods measuring 0.3–0.5 μm that take gram staining weakly, but Giemsa staining well. They reproduce by intracellular, transverse fission only. They can be cultured in hen embryo yolk sacs, in suitable experimental animals (mouse, rat, guinea pig) or in cell cultures.

Pathogenesis and clinical pictures. With the exception of *C. burnetii*, the organisms are transmitted by arthropods. In most cases, the arthropods excrete them with their feces and ticks transmit them with their saliva while sucking blood. The organisms invade the host organism through skin injuries. *C. burnetii* is transmitted exclusively by inhalation of dust containing the pathogens. Once inside the body, rickettsiae reproduce mainly in the vascular endothelial cells. These cells then die, releasing increasing numbers of organisms into the bloodstream. Numerous inflammatory lesions are caused locally around the destroyed endothelia. Ehrlichiae reproduce in the monocytes or granulocytes of membrane-enclosed cytoplasmic vacuoles. The characteristic morulae clusters comprise several such vacuoles stuck together.

Table 4.**13** summarizes a number of characteristics of the rickettsioses.

Diagnosis. Direct detection and identification of these organisms in cell cultures, embryonated hen eggs, or experimental animals is unreliable and is also not to be recommended due to the risk of laboratory infections. Special laboratories use the polymerase chain reaction to identify pathogen-specific DNA sequences. However, the method of choice is currently still the antibody assay, whereby the immunofluorescence test is considered the gold standard among the various methods. The Weil-Felix agglutination test (p. 295) is no longer used today due to low sensitivity and specificity.

Therapy. Tetracyclines lower the fever within one to two days and are the antibiotics of choice.

Epidemiology and prevention. The **epidemic form of typhus**, and earlier scourge of eastern Europe and Russia in particular, has now disappeared from Europe and occurs only occasionally in other parts of the world. **Murine typhus**, on the other hand, is still a widespread disease in the tropics and subtropics. **Spotted fevers** (e.g., Rocky Mountain spotted fever) occur with increased frequency in certain geographic regions, especially in the spring. **Tsutsugamushi fever** occurs only in Japan and Southeast Asia. The blood-sucking larvae of various mite species transmit its pathogen. **Q fever** epi-

Table **4.13** Pathogens and Clinical Pictures of the Rickettsioses and of Q Fever

Pathogen	Vector/host	Disease	Clinical picture
Typhus group			
Rickettsia prowazekii	Body louse/humans	Epidemic typhus (ET)	Incubation 10–14 days; high fever; 4–7 days after onset maculous exanthem; lethality as high as 20% if untreated
		Brill-Zinsser disease	Endogenous secondary infection by rickettsiae persisting in the RES; results from reduction of immune protection; milder symptoms than ET
R. typhi	Rat flea/rat	Murine typhus	Symptoms as in ET, but milder
Spotted fever group			
R. rickettsii	Hard tick/ rodents, tick	Rocky Mountain spotted fever (RMSF)	Incubation: 6–7 days; continuing fever 2–3 weeks; maculopapulous exanthem on extremities
R. conori	Hard tick/ rodents	Fièvre boutonneuse (Mediterranean fever)	Symptoms as in RMSF, necrotic lesions sometimes develop at bite locus
R. sibirica	Hard tick/ rodents	North Asian tick fever	Symptoms as in RMSF, necrotic lesions sometimes develop at bite locus
R. akari	Mite/rodents	Rickettsial pox	Fever; exanthem resembles that of chicken pox
Tsutsugamushi fever			
Orientia tsutsugamushi	Mite larvae/ rodents	Japanese spotted fever	Symptoms similar to ET plus local lesion at bite locus and lymphadenitis
Q fever (Query fever)			
Coxiella burnetii	Dust/sheep, cattle, goats, rodents	Q fever	Incubation 2–3 weeks; interstitial pneumonia (clinical picture often atypical); chronic Q fever (endocarditis) with onset years after primary infection, poor prognosis

Table 4.**14**   Pathogens and Clinical Picture of the Ehrlichioses

Pathogen	Vector/host	Disease	Clinical picture
Ehrlichia chaffeensis	Ticks/deer, dog	Human mono-cytotrophic ehrlichiosis (HME); monocytes are main target of pathogen	All ehrlichioses present as mild to occasionally severe mono-nucleosis-like multisystem disease with headache, fever, myalgias leukopenia, thrombo-cytopenia, anaemia, and raised transaminases. 20–30% show various symptoms in the gastro-intestinal tract and/or respiratory tract and/or CNS.
Ehrlichia ewingii and Anaplasma phagocytophi-lum	Ticks/dogs, horse, other animals	Human granulo-cytotrophic ehrlichiosis (HGE); granulo-cytes are main target of pathogen	Incubation time between 5–10 days. Antibiotics of choice are the tetracyclines.
Neorickettsia sennetsu	Host unknown; perhaps fish. Transmission from eating raw fish	Sennetsu fever; occurs in South-east Asia (Japan)	Cultivation from blood using cell cultures exhibits low sensitivity. Molecular techniques (PCR) better for pathogen detection. Use indirect immunofluores-cence for antibody titers.

4

demics are occasionally seen worldwide. The sources of infection are diseased livestock that eliminate the coxiellae in urine, milk, or through the birth canal. Humans and animals are infected by inhaling dust containing the pathogens. Specific preventive measures are difficult to realize effectively since animals showing no symptoms may be excreters. Active vaccination of persons exposed to these infections in their work provides a certain degree of immunization protection.

Until 1987, **ehrlichioses** were thought to occur only in animals. Tickborne *Ehrlichia* infections in humans have now been confirmed.

Bartonella and Afipia

Bartonella

Classification. The genus **Bartonella** includes, among others, the species *B. bacilliformis*, *B. quintana*, *B. henselae*, and *B. clarridgeia*.

Morphology and culture. *Bartonella* bacteria are small (0.6–1 µm), Gram-negative, frequently pleomorphic rods. Bartonellae can be grown on culture mediums enriched with blood or serum.

Table 4.**15** Pathogens and Clinical Pictures of Bartonelloses

Pathogen	Transmission/host	Disease	Clinical picture
Bartonella bacilliformis	Sand fly/humans	Oroya fever (Carrion's disease)	Incubation: 15–40 days; high fever; lymphadenitis; spleno-hepatomegaly; hemolytic anemia due to lysis of erythrocytes invaded by *B. bacilliformis*
		Verruga peruana phase of Oroya fever	Multiple, wartlike skin lesions on extremities, face, mucosa; onset either months after abating of Oroya fever or without an acute preceding infection
B. quintana	Lice/humans	Five-day fever (Wolhynian fever, trench fever)	Periodic relapses of fever (3–8) every 5 days, sepsis; bacillary angiomatosis (see below); also endocarditis
B. henselae	Cats to humans/cats	Cat scratch disease	Lymphadenopathy; fever; cutaneous lesion (not always present)
		Sepsis, bacillary angiomatosis	In patients with immune deficiencies (HIV); vascular proliferation in skin and mucosa (similar to verruga peruana)
		Bacterial peliosis hepatis/splenica	Cystic, blood-filled lesions in liver and spleen
B. clarridgeia		Cat scratch disease	See above

Diagnosis. Special staining techniques are used to render bartonellae visible under the microscope in tissue specimens. Growth in cultures more than seven days. Amplification of specific DNA in tissue samples or blood, followed by sequencing. Antibody assay with IF or EIA.

Therapy. Tetracyclines, macrolides.

Epidemiology and prevention. Oroya fever (also known as Carrion disease) is observed only in humans and is restricted to mountain valleys with elevations above 800 m in the western and central Cordilleras in South America because an essential vector, the sand fly, lives only there. Cat scratch disease, on the other hand, is known all over the world. It is transmitted directly from cats to humans or indirectly by cat fleas. The cats involved are usually not sick. Table 4.**14** lists the pathogens and clinical pictures for the various bartonelloses.

4

Afipia felis

The bacterial species *Afipia* (Armed Forces Institute of Pathology) *felis* was discovered several years ago. At first, it appeared that most cases of cat scratch disease were caused by this pathogen. Then it turned out that the culprit in those cases was usually either *B. henselae* or *B. clarridgeia* and that *Afipia felis* was responsible for only a small number. *Afipia felis* and *B. henselae* cat scratch infections present with the same clinical symptoms. Most cases of *A. felis* infections clear up spontaneously without antibiotic therapy. Should use of an antibiotic be clinically indicated, a tetracycline (or in severe cases a carbapenem or aminoglycoside) would be appropriate.

Chlamydia

■ Chlamydiae are obligate cell parasites. They go through two stages in their reproductive cycle: the elementary bodies (EB) are optimized to survive outside of host cells. In the form of the initial bodies (IB), the chlamydiae reproduce inside the host cells. The three human pathogen species of chlamydiae are *C. psittaci*, *C. trachomatis*, and *C. pneumoniae*. Tetracyclines and macrolides are suitable for treatment of all chlamydial infections.

C. psittaci is the cause of **psittacosis** or **ornithosis**. This zoonosis is a systemic disease of birds. The pathogens enter human lungs when dust containing chlamydiae is inhaled. After an incubation period of one to three weeks, pneumonia develops that often shows an atypical clinical course.

C. trachomatis is found only in humans. This species causes the following diseases: 1. **Trachoma**, a chronic follicular keratoconjunctivitis. The pathogens are transmitted by smear infection. 2. **Inclusion conjunctivitis** in newborn children and **swimming-pool conjunctivitis**. 3. **Nonspecific urogenital infections** in both men and women (urethritis, cervicitis, salpingitis, etc.). 4. **Lymphogranuloma venereum**, a venereal disease observed mainly in countries with warm climates.

C. pneumoniae is responsible for infections of the upper respiratory tract as well as for a mild form of **pneumonia**. There is current discussion in the literature concerning a possible role of *C. pneumoniae* in the pathogenesis of atherosclerotic cardiovascular disease.

4

Overview and General Characteristics of Chlamydiae

Definition and classification. The bacteria in the taxonomic family *Chlamydiaceae* are small (0.3–1 µm) obligate cell parasites with a Gram-negative cell wall. The reproductive cycle of the chlamydiae comprises two developmental stages: The elementary bodies are optimally adapted to survival outside of host cells. The initial bodies, also known as reticulate bodies, are the form in which the chlamydiae reproduce inside the host cells by means of transverse fission. Three human pathogen species of chlamydiae are known: *C. psittaci*, *C. trachomatis* (with the biovars *trachoma* and *lymphogranuloma venereum*), and *C. pneumoniae*.

Morphology and developmental cycle. Two morphologically and functionally distinct forms are known:

■ **Elementary bodies.** The round to oval, optically dense elementary bodies have a diameter of approximately 300 nm. They represent the infectious form of the pathogen and are specialized for the demands of existence outside the host cells. Once the elementary bodies have attached themselves to specific host cell receptors, they invade the cells by means of endocytosis (Fig. 4.**27**). Inside the cell, they are enclosed in an endocytotic membrane vesicle or inclusion, in which they transform themselves into the other form—initial bodies—within a matter of hours.

■ **Initial bodies**. Chlamydiae in this spherical to oval form are also known as reticular bodies. They have a diameter of approximately 1000 nm. The initial bodies reproduce by means of transverse fission and are not infectious while in this stage. At the end of the cycle, the initial bodies are transformed back into elementary bodies. The cell breaks open and releases the elementary bodies to continue the cycle by attaching themselves to new host cells.

Reproduction Cycle of Chlamydiae

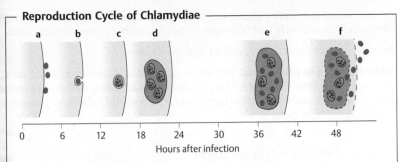

Fig. 4.**27** Two chlamydial stages: elementary body and initial body.
a Attachment of elementary body to cell membrane.
b Endocytosis.
c Transformation of elementary body into initial body inside the endosome.
d Reproduction of initial bodies by transverse fission.
e Transformation of some initial bodies back into elementary bodies.
f Lysis of inclusion vesicle and cell, release of initial and elementary bodies.

4

Culture. Chlamydiae exploit energy metabolism processes in their host cells that they themselves are lacking (ATP synthesis). For this reason, they can only be grown in special cell cultures, in the yolk sacs of embryonated hen eggs, or in experimental animals.

Chlamydia psittaci (Ornithosis, Psittacosis)

Pathogenesis and clinical picture. The natural hosts of *C. psittaci* are birds. This species causes infections of the respiratory organs, the intestinal tract, the genital tract, and the conjunctiva of parrots and other birds. Humans are infected by inhalation of dust (from bird excrements) containing the pathogens, more rarely by inhalation of infectious aerosols.

After an incubation period of one to three weeks, ornithosis presents with fever, headache, and a pneumonia that often takes an atypical clinical course. The infection may, however, also show no more than the symptoms of a common cold, or even remain clinically silent. Infected persons are not usually sources of infection.

Diagnosis. The pathogen can be grown from sputum in special cell cultures. Direct detection in the culture is difficult and only possible in specially equipped laboratories. The complement binding reaction can be used to identify antibodies to a generic antigen common to all chlamydiae, so that this test would also have a positive result in the presence of other chlamydial infections. The antibody test of choice is indirect microimmunofluorescence.

Therapy. Tetracyclines (doxycycline) and macrolides.

Epidemiology and prevention. Ornithosis affects birds worldwide. It is also observed in poultry. Diagnosis of an ornithosis in a human patient necessitates a search for and elimination of the source, especially if the birds in question are household pets.

Chlamydia trachomatis (Trachoma, Lymphogranuloma venereum)

C. trachomatis is a pathogen that infects only humans. Table 4.**16** lists the relevant diseases, biovars, and serovars.

Trachoma is a follicular keratoconjunctivitis. The disease occurs in all climatic zones, although it is more frequent in warmer, less-developed countries. It is estimated that 400 million people carry this chronic infection and that it has caused blindness in six million. The pathogen is transmitted by direct contact and indirectly via objects in daily use. Left untreated, the initially acute inflammation can develop a chronic course lasting months or years and leading to formation of a corneal scar, which can then cause blindness. The **laboratory diagnostics** procedure involves detection of *C. trachomatis* in conjunctival smears using direct immunofluorescence microscopy. The fluorochrome-marked monoclonal antibodies are directed against the MOMP (major outer membrane protein) of *C. trachomatis*. The pathogen can also

Table 4.**16** Human Infections Caused by *Chlamydia trachomatis*

Disease/syndrome	Biovar	Most frequent serovars *
Trachoma	*trachoma*	A, B, Ba, C
Inclusion conjunctivitis	*trachoma*	D, Da, E, F, G, H, I, Ia, J, K
Urethritis, cervicitis, salpingitis (pharyngitis, otitis media)	*trachoma*	B, C, D, E, F, G, H, I, K, L_3
Lymphogranuloma venereum (syn. lymphogranuloma inguinale, lymphopathia venerea, Favre-Durand-Nicolas disease)	*lymphogranuloma venereum*	L_1, L_2, L_2a, L_3

*   Determined with microimmunofluorescence.

be grown in cell cultures. The therapeutic method of choice is systemic and local application of tetracyclines over a period of several weeks.

Inclusion conjunctivitis. This is an acute, purulent papillary conjunctivitis that may affect neonates, children, and adults (swimming-pool conjunctivitis). Newborn children are infected during birth by pathogens colonizing the birth canal. Left untreated, a pannus may form as in trachoma, followed by corneal scarring. Laboratory diagnosis and therapy as in trachoma.

Genital infections. C. trachomatis is responsible for 30–60% of cases of non-gonococcal urethritis (NGU) in men. Possible complications include prostatitis and epididymitis. The pathogens are communicated by venereal transmission. The source of infection is the female sexual partner, who often shows no clinical symptoms.

In women, C. trachomatis can cause urethritis, proctitis, or infections of the genital organs. It has even been known to cause pelvioperitonitis and perihepatitis. Massive perinatal infection of a neonate may lead to an interstitial chlamydial pneumonia.

The relevant diagnostic tools include:

1. Detection under the microscope in smear material using direct immunofluorescence (see under trachoma).
2. Direct identification by means of amplification of a specific DNA sequence in smear material and urine.
3. Growing in special cell cultures.

Lymphogranuloma venereum. This venereal disease (syn. lymphogranuloma inguinale, lymphopathia venerea (Favre-Durand-Nicolas disease) not to be confused with granuloma inguinale, see p. 305) is frequently observed in the inhabitants of warm climatic zones. A herpetiform primary lesion develops at the site of invasion in the genital area, which then becomes an ulcus with accompanying lymphadenitis. Laboratory diagnosis is based on isolating the proliferating pathogen in cell cultures from purulent material obtained from the ulcus or from matted lymph nodes. The antibodies can be identified using the complement binding reaction or the microimmunofluorescence test. Tetracyclines and macrolides are the potentially useful antibiotic types.

Chlamydia pneumoniae

This new chlamydial species (formerly TWAR chlamydiae) causes infections of the respiratory organs in humans that usually run a mild course: influenza-like infections, sinusitis, pharyngitis, bronchitis, pneumonias (atypical). Clinically silent infections are frequent. C. pneumoniae is pathogenic in humans only. The pathogen is transmitted by aerosol droplets. These infections are probably among the most frequent human chlamydial infections. Serologica studies have demonstrated antibodies to *C. pneumoniae* in 60% of adults Specific laboratory diagnosis is difficult. Special laboratories can grow and identify the pathogen in cultures and detect it under the microscope using marked antibodies to the LPS (although this test is positive for all chlamydia infections). *C. pneumoniae*-specific antibodies can be identified with the microimmunofluorescence method. In a primary infection, a measurable titer does not develop for some weeks and is also quite low. The antibiotics of choice are tetracyclines or macrolides. There is a growing body of evidence supporting a causal contribution by *C. pneumoniae* to atherosclerotic plaque in the coronary arteries, and thus to the pathogenesis of coronary heart disease.

Mycoplasma

■ Mycoplasmas are bacteria that do not possess rigid cell walls for lack of a murein layer. These bacteria take on many different forms. They can only be rendered visible in their native state with phase contrast or dark field microscopy. Mycoplasmas can be grown on culture mediums with high osmotic pressure levels. *M. pneumoniae* frequently causes pneumonias that run atypical courses, especially in youths. Ten to twenty percent of pneumonias contracted outside of hospitals are caused by this pathogen. *M. hominis* and *Ureaplasma urealyticum* contribute to nonspecific infections of the urogenital tract. Infections caused by *Mycoplasmataceae* can be diagnosed by culture growth or antibody assays. The antibiotics of choice are tetracyclines and macrolides (macrolides not for *M. hominis*). Mycoplasmas show high levels of natural resistance to all betalactam antibiotics. ■

Classification. Prokaryotes lacking cell walls are widespread among plants and animals as components of normal flora and as pathogens. Human pathogen species are found in the family *Mycoplasmataceae*, genera *Mycoplasma* and *Ureaplasma*. Infections of the respiratory organs are caused by the species *M. pneumoniae*. Infections of the urogenital tract are caused by the facultatively pathogenic species *M. hominis* and *Ureaplasma urealyticum*. Other species are part of the apathogenic normal flora.

Morphology and culture. The designation mycoplasma is a reference to the many different forms assumed by these pathogens. The most frequent basic shape is a coccoid cell with a diameter of 0.3–0.8 μm. Long, fungilike filaments also occur. Mycoplasmas are best observed in their native state using phase contrast or dark field microscopy. Staining causes them to disintegrate. In contrast to all other bacteria, mycoplasmas possess no rigid cell wall. Flagellae, fimbriae, pili, and capsules are lacking as well. Due to their inherent plasticity, mycoplasmas usually slip through filters that hold back other bacteria. Since their cell wall contains no murein, mycoplasmas are completely insensitive to antibiotics that inhibit murein synthesis (e.g., betalactams).

Mycoplasmas can be cultured on special isotonic nutrient mediums. After two to eight days, small colonies develop resembling sunny-side-up eggs and growing partially into the agar.

Pathogenesis and clinical pictures.

■ **Infections of the respiratory organs.** The pathogen involved is *M. pneumoniae*. The organism is transmitted by aerosol droplets. The cells attach themselves to the epithelia of the trachea, bronchi, and bronchioles. The mechanisms that finally result in destruction of the epithelial cells are yet unknown. The infection develops into pneumonia with an inflammatory exudate in the lumens of the bronchi and bronchioles. The incubation period is 10–20 days. The infection manifests with fever, headache, and a persistent cough. The clinical pictures of the infection course is frequently atypical, i.e., the pneumonia cannot be confirmed by percussion and auscultation. A differential diagnosis must also consider viral pneumonias, ornithosis, and Q fever. Sequelae can set in during or shortly after the acute infection, including pericarditis, myocarditis, pancreatitis, arthritis, erythema nodosum, hemolytic anemias, polyneuritis, and others.

■ **Infections of the urogenital tract.** These infections are caused by *M. hominis* and *Ureaplasma urealyticum*. These facultatively pathogenic species also occur in healthy persons as part of the mucosal flora, so that their etiological role when isolated is often a matter of controversy. *U. urealyticum* is considered responsible for 10–20 % of cases of nongonococcal urethritis and prostatitis in men.

Diagnosis. These pathogens can be grown on special culture mediums. Commercially amplification tests are available for direct identification of *M. pneumoniae*. The CFT was formerly used to detect antibodies to *M. pneumoniae*; today this is done with IgM-specific EIAs. Antibody tests are of no diagnostic value in infections caused by *M. hominis* and *U. urealyticum*.

Therapy. The antibiotics of choice are tetracyclines and macrolides. *M. hominis* shows a natural resistance to macrolides, *U. urealyticum* to lincomycins. Concurrent partner treatment is recommended in urogenital infections.

Epidemiology and prevention. *M. pneumoniae* is found worldwide. Humans are the only source of infection. The pathogens are transmitted by droplet infection during close contact. Infections are frequently contracted in families, schools, homes for children, work camps, and military camps.

Incidence is particularly high between the ages of five and 15 years. About 10–20% of all pneumonias contracted outside hospitals are caused by this pathogen. *M. hominis* and *U. urealyticum* are transmitted either between sexual partners or from mother to neonate during birth. No specific prophylactic measures are available to protect against any of the mycoplasma infections.

Nosocomial Infections

■ Nosocomial infections occur in hospitalized patients as complications of their primary disease. Such infections are reported in an average of approximately 3.5% (Germany) to 5% (USA) of all hospitalized patients, in tertiary care hospitals in about 10% and in the intensive care units of those in about 15–20% of cases. The most frequent types of infection are urinary tract infections (42%), pneumonia (21%), surgical wound infections (16%), and sepsis (8%). The pathogen types most frequently involved are opportunistic, Gram-negative rods, staphylococci and enterococci, followed by fungi. The bacteria are often resistant to many different antibiotics. The hands of medical staff play a major role in transmission of the infections. Control of nosocomial infections requires a number of operational measures (disinfection, asepsis, rationalized antibiotic therapies, isolation), organizational measures (hygiene committee, recognition of infections, procedural guidelines, training programs), and structural measures. ■

Definition

The term **nosocomial infection** designates infections contracted by hospitalized patients 48 hours or more from the beginning of hospitalization. These are secondary infections that occur as complications of the primary diseases to be treated in the hospital.

Pathogens, Infections, Frequency

The significance of the different human pathogens in nosocomial infections varies widely:

■ **Subcellular entities.** Isolated cases of Creutzfeldt-Jakob disease due to unsterilized instruments have been described in the literature. Such accidents now no longer occur.

Table **4.17**   Relative Frequency of Causative Pathogens in Nosocomial Infections (arranged according to the pathogen frequency levels in the column "Total")[1]

Bacteria	UTI[2]	RTI[2]	PWI[2]	SEP[2]	Other[2]	Total
E. coli	40.5	9.9	23.3	13.2	15.6	22.40
Enterococci	19.8	29.5	27.2	0.0	11.7	14.75
Staphylococcus aureus	3.2	25.4	45.5	15.8	13.0	11.11
Coagulase-negative staphylo-cocci	4.5	9.9	14.8	34.2	10.4	8.01
Pseudomonas aeruginosa	5.4	46.5	26.0	0.0	1.3	7.65
Klebsiella sp.	4.1	20.8	15.0	10.5	3.9	6.01
Fungi	5.9	19.1	0.0	2.6	11.7	6.01
Streptococcus sp.	1.8	16.8	8.2	0.0	9.1	4.74
Proteus mirabilis	5.0	4.0	2.4	0.0	2.6	3.10
Enterobacter sp.	1.4	4.0	4.7	2.6	1.3	2.00
Serratia sp.	0.9	1.7	3.8	7.9	0.0	2.00
Other Enterobacteriaceae	1.9	6.3	9.7	2.6	3.9	2.00
Acinetobacter sp.	2.7	5.7	1.2	0.0	0.0	1.82
Anaerobes	0.5	0.0	4.8	0.0	0.0	1.46
Other Gram-positive bacteria	0.0	0.0	7.3	2.6	2.6	1.28
Morganella sp.	1.4	4.0	0.0	0.0	1.3	1.09
Providencia sp.	0.9	0.0	5.0	0.0	2.6	1.09
Pseudomonadaceae (exception: P. aeruginosa)	0.0	3.4	1.2	2.6	2.6	1.09
Other (under 1%)	0.5	0.0	5.0	2.6	1.3	3.48

4

[1] Data (modified) acc. to "*Nosokomiale Infektionen in Deutschland – Erfassung und Prevention (NIDEP–Studie)*." Vol. 56, Publication Series of the German Federal Health Office. Nomos Verlagsgesellschaft, Baden-Baden, 1995.
[2] UTI = urinary tract infections, RTI = lower respiratory tract infections, PWI = post-operative wound infections, SEP = primary sepsis, Other = all other infections.

There are no reliable figures available on viral nosocomial infections. A rough estimate puts viral nosocomial infections at less than 1% of the total. An example of a viral nosocomial infection is infectious hepatitis transmitted by blood or blood products.

■ **Bacteria** are the main pathogens involved in nosocomial infections. Most of the causative organisms are facultatively pathogenic (opportunistic) bacteria, which are frequently resistant to many different antibiotics. These bacteria have found niches in which they persist as so-called hospital flora. The resistance patters seen in these bacteria reflect the often wide variations between anti-infective regimens as practiced in different hospitals.

■ **Fungi.** Fungal nosocomial infections have been on the increase in recent years. It can be said in general that they affect immunocompromised patients and that neutropenic patients are particular susceptible.

Table 4.**17** lists the pathogens that cause the most significant nosocomial infections as determined in a prevalence study done in Germany (East and West) in 1995 (NIDEP Study).

Table 4.**18** shows the prevalence levels at which nosocomial infections occurred in 72 selected hospitals on a given date in the above study. The prevalence and pathogen data shown here approximate what other studies have found. Prevalence and incidence levels can vary considerably from hospital to

Table 4.**18**   Frequency (prevalence) of the Most Important Nosocomial Infection Types (%)[1]

Infection	Internal medicine	Surgery	Gyneco-logy	Intensive care	All patients
Urinary tract infections	1.57	1.45	0.91	2.35	1.46
Lower respiratory tract infections	0.63	0.30	0.09	9.00	0.72
Postoperative wound infections	0.03	1.34	0.05	1.37	0.55
Primary sepsis	0.31	0.15	0.14	2.15	0.29
Other infections	0.52	0.74	0.27	1.96	0.62
Patients with at least one infection	2.97	3.80	1.45	15.30	3.46

[1]   Figures from "*Nosokomiale Infektionen in Deutschland – Erfassung und Prevention (NIDEP–Studie).*" Vol. 56, Publication Series of the German Federal Health Office. Nomos Verlagsgesellschaft, Baden-Baden, 1995.

hospital. The prevalence of nosocomial infections increases with the size of the hospital. Within a particular hospital, the infection rate is always highest in the intensive care units.

Sources of Infection, Transmission Pathways

Nosocomial infections originate either from the patient's own flora (endogenous infections) or from external sources (exogenous infections). **Endogenous infections** are the more frequent type. In such cases, the patient may have brought the pathogens into the hospital. It is, however, frequently the case that a patient's skin and mucosa are colonized within one to two days by bacteria of the hospital flora, which often shows multiple resistance to antibiotics and replaces the patient's individual flora, and that most endogenous infections are then actually caused by the specific hospital flora. The source of infection for **exogenous infections** is most likely to lie with the medical staff. In most cases, the pathogens are transmitted from patient to patient during medical and nursing activities. Less frequently, the staff is either also infected or colonized by the hospital flora. Another important cause of nosocomial infections is technical medical measures that facilitate passage of the pathogens into the body. All invasive diagnostic measures present infection risks. The patient's surroundings, i.e., the air, floor, or walls of the hospital room, are relatively unimportant as sources of infection.

Control

The measures taken to control and prevent nosocomial infections correspond in the wider sense to the general methods of **infection control**. The many different individual measures will not be listed here. The infection control program varies depending on the situation in each particular hospital and can be summarized in three general groups:

Operational measures. This category includes all measures pertaining to treatment and care of patients and cleaning measures. This includes asepsis, disinfection, sterilization, and cleaning. Further precautionary operational measures include isolation of patients that would be sources of infection and the economical and specific administration of antibiotic therapies.

Organizational measures. The organization of hospital infection control must be adapted to the structure of each particular hospital. Realization of the necessary measures, which of course always involve working time and expense, is best realized by establishing an infection control committee charged with the following tasks: determination and analysis of the situation, definition of measures required to improve infection control by issuing binding guidelines, cooperation in the planning and acquisition of operational and structural facilities, cooperation on functional procedures in the various sections of the hospital, contributions to staff training in matters of hospital infection control. In order to carry out these tasks efficiently, the committee should have access to a working group of specialists. In larger hospitals, a hospital epidemiologist, and staff as required, are retained for these functions.

Structural measures.

These measures refer above all to new structures, which must be built in accordance with hygienic criteria. It is therefore the obligation of the planning architect to consult experts when planning the hygienically relevant parts of a construction measure. Hygienic aspects must of course also be considered in reconstruction and restoration of older building substance.

III
Mycology

Absidia corymbifera

5   General Mycology

F. H. Kayser

General Characteristics of Fungi

■ Fungi are eukaryotic microorganisms (domain eucarya) that occur ubiquitously in nature. Only about 200 of the thousands of species have been identified as human pathogens, and among these known pathogenic species fewer than a dozen are responsible for more than 90% of all human fungal infections.

The basic morphological element of filamentous fungi is the hypha and a web of intertwined hyphae is called a mycelium. The basic form of a unicellular fungus is the yeast cell. Dimorphic fungi usually assume the form of yeasts in the parasitic stage and the form of mycelia in the saprophytic stage. The cell walls of fungi consist of nearly 90% carbohydrate (chitin, glucans, mannans) and fungal membranes are rich in sterol types not found in other biological membranes (e.g., ergosterol). Filamentous fungi reproduce either **asexually** (mitosis), by hyphal growth and tip extension, or with the help of asexual spores. Yeasts reproduce by a process of budding. **Sexual** reproduction (meiosis) on the other hand, produces sexual spores. **Fungi imperfecti** or deuteromycetes are the designation for a type of fungi in which the fructification forms are either unknown or missing entirely.   ■

Definition and Taxonomy

Fungi are microorganisms in the domain eucarya (see. p. 5). They show less differentiation than plants, but a higher degree of organization than the prokaryotes bacteria (Table 5.1). The kingdom of the fungi (*Mycota*) comprises over 50 000 different species, only about 200 of which have been identified as human pathogens. Only about a dozen of these "pathogenic" species cause 90% of all human mycoses. Many mycotic infections are relatively harmless, for instance the dermatomycoses. In recent years, however, the increasing numbers of patients with various kinds of immune defects have resulted in more life-threatening mycoses.

Table **5.1**   Some Differences between Fungi and Bacteria

Properties	Fungi	Bacteria
Nucleus	Eukaryotic; nuclear membrane; more than one chromosome; mitosis	Prokaryotic; no membrane; nucleoid; only one "chromosome"
Cytoplasm	Mitochondria; endoplasmic reticulum; 80S ribosomes	No mitochondria; no endoplasmic reticulum; 70S ribosomes
Cytoplasmic membrane	Sterols (ergosterol)	No sterols
Cell wall	Glucans, mannans, chitin, chitosan	Murein, teichoic acids (Gram-positive), proteins
Metabolism	Heterotrophic; mostly aerobes; no photosynthesis	Heterotrophic; obligate aerobes and anaerobes, facultative anaerobes
Size, mean diameter	Yeast cells: 3–5–10 μm. Molds: indefinable	1–5 μm
Dimorphism	In some species	None

5

The taxonomy of the fungi is essentially based on their morphology. In medical mycology, fungi are classified according to practical aspects as dermatophytes, yeasts, molds, and dimorphic fungi. Molds grow in filamentous structures, yeasts as single cells and dermatophytes cause infections of the keratinized tissues (skin, hair, nails, etc.). Dimorphic fungi can appear in both of the two forms, as yeast cells or as mycelia (see the following pages).

Fungi are carbon heterotrophs. The saprobic or saprophytic fungi take carbon compounds from dead organic material whereas biotrophic fungi (parasites or symbionts) require living host organisms. Some fungi can exist in both saprophytic and biotrophic forms.

Morphology

Two morphological forms of fungi are observed (Fig. 5.1):

■ **Hypha:** this is the basic element of filamentous fungi with a branched, tubular structure, 2–10 μm in width.

Basic Morphological Elements of Fungi

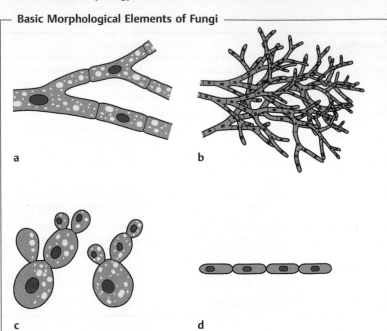

Fig. 5.1 There are two basic morphological forms: hypha and yeast.
a Hypha, septate, or nonseptate.
b Mycelium: web of branched hyphae.
c Yeast form, budding (diameter of individual cell 3–5 μm).
d Pseudomycelium.

■ **Mycelium:** this is the web or matlike structure of hyphae. Substrate mycelia (specialized for nutrition) penetrate into the nutrient substrate, whereas aerial mycelia (for asexual propagation) develop above the nutrient medium.

■ **Fungal thallus:** this is the entirety of the mycelia and is also called the fungal body or colony.

■ **Yeast:** the basic element of the unicellular fungi. It is round to oval and 3–10 μm in diameter. Several elongated yeast cells chained together and resembling true hyphae are called pseudohyphae.

■ **Dimorphism:** some fungal species can develop either the yeast or the mycelium form depending on the environmental conditions, a property called dimorphism. Dimorphic pathogenic fungi take the form of yeast cells in the parasitic stage and appear as mycelia in the saprophytic stage.

Metabolism

All fungi are carbon heterotrophs, which means they are dependent on exogenous nutrient substrates as sources of organic carbon, and with a few exceptions, fungi are obligate aerobes. Many species are capable of maintaining metabolic activity in the most basic of nutrient mediums. The known metabolic types of fungi include thermophilic, psychrophilic, acidophilic, and halophilic species. The metabolic capabilities of fungi are exploited in the food industry (e.g., in the production of bread, wine, beer, cheese, or single-cell proteins) and in the pharmaceutical industry (e.g., in the production of antibiotic substances, enzymes, citric acid, etc.). The metabolic activity of fungi can also be a damaging factor. Fungal infestation can destroy foods, wooden structures, textiles, etc. Fungi also cause numerous plant diseases, in particular diseases of crops.

Reproduction in Fungi

Asexual reproduction. This category includes the vegetative propagation of hyphae and yeasts as well as vegetative fructification, i.e., formation of asexual spores.

■ **Hyphae** elongate in a zone just short of the tip in which the cell wall is particularly elastic. This apical growth process can also include formation of swellings that develop into lateral hyphae, which can in turn also branch out.

■ **Yeasts** reproduce by budding. This process begins with an outgrowth on the mother cell wall that develops into a daughter cell or blastoconidium. The isthmus between the two is finally cut off by formation of a septum. Some yeasts propagate in both the yeast and hypha forms (Fig. 6.**2**, p. 362).

■ **Vegetative fructification.** A type of propagative form, the **asexual spores**, is formed in this process. These structures show considerable resistance to exogenous noxae and help fungi spread in the natural environment. Asexual spores come in a number of morphological types: **conidia, sporangiospores, arthrospores, and blastospores**. These forms rarely develop during the parasitic stages in hosts, but they are observed in cultures. The morphology of the asexual spores of fungi is an important identification characteristic.

Sexual fructification. Sexual reproduction in **fungi perfecti** (eumycetes) follows essentially the same patterns as in the higher eukaryotes. The nuclei of two haploid partners fuse to form a diploid zygote. The diploid nucleus then undergoes meiosis to form the haploid nuclei, finally resulting in the haploid sexual spores: **zygospores, ascospores, and basidiospores**. Sexual spores are only rarely produced in the types of fungi that parasitize human tissues.

Sexual reproduction structures are either unknown or not present in many species of pathogenic fungi, known as **fungi imperfecti** (deuteromycetes).

General Aspects of Fungal Disease

■ Besides fungal allergies (e.g., extrinsic allergic alveolitis) and mycotoxicoses (aflatoxicosis), fungal infections are by far the most frequent fungal diseases. Mycoses are classified clinically as follows:

— **Primary mycoses** (coccidioidomycosis, histoplasmosis, blastomycoses).
— **Opportunistic mycoses** (surface and deep yeast mycoses, aspergillosis, mucormycoses, phaeohyphomycoses, hyalohyphomycoses, cryptococcoses; penicilliosis, pneumocystosis).
— **Subcutaneous mycoses** (sporotrichosis, chromoblastomycosis, Madura foot (mycetoma).
— **Cutaneous mycoses** (pityriasis versicolor, dermatomycoses).

Little is known about fungal pathogenicity factors. The natural resistance of the macroorganism to fungal infection is based mainly on effective phagocytosis whereas specific resistance is generally through cellular immunity. Opportunistic mycoses develop mainly in patients with immune deficiencies (e.g., in neutropenia). Laboratory diagnostic methods for fungal infections mostly include microscopy and culturing, in order to detect the pathogens directly, and identification of specific antibodies. Therapeutics for treatment of mycoses include polyenes (above all amphotericin B), azoles (e.g., itraconazole, fluconazole, voriconazole), allylamines, antimetabolites (e.g., 5-fluorocytosine), and echinocandins (e.g., caspofungin). Antimycotics are often administered in combination. ■

Fungal Allergies and Fungal Toxicoses

Mycogenic Allergies

The spores of ubiquitous fungi continuously enter the respiratory tract with inspired air. These spores contain potent allergens to which susceptible individuals may manifest strong hypersensitivity reactions. Depending on the localization of the reaction, it may assume the form of allergic rhinitis, bronchial asthma, or allergic alveolitis. Many of these allergic reactions are certi-fied occupational diseases, i.e., "farmer's lung," "woodworker's lung," and other types of extrinsic allergic alveolitis.

Mycotoxicoses

Some fungi produce mycotoxins, the best known of which are the aflatoxins produced by the *Aspergillus* species. These toxins are ingested with the food stuffs on which the fungi have been growing. Aflatoxin B1 may contribute to primary hepatic carcinoma, a disease observed frequently in Africa and Southeast Asia.

Mycoses

Data on the general incidence of mycotic infections can only be approximate, since there is no requirement that they be reported to the health authorities. It can be assumed that **cutaneous mycoses** are among the most frequent in-fections worldwide. **Primary** and **opportunistic mycoses** are, on the other hand, relatively rare. Opportunistic mycoses have been on the increase in re-cent years and decades, reflecting the fact that clinical manifestations are only observed in hosts whose immune disposition allows them to develop. Increasing numbers of patients with immune defects and a high frequency of invasive and aggressive medical therapies are the factors contributing to the increasing significance of mycoses. Table 5.**2** provides a summary view of the most important human mycoses. The categorization of the infections used here disregards taxonomic considerations to concentrate on practical clinical aspects.

Host-pathogen interactions

The factors that determine the onset, clinical picture, severity, and outcome of a mycosis include interactions between fungal pathogenicity factors and host immune defense mechanisms. Compared with the situation in the field of bacteriology, it must be said that we still know little about the underlying causes and mechanisms of fungal pathogenicity.

Humans show high levels of nonspecific resistance to most fungi based on mechanical, humoral, and cellular factors (see Table 1.**6**, p. 22). Among these factors, phagocytosis by neutrophilic granulocytes and macrophages is the most important. Intensive contact with fungi results in the acquisition of spe-

Table **5.2** Overview of the Most Important Mycoses in Humans

Disease	Etiology	Remarks
Primary mycoses (do not occur endemic in Europe)		
Coccidioidomycosis	*Coccidioides immitis*	Pulmonary mycosis. Inhalation of spores. Southwestern US and South America
Histoplasmosis	*Histoplasma capsulatum*	Pulmonary mycosis. Inhalation of spores. Dissemination into RES. America, Asia, Africa
North American Blastomycoses	*Blastomyces dermatitidis*	Primary pulmonary mycosis. Secondary dissemination (dermal). North America, Africa
South American Blastomycoses	*Paracoccidioides brasiliensis*	Primary pulmonary mycosis. Secondary dissemination
Opportunistic mycoses		
Candidiasis (soor)	*Candida albicans*, other *Candida* sp.	Endogenous infection. Primary infection of mucosa and skin with secondary dissemination
Aspergillosis	*Aspergillus fumigatus* (90%); other *Aspergillus* sp.	Aspergilloses of the respiratory tract, endophthalmitis; aspergillosis of CNS; septic aspergillosis
Cryptococcosis	*Cryptococcus neoformans* (yeast; thick capsule)	Aerogenic infection. Pulmonary cryptococcosis. Secondary dissemination into CNS
Mucormycoses (zygomycoses)	*Mucor* spp.; *Rhizopus* spp.; *Absidia* spp.; *Cuninghamella* spp., and others	Rhinocerebral, pulmonary, gastrointestinal, cutaneous mucormycosis
Phaeohyphomycoses (caused by "dematious" or "black" fungi)	Over 100 species discovered to date, e.g., *Curvularia* spp.; *Bipolaris* spp.; *Alternaria* spp. Melanin integrated in cell wall	Subcutaneous infections, paranasal sinus infections, infections of the CNS, sepsis also possible
Pneumocystosis	*Pneumocystis carinii*	Defective cellular immunity

Table 5.2 *Continued: Overview of the Most Important Mycoses in Humans*

Disease	Etiology	Remarks
Hyalohyphomycoses (caused by colorless [hyaline] molds)	More than 40 species discovered to date, e.g., *Fusarium* spp.; *Scedosporium* spp.; *Paecilomyces lilacinus*	Infections of cornea and eye, pneumonia, osteomyelitis, arthritis, soft tissue infections, sepsis also possible
Yeast mycoses (except candidiasis)	*Torulopsis glabrata; Trichosporon beigelii; Rhodotorula* spp.; *Malassezia furfur*, and others	Infections of various organs in immunosuppressed patients. Sepsis also possible. *Malassezia furfur* in catheter sepsis in neonates and in intravenous feeding with lipids
Penicilliosis	*Penicillium marneffei*	Most frequent opportunistic infection in AIDS patients in Southeast Asia. Primary infection focus in lungs

Subcutaneous mycoses

Sporotrichosis	*Sporothrix schenckii*	Dimorphic fungus, ulcerous lesions on extremities
Chromoblastomycosis	*Phialophora verrucosa Fonsecea pedrosoi Cladosporium carrionii*, etc.	Black molds. Wartlike pigmented lesions on extremities. Tropical disease
Madura foot (mycetoma)	*Madurella mycetomi Scedosporium apiospermum*, etc.	Subcutaneous abscesses on feet or hands. Can also be caused by bacteria (see p. 273). In tropics and subtropics

Cutaneous mycoses

Pityriasis (or tinea versicolor)	*Malassezia furfur*	Surface infection; relatively harmless; pathogen is dependent on an outside source of fatty acids
Dermatomycoses Tinea pedis, T. cruris, T. capitis, T. barbae, T. unguinum, T. corporis	*Trichophyton* spp. *Microsporum* spp. *Epidermophyton* spp.	All dermatophytes are filamentous fungi (hyphomycetes). Anthropophilic, zoophilic, geophilic species. Always transmitted by direct or indirect contact

5

cific immunity, especially the cellular type. The role of humoral immunity in specific immune defense is secondary.

Diagnosis

The primary concern here is identification of the pathogen.

■ **Microscopy.** Native preparation: briefly heat material under coverslip with 10% KOH. Stained preparation: stain with methylene blue, lactophenol blue, periodic acid-Schiff (PAS), ink, etc.

■ **Culturing.** This is possible on universal and selective mediums. Sabouraud dextrose agar can contain selective agents (e.g., chloramphenicol and cycloheximide), this medium has an acid pH of 5.6. The main identifying structures are morphological, in particular the asexual and, if present, sexual reproductive structures. Biochemical tests are used mainly to identify yeasts and are generally not as important in mycology as they are in bacteriology.

■ **Serology.** By the identification of antibodies to special fungal antigens in patient's serum. The Interpretation of serological findings is quite difficult in fungal infections.

■ **Antigen detection.** By finding of specific antigens in the diagnostic material by direct means using known antibodies, possible in some fungal infections (e.g., cryptococcosis).

■ **Cutaneous test.** Cutaneous (allergy) tests with specific fungal antigens can be useful in diagnosing a number of fungal infections.

■ **Nucleic acid detection.** Combined with amplification, such tests are useful for rapid detection of mycotic diseases in immunocompromised patients.

Therapy

A limited number of anti-infective agents are available for specific treatment of fungal infections:

■ **Polyenes.** These agents bind to membrane sterols and destroy the membrane structure:
— Amphotericin B. Used In systemic mycoses. Fungicidal activity with frequent side effects. There are conventional galenic form and (new) various lipid forms.
— Nystatin, natamycin. Only for topical use in mucosal mycoses.

■ **Azoles.** These agents disrupt ergosterol biosynthesis. Their effect is mainly fungistatic with possible gastrointestinal side effects. Hepatic functional parameters should be monitored during therapy:
— Ketoconazole. One of the first azoles. No longer used because of side effects.
— Fluconazole. Oral or intravenous application. For the treatment of surface and systemic mycoses and cryptococcal meningitis in AIDS patients.
— Itraconazole. Oral and intravenous application. Use in systemic and cutaneous mycoses and also for the treatment of aspergillosis.
— Voriconazole. Oral and intravenous application. Good activity against *Candida* and *Aspergillus*. No acitivity against *Mucorales*.

■ **Antimetabolites.** 5-Fluorocytosine. Interferes with DNA synthesis (base analog). Given by oral application in candidiasis, aspergillosis, and cryptococcosis. It is necessary to monitor the course of therapy for the development of resistance. The toxicity of amphotericin B is reduced in combination with 5-fluorocytosine.

■ **Allylamines.** Terbinafine. By oral and topical application to treat dermatomycoses. Inhibition of ergosterol biosynthesis.

■ **Echinocandins. Caspofungin** has been approved as a salvage therapy in refractory aspergillosis. It is useful also in oropharyngeal and esophageal candidiasis. Inhibition of the biosynthesis of glucan of the cell wall.

■ **Griseofulvin.** This is an older antibiotic used in treatment of dermatomycoses. By oral application, therapy must often be continued for months.

5

6   Fungi as Human Pathogens

Primary Mycoses

■ Primary systemic mycoses include histoplasmosis (*Histoplasma capsulatum*), North American blastomycosis (*Blastomyces dermatitidis*), coccidioidomycosis (*Coccidioides immitis*), and South American blastomycosis (*Paracoccidioides brasiliensis*). The natural habitat of these pathogens is the soil. Their spores are inhaled with dust, get into the lungs, and cause a primary pulmonary mycosis. Starting from foci in the lungs, the organisms can then be transported, hematogenously or lymphogenously, to other organs including the skin, where they cause granulomatous, purulent infection foci. Laboratory diagnostics aim at direct detection of the pathogens under the microscope and in cultures as well as identification of antibodies. The therapeutics used to treat these infections are amphotericin B and azoles. All of the primary systemic mycoses are endemic to certain geographic areas, in some cases quite limited in extent. Central Europe is not affected by these diseases. They are not communicable among humans. ■

Histoplasma capsulatum (Histoplasmosis)

Histoplasma capsulatum is the pathogen responsible for histoplasmosis, an intracellular mycosis of the reticuloendothelial system. The sexual stage or form of this fungus is called *Emmonsiella capsulata*.

Morphology and culture. *H. capsulatum* is a dimorphic fungus. As an infectious pathogen in human tissues it always forms yeast cells (Fig. 6.**1**). The small individual cells are often localized inside macrophages and have a diameter of 2–3 µm.

    Giemsa and gram staining do not "take" on the cell walls of *H. capsulatum*, for which reason the cells often appear to be surrounded by an empty areola, which was incorrectly taken to be a capsule, resulting in the designation *H. capsulatum*. This species can be grown on the nutrient mediums normally used for fungal cultures. *H. capsulatum* grows as a mycelium in two to three weeks on Sabouraud agar at a temperature of 20–30 °C.

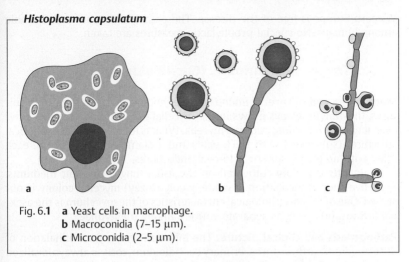

Histoplasma capsulatum

Fig. 6.**1** **a** Yeast cells in macrophage.
  b Macroconidia (7–15 μm).
  c Microconidia (2–5 μm).

6

Pathogenesis and clinical picture. The natural habitat of *H. capsulatum* is the soil. Spores (conidia) are inhaled into the respiratory tract, are taken up by alveolar macrophages, and become yeast cells that reproduce by budding. Small granulomatous inflammatory foci develop. The pathogens can disseminate hematogenously from these primary infection foci. The reticuloendothelial system (RES) is hit particularly hard. Lymphadenopathies develop and the spleen and liver are affected. Over 90 % of infections remain clinically silent. The clinical picture depends heavily on any predisposing host factors and the infective dose. A histoplasmosis can also run its course as a respiratory infection only. Disseminated histoplasmoses are also observed in AIDS patients.

Diagnosis. Suitable material for diagnostic analysis is provided by bronchial secretion, urine, or scrapings from infection foci. For microscopic examination, Giemsa or Wright staining is applied and yeast cells are looked for inside the macrophages and polymorphonuclear leukocytes. Cultures on blood or Sabouraud agar must be incubated for several weeks. Antibodies are detected using the complement fixation test and agar gel precipitation. The diagnostic value of positive or negative findings in a histoplasmin scratch test is doubtful.

Therapy. Treatment with amphotericin B is only indicated in severe infections, especially the disseminated form.

Epidemiology and prevention. Histoplasmosis is endemic to the midwestern USA, Central and South America, Indonesia, and Africa. With few exceptions,

Western Europe is free of the disease. The pathogen is not communicable among humans. No special prophylactic measures are taken.

Coccidioides immitis (Coccidioidomycosis)

Morphology and culture. *C. immitis* is an atypical dimorphic fungus. In cultures, this fungus always grows in the mycelial form; in body tissues, however, it neither buds nor produces mycelia. What is found in vivo are spherical structures (spherules) with thick walls and a diameter of 15–60 μm, each filled with up to 100 spherical-to-oval endospores.

C. immitis is readily cultivated on the usual fungus nutrient mediums. After five days of incubation, a white, wooly (fuzzy) mycelial colony is observed. One of the morphological characteristics of the mycelium is the asexual arthrospores seen as separate entities among the hyphae.

Pathogenesis and clinical picture. The infection results from inhalation of dust containing arthrospores. Primary coccidioidomycosis is always localized in the lungs, whereby the level of manifestation varies from silent infections (60% of infected persons) to severe pneumonia. Five percent of those infected develop a chronic cavernous lung condition. In fewer than 1%, hematogenous dissemination produces granulomatous lesions in skin, bones, joints, and meninges.

Diagnosis. The available tools are pathogen detection in sputum, pus, cerebrospinal fluid or biopsies, and antibody identification. The spherules can be seen under the microscope in fresh material. The fungus can be readily cultured on Sabouraud agar at 25 °C. The resulting arthrospores are highly infectious and must be handled very carefully. Antibodies can be detected using the complement fixation test, gel precipitation or latex agglutination. A coccidioidin skin test measuring any cellular allergy to components of the fungus is used as an initial orientation test if an infection is suspected.

Therapy. Amphotericin B can be used to treat the disseminated forms. An oral azole derivative will serve as an alternative, or for use, in clinically less severe forms.

Epidemiology and prevention. Coccidioidomycosis is endemic to desert areas of California, Arizona, Texas, New Mexico, and Utah and is only rarely observed elsewhere. The source of infection is the fungus-rich soil. Animals can also be infected. This disease is not transmitted among humans or from animals to humans.

Blastomyces dermatitidis
(North American Blastomycosis)

Blastomyces dermatitidis is a dimorphic fungus that causes a chronic granulomatous infection. The pathogens occur naturally in the soil and are transmitted to humans by inhalation.

The primary blastomycosis infection is pulmonary. Secondary hematogenous spread can lead to involvement of other organs including the skin. **Laboratory diagnostic** methods include microscopy and culturing to identify the fungus in sputum, skin lesion pus, or biopsy material. Antibody detection using the complement fixation test or agar gel precipitation is of limited diagnostic value. Amphotericin B is the **therapeutic agent** of choice. Untreated blastomycoses almost always have a lethal outcome.

Blastomycosis occurs mainly in the Mississippi Valley as well as in the eastern and northern USA. Infections are also relatively frequent in animals, especially dogs. Susceptible persons cannot, however, be infected by infected animals or humans. There are no prophylactic measures.

Paracoccidioides brasiliensis
(South American Blastomycosis)

6

Paracoccidioides brasiliensis (syn. *Blastomyces brasiliensis*) is a dimorphic fungus that, in living tissues, produces thick-walled yeast cells of 10–30 μm in diameter, most of which have several buds. When cultivated (25 °C), the fungus grows in the mycelial form.

The natural habitat of *P. brasiliensis* is probably the soil. Human infections are caused by inhalation of spore-laden dust. Primary purulent and/or granulomatous infection foci are found in the lung. Starting from these foci, the fungus can disseminate hematogenously or lymphogenously into the skin, mucosa, or lymphoid organs. A disseminated paracoccidioidomycosis progresses gradually and ends lethally unless treated. The **therapeutic agents** of choice are azole derivatives (e.g., itraconazole), amphotericin B, and sulfonamides. Therapy can prevent the disease from progressing, although no cases are known in which the disease is eliminated over the longer term. **Laboratory diagnostics** are based on detection of the pathogen under the microscope and in cultures as well as on antibody detection with the complement fixation test or gel precipitation.

Paracoccidioidomycosis is observed mainly among farmers in rural parts of South America.

Opportunistic Mycoses (OM)

■ Opportunistic mycoses (OM) that affect skin and mucosa as well as internal organs are caused by both yeast and molds. A precondition for development of such infections is a pronounced weakness in the host's immune defenses. Candidiasis is an endogenous infection. Other OMs are exogenous infections caused by fungi that naturally inhabit the soil or plants. These environmental fungi usually invade via the respiratory tract. The most important are aspergillosis, cryptococcosis, and the mucormycoses. Besides *Candida* and other yeasts, phaeohyphomycetes and hyalohyphomycetes, which are only very mildly pathogenic, can also cause systemic infections. All OMs have a primary infection focus, usually in the upper or lower respiratory tract. From this focus, the pathogens can disseminate hematogenously and/or lymphogenously to infect additional organs. Infection foci should be removed surgically if feasible. Antimycotic agents are used in chemotherapy. In infected immunocompromised patients, the prognosis is usually poor.   ■

6

Candida (Soor)

At least 70% of all human *Candida* infections are caused by *C. albicans*, the rest by *C. parapsilosis*, *C. tropicalis*, *C. guillermondii*, *C. kruzei*, and a few other rare *Candida* species.

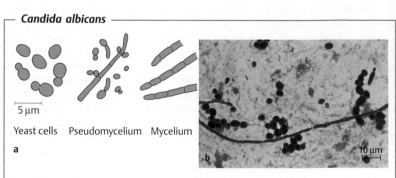

┌─ *Candida albicans* ─

5 μm

Yeast cells   Pseudomycelium   Mycelium

a

b   10 μm

Fig. 6.**2**   *Candida albicans.*
a Morphological forms.
b Gram staining of sputum: Gram-positive yeast cells and hyphae.
Clinical diagnosis: candidiasis of the respiratory tract.

Morphology and culture. Gram staining of primary preparations reveals *C. albicans* to be a Gram-positive, budding, oval yeast with a diameter of approximately 5 µm. Gram-positive pseudohyphae are observed frequently and septate mycelia occasionally (Fig. 6.**2**).

C. albicans can be grown on the usual culture mediums. After 48 hours of incubation on agar mediums, round, whitish, somewhat rough-surfaced colonies form. They are differentiated from other yeasts based on morphological and biochemical characteristics.

Pathogenesis and clinical pictures. *Candida* is a normal inhabitant of human and animal mucosa (commensal). *Candida* infections must therefore be considered endogenous. Candodoses usually develop in persons whose immunity is compromised, most frequently in the presence of disturbed cellular immunity. The mucosa are affected most often, less frequently the outer skin and inner organs (deep candidiasis). In oral cavity infections, a white, stubbornly adherent coating is seen on the cheek mucosa and tongue. Patho-

---

Clinical Forms of Candidosis

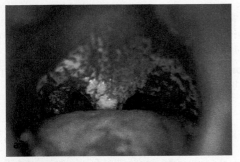

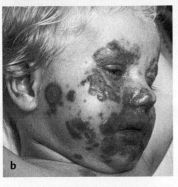

Fig. 6.**3** **a** Oral soor; surface infection of cheek mucosa and tongue by *Candida albicans* in an AIDS patient.
b Chronic mucocutaneous candidiasis in a child with a cellular immunodeficiency syndrome.

6

morphologically similar to oral soor is vulvovaginitis. Diabetes, pregnancy, progesterone therapy, and intensive antibiotic treatment that eliminate the normal bacterial flora are among the predisposing factors. Skin is mainly infected on the moist, warm parts of the body. *Candida* can spread to cause secondary infections of the lungs, kidneys, and other organs. Candidial endocarditis and endophthalmitis are observed in drug addicts. Chronic mucocutaneous candidiasis is observed as a sequel to damage of the cellular immune system (Fig. 6.**3**).

Diagnosis. This involves microscopic examination of preparations of different materials, both native and Gram-stained. *Candida* grows on many standard nutrient mediums, particularly well on Sabouraud agar. Typical yeast colonies are identified under the microscope and based on specific metabolic evidence.

Detection of *Candida*-specific antigens in serum (e.g., free mannan) is possible using an agglutination reaction with latex particles to which monoclonal antibodies are bound. Various methods are used to identify antibodies in deep candidiasis (agglutination, gel precipitation, enzymatic immunoassays, immunoelectrophoresis).

Therapy. Nystatin and azoles can be used in topical therapy. In cases of deep candidiasis, amphotericin B is still the agent of choice, often administered together with 5-fluorocytosine. Echinocandins (e.g., caspofungin) can be used in severe oropharyngeal and esophageal candidiasis.

Epidemiology and prevention. *Candida* infections are, with the exception of candidiasis in newborn children, endogenous infections.

Aspergillus (Aspergillosis)

Aspergilloses are most frequently caused by *Aspergillus fumigatus* and *A. flavus*. *A. niger*, *A. nidulans*, and *A. terreus* are found less often. Aspergilli are ubiquitous in nature. They are found in large numbers on rotting plants.

Morphology and culture. *Aspergillus* is recognized in tissue preparations, exudates and sputum by the filamentous, septate hyphae, which are approximately 3–4 μm wide with Y-shaped branchings (Fig. 6.**4**).

Aspergillus grows rapidly, in mycelial form, on many of the mediums commonly used in clinical microbiology. Sabouraud agar is suitable for selective culturing.

Pathogenesis and clinical pictures. The main portal of entry for this pathogen is the bronchial system, but the organism can also invade the body through injuries in the skin or mucosa. The following localizations are known for aspergilloses:

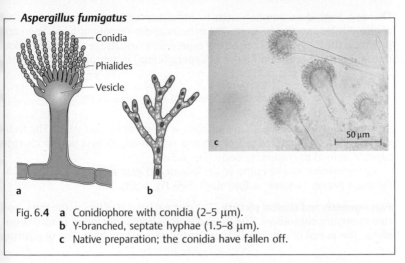

Aspergillus fumigatus

— Conidia
— Phialides
— Vesicle

50 μm

a b c

Fig. 6.4 **a** Conidiophore with conidia (2–5 μm).
        b Y-branched, septate hyphae (1.5–8 μm).
        c Native preparation; the conidia have fallen off.

6

■ **Aspergillosis of the respiratory tract.** An aspergilloma is a circumscribed "fungus ball" that usually grows in a certain space (e.g., a cavern). Another pulmonary aspergillosis is a chronic, necrotizing pneumonia. Acute, invasive pulmonary aspergillosis is seen in patients suffering from neutropenia or AIDS or following organ transplants and has a poor prognosis. Another aspergillosis of the respiratory tract is tracheobronchitis. Of all fungi, aspergilli are most frequently responsible for various forms of sinusitis. In persons with atopic allergies, asthma may be caused by an allergic aspergillus alveolitis.

■ **Other aspergilloses.** Endophthalmitis can develop two to three weeks after surgery or an eye injury and the usual outcome is loss of the eye. Cerebral aspergillosis develops after hematogenous dissemination. Less often, *Aspergillus* spp. cause endocarditis, myocarditis, and osteomyelitis.

Diagnosis. Since *Aspergillus* is a frequent contaminant of diagnostic materials, diagnosis based on direct pathogen detection is difficult. Finding the typically branched hyphae in the primary preparation and repeated culture growth of *Aspergillus* make the diagnosis probable. If the branched hyphae are found in tissue biopsies stained with methenamine silver stain, the diagnosis can be considered confirmed.

Using latex particles coated with monoclonal antibodies, *Aspergillus*-specific antigen (*Aspergillus* galactomannan) can be detected in blood serum in an agglutination reaction. Antibodies in systemic aspergilloses are best detected by immunodiffusion and ELISA. PCR-based methods detect *Aspergillus-DNA*.

Therapy. High-dose amphotericin B, administered in time, is the agent of choice. Azoles can also be used. The echinocandin caspofungin has been approved in the treatment of refractory aspergillosis as salvage therapy. Surgical removal of local infection foci (e.g., aspergilloma) is appropriate.

Cryptococcus neoformans (Cryptococcosis)

Morphology and culture. *C. neoformans* is an encapsulated yeast. The individual cell has a diameter of 3–5 μm and is surrounded by a polysaccharide capsule several micrometers wide (Fig. 6.**5a**).

C. neoformans can be cultured on Sabouraud agar at 30–35 °C with an incubation period of three to four days (See Fig. 6.**5b**).

Pathogenesis and clinical picture. The normal habitat of this pathogen is soil rich in organic substances. The fungus is very frequently found in bird droppings. The portal of entry in humans is the respiratory tract. The organisms

6

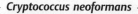
Cryptococcus neoformans

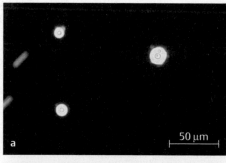
a

50 μm

Fig. 6.**5 a** Ink preparation from cerebrospinal fluid; negative image of thick, mucoid capsule surrounding the yeast cells. Clinical diagnosis: cryptococcal meningitis.
b Culture on Sabouraud agar: whitish, creamy colonies.

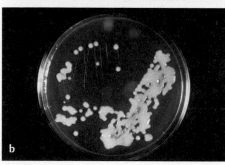
b

are inhaled and enter the lungs, resulting in a pulmonary cryptococcosis that usually runs an inapparent clinical course. From the primary pulmonary foci, the pathogens spread hematogenously to other organs, above all into the central nervous system (CNS), for which compartment *C. neoformans* shows a pronounced affinity. A dangerous meningoencephalitis is the result. Good preconditions for dissemination from the lung foci are provided especially by primary diseases that weaken the immune defenses. Malignancies and steroid therapy are other frequent predisposing factors. AIDS patients also frequently develop cryptococcoses.

Diagnosis. This is particularly important in meningitis. The pathogens can be detected in cerebrospinal fluid sediment using phase contrast microscopy. An ink preparation results in a negative image of the capsule (see Fig. 6.**5a**). Culturing is most successful on Sabouraud agar. *C. neoformans* can be differentiated from other yeasts and identified based on special metabolic properties (e.g., breakdown of urea). A latex agglutination test is available for detection of capsule polysaccharide in cerebrospinal fluid and serum (anticapsular antibodies coupled to latex particles). Identification of antibodies to the capsular polysaccharide is achieved by means of an agglutination test or an enzymatic immunosorbence test.

Therapy. Amphotericin B is the agent of choice in CNS cryptococcosis, often used in combination with 5-fluorocytosine.

Epidemiology and prevention. No precise figures are available on the frequency of pulmonary cryptococcosis. The incidence of the attendant meningoencephalitis is one case per million inhabitants per year. There are no specific prophylactic measures.

Mucor, Absidia, Rhizopus (Mucormycoses)

Mucormycoses are caused mainly by various species in the genera *Mucor*, *Absidia*, and *Rhizopus*. More rarely, this type of opportunistic mycosis is caused by species in the genera *Cunninghamella, Rhizomucor,* and others. All of these fungal genera are in the order *Mucorales* and occur ubiquitously. They are found especially often on disintegrating organic plant materials.

Morphology and culture. Mucorales are molds that produce broad, nonseptate hyphae with thick walls that branch off nearly at right angles (Fig. 6.**6**). Mucorales are readily cultured. They grow on all standard mediums, forming high, whitish-gray to brown, "fuzzy" aerial mycelium.

Culturing is best done on Sabouraud agar.

Pathogenesis and clinical pictures. *Mucorales* are typical opportunists that only cause infections in patients with immune deficiencies or metabolic dis-

6

Mucorales (Zygomycetes)

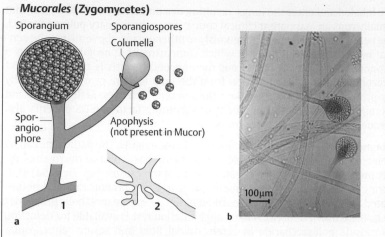

Fig. 6.6 **a** Morphological elements:
1 = sporangium (60–350 µm) with sporangiospores (5–9 µm),
2 = nonseptate hyphae (diameter 6–15 µm) with rhizoid (→ rootlike structure).
b *Absidia corymbifera*: lactophenol blue preparation. Material from culture.

orders (diabetes). The pathogens penetrate into the target organic system with dust. They show a high affinity to vascular structures, in which they reproduce, potentially resulting in thrombosis and infarction. The infections are classified as follows according to their manifestations:

■ **Rhinocerebral mucormycosis**, spreads from the nose or sinuses and may affect the brain. Most often observed as a sequel to diabetic acidosis.

■ **Pulmonary mucormycosis**, with septic pulmonary infarctions. Occurs most frequently in neutropenic malignancy patients under remission therapy.

■ **Gastrointestinal mucormycosis** (vary rare), seen in undernourished children and accompanied by infarctions of the gastrointestinal tract.

■ **Cutaneous mucormycosis**, manifests as a sequel to skin injuries, especially burns.

■ **Disseminated mucormycosis**, as a sequel to any of these forms, especially pulmonary mucormycosis.

Diagnosis. Confirmation of diagnosis is based on detection of tissue infiltration by morphologically typical fungal hyphae. Culturing can be attempted on

Sabouraud agar. Identification concerns solely the morphological characteristics of the fructification organs. There is no method of antibody-based diagnosis.

Therapy. Amphotericin B is the antimycotic agent of choice. Surgical measures as required. Control of the primary disease.

Phaeohyphomycetes, Hyalohyphomycetes, Opportunistic Yeasts, Penicillium marneffei

The list of clinically relevant fungi previously not categorized as classic opportunists has lengthened appreciably in recent years. These organisms are now being found in pathogenic roles in patients with malignancies, in AIDS patients, in patients undergoing cytostatic and immunosuppressive therapies, massive corticosteroid therapy, or long-term treatment with broad-spectrum antibiotics. The terms phaeohyphomycetes, hyalohyphomycetes, and opportunistic yeasts have been created with the aim of simplifying the nomenclature.

Phaeohyphomycoses. These are subcutaneous and paranasal sinus infections caused by "dematious" molds or "black fungi." To date, numerous genera and species have been described as pathogenic agents. Common to all is the formation of hyphae, which appear as a brownish black color due to integration of melanin in the hyphal walls. Examples of the genera include *Curvularia*, *Bipolaris*, *Exserohilum*, *Wangiella*, *Dactylaria*, *Ramichloridium*, *Chaetomium*, and *Alternaria*. The natural habitat of these fungi is the soil. They occur worldwide. Phaeohyphomycetes invade the body through injuries in the skin or inhalation of spores. Starting from primary foci (see above), the pathogens can disseminate hematogenously to affect other organs including the CNS. The clinical pictures of such infections most closely resemble the mucormycoses and aspergillosis. If feasible, surgical removal of infected tissues and administration of antimycotic agents is indicated. The prognosis is poor.

Hyalohyphomycoses. This collective term is used for mycoses caused by hyaline (melanin-free) molds. Examples of some of the genera are *Fusarium*, *Scopulariopsis*, *Paecilomyces*, *Trichoderma*, *Acremonium*, and *Scedosporium*. These fungi are also found all over the world. Pathogenesis, clinical pictures, therapy, and prognosis are the same as for the phaeohyphomycoses.

Opportunistic yeast mycoses. Other yeasts besides the most frequent genus by far, *Candida*, are also capable of causing mycoses in immunosuppressed patients. They include *Torulopsis glabrata*, *Trichosporon beigelii*, and species of the genera *Rhodotorula*, *Malassezia*, *Saccharomyces*, *Hansenula*, and others. These "new" mycoses are not endogenous, but rather exogenous infections. In

6

clinical and therapeutic terms, they are the same as candidiasis. *Malassezia furfur* occasionally causes catheter sepsis in premature neonates and persons who have to be fed lipids parenterally. Lipids encourage growth of this yeast.

Penicilliosis. This fungal infection is caused by the dimorphic fungus *Penicillium marneffei*, which probably inhabits the soil. *P. marneffei* infections are one of the most opportunistic infections most frequently seen in AIDS patients who either live in Southeast Asia or have stayed in that area for a while. The infection foci are located primarily in the lungs, from where dissemination to other organs can take place. The therapeutic of choice in the acute phase is amphotericin B, this treatment must be followed by long-term prophylactic azoles (itraconazole) to prevent remission.

Pneumocystis carinii (Pneumocystosis)

■ *Pneumocystis carinii* is a single-celled, eukaryotic microorganism that was originally classified as a protozoan, but is now considered a fungus. This pathogen can cause pneumonia in persons with defective cellular immune systems, in particular those showing AIDS. Extrapulmonary manifestations are also recorded in a small number of cases. Laboratory diagnostic methods include direct detection of the microbes under the microscope, by means of direct immunofluorescence or PCR. Appropriate anti-infective agents for therapy include cotrimoxazole, pentamidine, or a combination of the two. ■

Pneumocystis carinii is a single-celled, eukaryotic microorganism that was, until recently, classified with the protozoans. Molecular DNA analysis has revealed that it resembles fungi more than it does protozoans, although some of the characteristic properties of fungi, such as membrane ergosterol, are missing in *Pneumocystis carinii*. This microbe occurs in the lungs of many mammalian species including humans without causing disease in the carriers. Clinically manifest infections emerge in the presence of severe underlying defects in cellular immunity, as in AIDS.

Morphology and developmental cycle. Three developmental stages are known for *P. carinii*. The **trophozoites** are elliptical cells with a diameter of 1.5–5 µm. Presumably, the trophic form reproduces by means of binary transverse fission, i.e., asexually. Sexual reproduction does not begin until two haploid trophozoites fuse to make one diploid **sporozoite** (or precyst), which are considered to be an intermediate stage in sexual reproduction. After further nuclear divisions, the sporozoites possess eight nuclei at the end of their development. The nuclei then compartmentalize to form eight spores with a diameter of 1–2 µm each, resulting in the third stage of development, the **cyst**. The cysts then release the spores, which in turn develop into trophozoites.

Culture. *P. carinii* cannot be grown in nutrient mediums. It can go through a maximum of 10 developmental cycles in cell cultures. Sufficient propagation is only possible in experimental animals, e.g., rats. This makes it difficult to study the pathogen's biology and the pathogenic process and explains why all aspects of these infections have not yet been clarified.

Pathogenesis and clinical pictures. Humans show considerable resistance to *P. carinii* infections, which explains why about two-thirds of the populace are either carriers or have a history of contact with the organism. Disease only becomes manifest in the presence of defects in the cellular immune system. Of primary concern among the clinical manifestations is the **interstitial pneumonia**. Profuse proliferation of the pathogen in the alveoli damages the alveolar epithelium. The pathogens then penetrate into the interstitium, where they cause the pneumonia. Starting from the primary infection foci, the fungi spread to other organs in 1–2% of cases, causing extrapulmonary *P. carinii* infections (of the middle ear, eye, CNS, liver, pancreas, etc.).

Diagnosis. Suitable types of diagnostic material include pulmonary biopsies or bronchoalveolar lavage (BAL) specimens from the affected lung segments. Grocott silver staining can be used to reveal cysts and Giemsa staining shows up trophozoites and sporozoites. Direct immunofluorescence, with labeled monoclonal antibodies to a surface antigen of the cysts, facilitates detection

6

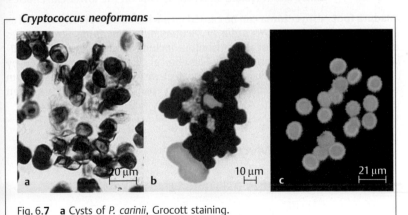

Cryptococcus neoformans

Fig. 6.7 **a** Cysts of *P. carinii*, Grocott staining.
b Yeast fungi, Grocott staining (for differential diagnosis).
c Cysts of *P. carinii*, detection with direct immunofluorescence and monoclonal antibodies.

(see Fig. 6.**7c**). Amplification of specific DNA sequences using the PCR has recently come to the fore as a useful molecular detection method.

Therapy. Acute pneumocystosis is treated with cotrimoxazole (oral or parenteral) or pentamidine (parenteral) or a combination of both of these anti-infective agents. Pentamidine can also be applied in aerosol form to reduce the side effects.

Subcutaneous Mycoses

Fungi that cause classic subcutaneous mycoses grow in the soil and on dying plants. They penetrate through skin injuries into the subcutaneous connective tissue, where they cause local, chronic, granulomatous infections. These infections are seen mainly in the tropics and subtropics.

Sporotrichosis is caused by *Sporothrix schenckii*, a dimorphic fungus that grows as yeast cells in host tissues. Sporotrichosis is characterized by an ulcerous primary lesion, usually on an extremity, and multiple nodules and abscesses along the lymphatic vessels.

Chromomycosis (also chromoblastomycosis) can be caused by a number of species of black molds. The nomenclature of these pathogens is not firmly established. Weeks or months after the spores penetrate into a host, wartlike, ulcerating, granulomatous lesions develop, usually on the lower extremities.

Madura foot or **mycetoma** can be caused by a wide variety of fungi as well as by filamentous bacteria (*Nocardia* sp., *Actinomadura madurae*, *Streptomyces somaliensis*). Potential fungal contributors include *Madurella* sp., *Pseudoallescheria boydii*, and *Aspergillus* sp. The clinical picture is characterized by subcutaneous abscesses, usually on the feet or hands. The abscesses can spread into the musculature and even into the bones. Fistulae are often formed.

Cutaneous Mycoses

Dermatophytes (Dermatomycoses or Dermatophytoses)

Dermatophytes are fungi that infect tissues containing plenty of keratin (skin, hair, nails).

Classification. Dermatophytes are classified in three genera: **Trichophyton** (with the important species *T. mentagrophytes, T. rubrum, T. schoenleinii, T. tonsurans*); **Microsporum** (*M. audouinii, M. canis, M. gypseum*); and **Epidermophyton** (*E. floccosum*). Some dermatophyte species are anthropophilic, others zoophilic. The natural habitat of the geophilic species *M. gypseum* is the soil.

Morphology and culture. The dermatophytes are filamentous fungi. They grow readily on fungal nutrient mediums at 25–30 °C. After 5–14 days, cultures with a woolly appearance, in different colors, usually develop (Fig. 6.**8**).

Pathogenesis and clinical pictures. Dermatomycoses are infections that are transmitted directly by human contact, animal-human contact or indirectly on inanimate objects (clothes, carpets, moisture, and dust in showers, swimming pools, wardrobes, gyms). The localization of the primary foci corresponds to the contact site. Thus feet, uncovered skin (hair, head, facial skin) are affected most frequently. Different species can cause the same clinical picture. Frequent dermatomycoses include:

— **Dermatophytes** —

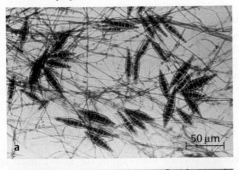

Fig. 6.**8** **a** *Microsporum canis*. Lactophenol blue preparation: large, fusiform macroconidia.
b *Trichophyton mentagrophytes*. Lactophenol blue preparation: thin-walled, cylindrical macroconidia; numerous microconidia, often in clumps; spiral hyphae.

50 μm

50 μm

6

■ **Tinea corporis (ringworm):** *Microsporum canis* and *Trichophyton mentagrophytes*. Affects hairless skin.

■ **Tinea pedis (athlete's foot):** *T. rubrum, T. mentagrophytes,* and *Epidermophyton floccosum*. Affects mainly the lower legs.

■ **Tinea capitis:** *T. tonsurans* and *M. canis*. Affects scalp hair.

■ **Tinea barbae:** *T. rubrum* and *T. mentagrophytes*. Beard ringworm.

■ **Tinea unguium:** *T. rubrum, T. mentagrophytes,* and *E. floccosum*.

■ **Onychomycosis (nail mycosis):** Various dermatophytes and Candida spp.

Diagnosis. Material suitable for diagnostic analysis include skin and nail scrapings and infected hair. The fungi are observed under the microscope in a KOH preparation. Identification is based on the morphology of the hyphae as well as on the macroconidia and microconidia in the fungal cultures.

Therapy. Dermatomycoses can be treated with locally applied antimycotic agents. In cases of massive infections of the hair, and above all of the nails, the oral allylamine terbinafine or azoles can be used. Griseofulvin is rarely used today.

Epidemiology and prevention. Dermatophytes occur naturally all over the world. The geophilic dermatophyte, *M. gypseum,* can cause infections in persons in constant, intensive contact with the soil (e.g., gardeners). Prophylactic measures for all dermatomycoses consist in avoiding direct contact with the pathogen. Regular disinfection of showers and wardrobes can contribute to prevention of athlete's foot, a very frequent infection.

Other Cutaneous Mycoses

Pityriasis (or **tinea**) **versicolor** is a surface infection of the skin caused by *Malassezia furfur.* This infection is observed mainly in the tropics but is known all over the world. It causes hypopigmentations. *M. furfur* is dependent for its metabolic needs on a source of long-chain fatty acids. This fungus is actually a component of the skin's normal flora. The pathogenesis of the infections has not yet been clarified.

Tinea nigra, which occurs mainly in the tropics, is caused by *Exophiala werneckii.* Infection results in brown to black, maculous efflorescences on the skin.

White and black piedras is an infection of the hair caused by *Trichosporon beigelii* or *Piedraia hortae.*

IV
Virology

Herpes simplex Virus

7   General Virology

K. A. Bienz

Definition

■ Viruses are complexes consisting of protein and an RNA or DNA genome. They lack both cellular structure and independent metabolic processes. They replicate solely by exploiting living cells based on the information in the viral genome.   ■

Viruses are **autonomous infectious particles** that differ widely from other microorganisms in a number of characteristics: they have no cellular structure, consisting only of proteins and nucleic acid (DNA or RNA). They have no metabolic systems of their own, but rather depend on the synthetic mechanism of a living host cell, whereby the viruses exploit normal cellular metabolism by delivering their own genetic information, i.e., nucleic acid, into the host cell. The host cell accepts the nucleic acid and proceeds to produce the

Table 7.1   Essential Characteristics of Viruses

Size	25 nm (picornavirus) to 250 × 350 nm (smallpox virus). Resolving power of a light microscope: 300 nm, bacteria: 500–5000 nm. The comparative sizes are illustrated in Fig. 7.**1**.
Genome	DNA or RNA. Double-stranded or single-stranded nucleic acid, depending on the species.
Structure	Viruses are complexes comprising virus-coded protein and nucleic acid; some viral species carry cell-coded components (membranes, tRNA).
Reproduction	Only in living cells. The virus supplies the information in the form of nucleic acids and in some cases a few enzymes; the cell provides the remaining enzymes, the protein synthesizing apparatus, the chemical building blocks, the energy, and the structural framework for the synthetic steps.
Antibiotics	Viruses are unaffected by antibiotics, but can be inhibited by interferon and certain chemotherapeutic agents.

—— **Comparative Sizes of Viruses and Bacteria** ——

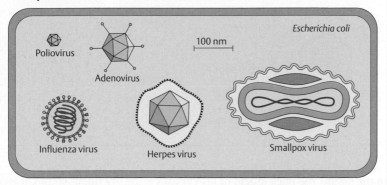

Fig. 7.**1**   Different virus species are shown here to scale inside an *E. coli* bacterium.

components of new viruses in accordance with the genetic information it contains. One thus might call viruses "vagabond genes."

Viruses infect bacteria (so-called bacteriophages), plants, animals, and humans. The following pages cover mainly the human pathogen viruses (see Fig. 7.**1**). Table 7.**1** lists the essential characteristics of viruses.

7

Morphology and Structure

■ A mature virus particle is also known as a **virion**. It consists of either two or three basic components:

— A **genome** of DNA or RNA, double-stranded or single-stranded, linear or circular, and in some cases segmented. A single-stranded nucleic acid can have plus or minus polarity.

— The **capsid**, virus-coded proteins enclosing the nucleic acid of the virus and determining its antigenicity; the capsid can have a cubic (rotational), helical or complex symmetry and is made up of subunits called capsomers.

— In some cases an **envelope** (Fig. 7.**2**) that surrounds the capsid and is always derived from cellular membranes.   ■

Genome. The viral genome is either DNA or RNA, and viruses are hence categorized as DNA or RNA viruses (see also p. 380). The nucleic acid of DNA viruses is usually double-stranded (ds) and linear or circular depending

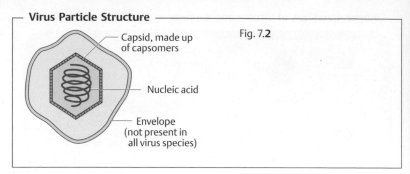

Virus Particle Structure

Fig. 7.**2**

Capsid, made up of capsomers

Nucleic acid

Envelope (not present in all virus species)

on the family; the nucleic acid of RNA viruses is usually single-stranded (ss), with the exception of the reoviruses, and is also segmented in a number of virus families. Viruses with ssRNA are divided into two groups: if the RNA of the genome has the same polarity as the viral mRNA and can thus function directly as messenger RNA it is called a plus-strand (or positive-strand) or "sense" RNA strand and these viruses are *sense* or *plus-strand* viruses. If the genome RNA has the polarity opposite to that of the mRNA, and therefore cannot be translated into proteins until it has first been transcribed into a complementary strand, it is called a minus-strand (or negative-strand) or "antisense" RNA strand and the viruses are *antisense* or *minus-strand* viruses.

Capsid. The capsid (Fig. 7.**2**) is the "shell" of virus-coded protein that encloses the nucleic acid and is more or less closely associated with it. The combination of these two components is often termed the nucleocapsid, especially if they are closely associated as in the myxoviruses. The capsid is made up of subunits, the capsomers, the number of which varies but is specific and constant for each viral species. These are spherical or cylindrical structures composed of several polypeptides. The capsid protects the nucleic acid from degradation. In all except enveloped viruses, it is responsible for the attachment of the viruses to the host cell ("adsorption," see the chapter on replication, p. 384) and determines specific viral antigenicity.

Envelope. The envelope (Fig. 7.**2**), which surrounds the capsid in several virus families, is always dependent on cellular membranes (nuclear or cell membrane, less frequently endoplasmic reticulum). Both cell-coded and viral proteins are integrated in the membrane when these elements are transformed into the envelope, frequently in the form of "spikes" (or peplomers, Fig. 7.**3**). Enveloped viruses do not adsorb to the host cell with the capsid, but rather with their envelope. Removing it with organic solvents or detergents reduces the infectivity of the viruses ("ether sensitivity").

Other Components of Viral Particles

Various **enzymes**. Viruses require a number of different enzymes depending on genome type and mode of infection. In several virus species enzymes are a component of the virus particle, for example the neuraminidase required for invasion and release of myxoviruses. Other examples include nucleic acid polymerases such as the RNA-dependent RNA polymerases in antisense viruses, the DNA polymerases in smallpox viruses and the RNA-dependent DNA polymerase ("reverse transcriptase") in hepatitis B viruses and retroviruses (see p. 385f.).

Hemagglutinin. Some viruses (above all myxoviruses and paramyxoviruses) are capable of agglutinating various different human or animal erythrocytes. These viruses bear a certain surface protein (hemagglutinin) in their envelope that enables them to do this. The hemagglutination phenomenon can be made use of for quantitative viral testing or—in the hemagglutination inhibition test—for virus identification and antibody identification (p. 405ff.). In biological terms, hemagglutinin plays a decisive role in adsorption and penetration of the virus into the host cell.

Structural Patterns

Cubic symmetry (rotational symmetry). Viruses with rotational symmetry are icosahedrons (polyhedrons with 20 equilateral triangular faces). The number of capsomers per virion varies from 32 to 252 and depends on the number of capsomers (two to six) making up one side of the equilateral triangle. The capsomers in a virion need not all be the same, either in their morphology, antigen make-up or biological properties. Purified icosahedral viruses can be crystallized, so that images of them can be obtained using the methods of radiocrystallography. A number of virus images have been obtained with this method at a resolution of 2 A.

Helical symmetry. Helical symmetry is present when one axis of a capsid is longer than the other. The nucleic acid and capsid protein are closely associated in the ribonucleoprotein (RNP), in which the protein is tightly arrayed around the nucleic acid strand. This RNA-protein complex is known as the nucleocapsid, which takes the form of a helix inside the viral envelope. Fig. 7.**3b** shows this in influenza virus the envelope of which has been partly removed and Fig. 7.**3a** illustrates these symmetries schematically.

Complex symmetry. Complex structural patterns are found in bacteriophages and the smallpox virus (see Fig. 7.**1**, right). T bacteriophages, for example, have an icosahedral head containing the DNA and a tubelike tail through which the DNA is injected into the host cell.

7

Viruses with Helical Symmetry

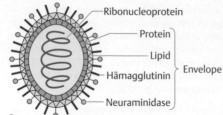

Fig. 7.**3** **a** Schematic structure of a myxovirus.
b Influenza viruses viewed with an electron microscope: The ribonucleoprotein spiral (nucleocapsid, NC) is visible inside the partially removed envelope (E). S = spikes.

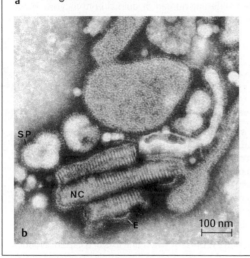

Classification

■ The taxonomic system used for viruses is artificial (i.e., it does not reflect virus evolution) and is based on the following morphological and biochemical criteria:

— **Genome:** DNA or RNA genome (important basic differentiation of virus types!) as well as configuration of nucleic acid structure: single-stranded (ss) or double-stranded (ds); RNA viruses are further subclassified according to plus and minus polarity (p. 383f.).

— **Capsid symmetry:** cubic, helical, or complex symmetry.

— Presence or absence of an **envelope**.

— **Diameter** of the virion, or of the nucleocapsid with helical symmetry.

The origins and evolution of the viruses are still largely in the dark. In contrast to the taxonomic systems used to classify the higher forms of life, we are therefore unable to classify viruses in such evolutionary systems. An international nomenclature committee groups viruses according to various criteria and designates these groups, analogously to the higher forms, as families, genera, and species. Despite this element of "artificiality" in the system now in use, the groups appear to make biological sense and to establish order in the enormous variety of known viruses (see Table 7.**2**, based on publications by the International Committee on Taxonomy of Viruses). ■

Replication

■ The steps in viral replication are as follows:
— **Adsorption** of the virus to specific receptors on the cell surface.
— **Penetration** by the virus and intracellular release of nucleic acid.
— **Proliferation** of the viral components: virus-coded synthesis of capsid and noncapsid proteins, replication of nucleic acid by viral and cellular enzymes.
— **Assembly** of replicated nucleic acid and new capsid protein.
— **Release** of virus progeny from the cell. ■

7

As shown on p. 376, viruses replicate only in living host cells. The detailed steps involved in their replication are shown below (Fig. 7.**4**). The reactions of the infected cell (cytopathology, tumor transformation, etc.) are described on p. 392.

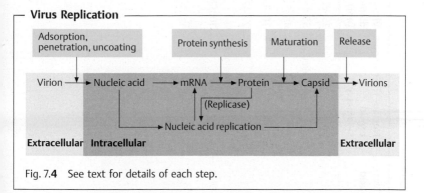

Virus Replication

Fig. 7.**4**   See text for details of each step.

Table 7.2 Taxonomy of the Viruses

Nucleic acid	Nucleo-capsid symmetry	Envelope	Virus diameter (nm)	ss/ds [1] (polarity)	Family	Genus	Exemplary important species
DNA	cubic	naked	19–25	ss	Parvoviridae	Erythrovirus	Parvovirus B19
			55	ds	Papillomaviridae	Papillomavirus	Human papilloma virus (HPV)
			45	ds	Polyomaviridae	Polyomavirus	BK virus, JC virus
			70–90	ds	Adenoviridae	Mastadenovirus	Adenoviruses
		envelope	27/42[2]	ss	Hepadnaviridae	Ortho-hepadnavirus	Hepatitis B virus
			100/200[2]	ds	Herpesviridae	Simplexvirus	Herpes simplex virus
						Varicellovirus	Varicella zoster virus
						Cytomegalovirus	Cytomegalovirus
						Roseolovirus	Human herpesvirus 6
						Lymphocrypto-virus	Epstein-Barr virus
	complex – envelope		230 × 350	ds	Poxviridae	Orthopox	Variola virus, vaccinia virus
						Parapox	Orf virus

RNA viruses classification

Symmetry	Envelope[2]	Size (nm)	Nucleic acid[1]	Family	Genus	Examples
cubic	naked	24–30	ss(+)	Picornaviridae	Enterovirus	Poliovirus, echovirus, coxsackie viruses
					Hepatovirus	Hepatitis A virus
					Rhinovirus	Rhinovirus 1–117
					Parechovirus	Parechoviruses
		30	ss(+)	Astroviridae	Astrovirus	Astroviruses
		33	ss(+)	Caliciviridae	Calicivirus	Hepatitis E virus
		60–80	ds segm.	Reoviridae	Coltivirus	Colorado tick fever virus
					Orthoreovirus	Reovirus 1–3
					Rotavirus	Rotaviruses
	envelope	60–70	ss(+)	Togaviridae	Alphavirus	Sindbis virus
					Rubivirus	Rubella virus
		40	ss(+)	Flaviviridae	Flavivirus	Yellow fever virus
					Hepacivirus	Hepatitis C virus
helical	envelope	80–220	ss(+)	Coronaviridae	Coronavirus	SARS virus
		80–120	ss segm.(–)	Orthomyxoviridae	Influenzavirus	Influenza A, B, C virus
		150–300	ss(–)	Paramyxoviridae	Pneumovirus	Human respiratory syncytial virus
					Paramyxovirus	Human parainfluenza virus 1 and 3
					Rubulavirus	Mumps virus
					Morbillivirus	Measles virus
		60 × 180	ss(–)	Rhabdoviridae	Lyssavirus	Rabies virus
		80 × filament.	ss(–)	Filoviridae	Filovirus	Marburg virus, Ebola virus
		100	ss segm. (–)	Bunyaviridae	Bunyavirus	Bunyamwera virus
					Nairovirus	Crimean-Congo hemorrhagic fever virus
					Phlebovirus	Phlebotomus fever virus
					Hantavirus	Hantaan virus
?	envelope	50–300	ss segm. (+/–)	Arenaviridae	Arenavirus	LCMV, Lassa virus
		100	ss segm. (+)	Retroviridae	HTLV-retrovirus	HTLV I and II
					Spumavirus	Spumaviruses
					Lentivirus	HIV 1 and 2

1 = Configuration of nucleic acid: ss = single-stranded, ds = double-stranded; 2 = without/with envelope

Adsorption. Virus particles can only infect cells possessing surface "receptors" specific to the particular virus species. When a virus encounters such a cell, it adsorbs to it either with the capsid or, in enveloped viruses, by means of envelope proteins. It is therefore the receptors on a cell that determine whether it can be infected by a certain virus.

Receptors

Some aspects of the nature of the receptors are known. These are molecules that play important roles in the life of the cell or intercellular communication, e.g., molecules of the immunoglobulin superfamily (CD4: receptor for HIV; ICAM-1: receptor for rhinoviruses), the complement (C3) receptor that is also the receptor for the Epstein-Barr virus, or glycoproteins the cellular functions of which are not yet known.

Practical consequences arise from this growing knowledge about the receptors: on the one hand, it aids in the development of antiviral therapeutics designed to inhibit the adsorption of the viruses to their target cells. On the other hand, the genetic information that codes for certain receptors can be implanted into cells or experimental animals, rendering them susceptible to viruses to which they would normally be resistant. An example of this application is the use in experimental studies of transgenic mice rendered susceptible to polioviruses instead of primates (e.g., on vaccine testing).

7

Penetration and uncoating. Viruses adsorbed to the cell surface receptors then penetrate into the cell by means of pinocytosis (a process also known as viropexis). In enveloped viruses, the envelope may also fuse with the cell membrane, releasing the virus into the cytoplasm. Adsorption of such an enveloped virus to two cells at the same time may result in cell fusion. The next step, known as uncoating, involves the release of the nucleic acid from the capsid and is apparently (except in the smallpox virus) activated by cellular enzymes, possibly with a contribution from cell membranes as well. The exact mechanism, which would have to include preservation of the nucleic acid in toto, is not known for all viruses.

Replication of the nucleic acid. Different processes are observed corresponding to the types and configurations of the viral genome (Fig. 7.**5**).

— **DNA viruses:** the replication of viral DNA takes place in the cell nucleus (exception: poxviruses). Some viruses (e.g., herpesviruses) possess replicases of their own. The smaller DNA viruses (e.g., polyomaviruses), which do not carry information for their own DNA polymerase, code for polypeptides that modify the cellular polymerases in such a way that mainly viral DNA sequences are replicated.

Hepadnaviruses: the genome consists of an ssDNA antisense strand and a short sense strand (Fig. 7.**5e**). The infected cell transcribes an RNA sense strand ("template strand") from the antisense strand. This template strand is integrated in virus capsids together with an RT DNA polymerase. The polymerase synthesizes a complementary antisense DNA and, to "seal off" the ends of the genome, a short sense DNA from the template strand.

- **RNA viruses:** since eukaryotic cells possess no enzymes for RNA replication, the virus must supply the RNA-dependent RNA polymerase(s) ("replicase"). These enzymes are thus in any case virus-coded proteins, and in some cases are actually components of the virus particle.

Single-stranded RNA: in *sense-strand viruses*, the RNA functions as mRNA "as is," meaning the information can be read off, and the replicase synthesized immediately. *Antisense-strand viruses* must first transcribe their genome into a complementary strand that can then act as mRNA. In this case, the polymerase for the first transcription is contained in the mature virion and delivered into the cell. In ssRNA viruses, whether sense or antisense strands, complementary strands of the genome are produced first (Fig. 7.**5a, b**), then transcribed into daughter strands. They therefore once again show the same polarity as the viral genome and are used in assembly of the new viral progeny.

Double-stranded RNA: a translatable sense-strand RNA is produced from the genome, which consists of several dsRNA segments (segmented genome). This strand functions, at first, as mRNA and later as a matrix for synthesis of antisense-strand RNA (Fig. 7.**5c**). Here as well, an RNA-dependent RNA polymerase is part of the virus particle.

Retroviruses also possess a sense-oriented RNA genome, although its replication differs from that of other RNA viruses. The genome consists of two single-stranded RNA segments with sense polarity and is transcribed by an enzyme in the virion (reverse transcriptase [RT]) into complementary DNA. The DNA is complemented to make dsDNA and integrated in the cell genome. Transcription into sense-strand RNA is the basis for both viral mRNA and the genomic RNA in the viral progeny (Fig. 7.**5d**).

Replication of the Viral Genome

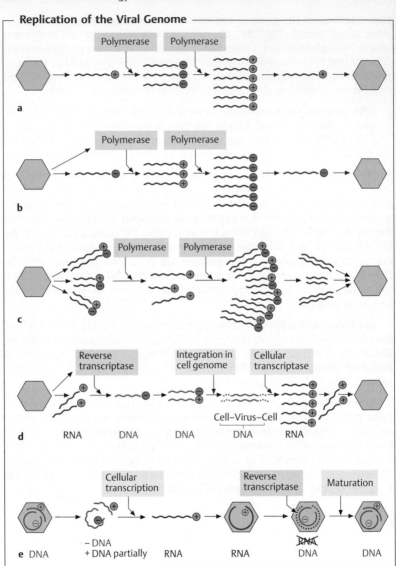

a — RNA, DNA, DNA, Cell–Virus–Cell, DNA, RNA

Viral Protein Synthesis

Production of viral mRNA. In a DNA virus infection, cellular polymerases transcribe mRNA in the nucleus of the host cell from one or both DNA strands, whereby the RNA is processed (splicing, polyadenylation, etc.) as with cellular mRNA. An exception to this procedure is the poxviruses, which use their own enzymes to replicate in the cytoplasm.

In *viruses with antisense-strand ssRNA and dsRNA* the transcription of the genomic RNA into mRNA is carried out by the viral polymerases, usually without further processing of the transcript.

In *sense-strand ssRNA viruses*, the genome can function directly as mRNA.

Certain viruses (arenaviruses, see p. 462f.) are classified as "*ambisense viruses.*" Part of their genome codes in antisense (–), another part in sense (+) polarity. Proteins are translated separately from subgenomic RNA and the antisense-coded proteins are not translated until the antisense strand has been translated into a sense strand.

Viral mRNA is produced for the **translation** process, based on both the genome of the invading virus and the nucleic acid already replicated.

◀ Fig. 7.**5** Schematic diagram of nucleic acid replication.

a Single-stranded RNA viruses with sense-strand genome: the virus-coded RNA polymerase transcribes the viral genome (+) into complementary strands (–) and these into new genomic RNA (+). The latter is then integrated in the viral progeny.

b Single-stranded RNA viruses with antisense-strand genome: the RNA polymerase in the virion transcribes the viral genome (–) into complementary strands (+), which a virus-coded polymerase then transcribes into new genomic RNA (–).

c Double-stranded RNA viruses: while still in the partially decapsidated virus particle, the virus-coded polymerase transcribes complementary strands (+) from the antisense strand of the (segmented) double-stranded viral genome; these complementary strands are complemented to make the new double-stranded viral genome.

d RNA replication in retroviruses: the reverse transcriptase (RT) carried by the virion transcribes the viral genome (two sense-RNA strands) into complementary DNA (–), which is complemented to produce dsDNA and integrated in the cell genome. The viral RNA is first degraded. Cellular enzymes produce new genomic RNA (+).

e DNA replication in hepadnaviruses: by means of cellular transcription, a sense-strand RNA is made from the viral genome (antisense DNA, partially double-stranded) and integrated in the new virion, where a virus-coded RT produces new genomic DNA (–) and destroys the RNA.

7

The actual protein synthesis procedure is implemented, coded by the viral mRNA, with the help of cellular components such as tRNA, ribosomes, initiation factors, etc. Two functionally different protein types occur in viruses:

■ The "noncapsid viral proteins" (NCVP) that do not contribute to capsid assembly. These proteins frequently possess enzymatic properties (polymerases, proteases) and must therefore be produced early on in the replication cycle.

■ The capsid proteins, also known as viral proteins (VP) or structural proteins, appear later in the replication process.

Protein Synthesis Control

Segmented genomes. A separate nucleic acid segment is present for each protein (example: reoviruses).

mRNA splicing. The correct mRNA is cut out of the primary transcript (as in the cell the exon is cut out of the hnRNA) (examples: adenoviruses, retroviruses, etc.).

"Early" and "late" translation. The different mRNA molecules required for assembly of so-called early and late proteins are produced at different times in the infection cycle, possibly from different strands of viral DNA (examples, papovaviruses, herpesviruses).

Posttranslational control. This process involves proteolytic cutting of the primary translation product into functional subunits. Viral proteases that recognize specific amino acid sequences are responsible for this, e.g., the two poliovirus proteases cut between glutamine and glycine or tyrosine and glycine. Such proteases, some of which have been documented in radiocrystallographic images, are potential targets for antiviral chemotherapeutics (example: HIV).

Viral maturation (morphogenesis). In this step, the viral capsid proteins and genomes (present in multiple copies after the replication process) are assembled into new, infectious virus particles. In some viral species these particles are also covered by an envelope (p. 378f.)

Release. The release of viral progeny in some cases correlates closely with viral maturation, whereby envelopes or components of them are acquired when the particles "bud off" of the cytoplasmic membrane and are expelled from the cell (Fig. 7.**6**). In nonenveloped viruses, release of viral progeny is realized either by means of lysis of the infected cell or more or less continuous exocytosis of the viral particles.

Release of Retroviruses from an Infected Cell

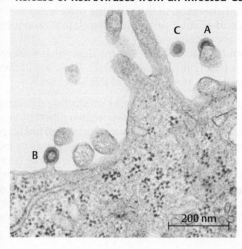

Fig. 7.**6** Electron microscope image of release of viral progeny. The process takes place in the order, A, B, C.

Genetics

7

■ Just as in higher life forms, viral genetic material is subject to change by mutation. Lack of a corrective replication "proofreading" mechanism results in a very high incidence of spontaneous mutations in RNA viruses, in turn greatly increasing the genotypic variability within each species ("viral quasispecies"). Furthermore, a potential for recombination of genetic material is also inherent in the replication process, not only material from different viruses but also from host cell and virus. This factor plays a major role in viral tumor induction and genetic engineering. Functional modifications arising from interactions between different viral species in mixed infections—e.g., phenotype mixing, interference, and complementation—have nothing to do with genetic changes. ■

Lasting genetic changes in viruses are caused, as in the higher life forms, either by mutation or recombination of genetic material. Temporary nongenetic interactions between viruses in some cases may mimic genetic changes.

Mutation. Mutations are changes in the base sequence of a nucleic acid, resulting in a more or less radical alteration of the resulting protein. So-called "silent mutations" (in the second or third nucleotide of a codon) do not influence the amino acid sequence of the protein.

Medically important are mutants with weakened virulence that have retained their antigenicity and replication capabilities intact. These are known as "attenuated" viruses. They are the raw material of live vaccines.

Recombination. The viral replication process includes production of a large number of copies of the viral nucleic acid. In cases where two different viral strains are replicating in the same cell, there is a chance that strand breakage and reunion will lead to new combinations of nucleic acid segments or exchanges of genome segments (influenza), so that the genetic material is redistributed among the viral strains (recombination). New genetic properties will therefore be conferred upon some of the resulting viral progeny, some of which will also show stable heritability. Genetic material can also be exchanged between virus and host cell by the same mechanism or by insertion of all, or part, of the viral genome into the cell genome.

Viruses as Vectors

The natural processes of gene transfer between viruses and their host cells described above can be exploited to give certain cells new characteristics by using the viruses as vectors. If the vector DNA carrying the desired additional gene integrates stably in the host cell genome (e.g., retroviruses, adenoviruses, or the adenoassociated virus), the host cell is permanently changed. This can become the basis for "gene therapy" of certain functional disorders such as cystic fibrosis or parkinsonism. Nonintegrating vectors (alphaviruses, e.g., the Sindbis virus, mengovirus, or vaccinia virus) result in temporary expression of a certain protein, which can be used, for instance, to immunize a host organism. By this means, wild foxes can be vaccinated against rabies using a vaccinia virus that expresses a rabies virus glycoprotein. Such experimental work must of course always comply with national laws on the release of genetically engineered microorganisms. It must also be mentioned here that only somatic gene therapy can be considered for use in humans. Human germline therapy using the methods of genetic engineering is generally rejected as unethical.

Nongenetic Interactions

In mixed infections by two (or more) viruses, various viral components can be exchanged or they may complement (or interfere with) each other's functions (phenotype mixing, complementation or interference). Such processes do not result in stable heritability of new characteristics.

In **phenotypic mixing**, the genome of virus A is integrated in the capsid of virus B, or a capsid made up of components from two (closely related) virus types is assembled and the genome of one of the "parents" is integrated in it. However, the progeny of such a "mixed" virus of course shows the genotype.

In phenotypic **interference**, the primary infecting virus (usually avirulent) may inhibit the replication of a second virus, or the inhibition may be mutual. The interference mechanism may be due to interferon production (p. 400) or to a metabolic change in the host cell.

In **complementation**, infecting viral species have genetic defects that render replication impossible. The "partner" virus compensates for the defect, supplying the missing substances or functions in a so-called helper effect. In this way, a defective and nondefective virus, or two defective viruses, can complement each other. Example: murine sarcoma viruses for which leukemia virus helpers deliver capsid proteins or the hepatitis D virus, which replicates on its own but must be supplied with capsid material by the hepatitis B virus (see Chapter 8, p. 429f.).

"Quasispecies." When viral RNA replicates, there is no "proofreading" mechanism to check for copying errors as in DNA replication. The result is that the rate of mutations in RNA viruses is about 10^4, i.e., every copy of a viral RNA comprising 10 000 nucleotides will include on average one mutation. The consequence of this is that, given the high rate of viral replication, all of the possible viable mutants of a viral species will occur and exist together in an inhomogeneous population known as quasispecies. The selective pressure (e.g., host immune system efficiency) will act to select the "fittest" viruses at any given time. This explains the high level of variability seen in HIV as well as the phenomenon that a single passage of the attenuated polio vaccine virus through a human vaccine recipient produces neurovirulent revertants.

Occurrence of "new" viral species. It appears to be the exception rather than the rule that a harmless or solely zoopathic virus mutates to become an aggressive human pathogen. In far more cases, changed environmental conditions are responsible for new forms of a disease, since most "new" viruses are actually "old" viruses that had reached an ecological balance with their hosts and then entered new transmission cycles as a result of urbanization, migration, travel, and human incursion into isolated biotopes (examples include the Ebola, Rift Valley fever, West Nile, pulmonary Hanta, and bat rabies viruses).

Host-Cell Reactions

■ Possible consequences of viral infection for the host cell:
— **Cytocidal infection (necrosis):** viral replication results directly in cell destruction (cytopathology, so-called "cytopathic effect" in cell cultures).
— **Apoptosis:** the virus initiates a cascade of cellular events leading to cell death ("suicide"), in most cases interrupting the viral replication cycle.
— **Noncytocidal infection:** viral replication per se does not destroy the host cell, although it may be destroyed by secondary immunological reactions.
— **Latent infection:** the viral genome is inside the cell, resulting in neither viral replication nor cell destruction.
— **Tumor transformation:** the viral infection transforms the host cell into a cancer cell, whereby viral replication may or may not take place depending on the virus and/or cell type involved. ■

Cell Destruction (Cytocidal Infection, Necrosis)

Cell death occurs eventually after initial infection with many viral species. This cytopathological cell destruction usually involves production of viral progeny. Virus production coupled with cell destruction is termed the "lytic viral life cycle." Cell destruction, whether necrotic or apoptotic (see below) is the reason (along with immunological phenomena) for the disease manifested in the macroorganism (see Pathogenesis, p. 396ff.).

Structural changes leading to necrosis: morphological changes characteristic of a given infecting virus can often be observed in the infected cell. The effects seen in virally infected cell cultures are well-known and are designated by the term "cytopathic effect" (CPE). These effects can also be exploited for diagnostic purposes (p. 405). They include rounding off and detachment of cells from adjacent cells or the substrate, formation of multinuclear giant cells, cytoplasmic vacuoles, and inclusion bodies. The latter are structures made up of viral and/or cellular material that form during the viral replication cycle, e.g., viral crystals in the nucleus (adenoviruses) or collections of virions and viral material in the cytoplasm (smallpox viruses). Although these structural changes in the host cell do contribute to necrotic cytopathy, their primary purpose is to support specific steps in viral synthesis. For example, RNA synthesis and viral assembly in picornavirus infections requires specific, new, virus-induced membrane structures and vesicles that subsequently manifest their secondary effect by causing a CPE and eventual cell death.

Shutoff Phenomena

Some viruses are able to block, more or less completely, steps in cellular macromolecule synthesis not useful to them. Herpesviruses, for example, which possess DNA polymerase of their own, block cellular DNA synthesis. DNA replication in adenoviruses, by contrast, is directly coupled to that of the cell. Such shutoff phenomena apparently contribute to rapid and efficient viral replication by eliminating competing cellular synthetic processes. In polioviruses, which inhibit both transcription and translation in the host cell, the shutoff processes are induced by viral proteins that interfere with the relevant regulatory mechanisms in order to inhibit transcription and to inactivate initiation factor eIF4GII, which is not required for translation of *Enterovirus* mRNA, in order to inhibit translation. These shutoff phenomena of course also have a pathogenic effect since they inhibit cellular metabolism, but not in such a way as to necessarily kill the host cell.

Apoptosis. Cells possess natural mechanisms that initiate their self-destruction (apoptosis) by means of predetermined cytoplasmic and nuclear changes. Infections with some viruses may lead to apoptosis. In rapidly replicating viruses, the viral replication process must be decelerated to allow the slow, energy-dependent process of apoptosis to run its course before the cell is destroyed by virus-induced necrosis. The body rapidly eliminates apoptotic cells before an inflammatory reaction can develop, which is apparently why virus-induced apoptosis used to be overlooked so often. Apoptosis can thus be considered a defense mechanism, although certain viruses are able to inhibit it.

Virus Replication without Cell Destruction (Noncytocidal Infection)

This outcome of infection is observed with certain viruses that do not cause any extensive restructuring of the host cell and are generally released by "budding" at the cell surface. This mode of replication is seen, for example, in the oncornaviruses and myxoviruses and in the chronic form of hepatitis B virus infection. However, cell destruction can follow as a secondary result of infection, however, if the immune system recognizes viral antigens on the cell surface, classifies it as "foreign" and destroys it.

Latent Infection

In this infection type, the virus (or its genome) is integrated in a cell, but no viral progenies are produced. The cell is accordingly not damaged and the macroorganism does not manifest disease. This form of infection is found, for instance, with the adenovirus group and in particular the herpesviruses, which can remain latent for long periods in the human body. Latency protects these viruses from immune system activity and thus is part of their survival strategy. However, a variety of initiating events (see Chapter 8, p. 419) can initiate a lytic cycle leading to manifest disease and dissemination of the virus. Repeated activation of a latent virus is termed recidivation (e.g., herpes labialis).

Tumor Transformation

Infections by a number of viruses do not result in eventual host cell death, but rather cause tumor transformation of the cell. This means the cell is altered in many ways, e.g., in its growth properties, morphology, and metabolism. Following an infection with DNA tumor viruses, the type of host cell infected determines whether the cell reaction will be a tumor transformation, viral replication or lytic cycle. The transformation that takes place after infection with an RNA tumor virus either involves no viral replication (nonpermissive infection) or the cell produces new viruses but remains vital (permissive infection).

Carcinogenic Retroviruses ("Oncoviruses")

Genome structure and replication of the oncoviruses. The genomes of all oncoviruses possess *gag* (group-specific antigen), *pol* (enzymatic activities: polymerase complex with reverse transcriptase, integrase, and protease), and *env* (envelope glycoproteins) genes. These coding regions are flanked by two control sequences important for regulatory functions called LTR (= long terminal repeats), Fig. 7.**7**. These sequences have a promoter/enhancer function and are responsible for both reverse transcription and insertion of the viral genome into the cell DNA. Certain oncoviruses possess a so-called "*onc* gene" instead of the *pol* region (*onc* gene = oncogene, refers to a cellular gene segment acquired by recombination, see below). These viruses also often have incomplete *gag* and/or *env* regions. Such viruses are defective and require a helper virus to replicate (complementation, see p. 391). An exception to this principle is the Rous sarcoma virus, which possesses both an *onc* gene and a complete set of viral genes and can therefore replicate itself.

Genomic Organization in Oncoviruses

a | LTR | gag | pol | env | LTR

b | LTR | (gag) | v-onc | (env) | LTR

Fig. 7.7 **a** Autonomously reproducing oncoviruses with the three replication genes *gag, pol, env*, flanked by the LTR regions.
b Defective oncoviruses contain an *onc* gene instead of the entire *pol* region and parts of the *gag* and *env* regions.

Oncogenes

Over 100 *onc* genes (so-called "oncogenes") have been found in the course of tumor virology research to date. These genes enable tumor viruses to transform their host cells into tumor cells. The various types of oncogenes are designated by abbreviations, in most cases derived from the animal species in which the virus was first isolated. Further investigation of these viral oncogenes have now shown that these genes are not primarily of viral origin, but are rather **normal, cellular genes** widespread in humans and animals and acquired by the oncoviruses in their host cells, which can be transferred to new cells (transduction). Such a cellular gene, not oncogenic per se, is called a **proto-oncogene**.

The normal function of the proto-oncogenes concerns the regulation of cell growth in the broadest sense. Their gene products are growth factors, growth factor or hormone receptors and GTP-binding or DNA-binding proteins. Proto-oncogenes are potential contributors to tumor development that have to be "**activated**" before they can actually have such effects. This can occur by way of several different mechanisms:
— Chromosomal translocation: proto-oncogenes are moved to different chromosomes and thus placed under the influence of different cellular promoters, resulting in a chronic overexpression of the corresponding protein.
— Mutation of the proto-oncogene.
— Transduction of the proto-oncogene by an oncovirus. The oncovirus promoter may induce overexpression of the proto-oncogene, resulting in a tumor.

Tumor induction by oncoviruses. Both types of carcinogenic retroviruses, i.e., those with no oncogene and intact replication genes (*gag, pol, env*, flanked by the LTR regions) and those that have become defective by taking on an oncogene, can initiate a tumor transformation. On the whole, oncoviruses play only a subordinate role in human tumor induction.

■ **Retroviruses without an oncogene:** LTR are highly effective promoters. Since the retrovirus genome is integrated in the cell genome at a random position, the LTR can also induce heightened expressivity in cellular proto-oncogenes ("promoter insertion hypothesis" or "insertion mutagenicity"), which can lead to the formation of tumors. This is a slow process (e.g., chronic leukemias) in which cocarcinogens can play an important role. The transformed cells produce new viruses.

■ **Retroviruses with an oncogene:** a viral oncogene always represents a changed state compared with the original cellular proto-oncogene (deletion, mutation). It is integrated in the cell genome together with the residual viral genome (parts) after reverse transcription, and then expressed under the influence of the LTR, in most cases overexpressed. This leads to rapid development of acute malignancies that produce no new viruses.

Overproduction of oncogene products can be compensated by gene products from antioncogenes. The loss or mutation of such a suppressor gene can therefore result in tumor formation.

DNA Tumor Viruses

Genes have also been found in DNA tumor viruses that induce a malignant transformation of the host cell. In contrast to the oncogenes in oncoviruses, these are genuine viral genes that have presumably developed independently of one another over a much longer evolutionary period. They code for viral regulator proteins, which are among the so-called early proteins. They are produced early in the viral replication cycle and assume essential functions in viral DNA replication. Their oncogenic potential derives among other things from the fact that they bind to the products of tumor suppressor genes such as *p53*, *Rb* (antioncogenes, "antitransformation proteins" see above) and can thus inhibit their functions. DNA viruses are more important inducers of human tumors than oncoviruses (example: HHV8, papovaviruses, hepatitis B viruses, Epstein-Barr viruses).

Pathogenesis

■ The term "pathogenesis" covers the factors that contribute to the origins and development of a disease. In the case of viruses, the infection is by a parenteral or mucosal route. The viruses either replicate at the portal of entry only (**local infection**) or reach their target organ hematogenously, lympogenously or by neurogenic spread (**generalized infection**). In both cases, viral replication induces degenerative damage. Its extent is determined by the extent of virus-induced cell destruction and sets the level of disease manifestation. Immunological responses can contribute to elimination of the viruses by destroying the infected cells, but the same response may also exacerbate the course of the disease.   ■

Transmission. Viruses can be transmitted horizontally (within a group of individuals (Table 7.**3**) or vertically (from mother to offspring). Vertical infection is either transovarial or by infection of the virus in utero (ascending or diaplacental). Connatal infection is the term used when offspring are born infected.

Portal of entry. The most important portals of entry for viruses are the mucosa of the respiratory and gastrointestinal tracts. Intact epidermis presents a barrier to viruses, which can, however, be overcome through microtraumata (nearly always present) or mechanical inoculation (e.g., bloodsucking arthropods).

Viral dissemination in the organism. There are two forms of infection:

■ **Local infection.** In this form of infection, the viruses spread only from cell to cell. The infection and manifest disease are thus restricted to the tissues in the immediate vicinity of the portal of entry. Example: rhinoviruses that reproduce only in the cells of the upper respiratory tract.

■ **Generalized infection.** In this type, the viruses usually replicate to some extent at the portal of entry and are then disseminated via the *lymph ducts* or *bloodstream* and reach their target organ either directly or after infecting a further organ. When the target organ is reached, viral replication and the resulting cell destruction become so widespread that clinical symptoms develop. Examples of such infection courses are seen with enteroviruses that replicate mainly in the intestinal epithelium, but cause no symptoms there.

7

Table 7.**3** Horizontal Transmission of Pathogenic Viruses

Mode of transmission	Examples
Direct transmission	
– fecal-oral (smear infection)	Enteroviruses
– aerogenic (droplet infection)	Influenza viruses
– intimate contact (mucosa)	Herpes simplex virus
Indirect transmission	
– alimentary	Hepatitis A virus
– arthropod vectors	Yellow fever virus
– parenteral	Hepatitis B virus

Clinical symptoms in these infections first arise in the target organs such as the CNS (polioviruses, echoviruses) or musculature (coxsackie viruses).

Another mode of viral dissemination in the macroorganism is neurogenic spread along the *nerve tracts*, from the portal of entry to the CNS (rabies), or in the opposite direction from the ganglions where the viruses persist in a latent state to the target organ (herpes simplex).

Organ Infections, Organotropism

Whether a given cell type can be infected by a given viral species at all depends on the presence of certain receptors on the cell surface (p. 384). This mechanism explains why organotropism is observed in viruses. However, the tropism is only apparent; it is more accurate to speak of susceptible and resistant cells (and hence organs). Another observation is that cells grown in the laboratory in cell cultures can completely change their sensitivity or resistance to certain viral species compared with their organ of origin.

Course of infection. The organ damage caused by viruses is mainly of a degenerative nature. Inflammatory reactions are secondary processes. The severity of the clinical symptoms depends primarily on the extent of virus-induced (or immunological, see below) cell damage. This means most of the viral progeny are produced prior to the occurrence of clinical symptoms, with consequences for epidemiology and antiviral therapies (p. 404). It also means that infections can go unnoticed if cell destruction is insignificant or lacking entirely. In such cases, the terms *inapparent*, silent, or subclinical infection are used, in contrast to *apparent* viral infections with clinical symptoms. Virus replication and release do take place in inapparent infections, as opposed to *latent* infections (p. 394), in which no viral particles are produced.

Immunological processes can also influence the course of viral infections, whereby the infection can be subdued or healed (p. 401ff.). On the other hand, the infection may also be exacerbated, either because immune complexes are formed with viruses or viral components (nephritis) or because the immune system recognizes and destroys virus-infected cells. This is possible if viral antigens are integrated in the cell membrane and thus expressed on the cell surface. These processes become pathologically significant in cases in which the viruses themselves cause little or no cell destruction (p. 393).

Antibody-Dependent Enhancement of Viral Infection

The disease process can also be worsened when viruses react with subneutralizing amounts or types of antibodies. The Fc fragment of the antibodies bound to the viruses can then react with the Fc receptors on specific cells. This makes it possible for cell types to be infected that are primarily resistant to the virus in question because they possess no viral receptors (but in any case Fc receptors). This process—called "antibody-dependent enhancement of viral infection" or ADE, reflecting the fact that the antibodies exacerbate the infection—has been experimentally confirmed with a number of virus types to date, including herpes virus, poxvirus, reovirus, flavivirus, rhabdovirus, coronavirus, bunyavirus, and HIV species.

Virus excretion. Excretion of newly produced viruses depends on the localization of viral replication. For example, viruses that infect the respiratory tract are excreted in expired air (droplet infection). It must be remembered that in generalized infections not only the target organ is involved in excretion, but that primary viral replication at the portal of entry also contributes to virus excretion (for example enteroviruses, which replicate primarily in the intestinal wall and are excreted in feces). Once again, since the symptoms of a viral disease result from cell destruction, production, and excretion of new virus progeny precede the onset of illness. As a rule, patients are therefore contagious before they really become ill.

7

Defense Mechanisms

■ The mechanisms available to the human organism for defense against viral infection can be classified in two groups. The **nonspecific immune defenses**, in which interferons play a very important part, come first. Besides their effects on cell growth, immune response, and immunoregulation, these substances can build up a temporary resistance to a viral infection. Interferons do not affect viruses directly, but rather induce cellular resistance mechanisms (synthesis of "antiviral proteins") that interfere with specific steps in viral replication. The **specific immune defenses** include the *humoral immune system*, consisting mainly of antibodies, and the *cellular immune system*, represented mainly by the T lymphocytes. In most cases, cellular immunity is more important than humoral immunity. The cellular system is capable of recognizing and destroying virus-infected cells on the surfaces of which viral antigens are expressed. The humoral system can eliminate only extracellular viruses. ■

Nonspecific Immune Defenses

The nonspecific immune defense mechanisms are activated immediately when pathogens penetrate the body's outer barriers. One of the most important processes in these basic defenses is phagocytosis, i.e., ingestion and destruction of pathogens. Granulocytes and natural killer cells bear most of the responsibility in these mechanisms. Changes in pH and ion balance as well as fever also play a role, for example, certain temperature-sensitive replication steps can be blocked. The most important humoral factor is the complement system. Interferons, which are described below, are also potent tools for fighting off viral infections. The other mechanisms of nonspecific immune defense are described in Chapter 2, (Principles of Immunology, p. 43ff.).

Interferons (IFN) are cell-coded proteins with a molecular weight of about 20 kDa. Three types are differentiated (leukocyte interferon = IFNα, fibroblast interferon = IFNβ, and immune interferon = IFNγ) of which the amino acid sequences are known and which, thanks to genetic engineering, can now be produced in practically unlimited amounts. Whereas the principal biological effects of interferons on both normal and malignant cells are antiviral and antimitotic, these substances also show immunomodulatory effects. Their clinical applications are designed accordingly. In keeping with the scope of this section, the following description of their antiviral activity will be restricted to the salient virological aspects (Fig. 7.8):

A number of substances can induce the production of interferon in a cell, for example double-stranded RNA, synthetic or natural polynucleotides, bacteria, various low-molecular compounds and, above all, viruses. All of these

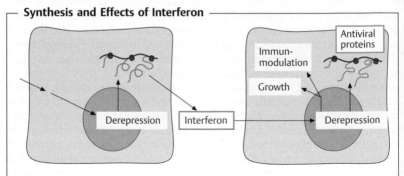

Synthesis and Effects of Interferon

Fig. 7.8 An interferon-inducing substance initiates production of interferon in the first cell. In the second cell, interferon induces, for instance, production of antiviral proteins.

substances have the same effect: they derepress the cellular *interferon* gene, inducing the cell to begin producing interferon precursors. Following glycosylation, the finished interferon is released into the surrounding area and binds to the interferon receptor of the nearest cell. The presence or lack of this receptor determines what effect the interferon will have. It also explains the more or less pronouncedly species-specific nature of the cell-to-interferon relationship. In principle, the effect of interferon is strongest within the species in which it was produced. Within the recipient or "target" cell the interferon induces the expression of the so-called *interferon-stimulated genes* (ISG) by means of a signal cascade, the result of which is to inhibit viral replication.

Interferon-Induced Proteins

(2'-5')(A)n synthetase. This cellular enzyme is first produced in an inactive form. It is then activated by double-stranded RNA, after which it can polymerize oligoadenylate out of ATP. This product then activates a cellular ribonuclease (RNase L), which inactivates viral (and cellular) mRNA.

P1/eIF-2 kinase. This cell-coded kinase is also inactive in its native state and must also be activated by dsRNA. It is then able to phosphorylate the ribosomal protein P1 and the initiation factor eIF-2, resulting in inhibition of protein synthesis initiation.

How viral and cellular protein synthesis are told apart in this kinase activation process is not quite clear. Perhaps the dsRNA needed to activate the enzyme is the key: this substance is lacking in noninfected cells and is only produced in cells infected by an (RNA) virus, so that the antiviral enzymes can only be activated in the infected cells.

Mx protein. The observation that certain mice are resistant to influenza viruses led to the discovery of the interferon-induced, 75–80 kDa Mx proteins coded for by dominant hereditary *Mx* genes. Mx proteins accumulate in mouse cell nuclei and inhibit the mRNA synthesis of influenza viruses. Mx$^-$ mice are killed by influenza. In humans, Mx proteins accumulate in the cytoplasm, but their mechanism of action is unknown.

Specific Immune Defenses

The specific, adaptive immune defenses include both the humoral system (antibody-producing B cells) and the cellular system (T helper cells and cytotoxic T lymphocytes). In general, viruses the antigens of which are expressed on the surface of the infected cells tend to induce a cellular immune response and viruses that do not change the antigenicity of their host cells tend to activate the humoral system.

Humoral immunity. Antibodies can only attack viruses outside of their host cells, which means that once an infection is established within an organ it can hardly be further influenced by antibodies, since the viruses spread directly from cell to cell. In principle, the humoral immune system is thus only capable of preventing a generalized infection, but only if the antibodies are present at an early stage (e.g., induced by a vaccination). Class IgG and IgM antibodies are active in the bloodstream (see Chapter 2) and class IgA is active on the mucosal surface. The effect of the antibodies on the viral particles ("neutralization") is based on steric hindrance of virus adsorption to the host cells by the antibodies attached to their surfaces. The neutralizing effect of antibodies is strongest when they react with the receptor-binding sites on the capsids so as to block them, rendering the virus incapable of combining with the cellular receptors (p. 384).

Cellular immunity. This type of immune defense is far more important when it comes to fighting viral infections. T lymphocytes (killer cells) recognize virus-infected cells by the viral antigens on their surfaces and destroy them. The observation that patients with defective humoral immunity generally fare better with virus infections than those with a defective cellular response underlines the fact that the cellular immune defense system is the more important of the two.

Prevention

■ The most important prophylactic measures in the face of potential viral infections are active vaccines. Vaccines containing inactivated viruses generally provide shorter-lived and weaker protection than live vaccines. Passive immunization with human immunoglobulin is only used in a small number of cases, usually as postexposure prophylaxis. ■

Value of the different methods. In general, vaccination, i.e., induction of immunity (*immune prophylaxis*) is the most important factor in prevention of viral infection. *Exposure prophylaxis* is only relevant to hygienic measures necessitated by an epidemic and is designed to prevent the spread of pathogens in specific situations. *Chemoprophylaxis*, i.e., administration of chemotherapeutic agents when an infection is expected instead of after it has been diagnosed to block viral metabolism, is now justified in selected cases, e.g., in immunosuppressed patients (see Chemotherapy, p. 404).

There are two basic types of vaccines:

Active immunization. In this method, the antigen (virus) is introduced into the body, either in an inactivated form, or with attenuated pathogenicity but still capable of replication, to enable the body to build up its own immunity.

■ **Inactivated vaccines.** The immunity that develops after so-called "dead vaccines" are administered is merely humoral and generally does not last long. For this reason, booster vaccinations must be given repeatedly. The most important dead vaccines still in use today are influenza, rabies, some flavivirus, and hepatitis A and B vaccines. Some inactivated vaccines contain the most important immunogenic proteins of the virus. These so-called split vaccines induce more efficient protection and, above all, are better tolerated. Some of them are now produced by genetic engineering methods.

■ **Live attenuated vaccines.** These vaccines confer effective and long-lasting protection after only a single dose, because the viruses contained in them are capable of replication in the body, inducing not only humoral, but sometimes cellular immunity as well, not to mention local immunity (portal of entry!). Such live vaccines are preferable when available. There are, however, also drawbacks and risks, among them stability, the increased potential for contamination with other viruses, resulting in more stringent testing and the possibility that a back-mutation could produce a pathogenic strain (see Variability and Quasispecies of Viruses, p. 391).

7

■ **Vaccines with recombinant viruses.** Since only a small number of (surface) viral proteins are required to induce protective immunization, viral vectors are used in attempts to express them in vaccine recipients (see p. 390). Suitable vectors include the least virulent virus strains among the picornaviruses, alphaviruses, and poxviruses. There must be no generalized immunity to the vector in the population so that it can replicate in vaccine recipients and the desired protein will at the same time be expressed. Such recombinant vaccines have not yet been approved for use in humans. A rabies vaccine containing the recombinant vaccinia virus for use in animals is the only practical application of this type so far (p. 390).

■ **Naked DNA vaccine.** Since pure DNA can be inserted into eukaryotic cells (transfection) and the information it carries can be expressed, DNA that codes for the desired (viral) proteins can be used as vaccine material. The advantages of such vaccines, now still in the trial phase, include ease of production and high stability.

Passive immunization. This type of vaccine involves the injection of antibodies using only human immunoglobulins. The protection conferred is of short duration and only effective against viruses that cause viremia. Passive immunization is usually administered as a postexposure prophylactic measure, i.e., after an infection or in situations involving a high risk of infection, e.g., to protect against hepatitis B and rabies (locally, bite wound). Table 1.**13** (p. 33) and Table 8.**7** (rabies, p. 470) list the most important vaccines.

Chemotherapy

■ Inhibitors of certain steps in viral replication can be used as chemotherapeutic agents to treat viral infections. In practical terms, it is much more important to inhibit the synthesis of viral nucleic acid than of viral proteins. The main obstacles involved are the low level of specificity of the agents in some cases (toxic effects because cellular metabolism is also affected) and the necessity of commencing therapy very early in the infection cycle. ■

Problems of chemotherapy. As described on p. 381, viral replication is completely integrated in cell metabolism. The virus supplies only the genetic in-

Table 7.**4** The Most Important Antiviral Chemotherapeutics

Chemotherapeutic agent	Effect/indication
Adamantanamin (amantadine)	Inhibition of uncoating in influenza viruses
Acycloguanosine (acyclovir, Zovirax)	Inhibition of DNA synthesis in HSV and VZV
Dihydropropoxymethylguanosine (DHPG, ganciclovir, Cymevene)	Inhibition of DNA synthesis in CMV
Ribavirin	Inhibition of mRNA synthesis and capping. Infections with Lassa virus and perhaps in severe paramyxovirus and myxovirus infections
Nucleoside RT inhibitors (NRTI)	Inhibition of RT in HIV (p. 454)
Phosphonoformate (foscarnet)	Inhibition of DNA synthesis in herpesviruses, HIV, HBV
Protease inhibitors	Inhibition of viral maturation in HIV
Neuraminidase inhibitors	Inhibition of release of influenza viruses
Antisense RNA	Complementary to viral mRNA, which it blocks by means of hybridization (duplexing)

formation for proteins to be synthesized by the cell. This close association between viruses and their host cells is a source of some essential difficulties encountered when developing virus-specific chemotherapeutics, since any interference with viral synthesis is likely to affect physiological cellular synthetic functions as well. Specific intervention is only possible with viruses that code for their own enzymes (e.g., polymerases or proteases), which enzymes also react with viral substrates. Another problematic aspect is the necessity of administering chemotherapeutics (Table 7.**4**) early, preferably before clinical symptoms manifest, since the peak of viral replication is then usually already past (p. 399).

Development of resistance to chemotherapeutics. Acyclovir-resistant strains of herpesviruses, in particular herpes simplex viruses, are occasionally isolated. Less frequently, cytomegaly viruses resistant to ganciclovir are also found. These viruses possess a thymidine kinase or DNA polymerase altered by mutation. Infections caused by resistant herpesviruses are also observed in immunodeficient patients; the pathogens no longer respond to therapy after long-term treatment of dermal or mucosal efflorescences.

There are, as yet, no standardized resistance tests for chemotherapy-resistant viruses, so that the usefulness of such test results is of questionable value in confirmed cases. Also, the results obtained in vitro unfortunately do not correlate well with the cases of resistant viruses observed in clinical settings.

7

Laboratory Diagnosis

■ The following methods can be used to obtain a virological laboratory diagnosis:

— **Virus isolation** by growing the pathogen in a compatible host; usually done in cell cultures, rarely in experimental animals or hen embryos.
— **Direct virus detection.** The methods of serology, molecular biology, and electron microscopy are used to identify viruses or virus components directly, i.e., without preculturing, in diagnostic specimens.
— **Serodiagnostics** involving assay of antiviral antibodies of the IgG or IgM classes in patient serum. ■

Indication and methods. Laboratory diagnostic procedures for virus infections are costly, time-consuming, and require considerable staff time. It is therefore important to consider carefully whether such tests are indicated in a confirmed case. The physician in charge of treatment must make this decision based on detailed considerations. In general, it can be said that

Table 7.5 Virological Laboratory Diagnostics

Diagnostic approach	Methods	Detection/identification of	Advantages/disadvantages
Isolation	Growing in cell cultures	Infectivity, pathogenicity	Slow but sensitive method
Direct detection	Electron microscopy, EIA, IF, hybridization, PCR	Viral particles, antigens, genome	Fast method, but may be less sensitive
Serology	EIA, IF, etc.	Antibodies	Retrospective method

laboratory diagnostics are justified if further treatment of the patient would be influenced by an etiological diagnosis or if accurate diagnostic information is required in the context of an epidemic or scientific research and studies.

There are essentially three different methods used in virological diagnostics (Table 7.5):

1. *Virus isolation* by growing the pathogen in a compatible host; usually done in cell cultures.
2. *Direct virus detection* in patient material; identification of viral particles using electron microscopy, viral antigens with the methods of serology, and viral genome (components) using the methods of molecular biology.
3. *Antibody assay* in patient serum.

General guidelines for viral diagnostics are listed below. Specific details on detection and identification of particular viral species are discussed in the relevant sections of Chapters 8 and 12.

Virus Isolation by Culturing

In this approach, the virus is identified based on its infectivity and pathogenicity by inoculating a host susceptible for the suspected virus—in most cases cell cultures—with the specimen material. Certain changes observed in the culture (cytopathic effect [CPE] p. 392f.) indicate the presence of a virus.

Cell Cultures

A great majority of viruses can be grown in the many types of human or animal cells available for culture. So-called primary cell cultures can be created with various fresh tissues. However, the cells in such primary cultures can only divide a limited number of times. Sometimes so-called cell lines can be developed from primary cultures with unlimited in-vitro culturing capacity. Well-known examples of this phenomenon are HeLa cells (human portio carcinoma cells) and Vero cells (monkey renal fibroblasts). For diagnostic purposes, the cell cultures are usually grown as "monolayers," i.e., a single-layer cell film adhering to a glass or plastic surface.

Viral replication in cell cultures results in morphological changes in the cells such as rounding off, formation of giant cells, and inclusion bodies (so-called CPE, see also p. 392f.). The CPE details will often suffice for an initial approximate identification of the virus involved.

Sampling and transport of diagnostic specimens. Selection of suitable material depends on the disease and suspected viral species (see Chapter 8). Sampling should generally be done as early as possible in the infection cycle since, as was mentioned on p. 399, viral replication precedes the clinical symptoms. Sufficiently large specimens must be taken under conditions that are as sterile as possible, since virus counts in the diagnostic material are almost always quite low. Transport must be arranged quickly and under cold box conditions. The half-life of viruses outside the body is often very short and must be extended by putting the material on ice. A number of virus transport mediums are commercially available. A particular transport medium should be selected after consulting the laboratory to make sure the medium is compatible with the laboratory methods employed. Such mediums are particularly important if the diagnostic material might otherwise dry out.

Information provided to the laboratory. The laboratory must be provided with sufficient information concerning the course and stage of the disease, etc. This is very important if the diagnostic procedure is to be efficient and the results accurate. Clinical data and tentative diagnoses must be provided so the relevant viruses can be looked for in the laboratory. Searching for every single virus potentially present in the diagnostic material is simply not feasible for reasons of cost and efficiency.

Laboratory processing of the material. Before the host is inoculated with the specimen material for culturing, contaminant bacteria must be eliminated with antibiotics, centrifugation, and sometimes filtering. All of these manipulations of course entail the risk of virus loss and reduction of test sensitivity, so the importance of sterile sampling cannot be overemphasized. In a few cases, virus enrichment is indicated, e.g., by means of ultracentrifugation.

Selection of a host system. The host system to be used is chosen based on the suspected (and relevant) virus infectors. Observation and incubation times, and thus how long a laboratory diagnosis will take, also depend on the viral species under investigation.

Identification of the viruses is based first on the observed cell changes, then determined serologically using known antibodies and appropriate methods such as immunoelectron microscopy, EIA, or the neutralization test (see p. 402 for the neutralization mechanism). Methods that detect the viral genome by means of in-situ or filter hybridization are now seeing increasing use.

Significance of results. The importance of virus isolation depends on the virus type. In most cases, isolation will be indicative of the etiology of the patient's disease. In some cases, (in particular the herpesvirus and adenovirus group, see Chapter 8), latent viruses may have been activated by a completely different disease. In such cases, they may of course be isolated, but have no causal connection with the observed illness.

Isolation is the most sensitive method of viral diagnostic detection, but it cannot detect all viruses in all situations. This means that a negative result does not entirely exclude a viral infection. Another aspect is that the methods of virus isolation, with few exceptions, detect only mature, infectious virions and not the latent viruses integrated in the cells. This renders diagnostic isolation useless during latency (e.g., herpes simplex between recidivations).

Amplification culture. In this method, the virus is grown for a brief period in a cell culture. Before the CPE is observed, the culture is tested using the antigen and genomic methods described. This is also known as a "shell vial assay" because the cells are grown on coverslips in shell vials (test tubes with screw caps). Using this arrangement, method sensitivity can be increased by centrifuging the diagnostic material onto the cell monolayer. The greatest amount of time is saved by detecting the virus-specific proteins produced early in the infection cycle, which is why the search concentrates on such so-called "early antigens" (see p. 388). Using this method, the time required to confirm a cytomegaly virus, for instance, can be shortened from four to six weeks to only two to five days with practically no loss of sensitivity compared to classic isolation methods.

Direct Virus Detection

In this diagnostic approach, the viruses are not identified as infectious units per se, but rather as viral particles or parts of them. The idea is to find the viruses directly in the patient material without prior culturing or replication. Viruses in serous fluids such as the contents of herpes simplex or varicella-zoster blisters can be viewed under the electron microscope (EM). It must be remembered, however, that the EM is less sensitive than virus isolation in cultures by a factor of 10^5. Viral antigens can be detected in secretions using enzyme immunoassay (EIA), passive agglutination, or in smears with immunofluorescence performed with known antibodies, for instance monoclonal antibodies. Analogously, the viral genome can be identified by means of filter hybridization, or in smears or tissue sections with in-situ hybridization using DNA or RNA complementary to the viral genome as a probe.

Sampling and transport of diagnostic specimens. Transport of patient material for these methods is less critical than for virus isolation. Cold box transport is usually not required since the virus need not remain infectious.
— Electron microscopy. For negative contrast EM, the specimen is transported to the laboratory without any additives (dilution!).
— Antigen assay. For an immunofluorescence antigen assay, slide preparations must be made and fixed immediately after sampling. Special extraction mediums are used in EIA. Since commercial kits are used in most cases, procedure and reagents should be correlated with the laboratory.
— Genome hybridization. Here as well, the specimen material must meet specific conditions depending on whether the viruses are to be identified by the in-situ method or after extraction. This must be arranged beforehand with the laboratory.

Significance of results. A positive result with a direct virus detection method has the same level of significance as virus isolation. A negative test result means very little, particularly with EM, due to the low level of sensitivity of this method. The antigen assay and genome hybridization procedures are more sensitive than EM, but they are selective and detect only the viruses against which the antibodies or the nucleic acid probe used, are directed. It is therefore of decisive importance to provide the laboratory with detailed information. (See p. 208f. for definitions of the terms *sensitivity* and *specificity*.)

7

Virus Detection Following Biochemical Amplification

Polymerase chain reaction (**PCR**, Fig. 7.**9**). This method provides a highly sensitive test for viral genomes. First, nucleic acid is extracted from the patient material to be analyzed. Any RNA virus genome present in the material is transcribed into DNA by reverse transcriptase (see p. 385f.). This DNA, as well as the DNA of the DNA viruses, is then replicated in vitro with a DNA polymerase as follows: after the DNA double strand has been separated by applying heat, two synthetic oligonucleotides are added that are complementary to the two ends of the viral genome segment being looked for and can hybridize to it accordingly. The adjacent DNA (toward each 5' end) is then

Polymerase Chain Reaction

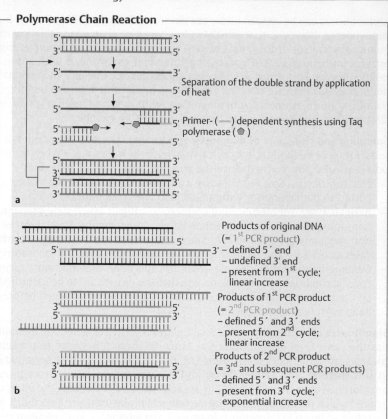

Separation of the double strand by application of heat

Primer-(—) dependent synthesis using Taq polymerase (⬠)

a

Products of original DNA
(= 1st PCR product)
– defined 5´ end
– undefined 3´ end
– present from 1st cycle;
  linear increase

Products of 1st PCR product
(= 2nd PCR product)
– defined 5´ and 3´ ends
– present from 2nd cycle;
  linear increase

Products of 2nd PCR product
(= 3rd and subsequent PCR products)
– defined 5´ and 3´ ends
– present from 3rd cycle;
  exponential increase

b

Fig. 7.9   **a** Two oligonucleotide primers are hybridized to the DNA double strands, which have been separated by heating. A heat-stable polymerase (e.g., *Taq* polymerase from **Thermus aquaticus**) is then added and extends these primers along the length of, and complementary to, the matrix strand. The resulting double strands are then once again separated by heat and the reaction is repeated.
b The DNA strands produced in the first cycle (1st generation) have a defined 5´ end (corresponding to the primer) and an undefined 3´ end. All of the subsequent daughter strands (2nd to nth generation) have a uniform, defined length.

copied with an added polymerase, whereby the oligonucleotides act as primers. The new and old strands are once again separated by heat and the reaction is started over again. Running several such cycles amplifies the original viral DNA by a factor of many thousands. Beginning with the second generation, the newly synthesized DNA strands show a uniform, defined length and are therefore detectable by means of gel electrophoresis. The specificity of the reaction is verified by checking the sequences of these DNA strands by means of hybridization or sequencing. The amplification and detection systems in use today for many viruses are increasingly commercially available, and in some cases are also designed to provide quantitative data on the "viral load."

Serodiagnosis

If a viral infection induces humoral immunity (see p. 48f. and 401), the resulting antibodies can be used in a serodiagnosis. When interpreting the serological data, one is confronted by the problem of deciding whether the observed reactions indicate a fresh, current infection or earlier contact with the virus in question. Two criteria can help with this decision:

Detection of IgM (without IgG) proves the presence of a fresh primary infection. IgM is now usually detected by specific serum against human IgM in the so-called capture test, an EIA (p. 128).

To test for IgM alone, a blood specimen must be obtained very early in the infection cycle. Concurrent detection of IgG and IgM in blood sampled somewhat later in the course of the disease would also indicate a fresh infection. It could, however, also indicate a reactivated latent infection or an anamnestic reaction (i.e., a nonspecific increase in antibodies in reaction to a nonrelated infection), since IgM can also be produced in both of these cases.

A **fourfold increase in the IgG titer** within 10–14 days early on in the course of the infection or a drop of the same dimensions later in the course would also be confirmation.

8   Viruses as Human Pathogen

K. A. Bienz

DNA Viruses

Viruses with Single-Stranded DNA Genomes

The groups of viruses with single-stranded DNA genomes are contained in only one family, the parvoviruses, with only a single human pathogen type. The *Geminiviridae, Circoviridae*, and many other families have circular single-stranded DNA, but infect only plants and, more rarely, animals.

Parvoviruses

■ This group's only human pathogen, parvovirus B19, is the causative virus in erythema infectiosum (also known as "slapped cheek syndrome" or the "fifth disease") in children and causes aplastic crisis in anemic patients. The virus also contributes to joint diseases, embryopathies, and tissue rejection following renal transplants. Diagnosis: serological (IgG and IgM) and PCR.   ■

Pathogen. The parvoviruses are among the smallest viruses with a diameter of 19–25 mm. They are icosahedral, nonenveloped, and their genome is in the form of single-stranded DNA (ssDNA). Some parvoviruses can only replicate in the presence of a helper virus (adenovirus or herpesvirus). Parvovirus B19, the only human pathogenic parvovirus identified to date, is capable of autonomic replication, i.e., it requires no helper virus. Some zoopathic strains also show this capability in rodents, dogs, and pigs.

Pathogenesis and clinical picture. Parvovirus B19 replicates in the bone marrow in erythrocyte precursor cells, which are destroyed in the process. In patients already suffering from anemia (sickle-cell anemia, chronic hemolytic anemia), such infections result in so-called aplastic crises in which the lack of erythrocyte resupply leads to a critical shortage. In otherwise healthy persons, these infections usually run an asymptomatic course. They can, however, also cause a harmless epidemic infection in children, erythema infectiosum ("slapped-cheek syndrome" or "fifth disease"). This childhood disease, which used to be classified as atypical measles, is characterized by sudden onset of exanthem on the face and extremities. Certain forms of arthritis are considered complications of a parvovirus B19 infection. The virus also appears to cause spontaneous abortions in early pregnancy and fetal damage in late pregnancy (hydrops fetalis).

Diagnosis. An enzyme immunoassay reveals antibodies of the IgG and IgM classes. During the viremic phase, at the onset of clinical symptoms, the virus can also be identified in the blood by means of electron microscopy or PCR. In-vitro culturing of the pathogen is not standard procedure.

Epidemiology and prevention. The transmission route of human parvovirus B19 is not known. Droplet infection or the fecal-oral route, analogous to other parvoviruses, is suspected. Blood and blood products are infectious, so that multiple transfusion patients and drug addicts are high incidence groups. No specific prophylactic measures are recommended.

Viruses with Double-Stranded DNA Genomes

Viruses with double-stranded DNA genomes are classified in six families: papillomavirus, polyomavirus, adenovirus, herpesvirus, poxvirus, and hepadnavirus. Carcinogenic types have been found in all groups except the poxviruses (see Chapter 7, DNA tumor viruses).

8

Papillomaviruses

■ The over 70 viral types in the genus *Papillomavirus* are all involved in the etiology of benign tumors such as warts and papillomas, as well as malignancies, the latter mainly in the genital area (cervical carcinoma). These organisms cannot be grown in cultures. Diagnosis therefore involves direct detection of the viral genome and histological analysis. Serology is less important in this group. ■

Pathogens. The papillomaviruses have a diameter of 55 nm and contain an 8 kbp dsDNA genome. There are two distinct regions within the circular genome: one that codes for the regulator proteins produced early in the replication cycle and another that codes for the structural proteins synthesized later. Over 70 papillomavirus types have been described to date, all of which induce either benign or malignant tumors in natural or experimental hosts.

Pathogenesis and clinical picture. Papillomaviruses infect cells in the outer layers of the skin and mucosa and cause various types of warts by means of local cell proliferation (Fig. 8.**1**). Specific virus types correlate with specific pathohistological wart types. Plantar and vulgar warts, flat juvenile warts, and juvenile laryngeal papillomas apparently always remain benign. By contrast, the genital warts caused by types 6 and 11 (condylomata acuminata) can show carcinomatous changes. Of all papillomavirus-caused cervical dysplasias, 50 % contain human papillomavirus (HPV) 16 and 20 % HPV 18.

All wart viruses induce primary proliferation of the affected cells with large numbers of viruses found in the cell nuclei. Whether a malignant degeneration will take place depends on the cell and virus type involved, but likely on the presence of cocarcinogens as well. In carcinomas, the viral DNA is found in integrated form within the host-cell genome, whereas in premalignant changes the viral genomes are found in the episomal state. Papillomaviruses possess oncogenes (*E5*, *E6*, and *E7* genes) that bind the products of tumor suppressor genes: E6 binds the *p53* gene product, E7 the *Rb* gene product (see p. 396f.).

Diagnosis. Human papillomaviruses cannot be cultivated in vitro. They are detected and identified by means of histological analysis and, in malignancies in particular, by means of in-situ hybridization. Antibody assay results have a low significance level and these procedures are not standard routine.

Epidemiology and prevention. Since viruses are produced and accumulate in wart tissues, papillomaviruses are transmissible by direct contact. Warts can also spread from one part of the body to another (autoinoculation). A certain level of prophylactic protection can be achieved with hygienic measures.

8

Warts Caused by Papillomaviruses

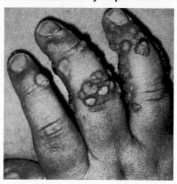

Fig. 8.**1**

Polyomaviruses

■ A medically important polyomavirus, the JC virus, causes progressive multifocal leukoencephalopathy (PML), a demyelinating disease that has become more frequent as a sequel to HIV infections, but is otherwise rare. The same applies to the BK virus, which affects bone marrow transplantation patients. Electron microscopy or PCR are the main diagnostic tools. ■

Pathogens. The polyomaviruses can be divided into two groups: in one group are the SV40 and SV40-like viruses (Fig. 8.2) such as human pathogen JC and BK viruses. In the other are the true polyomaviruses such as the carcinogenic murine polyomavirus. The designations JC and BK are the initials of the first patients in whom these viral types were identified. There are also a number of other zoopathic oncogenic polyomaviruses. The name *polyoma* refers to the ability of this organism to produce tumors in many different organs.

Pathogenesis and clinical picture. The JC and BK viruses are widespread: over 80% of the adult population show antibodies to them, despite which, clinical manifestations like PML are very rare. The viruses can be reactivated by a weakening of the immune defense system. The JC virus attacks the macroglia, especially in AIDS patients, to cause progressive multifocal PML, a demyelinating process in the brain with disseminated foci that is fatal

— Polyomaviruses (SV40) —————————————————

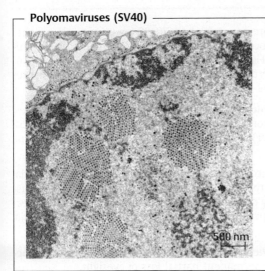

Fig. 8.2 Section through viral conglomerations in the nucleus of the host cell (TEM).

500 nm

8

within one year. The BK virus can cause hemorrhagic cystitis in bone marrow transplantation patients.

Diagnosis. The JC and BK viruses can be grown in cultures, albeit with great difficulty and not for diagnostic purposes. Both can be detected with PCR and the BK virus can be seen under the electron microscope in urine. Antibody assays are practically useless due to the high level of generalized contamination.

Epidemiology. Despite the high level of generalized contamination, the transmission routes used by the human polyomaviruses have not been clarified.

Adenoviruses

■ There are a total of 41 types of adenoviruses and they cause a wide variety of diseases. Influenza infections of the upper, less frequently the lower, respiratory tract and eye infections (follicular conjunctivitis, keratoconjunctivitis) are among the more significant clinical pictures. Intestinal infections are mainly caused by the only not culturable virus types 40 and 41. Diagnosis: antibody assay in respiratory adenovirus infections. Serology is not reliable in the eye and intestinal infections. It is possible to isolate the pathogens in cell cultures from eye infections. Enteral adenoviruses are detected in stool by means of electron microscopy, enzyme immunoassay, or passive agglutination. ■

Pathogens. Adenoviruses are nonenveloped, 70–90 nm in size, and icosahedral. Their morphogenesis occurs in the cell nucleus, where they also aggregate to form large crystals (Fig. 8.**3**). Their genome is a linear, 36–38 kbp double-stranded DNA. Adenoviruses got their name from the adenoidal tissues (tonsils) in which they were first identified.

Pathogenesis and clinical picture. Adenoviruses cause a variety of diseases, which may occur singly or concurrently. The most important are infections of the upper (sometimes lower) respiratory tracts, the eyes, and the intestinal tract.

■ Infections of the **respiratory tract** take the form of rhinitis or abacterial pharyngitis, depending on the virus type as well as presumably on the disposition of the patient. They may also develop into acute, influenzalike infections or even, especially in small children, into a potentially fatal pneumonia.

■ The **eye infections**, which may occur alone but are often concurrent with pharyngitis, range from follicular conjunctivitis to a form of keratoconjunctivitis that may even cause permanent partial loss of eyesight.

Adenoviruses

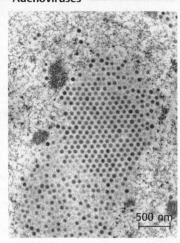

Fig. 8.**3**   Viral crystals in the nucleus of the host cell (TEM).

500 nm

■ An important aspect of the **intestinal infections** is that the primary gastroenteritis forms are caused by the viral strains 40 and 41, which are difficult to culture.

Adenoviruses can persist for months in the regional lymph nodes or tonsils until they are reactivated.

Diagnosis. Antibody assays in patient serum are the main approach taken in respiratory adenovirus infections. Serology is unreliable in the eye and intestinal infections, since hardly any antibodies are produced in response to such highly localized infections. It is possible to isolate the viruses that cause respiratory infections by inoculating cell cultures with pharyngeal material or bronchial secretion and with conjunctival smears in eye infections. Enteral adenoviruses, on the other hand, are hard to culture. The best approach to detecting them is therefore to subject stool specimens to electron microscopy, enzyme immunoassay, or passive agglutination methods.

Epidemiology and prevention. Humans are the source of infection. Susceptibility is the rule. Generalized contamination of the population begins so early in childhood that adenovirus infections play a more significant role in children than in adults. Transmission of respiratory adenoviruses is primarily by droplet infection, but also as smear infections since the virus is also excreted in stool. Eye infections can be contracted from bathing water or, in the case of adenovirus type 8 in particular, iatrogenically from insuffi-

8

ciently sterilized ophthalmological instruments. The enteral infections are also transmitted by the fecal-oral route, mainly by contact rather than in water or food. Adenoviruses are the second most frequent diarrhea pathogen in children after rotaviruses (p. 456f.).

Herpesviruses

■ The viruses in this family all feature a practically identical morphology, but show little uniformity when it comes to their biology and the clinical pictures resulting from infections. One thing shared by all herpesviruses is the ability to reactivate after a period of latency.

■ The **herpes simplex virus** (HSV, two serotypes) is the pathogen that causes a vesicular exanthem (fever blisters, herpes labialis, or genitalis), encephalitis, and a generalized infection in newborns (herpes neonatorum).

■ The **varicella-zoster virus** (VZV) causes the primary infection chickenpox, which can then recidivate as zoster (shingles).

■ **Cytomegalovirus** (CMV) infections remain inapparent or harmless in the immunologically healthy, but can cause generalized, fatal infections in immunocompromised individuals.

■ The **Epstein-Barr virus** (EBV) is the pathogen in infectious mononucleosis and is also implicated in lymphomas (including Burkitt lymphoma) and nasopharyngeal carcinomas.

■ **Human herpesvirus 6** (HHV 6) is the pathogen that causes three-day fever (exanthema subitum, roseola infantum).

Human herpesvirus 8 (HHV 8) causes the AIDS-associated Kaposi sarcoma.

Diagnosis. Isolation, amplification culture, or direct detection can be used to diagnose herpes simplex, varicella-zoster, and cytomegaloviruses; antibody assays can be used for Epstein-Barr, human herpes 6 and 8, and varicella-zoster viruses; PCR can detect herpes simplex, varicella-zoster virus, cytomegalovirus, and human herpesvirus 6.

Therapy. Effective and well-tolerated chemotherapeutics are available to treat herpes simplex, varicella-zoster virus, and cytomegalovirus (acyclovir, ganciclovir). ■

Biology of the Herpesviruses

Several hundred herpesvirus species have been described in humans and animals, all with the same morphology (Fig. 8.**4a**). They have dsDNA genomes. Replication of the DNA and the morphogenesis of the virus particle take place in the host-cell nucleus. The envelope (inner nuclear membrane) is then formed when the virus penetrates the nuclear membrane (Fig. 8.**4b**), whereby depending on the cell and viral type involved a more or less substantial number of viruses receive an envelope after reaching the cytoplasm, at the cell membrane or not at all. The envelope is the major determinant of viral infectivity (see Chapter 7, p. 378f.). Since the envelope contains mainly host-cell determinants, it can also be assumed that it provides a level of protection from host immune responses.

Common to all herpesviruses is a high level of generalized contamination (60–90 % carriers) and the ability to persist in a latent state in the body over long periods. The different viral species persist in different cells, whereby the cell type is the decisive factor determining latency or replication of the virus. Herpes simplex virus and varicella-zoster virus do not produce any virus particles during latency, although they do produce one, or a few, mRNA types and the corresponding proteins. Cytomegalovirus and Epstein-Barr virus appear to maintain continuous production of small numbers of viruses as well, so that fresh infection of a small number of new cells is an ongoing process. These viruses would appear to produce persistent, subclinical infections concurrently with their latent status (p. 394). Reactivation of these latent viruses is apparently initiated by a number of factors (psychological stress, solar irradiation, fever, traumata, other infections, immunosuppressive therapy), but the actual mechanisms that reactivate the lytic viral life cycle are unknown.

Human herpesviruses (with the exception of the varicella-zoster virus) and many zoopathic herpes species have also been implicated in the etiology of malignancies.

8

Eight human herpesviruses that infect different organs are known to date, e.g., the skin (herpes simplex virus types 1 and 2, varicella-zoster virus), the lymphatic system (Epstein-Barr virus, human herpesvirus type 6, cytomegaloviruses), and the CNS (herpes simplex virus, cytomegalovirus).

Herpes simplex Virus (HSV)

Pathogen, pathogenesis, and clinical picture. The viral genome codes for about 90 proteins, categorized as "immediate early" (regulatory functions), "early" (DNA synthesis), and "late" (structural) proteins. Herpes simplex viruses are classified in types 1 and 2, which differ both serologically and biologically (host-cell spectrum, replication temperature). Initial infection with **herpes simplex type 1** usually occurs in early childhood. The portal of entry is normally the oral mucosa ("oral type") and the infection usually manifests as a gingivostomatitis. The viruses then wander along axons into the CNS, where they persist in a latent state in the trigeminal (Gasseri) gang-

Herpesviruses

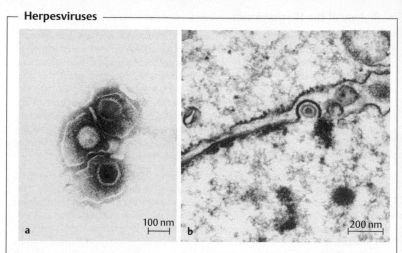

100 nm

200 nm

a   b

Fig. 8.**4**   **a** With envelope, **b** in the nucleus of the host cell; envelope formation at the nuclear membrane. The naked virion measures 100 nm and the virus with its envelope up to 200 nm.

lion. As with all herpesviruses, the pathogen remains in the macroorganism *permanently* after the primary infection. Following reactivation (endogenous recidivation), the viruses follow the same route back to the periphery, where they cause the familiar vesicular exanthem ("fever blisters," herpes labialis, Fig. 8.5). Despite established immunity, such recidivations can manifest repeatedly because the viruses wander within the nerve cells and do not enter

Herpes labialis

Fig. 8.**5**   Following the initial infection, herpes simplex viruses (HSV) persist in the latent state in nerve cells of the CNS. When reactivated, they travel down the axons of these cells to the periphery, where they cause the typical vesicular exanthem.

the intercellular space, thus remaining beyond the reach of the immune defenses. Possible complications include keratoconjunctivitis and a highly lethal form of encephalitis.

The initial infection with **HSV type 2** normally affects the urogenital area ("genital type") and can be contracted despite an existing HSV type 1 infection. HSV type 2 persists in the latent state in the lumbosacral ganglia or peripheral tissues, from where it causes episodes of manifest herpes genitalis. Neurological complications are very rare and more benign than in HSV type 1. On the other hand, infections of newborn children (herpes neonatorum), e.g., in cases of maternal genital herpes, are feared for their high lethality rate.

Diagnosis. Cultivating the pathogen from pustule contents is the method of choice in labial and genital herpes. In an HSV encephalitis, the cerebrospinal fluid will contain few viruses or none at all. In such cases, they can only be cultivated from tissues (biopsy or autopsy material). Virus detection by means of cerebrospinal fluid PCR is worth a try.

Direct detection of the viruses under an electron microscope is only practicable if the specimen contains large numbers of viruses, which in practice will normally only be the case in blister contents. The virus can also be detected directly in patient specimens using immunofluorescence or in-situ hybridization (p. 408), but the material must contain virus-infected cells, i.e., blister contents are not as suitable here as in electron microscopy and virus isolation.

Serological investigation results in HSV lack significance due to the high level of general contamination in the population.

Epidemiology, prevention, and therapy. HSV type 1 is transmitted by contact, and possibly by smear infection as well. Contamination with HSV therefore begins in early childhood. Transmission of HSV type 2 usually occurs during sexual intercourse, so that infections are generally not observed until after puberty. No immune prophylaxis (vaccination) is currently available for HSV. Acycloguanosine is used prophylactically in immunosuppressed patients (see Chapter 7, p. 404).

Specific therapy is possible with acycloguanosine. Used in time, this chemotherapy can save lives in HSV encephalitis.

Varicella-zoster Virus (VZV)

Pathogen, pathogenesis, clinical picture. The VZ virus differs substantially from HSV, both serologically and in many biological traits. For instance, it can only be grown in primate cell cultures, in which it grows much more slowly and more cell-associated than is the case with HSV. No subtypes have been described.

┌─ **Herpes zoster** ─────────────────────────────────

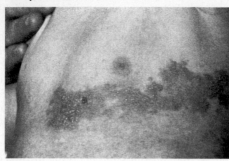

Fig. 8.6 The varicella zoster viruses (VZV) persist in the latent state in spinal ganglia cells. When reactivated, they cause dermal efflorescences in the corresponding dermatome.

└──

The initial infection with VZV manifests in the great majority of persons as chickenpox, an episodic papulous exanthem. The portals of entry are the nasopharyngeal space and the conjunctiva. From there, the virus undergoes a viremic phase in which it is transported by the blood to the skin, where the typical exanthem is produced. The disease confers an effective immunity. In immunodeficient patients, a VZV infection (or reactivation, see below) can affect other organs (lungs, brain) and manifest a severe, frequently lethal, course.

After the symptoms of chickenpox have abated, the VZV persists in the spinal ganglia and perhaps in other tissues as well. Following reactivation, zoster (shingles) develops (Fig. 8.6), whereby the virus once again spreads neurogenically and causes neuralgia as well as the typical zoster efflorescence in the skin segment supplied by the sensitive nerves. Reactivation is induced by internal or external influences and becomes possible when cellular VZV immunity drops off, i.e., after about the age of 45 assuming normal immune defenses.

Diagnosis. VZV can be detected with a wide spectrum of methods, namely PCR, isolation, direct viral detection by means of electron microscopy, detection of viral antigens using immunofluorescence in tissue specimens or cell smears, and serologically based on antibody titer increases or IgM detection.

Epidemiology, prevention, and therapy. VZV is highly contagious and is transmitted aerogenically. The primary infection, which manifests as chickenpox, is still almost exclusively a childhood disease today. A vaccine containing attenuated viruses is available for prevention of chickenpox and possibly zoster, but its use is currently a matter of controversy. In immunosuppressed patients, hyperimmunoglobulin can be used for passive immunization or postexposure immunity. Acycloguanosine is used both prophylactically and in treatment of VZV infections.

Cytomegalovirus (CMV)

Pathogen, pathogenesis, clinical picture. CMV is characterized by a narrow spectrum of hosts, slow replication, frequently involving formation of giant cells and late, slow development of cytopathology.

An initial infection with cytomegaly is inapparent in most persons, even in very early—perinatal or postnatal—infections. The virus apparently persists in the latent state in mononuclear cells. Reactivation can also run an asymptomatic course, but symptoms may also develop that are generally relatively mild, such a mononucleosislike clinical pictures, mild forms of hepatitis or other febrile illnesses. Droplet infection is the most frequent route of transmission, but smear infections and nursing infections are also possible. Generalized contamination with this pathogen (over 90% of the adult population is infected), frequent reactivation with, in some cases, months of continued excretion of viruses in saliva and urine and the wide variety of potential clinical pictures are all factors that often make it difficult to implicate CMV as the etiological cause of an observed illness. The virus infection can manifest as a sequel instead of a cause, for instance of a flulike illness. To labor the point somewhat, it could be said that the patient is not primarily ill due to a CMV infection, but rather has a florid CMV infection because he or she is ill.

The situation is different in AIDS, transplantation or malignancy patients, in whom a fresh CMV infection or reactivation—similarly to HSV and VZV—can result in severe generalized infections with lethal outcome. The liver and lungs are the main organs involved. Retinitis is also frequent in AIDS patients. In kidney transplant patients, a CMV infection of the mesangial cells can result in rejection of the transplant. Another feared CMV-caused condition is an intrauterine fetal infection, which almost always results from a primary infection in the mother: in 10% of cases the infection results in severe deformities.

Diagnosis. Amplification cultures (p. 408f.) from saliva, urine, buffy coat, tissue, or BAL (bronchoalveolar lavage) are a suitable method of confirming a florid CMV infection. In transplantation patients, the risk of a CMV manifestation can be estimated by immunocytochemical monitoring of the CMV-positive cell count in the peripheral blood ("antigenemia test"), since this count normally rises several days before clinical manifestations appear. Based on such an early warning, antiviral therapy can be started in time (ganciclovir, foscarnet). PCR results must be interpreted with a clear idea of how sensitive the method used can be, since the numbers of viruses found may be clinically insignificant. Hasty conclusions can result in "overdiagnosis," above all in CMV-positive transplant recipients.

Serological results are hardly useful in clarifying a florid infection due to the high level of generalized contamination. Added to this is the fact that the immunoincompetent patients in whom diagnosis of this infection would be particularly important are serologically problematical anyway. Serology does contribute to clearing up the CMV status of transplant recipients and donors.

Epidemiology, prevention, and therapy. CMV is transmitted by contact or smear infection, usually in childhood or adolescence. Immunosuppressed patients can be treated with hyperimmunoglobulin to provide passive immunity against infection or recidivation. Ganciclovir and foscarnet are therapeutically useful in transplantation, and particularly in AIDS patients, to combat CMV-induced pneumonia, encephalitis, and retinitis.

Epstein-Barr Virus (EBV)

Pathogen, pathogenesis, clinical picture. EBV infects only a narrow spectrum of hosts and replicates very slowly. It persists in a latent state in B lymphocytes and can lead to their immortalization and tumor transformation.

EBV enters the body through the mucosa. It replicates in epithelial cells of the oropharynx or cervix and enters B lymphocytes, where it continues to replicate. This results in the clinical picture of infectious mononucleosis (kissing disease or Pfeiffer disease), which is characterized by fever and a generalized but mainly cervical swelling of the lymph nodes, typically accompanied by tonsillitis, pharyngitis, and some cases of mild hepatic involvement. This virus also persists in latency, probably for the life of the patient, in (immortalized) B cells.

EBV and EBV-specific sequences and antigens are isolated in cases of Burkitt lymphoma and nasopharyngeal carcinoma. The higher incidence of Burkitt lymphoma in parts of Africa is attributed to a cofactor arising from the hyperendemic presence of malaria there. EBV exacerbates the B-cell proliferation resulting from a malaria infection. EBV has also been implicated in Hodgkin disease and T-cell lymphomas. These tumor forms also result from the interaction of EBV with other mechanisms of cell damage. In immunocompetent persons, the following lymphoproliferative diseases are sequelae of EBV infections:

— a benign polyclonal B-cell hyperplasia,
— its malignant transformation into a polyclonal B-cell lymphoma, and
— a malignant, oligoclonal or monoclonal B-cell lymphoma.

Diagnosis. Heterogenetic antibodies that agglutinate the erythrocytes of several animal species and antibodies to a variety of viral antigens are found in **acute** infectious mononucleosis:

— **VCA** (viral capsid antigen). Antibodies to VCA appear early and persist for life.
— **EA** (early antigen). Antibodies to EA are only detectable during the active disease.

— **EBNA** (Epstein-Barr nuclear antigen). Antibodies to EBNA are not produced until two to four weeks after disease manifestation, then persist for life.

Chronic mononucleosis is characterized by antibodies to VCA and EA.

The diagnostic procedures in lymphoproliferative diseases (see above) involve histology and cellular immunotyping.

Epidemiology, prevention, and therapy. EBV is excreted in saliva and pharyngeal secretions and is transmitted by close contact ("kissing disease"). As with all herpesviruses the level of generalized contamination is high, with the process beginning in childhood and continuing throughout adolescence. Neither immunoprophylactic nor chemoprophylactic measures have been developed as yet. Lymphoproliferative diseases involving viral replication can be treated with acyclovir and ganciclovir.

Human Herpesvirus (HHV) 6

Pathogen, pathogenesis, clinical picture. HHV-6 was isolated in 1986 in patients suffering from lymphoproliferative diseases and AIDS. The virus shows T-cell tropism and is biologically related to the cytomegalovirus. HHV-6 exists in two variants, HHV-6A and HHV-6B. The pathogenic implications of their reactivation have not yet been described.

HHV-6B is the causal pathogen in exanthema subitum (roseola infantum), a disease that is nearly always harmless, characterized by sudden onset with high fever and manifests as a typical exanthem in small children. Reports of HHV-6-caused illness in adults are rare and the clinical pictures described resemble mononucleosis (EBV-negative mononucleosis). Apparently, however, this virus can also cause severe infections in bone marrow transplant patients (pulmonary and encephalitic infections). HHV-6A has not yet been convincingly implicated in any clinical disease.

Diagnosis and epidemiology. HHV-6 can be cultured in stimulated umbilical lymphocytes. Potentially useful diagnostic tools include antibody assay and PCR.

Generalized contamination with HHV 6 begins in early childhood, eventually reaching levels exceeding 90% in the adult population. The virus persists in latent form in the salivary gland, so that mother-to-child transmission is most likely to be in saliva.

Human Herpesvirus (HHV) 8

Pathogen, clinical picture. HHV 8 has recently been identified as a decisive cofactor in induction of Kaposi sarcoma. The classic, sporadic form of this malignancy was described in 1872 in the Mediterranean area. It also occurs

8

following organ transplantations and is a significant cause of death in AIDS patients (12%).

The contribution of HHV 8 to the pathogenesis of Kaposi sarcoma appears to lie in dysregulation of cytokine and hormone production. In transplantation-association Kaposi sarcoma the virus can also be transmitted by the transplant.

Diagnosis. Antibody assay (EIA, IF, Western blot).

Poxviruses

■ The variola virus, which belongs to the genus *Orthopoxvirus* and is the causative agent in smallpox, was declared eradicated in 1980 after a WHO vaccination campaign. The **vaccinia virus**, used at the end of the 18th century by E. Jenner in England as a vaccine virus to protect against smallpox, is now used as a vector in molecular biology and as a hybrid virus with determinants from other viruses in experimental vaccines. Among the other orthopoxviruses found in animals, the monkeypox viruses are the main human pathogens. The animal pathogens **parapoxviruses** (milker's nodules, orf) are occasionally transmitted to humans, in whom they cause harmless exanthems.

The molloscum contagiosum virus affects only humans and causes benign tumors.

Diagnosis. Orthopoxviruses and parapoxviruses: electron microscopy. Molloscum contagiosum: histology. ■

8

── **Brick-Shaped Orthopoxvirus** ──────────

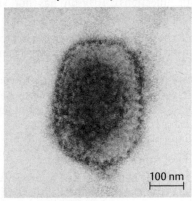

Fig. 8.**7** Poxviruses measure 200–350 nm, putting them just within the resolution range of light microscopes (TEM).

100 nm

Vaccinia Viruses

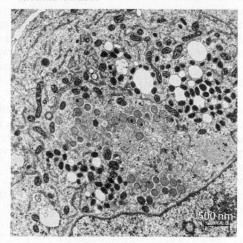

Fig. 8.8 The vaccinia viruses are the dark, electron-dense inclusions readily visible here. They replicate in a discrete cytoplasmic region (TEM).

500 nm

Pathogens. The viruses of the pox group are the largest viruses of all. At 230 × 350 nm they are just within the resolution range of light microscopes. They have a complex structure (Fig. 8.7) and are the only DNA viruses that replicate in a defined area within the host-cell cytoplasm, a so-called "virus factory" (Fig. 8.8).

The diseases smallpox (variola major) and the milder form alastrim (variola minor) now no longer occur in the human population thanks to a worldwide vaccination program during the 1970s. The last person infected by smallpox was registered in Somalia in 1977 and eradication of the disease was formally proclaimed in 1980. Since then, populations of the virus have been preserved in two special laboratories only.

8

The Family *Poxviridae*

This virus family comprises several genera:
■ the **orthopox**viruses include the variola and alastrim viruses, the vaccinia virus used in smallpox vaccines, the closely related (but not identical) cowpox viruses as well as the monkeypox, mousepox, and rabbitpox viruses.

Other genera with human pathogen strains include:
■ the **parapox**viruses including the orf virus and the milker's nodule virus (not to be confused with cowpox), transmitted to humans by sheep and cows, respectively;
■ the **molluscipox**viruses, i.e., the molluscum contagiosum virus.

Pathogenesis and clinical picture. Variola viruses are transmitted aerogenically. The mucosa of the upper respiratory tract provides the portal of entry. From there, the pathogens enter the lymphoid organs and finally penetrate to the skin, where typical eruptions form and, unlike varicella pustules, all develop together through the same stages (Fig. 8.9). The mucosae of the respiratory and intestinal tracts are also affected. Lethality rates in cases of smallpox (variola major) were as high as 40%. In alastrim (variola minor) the level was 2%, whereby the cause of death was often a bronchopneumonia.

The vaccinia virus is a distinct viral type of unknown origins, and not an attenuated variola virus. It was formerly used as a vaccine virus to protect against smallpox. The vaccination caused a pustular exanthem around the vaccination site, usually accompanied by fever. Encephalitis, the pathogenesis of which was never completely clarified, was a feared complication. It is assumed that an autoimmune reaction was the decisive factor. Other complications include generalized vaccinia infection and vaccinial keratitis. Vaccinia infections and their complications disappeared for the most part when smallpox was eradicated by the WHO vaccination campaign. Vaccinia viruses are still frequently used as vectors in molecular biology laboratories. The inherent pathogenicity of the virus should of course be kept in mind by experimenters.

Infections with *cowpox*, *orf*, and *milker's nodule* viruses are rare and usually harmless. The lesions remain localized on the skin (contact site), accompanied by a local lymphadenitis. These are typical occupational infections (farmers, veterinarians). The *molluscum contagiosum* virus is unusual in that in-vitro culturing of the virus has not succeeded to date. Infections with this virus do not confer immunity. The infection causes epidermal, benign tumors ("molluscum contagiosum warts").

Smallpox (Variola)

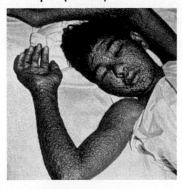

Fig. 8.**9** In contrast to the lesions in varicella infections, all smallpox pustules are at the same developmental stage.

Diagnosis. The poxviruses group are relatively easy to recognize under an electron microscope in pustule contents, provided the pustules have not yet dried out or been superinfected with bacteria. Orthopoxviruses and parapoxviruses can be differentiated morphologically, but the viruses within each genus share the same morphology. Molluscum contagiosum is diagnosed histologically.

Epidemiology and prevention. Diseased humans were the sole viral reservoir of variola and alastrim. Transmission was direct and aerogenic and, although the virus is highly resistant even when desiccated, less frequent via contaminated objects (bed linens). The vaccinia virus does not occur in nature and any human infections are now accidental (laboratory infections).

The zootropic poxviruses are transmitted solely by means of contact with infected animals. Molluscum contagiosum is transmitted by interhuman contact.

Hepadnaviruses: Hepatitis B Virus and Hepatitis D Virus

■ A hepatitis B virus (HBV) infection (see p. 385ff., replication) of the liver cells results in expression of viral antigen on the cell surface, followed by immunological cell damage with acute, possibly fulminant, chronic persistent or chronic aggressive hepatitis. The final stages can be liver cirrhosis or hepatocellular carcinoma. A concurrent or later superinfection by a defective, RNA-containing and HBV-dependent hepatitis D virus (HDV, delta agent) normally exacerbates the clinical course. Both viruses are transmitted in blood or body fluids, whereby even a tiny amount of blood may be enough to cause an infection.

Diagnosis: immunological antigen or antibody assay in patient serum. The antigen or antibody patterns observed provide insights on the stage and course of the disease.

Prevention: active immunization with HBV surface (HBs) antigen; concurrent postexposure passive immunization. ■

Hepatitis B pathogen. The *hepatitis B virus* (*HBV*) is the main representative of the family of hepadnaviruses, *Hepadnaviridae*. The name of the family is an acronym of the disease caused by the virus and its genomic type. It causes a sometimes chronic form of liver inflammation (hepatitis) and its genome consists of partially double-stranded DNA (hepadnavirus = hepatitis DNA virus). The replication cycle of the HBV includes a transient RNA phase (for details see Chapter 7, p. 385). The HBV possess an envelope made up

Hepatitis B Virus

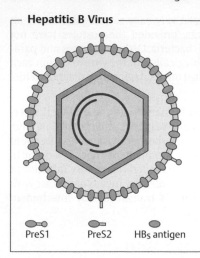

PreS1   PreS2   HBs antigen

Fig. 8.**10**   The capsid, which consists of Hbc and Hbe antigens, encloses the entire DNA antisense strand, the incomplete sense strand, and the reverse transcriptase (not shown here). The envelope contains the three forms of the Hbs antigen: PreS1 = complete protein, PreS2 = shortened form of PreS1, HBs antigen = HB surface antigen in the proper sense, shortened form of PreS2.

of a cellular double lipid layer in which are integrated the hepatitis B surface (HBs) antigen, a 25 kDa polypeptide, and its precursor stages PreS1 (40 kDa) and PreS2 (33 kDa). (Fig. 8.**10**). This envelope encloses the actual capsid, which consists of the hepatitis B core (HBc) antigen with 21 kDa and contains the genome together with the DNA polymerase (a reverse transcriptase, p. 385). The complete, infectious virion, also known as a Dane particle after its discoverer, has a diameter of 42 nm, the inner structure 27 nm. The virus replicates in liver cells. The Dane particles and the HBs antigen, but not the HBc antigen, are released into the bloodstream, whereby the HBs antigen is present in two different forms, a filamentous particle approximately 22 × 100 nm and a spherical form with a diameter of about 22 nm. A further viral protein is the HBe antigen, which represents a posttranslational, truncated form of the HBc antigen and is no longer capable of spontaneous capsid formation. It is also released from the hepatic cells into the blood.

Hepatitis B Mutants

Using molecular biological methods refined in recent years, more and more HBV mutants have been found with one or more amino acid exchanges in certain proteins. HBs or PreS mutants are so-called "escape" mutants that can cause a new infection or recidivation despite immune protection by antibodies to HBs. Similarly, pre-HBVc or HBVc mutants can lead to a reactivation of HBV replication and thus to a chronic hepatitis, since they block formation of the HBe antigen and thus the point of attack for the cellular immune defenses. These HBc mutants are frequently observed under interferon therapy.

Hepatitis D pathogen. A certain percentage of HBV-infected persons, which varies geographically, are also infected by a second hepatitis virus discovered at the end of the seventies in Italy, the *delta agent* or *hepatitis D virus* (*HDV*). It was originally thought to be a new HBV antigen. In fact, it is an unclassified RNA virus that codes for the delta antigen. Its capsid consists of HBs antigen, i.e., HBV-coded material. For this reason, the virus can only replicate in persons infected with HBV (in this case the "helper virus").

The delta agent is 36 nm in size and possesses a very short viral RNA containing 1683 nucleotides. This RNA is circular, has antisense (minus) polarity and is reminiscent in size and structure of the RNA in plant viroids (p. 472f.). Its transcription and replication take place in the cell nucleus by means of a cellular polymerase. The resulting RNA sense strand contains, in contrast to viroids, a protein-coding segment comprising about 800 nucleotides, which the cell processes into an mRNA. The HDV codes for two proteins with 27 and 29 kDa (delta antigen). The shorter protein with 195 amino acids, which promotes RNA replication, is produced earlier in the replication cycle. Later, after the stop codon UAG of the mRNA has been transformed (enzymatically?) into UGG, the longer protein with 214 amino acids is synthesized; it inhibits replication and controls the encapsidation of the HDV RNA in the HBs antigen.

Pathogenesis and clinical picture. The incubation period of hepatitis B is four to 12 weeks, followed by the acute infection phase, icteric, or anicteric course, once again with a variable duration of two to 12 weeks. The hepatic cell damage resulting from an HBV infection is not primarily due to cytopathic activity of the virus, but rather to a humoral and cellular immune response directed against the virus-induced membrane antigens (HBs, HBc) on the surface of the infected hepatocytes: 0.5–1% of those infected experience a fulminant, often lethal, hepatitis. In 80–90% of cases the infection runs a benign course with complete recovery and elimination of the HBV from the body. A chronic infection develops in 5–10% (see p. 393, persistent viral infections). Three forms are differentiated, but mixed forms are possible:
— healthy HBV carriers,
— chronic persistent hepatitis (CPH) without viral replication, and finally
— chronic aggressive hepatitis (CAH) with viral replication and a progressive course.

A chronic infection can result in development of a carcinoma (hepatocellular carcinoma, HCC) or cirrhosis of the liver, with incidence varying widely from one geographic area to another. The delta agent appears to have an unfavorable influence on the clinical course, usually making the disease more aggressive, increasing the number of complications and worsening the prognosis.

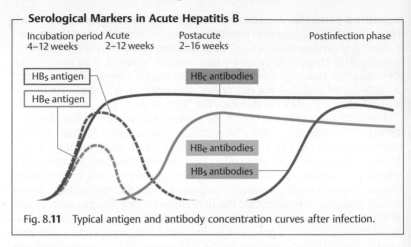

Fig. 8.11 Typical antigen and antibody concentration curves after infection.

Diagnosis. Hepatitis B is diagnosed by identifying the various HBV antigens or the antibodies directed against them. Both antigens and antibodies can be detected in patient blood using a solid phase test (enzyme immunoassay). The individual components manifest in specific patterns. Fig. 8.11 shows the sequence of phases in an uncomplicated hepatitis B infection, upon which the guiding principles in laboratory diagnosis of HBV infections are based (Table 8.1).

The hepatitis D virus is diagnosed by detection of delta antigen or possibly antibodies to delta (IgM) in the blood.

Tab. 8.1 Laboratory Diagnostics in HBV Infections

Status	Diagnostic test
Acute infection	HBc-IgM, HBs-Ag
Vaccine immunity	HBs-IgG
Recovered, healed	HBs-IgG, HBc-IgG
Chronic, patient infectious	HBe and HBs-Ag, PCR
Exclusion of HBV	HBc-IgG negative
Serology inconclusive, mutants, therapeutic monitoring	Quantitative PCR

Chronic hepatitis B

Development of a chronic hepatitis B infection is revealed by a changed antigen-antibody profile: the two antigens HBs and HBc (and raised transaminases) persist for over six months, whereby antibodies to HBe and HBs are not produced. A subsequent "late seroconversion" of HBe antigen to anti-HBe antibodies supports a better prognosis. Thorough clarification of chronic cases must include either immunohistological testing for HBV antigens in liver biopsies or PCR testing for the presence of viral DNA, and thus Dane particles, in patient serum.

Epidemiology and prevention. Humans are the sole reservoir of HBV. Transmission is parenteral, either with blood or body fluids containing HBV (sexual intercourse) that come into contact with mucosa, lesions, or microlesions in the skin. In transmission by blood, the tiniest amounts contaminating syringe needles, ear-piercing needles, tattooing instruments, etc. suffice to produce an infection. Hepatitis B infections from blood transfusions have been greatly reduced by thorough screening of blood donors for HBs antigens, despite which patients receiving multiple transfusions or dialysis remain a high-risk group.

Another high-risk group includes all healthcare workers with regular blood contact. All blood samples must be considered potentially infectious and handled only with disposable gloves. Addicts who inject drugs with needles are also obviously exposed to a very high level of risk.

Since no effective chemotherapy against HBV has been developed to date, the WHO recommends general hepatitis B prophylaxis in the form of active immunization with HBs antigen. In response to a sudden high-level infection risk (accidental inoculation with infectious material), persons whose immune status is uncertain should also be passively immunized with human anti-HBs antiserum—if possible within hours of pathogen contact.

It has not yet proved feasible to grow HBV in vitro. The antigen used in vaccinations can be isolated from human blood. Fear of AIDS infections has resulted in emotionally based, unjustifiable rejection of this vaccine. An alternative vaccine is now available based on developments in genetic engineering: the HBs antigen can now be synthesized by a yeast fungus.

Prevention: hepatitis B booster vaccines. Periodic booster shots, especially for persons at high risk, were recommended for some time to maintain sufficient immune protection. However, since all successfully vaccinated persons build up immunity rapidly following renewed contact with the pathogen ("immunological memory," see p. 94), this recommendation has been replaced in a number of countries by the following scheme:

Following immunization on the classic model (0, 1, and 6 months), the anti-HBs antibody titer is measured within one to three months. Responders (titer 100 IU/l) require no booster. In hyporesponders and nonresponders (ti-

8

ter <100 IU/l), an attempt should be made to reach a titer of 100 IU/l with a maximum of three further vaccinations.

RNA viruses

Viruses with Single-Stranded RNA Genomes, Sense-Strand Orientation

To date, six viral families with single-stranded RNA genomes in sense-strand orientation are known: picornavirus, calicivirus, togavirus, coronavirus, flavivirus, and retrovirus (common orthography: picornavirus, retrovirus, etc.).

Picornaviruses

■ The important human pathogenic genera of picornaviruses are:
- **Enteroviruses** with the polioviruses (poliomyelitis), cocksackieviruses and echoviruses.
- **Parechoviruses** types 1 and type 2.
- **Hepatoviruses** with the hepatitis A virus.
- **Rhinoviruses**, common cold viruses (rhinitis).

Transmission of enteroviruses, parechoviruses, and hepatoviruses is by the fecal-oral route. The viruses first replicate in the intestine, from which location they reach their target organ with the bloodstream. Large numbers of inapparent infections are typical of this group.

Rhinoviruses are transmitted by droplet infection and remain restricted to the upper respiratory mucosa.

Diagnosis: enteroviruses and parechoviruses are diagnosed by isolation in cell cultures or with PCR, hepatitis A serologically (IgM) and rhinoviruses, if at all, by isolation.

Prevention: basic polio immunization with dead or live vaccine; hepatitis A with dead vaccine; exposure prophylaxis with rhinoviruses. ■

The picornaviruses (Fig. 8.**12**: polioviruses) are among the most thoroughly studied viruses of all. The name *picorna* is an abbreviation that stands for two characteristics of this family: they are small (*pico*) viruses with an RNA genome (*rna*). The RNA is polyadenylated at its 3' end and has no cap at the 5' end, but instead a virus-coded, basic protein about 2 kDa in size, the VPg

--- Poliovirus ---------------------------------

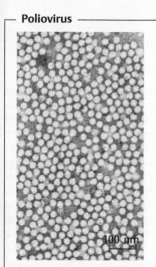

Fig. 8.**12**   Polioviruses are 24–30 nm in size and cause poliomyelitis.

(**v**irus **p**rotein, **g**enome-linked). It consists of approximately 7500 bases forming 2207 coding triplets (in the poliovirus). The combination of the ribosomes with the RNA is not, as in cellular mRNA, at the cap of the 5' end ("scanning model") but rather internally in the nontranslated region (NTR), which is about 750 nucleotides long and is positioned before the coding segment. The translation product of this RNA is a precursor polyprotein about 250 kDa in size, which is proteolytically divided into about 20 individual, functional proteins during or immediately after its synthesis. The N-terminal end of the polyprotein contains the capsid proteins, the middle region proteins that contribute to the expression of the structures required for RNA replication and formation of the CPE (p. 392f.) and the C-terminal segment includes proteins of an enzymatic character (protease for proteolytic cleavage of the primary translation product, see above, and the RNA-dependent RNA polymerase, see p. 385) as well as VPg, which functions as a primer for RNA synthesis.

The different human pathogenic genera of picornaviruses are the enteroviruses, parechoviruses, hepatoviruses, and rhinoviruses.

Enteroviruses (Poliovirus, Coxsackievirus, Echovirus) and Parechoviruses

Pathogen. The genus *Enterovirus*, isolated from the intestinal tract, includes these species:
— Poliovirus (poliomyelitis pathogen) with three serotypes.
— Coxsackievirus, group A, with 22 serotypes.

8

— Coxsackievirus, group B, with six serotypes.
— Echovirus with 34 serotypes.
— Enteroviruses numbers 68–71.

The genus *Parechovirus* includes the species parechovirus types 1 and 2.

Pathogenesis and clinical pictures. The enteroviruses and parechoviruses are transmitted per os and replicate at first in the lymphoid tissue of the pharyngeal space, later mainly in the intestinal wall. They then reach their "target organs" via the bloodstream (e.g., CNS, muscles, heart, liver), followed by manifest organ infection, which, however, only develops in a small percentage of cases. Most infections run an asymptomatic course. Viremia is always present, so that even asymptomatic enterovirus and parechovirus infections confer effective immunity. The cases of manifest infection frequently run atypical courses with mild clinical symptoms. The same viral type can cause different symptoms and several different viral types can cause a given clinical symptom. Recently, severe complications have been described, mainly as a sequel to hand, foot, and mouth disease (HFMD, Table 8.2) in Southeast Asia.

The following clinical pictures have been described for enteroviruses and parechoviruses (Table 8.2):

Diagnosis. The available laboratory diagnostic tools include PCR or isolation of the virus from cerebrospinal fluid, pharyngeal smear, or lavage, with the best chances of success from stool. Serodiagnosis plays only a minor role.

Epidemiology and prevention. Humans are the reservoir of the enteroviruses. Transmission is either direct (smear infection) or in food and water.

8

Table 8.**2**   Enteroviruses and Parechoviruses: Clinical Syndromes

Virus type	Important syndromes
Polioviruses	Poliomyelitis, paralysis, aseptic meningitis, encephalitis
Coxsackie viruses A & B, echoviruses, enterovirus 68–70	Meningitis, paralysis, pharyngitis (herpangina), pneumonia, hepatitis, maculous and vesicular exanthems, including hand, foot, and mouth disease (HFMD)
Coxsackie virus B	In addition to the above: myalgia, pleurodynia (Bornholm disease), pericarditis and myocarditis, pancreatitis, diabetes
Enterovirus 71	Acute hemorrhagic conjunctivitis, HFMD
Parechovirus 1 and 2	Respiratory and gastrointestinal ("summer diarrhea") infections

Where hygienic standards are high, droplet infections also play a significant role. Special prophylactic measures to prevent infections with coxsackieviruses or echoviruses are neither practicable nor generally necessary.

Salk introduced a dead vaccine in 1954 for poliomyelitis prophylaxis (IPV, inactivated polio vaccine) consisting of three poliovirus types inactivated by formalin. Five years later, the live vaccine (OPV, oral polio vaccine according to Sabin) was introduced, which contains three live but no longer neurovirulent poliovirus strains, either singly or in combination. The WHO plan to eradicate poliomyelitis worldwide would seem feasible with this vaccine as demonstrated by its eradication in several countries including all of South America.

Polio Vaccines: Pros and Cons

The **dead or inactivated vaccine** has the advantage of a long stability period and practically foolproof application safety. The disadvantages of this vaccine form are its high cost, the requirement for three injections and weaker or at least shorter-lived protection than is provided by the attenuated form. Work is ongoing on development of enhanced (eIPV) vaccines of this type.

The advantages of the **live vaccine** are its oral application route, low price and high level of efficiency. One disadvantage is its thermolability, resulting in reduced numbers of seroconversions (more nonresponders) in tropical countries. Another difficulty is presented by the (1 in 1×10^6) cases of paralysis (vaccination-associated paralytic poliomyelitis, VAPP) resulting from a vaccination. VAPP shows a higher level of incidence than infections by the wildtype poliovirus in industrialized countries, which has led practically all these countries to return to using IPV.

Hepatoviruses (Hepatitis A Virus)

8

Pathogen. The hepatitis A virus differs in some characteristics from enteroviruses, to which group it was long considered to belong. Growth in cell cultures requires long adaptation. Only one serotype is known to date.

Pathogenesis and clinical picture. The clinical picture of hepatitis A, so-called epidemic or infectious hepatitis, differs in no major particulars from that of hepatitis B (p. 429). The disease nearly always takes a benign course. Only a small number of fulminant (and sometimes lethal) or chronic courses have been described. The pathogenic process at first corresponds to that of the enteroviruses, whereby hepatitis A replicates in the intestine and then, after a brief viremic episode, attacks its target organ, the liver. Disease manifestation with this pathogen, unlike most of the enteroviruses but similar to hepatitis B, involves immunological processes.

Diagnosis is based on IgM detection due to the early presence of these antibodies in patient serum, in fact so early that a lack of hepatitis A antibodies at the onset of clinical manifestations excludes hepatitis A.

Epidemiology and prevention. Transmission is by food and water or in the form of smear infections. Infection with hepatitis A shows a clear north–south gradient: it has become virtually a travelers' disease in central Europe. Imported cases frequently cause minor outbreaks in families or schools. Active immunization with an inactivated HAV vaccine is available.

Rhinoviruses

Pathogens. The genomic organization and replication system of the rhinoviruses (117 serotypes found to date) generally match those of the enteroviruses, although they differ in that they are acid-sensitive and slightly denser.

Pathogenicity and clinical picture. The rhinoviruses, the causative pathogens of the common cold, infect the mucosa of the nasopharyngeal space (nose and throat). They remain strictly localized there and do not cause generalized infections. In rare cases, mainly in children, they are known to cause bronchitis or bronchopneumonia as well. The clinical picture is often worsened by bacterial superinfection.

Diagnosis. Laboratory diagnostics are only required in special cases of rhinovirus infection. The viruses can be grown in cell cultures.

Epidemiology and prevention. Rhinoviruses are transmitted directly, for example by contaminated hands, and partly by droplet infection as well. Infective contacts between humans appear to involve mechanical inoculation (introduction into the nasopharyngeal space with fingers). Rhinoviruses occur worldwide, with pronounced proliferation in the winter months. The fact that everyone comes down with colds repeatedly is explained by the very brief immunity conferred by infection and the many different viral types involved. Experiments have shown that the infections are always exogenous, i.e., not reactivations due to cold, wetness, etc. The only conceivable prophylactic measure is to avoid large groups of people.

Astrovirus and Calicivirus; Hepatitis E

■ Astroviruses, measuring 28–30 nm and caliciviruses, 30–35 nm, are enteritis pathogens in small children. Human pathogens in these groups include the Norwalk virus and hepatitis E virus (HEV). The latter occurs epidemically and endemically in Asian, Central American, and African countries. It is transmitted by the fecal-oral route, above all via drinking water, and causes relatively benign infections except in pregnant women. Hepatitis E is considered a traveler's disease. ■

Isolated cases and minor outbreaks of enteritis are typically attributed to unspecified viral infections. Besides unidentified bacterial infections, the viral pathogens that can cause such infections include adenovirus, rotavirus, astrovirus, and calicivirus, whereby the taxonomy of the latter two have not been confirmed.

Astroviruses

Pathogen. The astrovirus is 28–30 nm in size and owes its name to its starlike appearance. It contains sense RNA with approximately 7 500 nucleotides and appears to have a replication strategy similar to that of the picornaviruses.

Pathogenesis and clinical picture. Astroviruses that are animal and human pathogens are associated with episodes of diarrhea that nearly always run a harmless course. The etiological role of these viruses has still not been clarified. Astroviruses appear to possess only a low level of pathogenicity. It should be mentioned at this point that the role of viruses in enteritis is frequently exaggerated.

Diagnosis. Detection by means of electron microscopy.

Epidemiology. Astroviruses occur worldwide. They tend to infect young children and older persons weakened by other diseases.

Caliciviruses

Pathogen. Caliciviruses are 30–35 nm, possess only one capsid protein and a polyadenylated, 7500-nucleotide RNA with a VPg at the 5′ end. The surface of the viruses has a characteristic structure with small, regular, calyxlike concavities that give the capsid the form of a Star of David.

Caliciviruses are classified based on genomic similarities as either human caliciviruses (HuCV) or "small, round-structured viruses," SRSV. This designation stems from their initial identification under the electron microscope as "small, round, virus particles." The SRSV are grouped in two subtypes, I and II. Type I includes the Norwalk virus and a number of similar viruses named for their geographic venues, some with antigenicity differing from the Norwalk type.

Clinical picture. Caliciviruses cause enteritis. Together with rotaviruses (p. 456) and adenoviruses (p. 416), they are the most frequent viral enteritis pathogens in children, often causing minor epidemics during the winter months ("winter vomiting disease").

8

Diagnosis. Detection by means of electron microscopy or antigen assay in stool.

Epidemiology. Two-thirds of the adult population in the temperate zone carry antibodies to the Norwalk virus. SRSV are regularly implicated in minor epidemics and family outbreaks. The transmission route of the Norwalk virus has been described: in addition to the fecal-oral route, water and uncooked foods are involved.

Hepatitis E Viruses

Pathogen. An infectious inflammation of the liver endemic to Asia, Central America, and parts of Africa is apparently transmitted by the fecal-oral route. The RNA genome of the culprit agent has now been sequenced and the virus in question, the hepatitis E virus, has been classified with the caliciviruses. It occurs in at least 13 variants divided into three groups. In-vitro culturing of HEV has not succeeded to date.

Pathogenesis and clinical picture. The clinical course of hepatitis E infections tends to be benign and resembles that of hepatitis A. It shows no chronicity. However, infections in the third trimester of pregnancy have a lethality rate of 10–40%.

Diagnosis. The antibodies can be detected by means of an enzyme immunoassay. Apparently due to cross-reactions with other caliciviruses, the specificity of the results is uncertain. A diagnosis is often arrived at based on clinical evidence and medical history (travel to endemic areas).

Epidemiology. HEV causes repeated outbreaks of considerable dimensions in the parts of the world mentioned above. The infections can be traced to contaminated drinking water. Hepatitis E is imported to central Europe as a traveler's infection, although apparently less frequently than hepatitis A. No specific prophylactic measures exist.

Togaviruses

■ The togavirus family (*Togaviridae*) comprises two genera. ***Alphavirus*** infections are transmitted by arthropods and are imported to central Europe mainly by travelers to tropical and subtropical countries. Their clinical pictures are variable, but almost always include joint pain (arthralgias). The most important representative of the genus ***Rubivirus*** is the rubella virus, the causative agent in German measles. This normally harmless childhood disease can cause severe embryopathies during the first trimester of pregnancy. ■

Pathogen. The term togaviruses formerly included a variety of viruses, including what we now classify as the flaviviruses. As defined today, the togaviruses include the zoopathic pestiviruses, one species of rubivirus, the rubella virus and the alphaviruses with 25 species. The alphaviruses most important to travelers are the Chikungunya virus (Africa, Asia), the Sindbis virus (Africa, Asia, Australia), the Ross River virus (Australia, Oceania), and the Mayaro virus (South America), which are transmitted to humans by bloodsucking mosquitoes.

Togaviruses possess an icosahedral capsid and a closefitting envelope. The capsid measures 35–40 nm and the entire virion 60–65 nm. The genome of the togaviruses is a single-stranded, polyadenylated, sense RNA. Replication not only produces new 40S genomic RNA, but a subgenomic 26S RNA fragment as well, which codes for the capsid proteins. Viral progeny are released by "budding" at the cell surface.

Pathogenesis and clinical picture. The arthropodborne alphaviruses, zoonoses of the tropical and subtropical regions, frequently cause asymptomatic or benign infections with fever, exanthem, and joint pain. Occasionally, however, persistent arthralgia and polyarthritis (lasting months or even years) do occur, sometimes involving joint destruction. Even rarer, sequelae include encephalitis and meningoencephalitis with high lethality rates.

"German measles" is a harmless exanthemous infection in children and youths, caused by a rubivirus, the rubella virus, and transmitted by direct contact. The infections remain inapparent in nearly half the cases. The virus at first replicates in lymphoid organs at the portal of entry and in the nasopharyngeal space, after which a viremia develops before the exanthem manifests. In pregnant women, the virus takes this route through the placenta to the embryo, where it can cause congenital deformities or embryonic death, especially in the first three months of pregnancy. The organs in the developmental stage in this trimester are most seriously affected by the rubella infection. The most frequent congenital deformities are deafness, cataracts, cardiac defects, microcephaly, and spina bifida. In intrauterine embryo deaths due to rubella infections the immediate cause of death is usually myocardial damage. A measles infection confirmed by IgM detection or a raised antibody count is therefore an indication for a first-trimester abortion.

8

Diagnosis. Serodiagnosis is the method of choice in suspected alphavirus and rubivirus infections. EIA methods are also available for IgM detection.

Prevention. There are vaccines to protect against alphavirus infections and rubella. The main aim of rubella prophylaxis is to prevent rubella-caused embryopathies. Since 10–15 % of young adults are still susceptible to rubella infections and a live vaccine with few side effects that confers reliable immunity is available, serial vaccination of children (boys and girls!) is done before puberty. The vaccine is tolerated so well that prior immune status checks are not required.

Arboviruses

The term "arbovirus" (arthropodborne virus) was originally used as a synonym for togavirus. It is now no longer an official taxon since it refers only to the arthropod vectors, whereas the variety of virus types transmitted by this route is much greater, including for instance togavirus as well as flavivirus types.

Flaviviruses

■ Viruses in the flavivirus family (*Flaviviridae*) include the genera *Flavivirus*, *Hepacivirus*, and *Pestivirus*. **Flaviviruses** (the prototype being the yellow fever virus [Latin: *flavus*, yellow]) are transmitted by arthropods. They cause a biphasic infection that can have serious consequences (hemorrhagic fever with a high lethality rate). In southern and eastern countries, these viruses are significant human pathogens. Only one representative of this family, the tick-borne encephalitis pathogen, is encountered in Europe.

The **hepaciviruses** (**hepatitis C** [HCV] and **hepatitis G viruses**) are not arthropodborne. HCV is transmitted mainly in blood (transfusions, blood products, intravenous drug use) and is a frequent cause of chronic disease (70% of cases), including cirrhosis of the liver and hepatocellular carcinoma. The hepatitis G virus (HGV) is related to HCV and has not been characterized in detail as yet.

Pestiviruses are only important in veterinary medicine.   ■

Flaviviruses show morphological uniformity with an icosahedral capsid and closefitting, spiked envelope. The size of the capsid is about 30 nm and the whole virion measures 45 nm. The genome of the flaviviruses is a single-stranded sense RNA about 10 kb in size. It codes for three structural and seven nonstructural proteins. Both cotranslational and posttranslational protein processing (cleavage, p. 388), similar to what is seen in the picornaviruses, has been described. The morphogenesis of the virus occurs at the endoplasmic reticulum, into the lumen of which the finished viruses bud. These characteristics have not been directly demonstrated for the hepatitis C virus, which cannot be cultured in vitro.

The pestiviruses cause severe animal epidemics (e.g., swine fever). They are not transmitted by arthropods.

Flavivirus (Arthropodborne Yellow Fever Type)

Pathogen. The flavivirus family includes 63 species, among them the proto-typic virus of the family, the yellow fever virus, and the pathogen that causes European tickborne encephalitis (spring-summer meningoencephalitis, SSME). Table 8.3 lists the flaviviruses that cause significant travelers' diseases.

Pathogenesis and clinical picture. The arthropodborne flaviviruses cause diseases of different levels of severity. The infections are typically biphasic with an initial, not very characteristic phase including fever, headache, muscle pain, and in some cases exanthem (Denguelike disease). This phase in-

Table 8.**3** Overview of the Most Important Flaviviruses (arthropodborne)

Viral species	Transmitting vector	Geographic spread	Syndrome
Dengue	Mosquito (*Aedes, Stegomyia*)	West Africa, Pacific, South and Southeast Asia, Caribbean, Venezuela, Colombia, Brazil	Dengue syndrome, DHF, DSS
Yellow fever	Mosquito (*Aedes*)	West and Central Africa, South and Central America	Hemorrhagic fever
Japanese B encephalitis	Mosquito (*Culex*)	East, Southeast and South Asia, western Pacific	Encephalitis
St. Louis encephalitis	Mosquito (*Culex*)	North and Central America, Brazil, and Argentina	Encephalitis
West Nile fever	Mosquito (*Culex*), ticks (*Argasidae*)	East and West Africa, South and Southeast Asia, Mediterranean countries, recently USA as well	Dengue syndrome, encephalitis
Tickborne encephalitis (Central European* and Russian)	Ticks (*Ixodes*)	Central Europe, Russia	Encephalitis

* Syn. spring-summer meningoencephalitis (SSME)

8

cludes a pronounced viremia. The illness, in this stage often not recognized as a flavivirus infection, may then be over or it may progress after one to three days to a second, severe clinical picture: a hemorrhagic fever with a high lethality rate involving hemorrhages and intravasal coagulation. In Dengue fever, this form is becoming more and more frequent and is called Dengue hemorrhagic fever (DHF) or Dengue shock syndrome (DSS) depending on the predominant characteristics.

▬ Dengue Hemorrhagic Fever (DHF) or Dengue Shock Syndrome (DSS) ▬

One reason for the manifestation of more severe Dengue courses is the increasing mobility of the populace. This leads to the phenomenon of people overcoming one Dengue infection, then traveling to an area where a different Dengue serotype is endemic. What happens if they are infected again is known as an "antibody-dependent enhancement of viral infection" or ADE, see p. 399). Antibodies from the first infection attach to the viruses of the fresh infection, which are, however, not neutralized, but instead allowed entrance into cells via Fc receptors, resulting in DHF and DSS. Children still carrying antibodies from their mother during the first year of life can also experience these severe infection courses due to the same mechanism.

Diagnosis. A flavivirus infection always involves viremia (transmission by bloodsucking arthropods!). The viruses can be isolated from blood by inoculating cell cultures or newborn mice. In autopsies of fatal cases they can be isolated from liver tissue. The viruses are labile by nature and identification can take time, for which reason the diagnostic focus is on serology (titer rise or IgM detection).

Epidemiology and prevention. A cycle of infection involving a vertebrate host (mammals, birds) and a transmitting vector (bloodsucking mosquitoes and flies, ticks) has developed for most flavivirus infections. The cycles are efficient for the virus and relatively harmless for the host. The vertebrate host frequently shows few signs of disease and recovers from the infection after a brief viremia. During this period, the bloodsucking vector is infected, which thereafter remains a lifelong salivary secretor and thus infectious. In ticks, transovarian transmission of the virus is also possible. The human host is a dead end for the virus, not a normal component of the cycle. Exceptions to this are Dengue fever and urban yellow fever.

Humans are the only known main hosts for the Dengue virus. There are two forms of yellow fever: rural or jungle ("sylvatic") yellow fever with a monkey-mosquito-monkey (sometimes human) cycle and urban yellow fever with humans as the main hosts and *Aedes* mosquitoes as the transmitting vectors. This form is on the upswing due to increasing numbers of breeding places (e.g., empty tin cans in garbage piles) for the vector. Another "new" (more accurately: revived) infectious disease is the West Nile viral infection, observed for the first time in the USA (New York) in 1999, apparently introduced into the area by migrating birds. It is still not known why the geographic distribution of the virus or infected birds changed.

Vaccines are available against yellow fever (live vaccine) and European tickborne encephalitis (dead vaccine).

Hepaciviruses (Hepatitis C and G)

Pathogen. A series of hepatitis infections following blood transfusions was observed that could not be identified as either hepatitis A (p. 437) or hepatitis B (p. 429), and were therefore designated as "non-A-non-B (NANB) hepatitis." The discovery of the hepatitis C virus (HCV) by molecular biological means in 1988 was an elegant piece of work: RNA was extracted from the plasma of an infected chimpanzee, from which cDNA was produced using reverse transcriptase. The cDNA was then cloned and the corresponding proteins expressed. About one million clones were tested for reactivity with sera from patients suffering from chronic NANB hepatitis. A protein was found by this method that reacted with antibodies to NANB, whereupon the corresponding cloned DNA was used as a probe to identify further overlapping gene segments. They belong to a flavivirus with approximately 10 kb sense RNA and several genotypes. A similar strategy led to identification of a further flavivirus that also causes hepatitis, now known as the hepatitis G virus (HGV).

Pathogenesis and clinical picture. Hepatitis C resembles hepatitis B in many respects. One major difference is that it much more frequently produces a persistent infection (85%) and, in 70% of cases, develops into a chronic hepatitis, resulting in cirrhosis of the liver within 20 years and a hepatocellular carcinoma (HCC) in a further 10 years. The reason for the high level of viral persistence is thought to be a pronounced mutability facilitating evasion of the immune defenses (quasispecies of RNA viruses, p. 391).

Diagnosis of hepatitis C is done with antibody EIA using genetically engineered viral proteins. Western blot can be used to confirm the result. The RNA can be detected by means of RT-PCR and the course of therapy can be monitored with quantitative PCR.

Epidemiology and prevention. The incidence of HCV in Europe is about 0.3%, with a decreasing tendency in the younger segment of the population. About 50% of acute hepatitis cases are HCV infections. Transmission is by blood and blood products. High-risk persons include dialysis patients, healthcare staff, and needle-sharing drug consumers. Perinatal transmission is possible, but sexual contact does not appear to be a risk factor. The transmission route is not apparent in many cases, giving rise to the expression "community-acquired infection." Feasible protective measures are the same as in hep-

8

atitis B; no immunization by vaccine is available. Especially in combination with ribavirin (Table 7.**5**), therapeutic use of interferon can lead to elimination of the virus in persistent infections and thus to prevention of cirrhosis of the liver and HCC.

Coronaviruses

■ Infections with coronaviruses are widespread in humans and animals. Human pathogens include causative agents of rhinitislike infections and the virus of the "severe acute respiratory syndrome" (SARS), which first erupted in China in 2002.

Diagnosis: serology or electron microscopy for common cold strains; PCR or isolation for SARS. ■

Pathogen. The *Coronaviridae* family includes several viral species that can infect vertebrates such as dogs, cats, cattle, pigs, rodents, and poultry. The name (corona, as in wreath or crown) refers to the appearance of the viruses (Fig. 8.**13**). One coronavirus species (human coronavirus, HuCV) is known since some time to be a human pathogen. It has at least two serotypes and probably a number of serological variants. In November 2002, a new coronavirus emerged in China and, after originally being mistaken as a new influenza recombinant, was identified as the causative agent of severe acute respiratory syndrome, or SARS, in spring 2003. Its origin, possibly from animals, is not known to date.

8

— Coronavirus ——————————————————

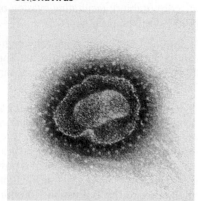

Fig. 8.**13** "Spikes" with club or drumstick-like swellings are located at regular, relatively generous intervals on the pleomorphic envelope, which measures 80–220 nm in diameter.

Coronavirus Replication and Viral Maturation

The coronavirus genome consists of the longest known, sense RNA strand exceeding 30 kb, which is integrated in the envelope in the form of a helical ribonucleoprotein. A hallmark of coronaviral RNA replication is the production of seven subgenomic mRNAs, each of which codes for one viral structural protein. The synthesis of progeny viral RNA takes place in association with specialized membrane structures, characterized as double-membrane vesicles. Viral maturation takes place in the rough endoplasmic reticulum after replacement of cellular proteins by viral proteins in the membranes. The viruses are then transported to the Golgi apparatus. The ensuing virus release mechanism is unknown. Recently, the receptor involved in the entry of the SARS virus into the cell was reported to be the angiotensin-converting enzyme 2 (ACE2).

Pathogenesis and clinical picture. *Common cold*-coronaviruses cause an everyday variety of respiratory infections, which are restricted to the ciliated epithelia of the nose and trachea. They are responsible for about 30% of common cold infections.

The immunity conferred by infection, apparently IgA-dependent, is short-lived. Reinfections are therefore frequent, whereby the antigenic variability of the virus may be a contributing factor. Various enteral coronaviruses with morphologies similar to the respiratory types have also been described in humans. Their pathogenicity, and hence their contribution to diarrhea, has not been clarified.

The *SARS virus* is transmitted aerogenically with an incubation time of two to 10 days. Clinically, fever and a marked shortness of breath is noted, developing into a severe atypical pneumonia with new pulmonary infiltrates on chest radiography. Shedding of virus is by respiratory discharges. Whether the virus present in other body fluids and excreta plays a decisive role for virus transmission is not yet clear.

Diagnosis. The *common-cold coronavirus* can be grown in organ cultures of human tracheal tissue or in human diploid cells. Isolating the viruses for diagnostic purposes is not routine. Serodiagnosis (complement-binding reaction, immunofluorescence or enzyme immunoassay) and electron microscopy are feasible methods.

The SARS virus can be identified by PCR or isolated in the Vero cell line.

Epidemiology and prevention. In November 2002, an outbreak of atypical pneumonia, later termed SARS, occurred in the southern Chinese city of Guangzhou (Guangdong Province). Only in February of 2003, the world was alerted about the lung disease, shortly before it escaped China, when a Guangdong resident in a Hong Kong hotel transmitted it to other guests who spread it to Toronto, Hanoi, Singapore, and elsewhere. Transmission of the virus is by droplets, but close contact ("household transmission")

8

with possibly other routes of transmission seems important. The only preventive measure to date is exposure prevention. Under therapy with ribavirin and intensive care, mortality of SARS is around 10%.

Retroviruses

■ Retroviruses possess an enzyme, reverse transcriptase, that can transcribe ssRNA into double-stranded DNA. This activity is reflected in the designation "retroviruses." Integration of the DNA thus derived from the viral genome in the host-cell genome is a precondition for viral replication. Certain retroviruses are also capable of **onco**genic cell transformation. Due to this potential and their **RNA** genome, these viruses are also called **oncorna**viruses (see Chapter 7).

Human pathogen retroviruses known to date include the types HTLV (human T-cell leukemia virus) I and II and HIV (human immunodeficiency virus) 1 and 2. The former are T-cell malignancy-causing pathogens, the latter cause acquired immune deficiency syndrome—AIDS.

AIDS manifests as a reduction of T helper cells after an average incubation time of 10 years. The collapse of cellular immunity results in occurrence of typical opportunistic infections (*Pneumocystis carinii* pneumonia, fungal and mycobacterial infections, CMV, and other viral infections) as well as lymphomas and Kaposi sarcoma. Transmission is by sexual intercourse, blood and blood products, as well as prenatal and perinatal infections.

Diagnosis: HIV infections are routinely detected by serology (antibodies or viral antigen). The circulating virus count (viral load) is determined by means of quantitative RT-PCR. The AIDS diagnosis is a clinical procedure that presupposes positive confirmation of HIV infection.

Therapy: inhibitors of reverse transcriptase and protease.

Prevention: exposure prophylaxis when contact with blood is involved (drug addicts, healthcare staff) and sexual intercourse. Postexposure prophylaxis and prophylaxis in pregnancy with chemotherapeutics. ■

Pathogen. The *Retroviridae* family is the classification group for all RNA viruses with reverse transcription of RNA to DNA in their reproductive cycles (RNA-dependent DNA synthesis) (p. 385). Only zoopathic retroviruses were known for many years. These viruses cause various kinds of tumors in animals. In 1980, retroviruses were also discovered in humans. This virus family includes seven genera, three of which play significant roles in human medicine:

— **HTLV-BLV retroviruses**, including HTL viruses types I and II and the bovine leukemia virus.
— **Spumaviruses**, which only occur in animals, two of which are (probably) from humans.
— **Lentiviruses**, with the human pathogens HIV 1 and 2, maedivirus (pneumonia), and visnavirus (encephalomyelitis) in sheep, viruses affecting goats and horses, and animal immune deficiency viruses.

A human pathogen retrovirus was isolated for the first time in 1980 from adults suffering from T-cell leukemias. It was designated as HTLV I (human T-cell leukemia virus). A short time later, a virus was isolated from hairy cell leukemia patients and named HTLV II.

HTLV I is found in adults with T-cell malignancy as well as in patients with neurological diseases (myelopathies). HTLV II appears to be associated with T-cell malignancy and other lymphoproliferative diseases. Its own etiological role is still under discussion.

Here is a summary of the human pathogenic aspects of HIV including its relation to acquired immune deficiency syndrome (AIDS).

The viral RNA genome, which is integrated in the genome of the host cell, contains the following genes and regulatory sequences (see. Fig. 8.**14**):

Genes essential to viral replication:

— *tat* gene: "transactive transcription," enhances the transcription and thus the expression of viral proteins by binding to the TAR (transactivation responsive region) in the LTR.
— *rev* gene: posttranscriptional activator for splicing and transport of viral mRNA (production of structural proteins).
— *LTR* sequence: promoter and enhancer elements.

Structural genes:

— *gag* gene: group-specific antigen.
— *pol* gene: codes for the reverse transcriptase, a protease and the integrase.
— *env* gene: envelope glycoprotein (gp).

Genes not essential to viral replication:

— **Virus infection factor (*vif*)**: makes the virus more infectious.
— **"Negative" factor (*nef*)**: inhibits or activates viral transcription as required, influences T-cell activation, reduces CD4 expression.
— *vpr*: controls rate of replication.
— *vpx*: only in HIV 2, controls rate of replication.
— *vpu*: only in HIV 1, contributes to viral release, increases CD4 turnover.

8

Structure and Genomic Organization of HIV

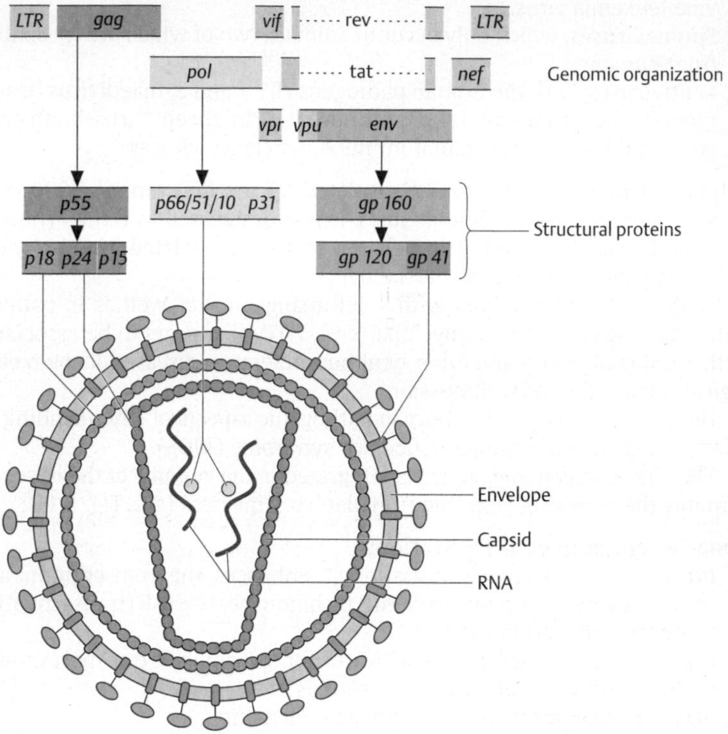

Fig. 8.**14**

Gene	Gene product	Function
Structural genes:		
gag	p55	p55 Nucleocapsid, precursor of p18, p24, p15
	p18	Matrix protein
	p24	Capsid protein
pol		Polymerase region
	p66/51/10	Reverse transcriptase/RNase/protease
	p31	Integrase
env	gp160	Glycoprotein, precursor of gp120, gp41
	gp120	Surface protein (binds to CD4 molecule of host cell)
	gp41	Transmembrane protein
Regulatory genes, see text.		

Human Immune Deficiency Virus (HIV)

HIV replication

HIV can infect T4 lymphocytes and other cells bearing the CD4 marker on their surface. The CD4 molecule is the main receptor for HIV, or more precisely for its gp120 (Fig. 8.**14**). In addition, either the chemokine receptor CCR5 (macrophage-tropic R5 HIV strains) or CXCR4 (T cell-tropic X4 strains) is used as a coreceptor. Persons with (homozygotic) missing CCR5 are highly resistant to HIV infection. A number of other coreceptors are also active depending on the viral strain involved. HIV is then taken in by the cell. After uncoating, reverse transcription takes place in the cytoplasm. The rest of the viral replication process basically corresponds to the description of retroviral replication on p. 385. The interaction of the many different contributing control genes is responsible for the long latency period and subsequent viral replication (see also Fig. 8.**14**).

Replication of HIV takes the form of a lytic cycle, i.e., it results in destruction of the host cell, making it an exception among retroviruses. It must also be noted that the cell destruction mechanism has not been completely explained. Cell fusions are induced by X4 strains (syncytial formation). These processes occur late in the infection cycle and are associated with progression to AIDS. R5 strains do not induce syncytia, are present early in the course of the infection, and are mainly responsible for transmission of HIV. Besides virus-induced cell destruction (p. 392), apoptosis also appears to play an important role in the elimination of CD4$^+$ cells.

Pathogenesis and clinical picture. AIDS was described as a discrete pathology of the immune system in 1981. The pathogenicity of the disease is based on suppression of cellular immunity as a result of the loss of the CD4$^+$ T helper cells.

The primary infection either remains inapparent or manifests as "acute retroviral syndrome" with conjunctivitis, pharyngitis, exanthem, and lymphadenopathy, as well as a transitory meningoencephalitis in some cases. p24 antigen (Fig. 8.**14**) is detectable in serum after about 14 days, i.e., before the antibodies. This stage is followed by a long period of clinical latency (the incubation period is described as 10 years), during which the carrier is clinically normal but may be infectious. The HI virus can persist in a latent state in CD4$^+$ T lymphocytes, macrophages, and the Langerhans cells in the skin. Apparently, viral replication continues throughout this period, especially in lymphoid organs.

The drop in CD4$^+$ lymphocytes and the rise in the virus count (viral load, see below) in peripheral blood is followed by the lymphadenopathic stage. Opportunistic infections then set in, frequently combined with lymphomas, the otherwise rare Kaposi sarcoma, or so-called AIDS encephalopathy (subacute AIDS encephalitis, AIDS dementia complex). Similar neurological symptoms may also be induced because of HIV-induced immunosuppression,

8

Table 8.**4**   Diagnostic Definitions for AIDS in Adults

CD4$^+$ T cells/µl	Clinical categories		
	A	B	C
>500	A1	B1	C1
200–499	A2	B2	C2
<200	A3	B3	C3

A3, B3, and C1–3 confirm AIDS diagnosis

Clinical categories

A: Asymptomatic or acute (primary) HIV infection; persistent generalized lymphadenopathy (LAS)

B: Symptoms indicative of weakened cellular immune defenses, but no AIDS-defining diseases.

C: AIDS-defining diseases:

>*Viruses*
>HSV: chronic ulcer, esophagitis, bronchitis, pneumonia
>VZV: generalized zoster
>CMV: retinitis, encephalitis, pneumonia, colitis
>JC virus: progressive multifocal leukoencephalopathy
>HIV: encephalitis
>HIV: wasting syndrome
>
>*Bacteria*
>Recurrent salmonellar septicemia
>Recurrent pneumonia
>Mycobacterial tuberculosis, pulmonary and extrapulmonary forms
>Opportunistic mycobacteria (*M. avium*, etc.), disseminated or extrapulmonary
>
>*Protozoans*
>*Cryptosporidium*: chronic diarrhea
>*Isospora belli*: chronic diarrhea
>*Toxoplasma gondii*: encephalitis
>
>*Fungi*
>*Candida*: esophagitis, pneumonia, bronchitis
>*Histoplasma, Cryptococcus neoformans*, coccidiosis: extrapulmonary, disseminated
>*Pneumocystis carinii*: pneumonia
>
>*Malignomas*
>Kaposi sarcoma
>Invasive cervical carcinoma
>B-cell lymphoma EBV-positive

8

Toxoplasma or papovaviruses (PML, see p. 415), or lymphomas. Table 8.**4** presents the CDC (Centers for Disease Control) classification of the stages in the course of HIV infection. The number of CD4+ T cells and the occurrence of so-called AIDS-defining diseases determine whether an HIV-positive patient is categorized as a case of AIDS (Table 8.**4**). The probability that an AIDS-defining disease will occur rises precipitously at CD4+ cell counts below 200.

Laboratory diagnosis. The following diagnostic tools are currently available for confirmation of an HIV infection (not the same as manifest AIDS, see above):

■ **HIV antibody detection.** EIA screening tests are now available using genetically engineered or synthesized viral antigens (first to third generation of screening tests). Every positive result requires confirmation by an alternative test (Western blot, see p. 123 and Fig. 2.**24**, p. 125, p24 antigen detection). The fourth-generation screening tests simultaneously detect antibodies to HIV 1 and 2 and p24 antigen (combination test) and are thus capable of detecting primary infections that are still antibody-negative.

■ **HIV antigen detection.** In this test, a viral protein is detected in serum, usually capsid protein p24. The p24 antigen is detectable in serum as early as two weeks after infection and disappears again after eight to 12 weeks. Following a clinically stable latency period, HIV antigen can become detectable months or years later (transitory or persistent). This renewed appearance of HIV antigen is usually followed by manifest AIDS and is therefore a negative prognostic sign.

■ **Rapid HIV test.** Antibody-based tests are available for rapid diagnosis in medical practices, hospitals, and health centers. Their specifications are equivalent to the third-generation screening tests.

■ **PCR.** The most important application of the polymerase chain reaction (PCR, see p. 409) today is to determine the so-called viral load, whereby a commercially available quantitative RT-PCR (reverse transcriptase PCR) is used to determine the number of viral RNA molecules per ml of blood, taking into account the added standard amounts of HIV RNA (quantification standard). This test provides a prognostic estimate of how great the risk of progression to AIDS is (manifestation of an AIDS-defining disease). It can also be used to monitor the success of therapy with RT and protease inhibitors.

The following HIV diagnostic procedure is now recommended: an HIV antibody screening test should first be performed to diagnose an HIV infection. If the test result is positive, a second serum specimen should be tested to confirm the result and exclude confusion of sera. If the initial screening test is negative, but a (primary) HIV infection is justifiably suspected, HIV antigen can be tested, for instance using the combination test.

8

Epidemiology and prevention. HIV is transmitted by blood, blood products, and sexual intercourse. The virus can also be transmitted from mother to child in intrauterine infection, perinatal transmission, or the mother's milk. Infection via saliva or insect bite has not been confirmed. Accordingly, three rules of behavior are now propagated to prevent the spread of HIV: use a good-quality condom for each act of sexual intercourse. For i.v. drug consumption use only sterile syringes and needles; never share or pass on these injection utensils. Couples one of whom is HIV-positive should avoid an unplanned pregnancy.

Intensive efforts are being made to develop a vaccine (active immunization) and several vaccines will soon be ready for field trials. The types under consideration include split vaccines (p. 403), genome-free particles, attenuated viruses, naked DNA, and inactivated virions. It is not practicable to cover this field of research in detail here due to the fast-moving, and the necessarily tenuous, nature of the ongoing work.

Therapy. The recommended therapeutic procedure is also subject to rapid changes, whereby the common goal is to reduce the number of viruses as far as possible (<50 RNA copies per ml) and as soon as possible. Doing so can delay the occurrence of clinical symptoms, eliminate existing symptoms and slow or stop the development of resistance in the HI viruses.

In general, therapy is considered in reaction to the initial retroviral syndrome. Therapy is recommended in the first, asymptomatic stage at CD4+ cell counts below 350, and if the count is higher than 350 only if the viral load is raised (consider therapy at 5000, therapy recommended at >30 000 RNA copies/ml). Pregnancy in an HIV-positive woman is a further therapeutic indication.

Three classes of substances are available for HIV therapy (see also p. 404f.):
- **Nucleosidic (or nucleotidic) reverse transcriptase inhibitors** (NRTI) (for example: azidothymidine, AZT; lamivudine, 3TC; didanosine, ddI, etc.). These are nucleoside analogs that bind to the active center of the enzyme are integrated in the DNA strands, resulting in "chain termination."
- **Nonnucleosidic reverse transcriptase inhibitors** (NNRTI) (for example: efavirenz, EFV; nevirapine, NVP, etc.). This class of substances also inhibits the production of viral cDNA by reverse transcriptase, but does not prevent viral production by infected cells.
- **Protease inhibitors** (PI) (for example: indinavir, IDV; ritonavir, RTV; saquinavir, SQV, etc.): PIs inhibit viral protease and thus viral maturation.

8

■ **Combination Treatments of HIV Infections:** ■

To avoid development of resistant HIV variants, a combination of at least three drugs from at least two substance classes is usually administered. The following combinations are currently established practice:

a) One PI and two NRTIs

b) One NNRTI and two NRTIs

c) Two PIs and one or two NRTIs

d) One PI and one NNRTI, alternatively with one or two NRTIs as well;

e) Three NRTIs

a) and b) appear to produce the best long-term results.

Standard vaccines can be used to prevent other infections, for example opportunistic infections in HIV-positive persons, especially children showing no symptoms. The dead vaccine type is recommended for polio. Live vaccine materials should generally not be used in persons showing AIDS symptoms.

■ **Precautions for Healthcare Staff** ■

All personnel in medical professions should know that HIV is not highly contagious and that precautions, as they apply to hepatitis B, are considered sufficient: wear protective gloves in all situations involving possible contact with blood. If blood droplets could be spattered or sprayed, masks and goggles should also be worn.

If exposure has occurred despite precautions (accidental injection, stab wound, contamination of a wound or mucosa with material containing HIV), immediate commencement of a combination therapy with one PI and two NRTIs for two to four weeks is indicated in addition to a thorough wound toilet and disinfection.

8

Viruses with Double-Stranded RNA Genomes

Reoviruses

■ Reoviruses possess a segmented, double-stranded RNA genome. Among the reoviruses, the rotaviruses are the most significant human pathogens. They cause diarrhea in small children and the elderly and can also produce severe sequelae in immunosuppressed patients.

Diagnosis: reovirus—isolation; rotavirus—antigen detection or electron microscopy. Isolation of this viral type in cell cultures is not a routine method. ■

Pathogen. The name *reo*virus is derived from the abbreviation for respiratory enteric orphan virus, recalling that no diseases were associated with the virus upon its discovery (hence "orphan virus"). The family *Reoviridae* includes, in addition to phytopathogenic and zoopathogenic strains, three genera in which human pathogens are classified:

— **Coltiviruses** include a large number of pathogens significant in veterinary medicine as well as the human pathogen virus that causes Colorado tick fever.
— **Reoviruses** in the narrower sense, with three serogroups.
— **Rotaviruses**, groups A to F, further subdivided into subgroups, serotypes, and electropherotypes (see below). The rotaviral genome consists of eleven segments of double-stranded RNA. Each segment codes for one viral protein. Some segments in other reoviruses code for two or three proteins.

Pathogenesis and clinical picture.

— **Coltiviruses.** Colorado tick fever usually runs a mild course with fever, myalgias, nausea, and vomiting, rarely encephalitis.
— **Reoviruses.** Implication of these viruses in diseases is still uncertain. It appears they are capable of infecting the respiratory and intestinal tracts of children. The fact that they are also found very frequently in asymptomatic persons makes it difficult to correlate them with specific clinical pictures.
— **Rotaviruses**. In the mid-seventies these viruses were recognized as diarrhea-causing viruses in infants and small children (Fig. 8.**15**). They are the most frequent cause of diarrhea in children aged six months to two years. It was recently discovered that they also play a role in infections of the elderly, and above all in immunosuppressed patients (e.g., bone marrow transplant patients), and can cause severe clinical pictures in these groups. Rotaviruses enter the body per os or by droplet infection, replicate in the villi of the small intestine and cause diarrhea, potentially resulting in exsiccosis.

Diagnosis. Colorado tick fever can be diagnosed serologically. Reovirus infections can be diagnosed by isolating the pathogens in cell cultures. Rotaviruses do not readily grow in cell cultures for diagnostic purposes. They can be detected more readily under an electron microscope or in antigen assays using commercially available solid phase tests (EIA) or passive agglutination. An elegant typing method for the different rotavirus strains involves analysis of the electrophoretic mobility of the 11 dsRNA strands of the viral genome.

Epidemiology. Humans are the sole natural reservoir of the infant pathogen rotaviruses. Generalized contamination is practically 100% when children reach school age, but carriers and reinfections are still possible despite immunity. Diarrheal infections are among the most important causes of death in

Rotaviruses

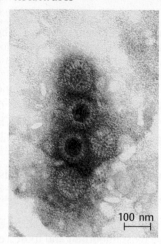

Fig. 8.**15** TEM image of rotaviruses in stool from an infant suffering from diarrhea. All of the viruses in the family Reoviridae possess a double icosahedral capsid. The outer capsid has a diameter of approximately 70 nm, the inner capsid approximately 40 nm. It contains the segmented RNA genome, comprising from 10 to 12 double-stranded subunits depending on the species.

100 nm

small children in developing countries; 20% of these infections are due to rotaviruses. In the temperate zone, rotaviruses are implicated in fewer individual infections; here they more frequently cause winter outbreaks in hospitals and homes for small children. Rotaviruses remain viable for long periods on objects and skin (hands!) and are therefore spread rapidly by infected persons and healthy carriers. The most effective prophylactic approach is to practice stringent hygiene.

8

Viruses with Single-Stranded RNA Genomes, Antisense-Strand Orientation

Six viral families have an antisense RNA genome: the *Orthomyxoviridae*, the *Bunyaviridae*, the *Arenaviridae*, the *Paramyxoviridae*, the *Rhabdoviridae*, and the *Filoviridae*. Just like all other RNA viruses, they require a RNA-independent RNA polymerase, which enters the cell within the viral particle in the infective process.

Orthomyxoviruses

■ The representatives of this family are the different influenza A viruses. The A type is the most important of the three. It is the pathogen responsible for epidemics and pandemics, since its antigenicity structure changes within a narrower range due to point mutations (more frequent) and within a broader range due to recombination (less frequent). Type B tends to be endemic and type C is very rare. Influenza viruses are the classic flu pathogens, whereby the clinical picture is often characterized by bacterial superinfections as well.

Diagnosis: isolation in cell cultures, serology later in the course of the infection.

Prevention: dead vaccine for high-risk persons, e.g., with circulatory diseases.   ■

Pathogen. This family has one genus, *Influenza virus*, with the three types influenza A, B, and C. Influenza A is by far the most important and most frequently observed influenza virus. It repeatedly causes epidemics and even pandemics at greater intervals, in contrast to influenza B, which tends to persist in endemic form and causes few outbreaks. Influenza C is rarely isolated, most frequently in youths. It plays on a minor role as an infective pathogen.

Structure and Replication

All influenza viruses show the same structure (see Fig. 7.**3**, p. 380) and a pronounced pleomorphism. In human tissues and fresh isolates, some filamentous forms several micrometers long are found, with increasingly round forms dominating after several laboratory passages. The genome of the influenza viruses is segmented and comprises eight separate antisense RNA strands, each of which codes for one specific protein. Together with the nucleoprotein, they form the helical nucleocapsid. Closely association with this structure is the RNA polymerase complex, which consists of three high-molecular-weight proteins with different functions. The nucleocapsid itself is embedded in a protein (so-called membrane or matrix protein). The virus is enclosed by an envelope made of cell membrane lipids with viral protein inclusions (hemagglutinin and neuraminidase, responsible for infectivity and viral progeny release). Both proteins are seen under the electron microscope as protrusions ("spikes") on the virus surface.

Replication of the influenza viruses proceeds as described on p. 385 for the antisense-strand viruses, whereby the **cap** of the viral mRNA is acquired by way of a unique mechanism. First, a protein of the polymerase complex separates the cap, together with 10–13 nucleotides, from the cellular RNA molecules by cleavage. This short, cap-bearing sequence serves as the primer in the synthesis of viral mRNA, which therefore begins with a cellular cap and a small piece of cellular RNA.   ▶

Continued: **Structure and Replication**

The close association of cellular and viral transcription is also reflected in the fact that RNA synthesis in the myxoviruses takes place in the nucleus of the host cell and not, as in other RNA viruses, in the cytoplasm.

Pathogenesis and clinical picture. The aerogenically transmitted influenza viruses normally replicate in the mucosa of the nasopharynx, resulting in a pharyngitis or at most a tracheobronchitis, after an incubation period of 24–72 hours. Pulmonary dissemination of the infection can result from an upper respiratory infection or manifest without one, whereby the prognosis in the latter case is less favorable. Pneumonia caused solely by the influenza virus is rare. As a rule, bacterial superinfections with staphylococci, streptococci, pneumococci, or *Haemophilus* bacteria are responsible. These infections, which used to be the normal cause of influenza deaths (*Haemophilus influenzae* in the "Spanish flu" of 1918), can be controlled with antibiotics.

Diagnosis. Influenza viruses can be grown and isolated in cell cultures if the diagnostic specimen is obtained very early, i.e., in the first one or two days of the infection. Throat lavages and swabs provide suitable material. The latter must be placed in a suitable transport medium without delay to prevent them from drying out. Identification of the cultured viruses is achieved based on the hemagglutinating properties of the myxoviruses in the hemagglutination inhibition test or by means of immunofluorescence.

If the specimen was obtained too late for virus isolation, a diagnosis can be arrived at by serological means, whereby a rise in the antibody titer of patient serum proves infection.

8

Table 8.**5** Classification and Antigen Structure of Influenza A Viruses

Viral prototype	Predominance	Antigen formula	
		Hemagglutinin (H)	Neuraminidase (N)
A/WS/33 A/PR8/34	1932–1946	HO	N1
A/Cambridge/46 A/F/M1/47	1946–1957	H1	N1
A/Singapore/57	1957–1968	H2	N2
A/Hong Kong/68	1968	H3	N2
A/USSR/77	1977	H1	N1

Epidemiology. Influenza A viruses are genetically variable. Slight antigenic changes are the general rule (antigenic drift, quasispecies, p. 391) and are explained by selection of point mutants in the hemagglutinin under immunological pressure. More profound changes (antigenic shifts) explain the periodic occurrence of influenza A epidemics and pandemics (Table 8.5).

■ Antigenic Shift ▬▬▬▬▬▬▬▬▬▬▬▬▬▬▬▬▬▬▬▬▬▬▬▬

It is assumed that an antigenic shift occurs when gene segments are exchanged between different influenza strains as follows: there are two major reservoirs of influenza A viruses, humans and certain (aquatic) bird species whereby, in the latter, influenza viruses occur with 13 hemagglutinin types and nine neuraminidase types in nearly all possible combinations. Mixed infections with avian and human virus strains are observed in pigs, made possible by certain farming practices, e.g., in Asia where duck and/or pig husbandry are practiced together with fish breeding. This makes it possible for different viral strains to infect the same host and for two strains to infect the same host cell, which can result in a recombination of gene elements from different influenza A strains. Table 8.5 shows antigenic changes in hemagglutinin and neuraminidase observed in the human influenza A virus since the 1930s.

Prevention and therapy. An inactivated adsorbate vaccine and some split vaccines (new: intranasal application) are available for influenza prophylaxis. The vaccine is recommended especially for persons whose occupation exposes them to such infections as well as persons with cardiovascular problems in their medical histories.

The therapeutic options include amantadine, which inhibits the viral uncoating process, and more recently neuraminidase inhibitors. These substances shorten the duration of illness by blocking the release of the viruses from the host cells and their further dissemination in the body.

Bunyaviruses

■ The **bunyavirus and phlebovirus species** are transmitted by arthropods. They cause benign, febrile infections, more rarely infections of the CNS and hemorrhagic fever. All bunyaviruses feature a single-stranded antisense RNA genome with three segments. Certain types of hantaviruses are the pathogens responsible for "hemorrhagic fever with renal syndrome" (HFRS), other types cause the "hantavirus pulmonary syndrome" (HPS). The hantavirus species are transmitted from mouse species to humans aerogenically.

Diagnosis: serological.

Prevention: exposure prophylaxis.

Pathogen. The family *Bunyaviridae* comprises over 200 viral species, among them four human pathogen genera: *Bunyavirus*, *Nairovirus*, *Phlebovirus*, and *Hantavirus*. The bunyaviruses are spherical, 80–110 nm in size, and posses envelopes with spikes formed on membranes of the smooth endoplasmic reticulum. The genome consists of three antisense-strand RNA segments, whereby each segment produces a separate ribonucleoprotein complex, resulting in a unique feature of the virion: it contains three helical nucleocapsids.

Pathogenesis and Clinical Picture.

■ **Genus *Bunyavirus*:** these viruses are transmitted by arthropods. They cause benign forms of encephalitis such as California encephalitis and La-Crosse virus infections, both endemic to the USA, and the Oropouche virus in Brazil.

■ **Genus *Nairovirus*:** the main human pathogen in this group is the Crimean-Congo hemorrhagic fever virus, with a lethality rate as high as 50%. The virus is endemic to southeastern Europe, Central Asia, China, Saudi Arabia, and Africa and is transmitted by ticks as well as by direct contact with infected animals or patients.

■ **Genus *Phlebovirus*:** this group includes the pathogens that cause the benign Pappataci or phlebotomus fever ("sandfly fever"), which occurs in Europe (Italy, Yugoslavia), North Africa, Asia, and South America and is transmitted by the phlebotomus sandfly.

Rift Valley fever (RVF), an acute, febrile disease, rarely also involving hemorrhagic fever, is transmitted by mosquitoes and is endemic to Africa, usually following epizooties in livestock, in which case aerosol infection occurs (slaughtering). Epidemics have been reported with over 200 000 cases in Egypt and 25 000 cases in Senegal. Further epidemics have occurred in Somalia, Kenya, and Sudan.

8

■ **Genus *Hantavirus*:** this genus includes several viral species (or serotypes) (Table 8.**6**) that can be classified in two groups according to the clinical symptoms they cause:

■ the pathogens of **nephropathica epidemica** (NE) and **hemorrhagic fever with renal syndrome** (HFRS),

■ and the **hantavirus pulmonary syndrome** (HPS).

The sources of infection are rodents (mice and rats). The infection is acquired by inhaling aerosols of urine, feces, and animal saliva. In NE and HFRS a renal dysfunction follows the influenzalike symptoms. HPS infection results in a rapidly progressive, acute dyspnea with pulmonary edema and is lethal in 60% of cases.

Table 8.**6** Serotypes of Hantaviruses

Serotype	Syndrome	Geographic dissemination
Hantaan	HFRS, severe form	Asia, southeastern Europe
Belgrade	HFRS, severe form	Southeastern Europe
Puumala	NE	Central and northern Europe
Seoul	HFRS, mild form	Worldwide
Sin Nombre, etc.	HPS	US, Canada

Diagnosis. It is possible to isolate the virus from blood, but the procedure is too drawn-out and costly for routine diagnostics. Serology (IgM detection) is the method of choice, although the results can be difficult to interpret with bunyaviruses due to the rapidly changing antigenic variants produced in many of the viral species.

Epidemiology and prevention. The bunyaviruses and phleboviruses are transmitted by bloodsucking arthropods, whereby the cycle involves either human and vector only or, as with the togaviruses and flaviviruses, a mammal-arthropod-mammal cycle actually independent of humans, and in which human victims represent a dead end for the infectious agent. Hantaviruses are transmitted aerogenically to humans from rodents, in which the viruses persist apathogenically for the lifespan of the animal. The most recent isolates of the HPS pathogens have also apparently persisted in the reservoir animals for a long time, with occasional human infections as shown by retrospective analysis of blood and tissue specimens. Viral outbreaks are explained by sudden plagues of mice. Preventive measures include exposure prophylaxis (avoidance of insect bites and contact with rodents). An active vaccination is available for protection against Rift Valley fever.

Arenaviruses

■ The arenaviruses are "ambisense" viruses, meaning they possess genomic elements with minus (antisense) as well as plus (sense) polarity. It is quite possible for both coding orientations to occur on one and the same segment (of the segmented genome). Rodents are the natural reservoir of these viruses, from which they can infect humans. An infection with the LCM (lymphocytic choriomeningitis) virus is normally harmless. By contrast, infections by the African Lassa and the South American Junin and Machupo viruses show high lethality rates (hemorrhagic fevers).

Diagnosis: Lassa: virus isolation in special laboratories (biosafety level 4). LCM: serology.

Pathogen. Most members of the *Arenaviridae* family were first identified in the 1960s. The protoype arenavirus, the pathogen that causes lymphocytic choriomeningitis (LCM), was identified 30 years earlier. Studies involving this virus have contributed a great deal to our understanding of cellular immunity in general and infection-related immunopathology in particular.

The human pathogens among the arenaviruses are the LCM virus (Europe, America), the Lassa virus (Africa), and the Junin and Machupo viruses (South America). All arenaviruses are spherical to pleomorphic and 50–300 nm in size (on average 110–130 nm). They consist of a "spiked" envelope derived from the plasma membrane, with an inner structure that appears to be granulated when viewed in ultrathin sections. It is to these granula the viral family owes its name (*arenosus* = sandy). They are considered to be host-cell ribosomes. The virion contains at least three strands of host RNA in addition to two viral RNA segments.

Ambisense Genome

The genome of the arenaviruses contains genomic components with sense (plus) polarity and others with antisense (minus) polarity (ambisense viruses, see p. 387) and is structured as follows: the smaller S part (S = small) codes in the 3′ part as an antisense-strand RNA for the nucleocapsid protein (NP) and in the 5′ part as sense-strand RNA for a viral glycoprotein. Each protein is translated separately from the subgenomic RNA; the NP, coded with the antisense orientation, is first transcribed into a sense-strand RNA. The L part (l = large) codes at the 3′ end in antisense-strand orientation for the viral polymerase and at the 5′ end in sense-strand orientation for a regulatory RNA-binding protein.

8

Pathogenesis and clinical picture. The source of nearly all human arenavirus infections is to be found in rodents. The virus enters the body per os, aerogenically or possibly also by skin contact. A pronounced viremia develops at first, followed by organ manifestations. In the case of LCM these are normally harmless and flulike, although they can also develop into meningitis or encephalitis, in rare cases with a lethal outcome. The Lassa virus is pantropic. It causes a hemorrhagic fever affecting nearly all inner organs and has a high rate of lethality. Death results from shock and anoxia. The clinical picture resulting from Junin and Machupo virus infections is similar. Compared to Lassa infections, CNS involvement is more frequent and the lethality rate is somewhat lower with these two viruses.

Diagnosis. In the acute stage, arenaviruses can be isolated from the patient's blood. Postmortem isolation is best done from liver tissue. In the hemorrhagic fevers, especially Lassa fever, the blood is highly infectious and handling it requires proper precautions and utmost care (aerosol formation!). Isolation of the virus is relatively easy in cell cultures. For reasons of safety, only special high-security laboratories are qualified to handle these organisms (e.g., at the Centers for Disease Control and Prevention in Atlanta, GA, USA).

Serodiagnosis is also feasible using standard serological techniques.

Epidemiology and prevention. All arenaviruses are endemic to rodents and are transmitted to humans by these animals.

No specific immunoprophylactic tools have been developed for any of these viruses. As far as exposure prophylaxis is concerned, it must be remembered that the LCM, Junin, and Machupo viruses are not transmitted among humans, but that the Lassa virus *is* transmitted by this route. The most stringent precautions are therefore called for when treating Lassa patients. Healthcare staff must wear special clothing and facemasks and special reduced-pressure plastic tents are recommended as patient cubicles. The therapeutic tools available for treatment are ribavirin and human immunoglobulin.

Paramyxoviruses

■ This family includes the genera:

■ *Parmyxovirus* with the parainfluenza viruses.

■ *Rubulavirus* with the mumps virus.

■ *Morbillivirus* with the measles virus.

■ *Pneumovirus* with the respiratory syncytial virus (RS).

■ **Nonclassified paramyxoviruses** (Hendra, Nipah).

The clinical manifestations include respiratory infections (parainfluenza, pseudocroup, mumps, RS, Nipah, Hendra), parotitis, and infections of other glandular organs (mumps), exanthem (measles), and CNS infections (mumps, measles, Nipah, Hendra).

Prevention: live vaccines are used to protect against measles and mumps; no immunoprophylactic tools are available against the other paramyxoviruses. ■

Pathogen. The family *Paramyxoviridae* is a heterogeneous one, both in its biology and pathogenic properties. It is divided into two subfamilies:

■ *Paramyxovirinae* with the genera:
— *Paramyxovirus* with the human pathogen species parainfluenza virus types 1 and 3.
— *Rubulavirus* with the mumps virus and parainfluenza virus types 2 and 4.
— *Morbillivirus* with the human pathogen measles virus and several zoopathic species that cause severe respiratory infections in various animal species (dogs [canine distemper], cats, cattle, seals, dolphins, turtles).
— The nonclassified, closely related zoopathic and human pathogen *Hendra* and *Nipah* viruses.

■ *Pneumovirinae*, genus *Pneumovirus*, probably with several types of RS virus (respiratory syncytial virus).

Structure of the Paramyxoviruses

All paramyxoviruses have a similar structure (Fig. 8.**16**). They are pleomorphic. The smallest forms are 120–150 nm in size (with the exception of the somewhat smaller RS virus). They also possess an envelope that encloses the nucleocapsid. The genome consists of a continuous, single-stranded antisense RNA. The envelope is derived from the cell membrane. Various viral proteins are integrated in the envelope, visible in the form of spikes. The generic taxons are based on these spikes: parainfluenza and mumps viruses have two types of spikes, one containing the hemagglutinin (i.e., possessing hemagglutination activity) coupled with neuraminidase (HN protein), and the other the so-called fusion (F) protein, responsible for fusion of the envelope with the cell membrane. Measles viruses contain no neuraminidase and pneumoviruses possess only the F protein.

Parainfluenza Virus

8

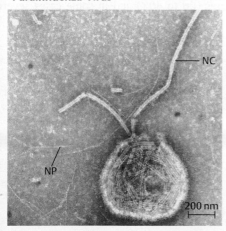

Fig. 8.**16** The envelope here is torn open, allowing the helical nucleocapsid (NC) to escape. NP: primary nucleoprotein helix (TEM).

Pathogenesis and clinical picture.

■ The **parainfluenza viruses** cause flulike infections, mainly in small children, which occasionally progress to bronchitis or even pneumonia. Occasionally, a dangerous croup syndrome develops. Bacterial superinfections are frequent, as are the usually harmless reinfections.

■ In **mumps virus** infections the virus first replicates in the respiratory tract, then causes a viremia, after which a parotitis is the main development as well as, fairly frequently, mumps meningitis. Complications include infection of various glandular organs. Orchitis can occur in postpuberty boys who contract mumps.

■ **Measles.** The pathogenesis of measles has not been fully explained. It is assumed that the virus, following primary replication in lymphoid tissues, is distributed hematogenously in two episodes. Thereafter the oral mucosa displays an enanthem and the tiny white "Koplik's spots." Then the fever once again rises and the typical measles exanthem manifests (Fig. 8.**17**). Possible complications include otitis in the form of a bacterial superinfection as well as pneumonia and encephalitis. A rare late sequel of measles (one case per million inhabitants) is subacute sclerosing panencephalitis (SSPE) in which nucleocapsids accummulate in brain cells, whereby few or no viral progeny are produced for lack of matrix protein. This disease occurs between the ages of one and 20, involves loss of memory and personality changes, and usually results in death within six to 12 months.

■ **Nipah and Hendra virus** infections are zoonoses endemic to Southeast Asia (Nipah) or Australia (Hendra). Both infections result in encephalitis with relatively high lethality rates (up to 40%) and in some cases severe interstitial pneumonias.

8

— **Measles Exanthem** —————————————————————

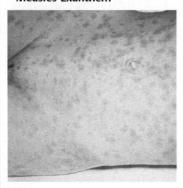

Fig. 8.**17** The typical exanthem manifests during what is presumably the second hematogenous disseminative episode of the morbilliviruses.

■ **RS viruses** cause bronchiolitis or pneumonia, mainly in children up to six months of age, or rarely up to two years. Immune status appears to play an important role in the course of the infection. It has been determined that the course of the disease is more severe in children who have received dead vaccine material (similarly to measles). This is presumably due to antibodies, in the case of small children the mother's antibodies acquired by diaplacental transport. Immunosuppressed patients, for instance, bone marrow recipients, are also at risk for RSV.

Diagnosis. In addition to serodiagnostic methods, direct detection tests based on immunofluorescence or enzyme immunoassay are available for paramyxoviruses, some of them quite sensitive. Paramyxoviruses replicate readily in cell cultures from human tissues.

Epidemiology. Paramyxoviruses are transmitted by droplet infection. Generalized contamination levels in the population (except for Nipah and Hendra) are already very high in childhood (90% in 10-year-old children for parainfluenza virus types 1–3).

Nipah and Hendra viruses are zoonoses that are transmitted to humans from animals (Nipah: pigs, Hendra: horses). Various different animals can be infected by these pathogens, but bats (*Pteropus*) appear to be the natural reservoir for both viruses.

Prevention. Attenuated live vaccines are available for measles and mumps. The **dead** vaccine should not be used due to the aggravating effect mentioned above. No vaccines have as yet been developed for the other parainfluenza viruses.

Rhabdoviruses

8

■ Among the rhabdoviruses, the lyssaviruses, genotypes 1–7, are human pathogens. They are transmitted by the bite of an infected animal in its saliva and infections, once fully manifest, are always lethal (rabies, hydrophobia). The reservoir for type 1 is provided by wild animals in general (foxes, etc.), bats (sylvatic rabies), and, in Asia, dogs (urban rabies). Types 2–7 are restricted to Europe, Asia, Africa, and Australia with their main reservoir in bats.

Diagnosis: direct detection with IF in cornea cells and skin biopsies, postmortem isolation from brain tissues.

Prevention: due to the week-long and even month-long incubation period (except in types 2–4), postexposure prophylactic vaccination with combined active (dead vaccine) and passive (human immunoglobulin) vaccines is possible. Pre-exposure prophylaxis in the form of dead vaccine is administered to persons at high risk. ■

Pathogen. The rhabdoviruses of significance in human medicine are classified in seven genotypes. Type 1 is the classic, worldwide type that occurs in two forms: the "street virus" isolated from humans and animals and the "virus fixe" according to Pasteur. In 1882, Pasteur had transmitted the virus intracerebrally to rabbits. Following repeated passages of the virus in the rabbits, he had developed a dead vaccine type. Due to the brain-to-brain passages in the laboratory animals, the "virus fixe" became so highly adapted to brain tissue that it was unable to replicate in extraneural tissues. Types 2–4 were isolated from African bats, types 5 and 6 from European bats, and type 7 from Australian bats.

Rhabdoviruses are rodlike, 60 × 180 nm in size, with one end flat and one end rounded ("bulletshaped") and a spiked envelope surrounding a nucleocapsid similar to that of the myxoviruses. The genome consists of antisense-strand RNA.

Pathogenesis and clinical picture. Rabies viruses are almost always transmitted by the bite, sometimes also the scratch, of a rabid animal (exceptions, see below). The virus at first replicates at the portal of entry in muscle and connective tissue, then wanders along the nerve cells into the CNS, where more viral replication takes place. Using the same route, the virus then disseminates from the CNS into peripheral organs, above all the salivary glands, cornea, and kidneys. The primary clinical picture is an encephalitis with lethal outcome for humans and animals once it has broken out.

Clinical Course of Rabies

The disease goes through three stages. The initial, or prodromal, stage involves itching and burning at the portal of entry (bite wound), nausea, vomiting, and possibly a melancholy mood. In the second or excitative stage, cramps and spasms of the pharynx and larynx are the main symptoms, rendering swallowing very painful. The spasms can be induced by the mere sight of water ("hydrophobia"). Other mild acoustic and visual stimuli may elicit exaggerated reactions including attacks of cramps and violent anger, hitting, biting, and screaming. Death occurs within three to four days at the earliest. The third, paralytic, stage may develop instead of early death, with ascending paralysis and asphyxia, leading to exitus. Therapy is exclusively symptomatic. Since the patient experiences the disease in a fully conscious state, most of the medication serves to alleviate the pain and anxiety states. The disease runs essentially the same course in humans and animals, whereby the behavior of animals is often radically altered: wild animals lose their fear of humans and tame pets become aggressive. Rabies with the excitative stage is known as "furious rabies," without it as "dumb rabies."

Diagnosis. An intra-vitam laboratory diagnosis is established by examining an impression preparation from the cornea or skin biopsies with immunofluorescence. Postmortem, rabies viruses can be found in the brain tissue of humans and animals by inoculating newborn mice or cell cultures with brain tissue or saliva.

Because antibody production begins so late, serodiagnosis is not practicable. Serological analysis is used to check for vaccine protection. Useful technical tools include an EIA or neutralization test (RFFIT, **r**apid **f**luorescent **f**ocus **i**nhibition **t**est in cell cultures). Special laboratories are used for the diagnostic testing.

Epidemiology. Lyssavirus type 1 is endemic to North America and Europe in wild animals (sylvatic rabies) and in certain tropical areas in domestic pets as well, in particular dogs (urban rabies). The reservoir for the remaining lyssavirus types are bloodsucking (hemovorous) as well as fructivorous and insectivorous bats.

The virus is excreted with the saliva of the diseased or terminal incubator animal and enters other animals or humans through scratch or bite wounds. The virus is highly labile, so transmission on contaminated objects is very rare. Human-to-human transmission has not been confirmed with the exception of cases in which rabies in corneal donors had gone unnoticed.

Prevention. The long incubation period of the rabies virus—in humans several weeks to several months, depending on the localization and severity of the bite wound—makes postexposure protective vaccination feasible. Development of the vaccine originated with Pasteur, who used a dead vaccine from the neural tissues of infected animals. Use of this original rabies vaccine often resulted in severe side effects with allergic encephalomyelitis. The vaccine types in use today are produced in diploid human embryonal cells (HDCV = **h**uman **d**iploid **c**ell **v**accine), hen fibroblasts or duck embryos. No further adverse reactions have been described with these vaccines, so that earlier apprehensions about the rabies vaccine are no longer justified.

The postexposure procedure depends on the type of contact, the species and condition of the biting animal and the epidemiological situation (Table 8.**7**). Exposure is constituted by a bite, wound contamination with saliva or licking of the mucosa, but not by simple petting. In endemic regions, any animal that bites unprovoked must be suspected of being rabid.

Postexposure prophylaxis begins with a rigorous wound toilet, the most important part of which is thorough washing out of the wound with soap, water, and a disinfectant agent. Passive immunization with 20 IU/kg human rabies immunoglobulin (RIG) is then begun, whereby half of the dose is instilled around the wound and the other half is injected i.m. Concurrently, active immunization is started with six doses of HDVC injected i.m. on days 0, 3, 7, 14, 30, and 90. The current therapeutic measures are summarized in Table 8.**7**.

Important: postexposure vaccination is apparently ineffective against the African viral strains (types 2–4).

Table 8.7 Rabies: Postexposure Prophylaxis (according to WHO recommendations issued in Geneva, 1992)

Animal species, epidemiological situation	Condition of animals	Treatment of exposed person[1]
Domestic pet Endemic area	–	HDCV and RIG[2]
Not from endemic area: Dog, cat	Healthy, can be observed for 10 days	None; if animal develops rabies within 10 days, begin immediately with HDCV/RIG
	Suspected rabies or rabid, unknown, escaped	HDCV and RIG
Other pets	–	Depends on epidemiological situation
Wild animal Wild carnivore, bats	Always consider rabid pending negative lab results	HDCV and RIG
Other wild animals: From endemic area	–	HDCV and RIG
Not from endemic area	–	Depends on epidemiological situation

HDCV: human diploid cell vaccine (active vaccination); RIG: rabies immunoglobulin from human source (passive vaccination).
[1] Treatment comprises administration of RIG and HDCV (see text). WHO recommendations also allow use of HDCV alone in cases of minor exposure (licking of skin).
[2] Discontinue treatment if animal under observation remains healthy for 10 days.

Persons exposed to an increased risk of contracting rabies can also be given pre-exposure protection with three doses of HDCV. Postexposure treatment is then limited to the wound toilet and HDCV injections.

Postexposure prophylaxis is impracticable in animals. Dogs and cats in particular must be vaccinated with living vaccine grown in duck embryos. In wild animals (foxes), oral bait vaccination programs have been successful. If the bait contains the attenuated rabies virus, exposure to it must be considered rabies exposure and the postexposure prophylactic procedure must be carried out. This does not apply to use of the recombinant vaccinia virus. However, see p. 428 on the pathogenicity of the vaccinia virus.

Filoviruses (Marburg and Ebola Viruses)

■ Two related African viruses are subsumed under the name filoviruses, Marburg and Ebola. These pathogens cause hemorrhagic fevers with high lethality rates. The few described Marburg virus outbreaks apparently involve monkey populations. Ebola outbreaks are apparently becoming more frequent. The natural reservoir of the filoviruses is unknown.

Diagnosis: by antigen assay, EM, and isolation.　　　　　■

Pathogen. The Marburg virus was isolated for the first time in 1967 as a result of three simultaneous outbreaks among laboratory staff in Marburg, Frankfurt, and Belgrade. The infection victims had been processing the organs of *Cercopithecus* (African green monkeys) from Uganda. Both the Marburg and Ebola viruses are threadlike, 14 μm-long viral particles, in some cases branched and 80 nm thick in diameter. Their surface consists of an envelope of host-cell membrane with viral spikes. The genome consists of antisense-strand RNA in a helical nucleocapsid 50 nm in diameter.

Pathogenesis and clinical picture. The Marburg and Ebola viruses cause so-called hemorrhagic fevers. The clinical picture first manifests with fever, headache, and neck pain, conjunctivitis and diarrhea, followed by hepatic, renal, and CNS involvement and finally, as a result of consumption coagulopathy, leads to extensive hemorrhaging and terminal shock. In terms of the anatomical pathology, nearly all organs show hemorrhages and fibrin deposits.

Diagnosis. Only designated laboratories with special safety facilities can undertake isolation work on these viruses. Detection is either in blood with an electron microscope or using immunofluorescence on tissue specimens. The pathogens can be grown in cell cultures. Serodiagnosis is also possible.

Epidemiology and prevention. The reservoir of the Marburg and Ebola viruses is unknown. Subsequent to the Marburg outbreak in 1967 among lab personnel in Europe, Marburg viruses have only been found in Africa. The Ebola virus, named after a river in Zaire, has caused several outbreaks in Africa since 1976 in which lethality rates of 50–90% were observed. Imported Ebola infections have also been seen in monkey colonies in the USA and Italy.

　　Protective suits and vacuum-protected plastic tents are no longer recommended for healthcare workers in contact with Marburg and Ebola patients (as with Lassa fever), since interhuman transmission is by excretions (smear infection) and in blood, but not aerogenic. Despite this fact, the high level of infectivity of any aerosols from patient material must be kept in mind during laboratory work and autopsies.

8

Subviral Pathogens: Viroids and Prions

■ **Viroids** are phytopathologically significant, noncoding RNA molecules that interfere with cellular regulation as antisense RNA. The hepatitis D virus has some structural similarity to viroids.

Prions consist of a cell-coded protein (PrP: prion protein) altered in its conformation and by point mutations. They are infectious and can cause normal cellular PrP to assume the pathological configuration. They cause the spongiform encephalopathies (Creutzfeldt-Jakob disease, CJD) in the classic and new variants (nvCJD), the Gerstmann-Sträussler-Scheinker (GSS) syndrome, and animal diseases (scrapie, BSE) characterized by neuronal vacuolization and loss and so-called amyloid plaques.

Prevention: exposure prophylaxis (iatrogenic and alimentary transmission). ■

Viroids

Viroids were discovered at the end of the sixties during investigations of plant diseases. They consist of infectious, naked ssRNA in closed circular form with extensive base-pairing to form a rod-shaped strand 50 nm long. This RNA is 10 times smaller than the smallest viral nucleic acid and comprises, depending on the type, only 250–350 nucleotides. It does not function as mRNA and does not code for proteins. Its mode of replication is unknown, but certainly involves cellular enzymes.

Viroids cause a number of plant diseases with considerable economic impact. The following hypothesis is currently under discussion to explain their pathogenicity mechanism: viroids possess complementary sequences to cellular 7S RNA, comprising, together with six proteins, the "signal recognition particle." This particle controls the posttranslational membrane insertion of proteins. Viroids can thus interfere as "antisense (or interfering) RNA" with the function of 7S RNA and thus with membrane formation.

The only significant human pathogen structurally related to the viroids is the hepatitis D pathogen (HDV, delta agent, see p. 429). HDV consists of a viroidlike, also circular, RNA into which an antisense RNA coding for the delta agent is inserted.

Prions

Pathogen. Attention was first drawn to certain encephalopathic agents whose physical properties differed greatly from those of viruses. For instance, they showed very high levels of resistance to sterilization and irradiation procedures. It was later determined that these pathogens—in complete contrast to viruses and viroids—require only protein, and no nucleic acid, as the basis of their infectivity and pathogenicity. This gave rise to the term "prion" for "proteinaceous infectious particle." An intensive search for nucleic acid in the "particles" was fruitless.

Prions are misfolded forms of a cellular protein. They consist of only a single protein (PrP, prion protein), which naturally occurs, for example, on the surface of neurons. The region coding for this protein of approx. 35 kDa is located in a single exon and is derived from a cellular gene expressed in both healthy and diseased brains. Disease-associated PrP (the best-known prion is the scrapie pathogen, the protein of which is called PrP^{sc} [sc for scrapie]), is a mutant, slightly shortened (27–30 kDa) form of the normal PrP^c (c for cell). It differs from normal PrP^c in its altered configuration, its nearly complete resistance to proteases and in the fact that it tends to accumulate inside the cell.

Pathogenesis. Infectious PrP^{sc} can transform naturally occurring PrP^c into PrP^{sc}, resulting in an autocatalytic chain reaction in which mainly the pathological protein is produced. This is why mice lacking the gene for PrP (genetically engineered "knockout mice") cannot be infected with the pathological PrP^{sc} prion. Deposits of large amounts of the pathological protein in the form of so-called amyloid plaques are visible under a microscope in brain tissue from infected humans and animals.

Clinical picture. The following encephalopathies are considered to be caused by prion infections:

In humans:
- Creutzfeldt-Jakob disease (CJD)
- New variant CJD (nvCJD or vCJD)
- Gerstmann-Sträussler-Scheinker (GSS) syndrome
- Kuru

In animals:
- Scrapie (sheep, goats)
- Transmissible mink encephalopathy (TME)
- Wasting disease (deer)
- Bovine spongiform encephalopathy (BSE, "mad cow disease")

8

All of these diseases are designated as transmissible encephalopathies characterized by incubation periods of a number of years, long durations of disease (one to several years in humans) and lethal courses with motor disturbances (animals) and progressive dementia (humans). Histologically, the brain shows no inflammation, but rather vacuolization of neurons, loss of neurons, proliferation of glial cells, and amyloid plaques (see above).

Diagnosis. The diagnostic procedure is histological. Since there is no immune response to the pathological PrP, serodiagnostic methods are useless. The pathological protein can, however, be detected in lymphoid tissue biopsies using monoclonal antibodies.

Epidemiology. CJD, which occurs sporadically (one case per million inhabitants per year) is produced anew in every case by mutations in PrP^c. The disease can be transmitted iatrogenically (brain electrodes, corneal transplants). The pathogenicity of the GSS prion (PrP^{gss}) is based on a single amino acid change. Genetic factors also appear to have a predisposing effect in view of the existence of familial forms of GSS. Kuru is a disease that was spread in New Guinea by cannibalistic rites, probably originating with a case of CJD. Kuru no longer occurs today.

Alimentary transmission is possible in animals. PrP^{sc} was transmitted to cattle by feeding them animal meal made from scrapie-infected sheep remains, resulting in BSE. Despite the fact that transmission of prions from one species to another is not a simple process in principle, BSE prions were transmitted to humans by the alimentary route, resulting in nvCJD. This route of transmission was confirmed by structural analyze of the BSE and nvCJD prions.

From 1995, when the first nvCJD patient died, to the end of 2000, 51 cases of CJD with lethal outcome have been described. In contrast to classic CJD, these infections occurred in young people, whereby the incidence of nvCJD in older persons can be masked by dementias from other causes. The expected outbreak of nvCJD because of the BSE epidemic is currently a topic of extensive discussion.

As a result of this new disease threat, some countries have now prohibited the feeding of animal meal to certain kinds of livestock (in particular ruminants).

V
Parasitology

Trichinella spiralis

9 Protozoa

J. Eckert

General information on parasites. A parasite (from the Greek word *parasitos*) is defined as an organism that lives in a more or less close association with another organism of a different species (the host), derives sustenance from it and is pathogenic to the host, although this potential is not always expressed. In the wider sense, the term parasite refers to all organisms with such characteristics. In medicine the term is used in a narrower sense and designates eukaryotic pathogens, which belong to the protozoa (unicellular organisms Chapter 9) and metazoa, including helminths (parasitic "worms," Chapter 10), arthropods (Chapter 11), and some other groups of lower medical significance (Annelida, Pentastomida, not covered in this book). Parasites cause numerous diseases (parasitoses) in humans, some being of extraordinary significance (e.g., malaria). Of practical concern in central Europe are both autochthonous and imported (tropical and travelers') parasitic infections.

A uniform disease nomenclature has been adopted in this book with the sole use of the suffix *-osis* (plural *-oses*)—for example trypanosomosis and not trypanosomiasis. This system, based on the Standardized Nomenclature of Parasitic Diseases (SNOPAD) (originally published in 1988 and recommended by the International Society of Parasitologists) avoids the inconsistent usage of disease names, such as leishmaniasis on the one hand and toxoplasmosis on the other.

A selection of the most important parasitoses is presented in the following chapters. In Table 1.**10** (p. 28) zoonoses caused by parasites are listed.

Parasitic protozoa are eukaryotic, single-celled microorganisms about 1–150 µm in size and enclosed by a trilaminated cell membrane. They possess one, rarely two nuclei (and multinuclear reproductive forms). Reproduction is asexual by binary or multiple fission of the cell, or sexual. The cellular construction of the protozoa is generally the same as in other eukaryotes but they also exhibit some special features. For example, during the course of evolution some protozoa (*Giardia*, *Entamoeba*) have lost the mitochondria secondarily, except several genomic traits that were laterally transferred to the nuclei. The apicoplast present in some species of Apicomplexa (see *Toxoplasma*) is a residual of a former plastid typical for their ancestors. Some protozoa contain specialized organelles, such as glycosomes (exclusively in trypanosomatids), hydrogenosomes (trichomonads and protozoa

Table 9.1 Provisional Classification of the Protozoa Mentioned in the Text

Phylum ▪ Subphylum	Class	Order	Genus
Metamonada	Diplomonadea	Diplomonadida Enteromonadida Retortamonadida	*Giardia* *Enteromonas* *Chilomastix,* *Retortamonas*
Axostylata	Parabasalea	Trichomonadia	*Trichomonas,* *Pentatrichomonas,* *Dientamoeba*
Euglenozoa ▪ Kinetoplasta	Trypanosomatidea	Trypanosomatida	*Trypanosoma,* *Leishmania*
Amoebozoa	Lobosea	Amoebida	*Entamoeba,* *Iodamoeba,* *Endolimax,* *Acanthamoeba,* *Hartmanella,* *Balamuthia*
Heterolobosa	Schizopyrenidea	Schizopyrenida	*Naegleria*
Alveolata ▪ Apicomlexa	Coccidea	Eimeriida	*Toxoplasma,* *Isospora,* *Cyclospora,* *Sarcocystis,* *Cryptosporidium*
	Haematozoa	Haemosporida	*Plasmodium*
	Piroplasmea	Piroplasmida	*Babesia*
▪ Ciliophora	Litostomatea	Vestibuliferida	*Balantidium*
Microspora[1]	Microsporea	Microsporida	*Brachiola,* *Encephalitozoon,* *Enterocytozoon,* *Microsporidium,* *Nosema, Vittaforma*
		Pleistophorida	*Pleistophora,* *Trachipleistophora*
Incerta[2]			*Blastocystis*

[1] Closely related to fungi. [2] Taxonomy uncertain.

of other groups), and mitosomes (*Entamoeba*) (see under specific protozoan groups). Motile stages of the parasitic protozoa mostly move by means of flagella, cilia, or pseudopodia. Some species produce resistant stages (cysts, oocysts) in which the parasites can survive outside of their hosts for longer periods.

According to current theories, the protozoa are a heterogeneous group consisting of different phyla within the regnum of Eukaryota. The term protozoa has no phylogenetic significance but is still used as a collective name for the various eukaryotic unicellular organisms. The classification of the protozoa is highly controversial. Therefore, all classification systems have to be regarded as provisional (Table 9.**1**).

Giardia intestinalis

Causative agent of giardiosis, lambliosis

■ *Giardia intestinalis* (syn. *Giardia lamblia, G. duodenalis*), a parasite of worldwide distribution, occurs also in Europe with relatively high frequency. It is a parasite of the small intestine of humans that can cause enteritis. Infection occurs by peroral ingestion of *Giardia* cysts. Various species of mammalian animals are reservoir hosts.   ■

Occurrence. *G. intestinalis* has a worldwide distribution with prevalence rates of 2–5% in industrialized countries and very high rates, up to 50%, in developing countries. Children up to the age of five are frequently infected.

Parasite and life cycle. *Giardia* exists in two morphological forms: a motile vegetative stage, the trophozoite, and a cyst stage. The trophozoites live on the small intestine mucosa (less frequently on the gallbladder mucosa as well). They resemble a pear split lengthwise, are 9–21 μm long and 5–12 μm wide and possess eight flagella, two nuclei—one on each side of the longitudinal axis—and two claw-shaped median bodies (Figs. 9.**1** and 9.**11a**). Their dorsal side is convex, the anterior part of the ventral side forms a concave adhesive disk. Reproduction is by means of longitudinal binary fission of the trophozoites, which are able to produce variant specific surface proteins. *G. intestinalis* produces oval cysts (8–18 × 7–10 μm) with four nuclei, flagella, and claw-shaped median bodies. The cysts (and, less frequently, trophozoites) are excreted in stool. Fig. 9.**1** illustrates the life cycle of *G. intestinalis*.

Epidemiology. The genus *Giardia* includes several species (*G. intestinalis*, *G. muris*, *G. agilis*, etc.) that show morphological, biological, and genetic differences. *Giardia* isolates obtained from humans and various species of

– Giardia intestinalis: Life Cycle –

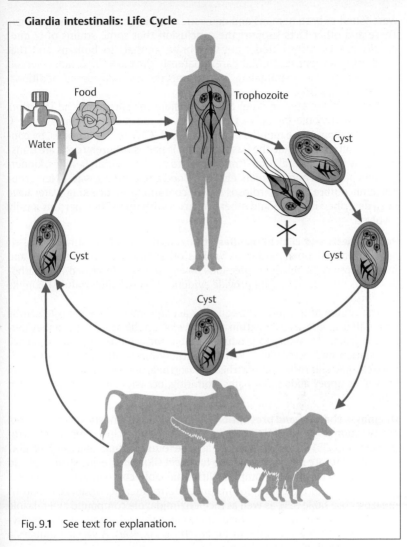

Fig. 9.**1** See text for explanation.

domestic and wild mammals are morphologically uniform and correspond to *G. intestinalis*. However, this is a genetically heterogeneous species, i.e., it comprises a number of different genotypes that can be differentiated by means of isoenzymatic and DNA analysis. Several identical genotypes were found in both humans and domestic animals (e.g., cattle, sheep, dogs). These and other facts support the conclusion that some strains of *G. duodenalis* can be transmitted from vertebrate animals to humans and that giardiosis is a zoonosis. Humans are apparently the most important reservoir hosts and certain mammalian animal species are considered additional sources of infection.

The cysts excreted in stool are responsible for spreading the infection. They remain viable for up to three weeks in moist surroundings at 21 °C and up to about three months in cool water (8 °C). The trophozoites, by contrast, die off soon outside the host. Infection is per os, whereby cysts are transmitted by the fecal-oral route from person to person (within families, kindergartens, between homosexuals, etc.) or in food and drinking water. Numerous epidemic outbreaks of giardiosos due to contaminated drinking water have been described in the US and other countries with up to 7000 persons locally involved.

Pathogenesis and clinical manifestations. In the small intestine, *G. intestinalis* can cause inflammation as well as other morphological changes and malabsorption. Gallbladder infections have also been described. The pathogenesis is unclear; new data provide evidence that *Giardia* produce toxinlike proteins.

The course of infection is frequently asymptomatic. The parasite can be eliminated spontaneously within a few weeks; on the other hand, it may persist for years. The ability to produce variable surface proteins may influence elimination and persistence. Patients with symptomatic infections experience chronic and recurrent diarrhea, steatorrhea, and signs of malabsorption as well as upper abdominal pains, vomiting, occasionally fever, and weight loss.

Diagnosis, therapy, and prevention. The standard diagnostic method is stool examination using the SAFC technique to detect cysts and (more rarely) trophozoites (p. 621). Trophozoites can also be found in duodenal aspirate. IFAT and ELISA kits are now also available to detect *Giardia*-specific structural and soluble antigens in stool samples. Nitroimidazole compounds are used for chemotherapy of infections, for instance metronidazole, ornidazole, and tinidazole (see Table 9.**5**), as well as the benzimidazole compound albendazole and the recently introduced nitazoxanide (nitrothiazole compound). Prophylactic measures are the same as for amebosis (p. 499). A vaccine induces a reliably protective effect in dogs and cats.

Trichomonas vaginalis

Causative agent of trichomonosis

■ *Trichomonas vaginalis* is a frequent flagellate species that occurs world-wide and is transmitted mainly by sexual intercourse. It causes vaginitis in women and urethritis in men. ■

Occurrence. The number of new cases is estimated at 170 million annually (WHO, 1998). In average populations of developed countries, infection rates are about 5–20% in women and usually below 5% in men.

Parasite, life cycle, and epidemiology. *Trichomonas vaginalis* is a pear-shaped protozoon about 10–20 μm long and 2–14 μm wide (Fig. 9.**2**). Five flagella emerge from a basal body at the anterior pole, four freely extend forwards and one extends backwards, forming the outer edge of the undulating membrane, which reaches back only just beyond the middle of the cell. An axial rod made up of microtubules (the axostyle) protrudes with its free tip from the posterior end of the cell. The oval cell nucleus lies near the upper pole of the protozoon. Trichomonads are anaerobic protozoa that possess hydrogenosomes, which are specialized organelles producing H_2 as a metabolite.

T. vaginalis colonizes the mucosa of the urogenital tract and reproduces by longitudinal binary fission. Trichomonads do not encyst, although rounded, nonmotile forms are observed which are degenerated stages without epidemiological significance.

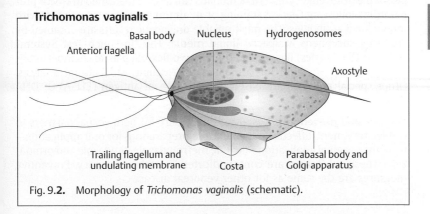

Fig. 9.**2.** Morphology of *Trichomonas vaginalis* (schematic).

Humans are the sole reservoir of *T. vaginalis*. The parasites are transmitted mainly during sexual intercourse. About 2–17% of female neonates born of infected mothers contract a perinatal infection.

T. vaginalis is highly labile outside of a host. Nonetheless, a few trophozoites can survive for up to five hours in the water of nonchlorinated thermal baths and for five minutes to 24 hours in tap water with standard chlorination; they are killed within a few minutes in swimming-pool water with high chlorine concentrations (44 mg/l). It is conceivable that infections could be transmitted by wet bathing suits, sponges, towels, etc. as well as acquired from nonchlorinated thermal baths and poorly maintained swimming pools, but there is no evidence showing that these are significant sources of infection.

Clinical manifestations. In women, *T. vaginalis* primarily colonizes the vaginal mucosa, more rarely that of the cervix. In about 20–50% of cases the infection is asymptomatic, but vaginitis can develop after an incubation period of two to 24 days. The infection results in production of a purulent, thin, yellowish discharge in which trichomonads, pus cells, and bacteria are found. The parasites also enter the urethra in about 75–90% of cases, where they can also cause an inflammation, but only rarely infect the urinary bladder or uterus. Infections in men are for the most part asymptomatic (50–90%), but they may also cause a symptomatic urethritis, more rarely involving the prostate gland and seminal vesicles as well. Infection does not confer effective immunity.

Diagnosis. A fresh specimen of vaginal or urethral secretion is mixed with physiological saline solution and examined under a microscope for trichomonads. The trichomonads are readily recognized by their typical tumbling movements. The round trichomonad forms, by contrast, are hardly distinguishable from leukocytes. Trichomonads can also be identified in smear preparations following Giemsa staining or in an immunofluorescence test with monoclonal antibodies. The most reliable diagnostic results are obtained by culturing specimens in special liquid media. The "In-Pouch Test System" (BioMed Diagnostics) has proved useful: two flexible plastic chambers containing culture medium for combined microscopic and cultural analysis. Other special methods are based on detection of antigen (ELISA) or DNA (PCR).

Therapy and prevention. It is always necessary for both sexual partners to receive treatment. Effective nitromidazole preparations for oral application—in women vaginal application—include metronidazole, tinidazole and ornidazole. These substances are contraindicated in early pregnancy. Preventive measures are the same as for other venereal diseases.

Trypanosoma

Causative agents of African trypanosomosis (sleeping sickness) and American trypanosomosis (Chagas disease)

■ *Trypanosoma brucei gambiense* and *Trypanosoma brucei rhodesiense* cause African trypanosomosis (sleeping sickness) in humans, which presents inter alia as fever and meningoencephalitis. In a chronic form (*T. gambiense*) the disease occurs mainly in western and central Africa, whereas the acute form (*T. rhodesiense*) is predominately distributed in eastern and southeastern Africa. The trypanosomes are transmitted by the bites of tsetse flies (*Glossina*). Antelopes and other wild or domestic animals serve as reservoir hosts of varying significance. *Trypanosoma cruzi*, the causative agent of American trypanosomosis (Chagas disease) occurs in humans and many vertebrate animals in Central and South America. It is transmitted in the feces of bloodsucking reduviid bugs. In recent years, considerable progress has been made in the control of Chagas disease. ■

General. The genus *Trypanosoma* (from *trypanon*: borer and *soma*: body) belongs to the family *Trypanosomatidae* (subphylum *Kinetoplasta*) (Table 9.**1**). One feature of this family is that various forms develop during the life cycle in vertebrates and vectors (insect) involved. The morphologically differentiated forms include spindly, uniflagellate stages (trypomastigote, epimastigote, promastigote) and a rounded, amastigote form (Fig. 9.**3b**). The trypomastigote form of the genus *Trypanosoma* has the following characteristic features: a central nucleus, an elongated mitochondrion containing the kinetoplast in its posterior section, an area free of cristae with especially densely packed DNA (Fig. 9.**3a**). Close to, but outside of the mitochondrion is the base of the flagellum, which originates in the plasmatic basal body. The flagellum is at first enclosed by the flagellar pocket, and then emerges onto the surface of the organism and runs to the anterior end of the organism as a pulling flagellum. The flagellar adheres locally to the cell surface so that an "undulating membrane" is folded out during movement—visible under a light microscope. Special organelles of the kinetoplastids are the membrane-enclosed glycosomes, which contain glycolytic enzymes. The cell is enclosed by an elementary membrane, which in the bloodstream stages is covered by a surface coat or glycocalyx (see below). Spiral microtubules forming a cytoskeleton are arranged along the inner cell membrane (see Fig. 9.**3a** for more cell organelles). In the epimastigote and promastigote forms, the kinetoplast and base of the flagellum are near the nucleus or more toward the anterior end. In the amastigote form, a reduced flagellum is visible by electron microscopy, but it does not emerge onto the cell surface (Fig. 9.**3b**).

9

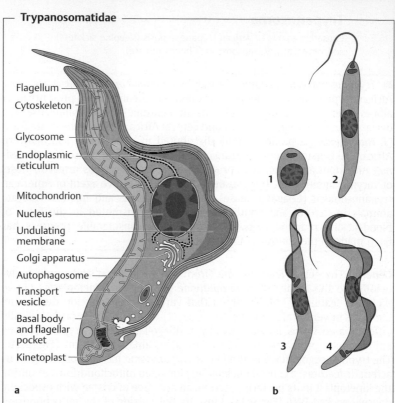

Flagellum
Cytoskeleton

Glycosome
Endoplasmic
reticulum

Mitochondrion
Nucleus
Undulating
membrane
Golgi apparatus
Autophagosome
Transport
vesicle
Basal body
and flagellar
pocket
Kinetoplast

a

b

Fig. 9.3 **a** Ultrastructure of *Trypanosoma* (trypomastigotic form) (according to Warren KS ed. *Immunology and Molecular Biology of Parasitic Infections*. 3rd ed. Boston: Blackwell; 1993). **b** Developmental forms: **1** amastigote, **2** promastigote, **3** epimastigote, **4** trypomastigote.

Trypanosomatidae multiply by longitudinal binary fission. In *Trypanosoma brucei brucei* (see below) there is evidence of genetic exchange during development within the vector (sexual reproduction).

Trypanosoma brucei gambiense and Trypanosoma brucei rhodesiense

Causative agents of African trypanosomosis (sleeping sickness)

Parasite species and occurrence. The causative agents of sleeping sickness are considered to be a subspecies of *Trypanosoma brucei* and therefore their taxonomically correct designations are *Trypanosoma brucei gambiense* and *Trypanosoma brucei rhodesiense*. In the following text they will be designated as *T. gambiense* and *T. rhodesiense*. Morphologically, these two subspecies differ neither from one another nor from *Trypanosoma brucei brucei*, one of the causative agents of the nagana in domestic animals that does not infect humans. These subspecies can be differentiated by means of biological criteria (e.g., host specificity, sensitivity to human serum) as well as isoenzymatic and DNA analysis.

Sleeping sickness occurs only in sub-Saharan Africa in regions between 14° north and 20° south latitude where the vectors (tsetse flies) are endemic (Fig. 9.**4**). Currently between 300 000 and 500 000 persons are infected in the heterogeneously distributed endemic areas in 36 African countries. The official numbers of new cases diagnosed annually (1999: 45 000) are unrealistically low because of the large numbers of unregistered cases (WHO, 2000). In some areas, sleeping sickness has occurred in increased,

Distribution of Sleeping Sickness in Africa

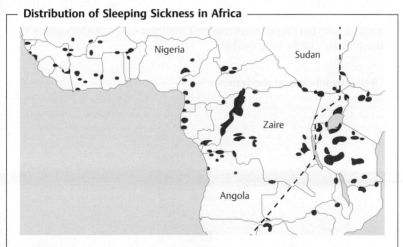

Fig. 9.**4** West of the dotted line preponderance of *Trypanosoma gambiense*, east of the line *T. rhodesiense* (according to *WHO Tech. Ser. 881*, Geneva: World Health Organization; 1998).

even epidemic proportions in recent years. The risk of infection for travelers staying briefly in endemic areas is low, but infections do occur on a regular basis.

Life cycle. *T. gambiense* and *T. rhodesiense* parasitize extracellular in the blood plasma or in other body fluids of vertebrates (Fig. 9.**5**). The trypomastigote forms are pleomorphic in human blood (Fig. 9.**6**): with increasing parasitemia they transform to slender, 25–40 µm-long forms with the flagellar tip extending beyond the anterior end which reproduce by longitudinal binary fission. With decreasing parasitemia, they appear as short, "stumpy" approximately 12–25 µm long forms without a free flagellar end. These forms do not divide in blood but are infective for *Glossina* (tsetse flies). Under a light microscope in a Giemsa-stained blood smear the trypanosomes present as spindly organisms with a central nucleus, a kinetoplast at the posterior end (both stained violet) and an undulating membrane (Fig. 9.**5**). The cell surface of the bloodstream forms is covered with a uniform layer (about 10–15 nm thick) of a specific glycoprotein, which can be replaced by another glycoprotein. These glycoproteins are denominated as variant specific surface antigens (VSSA), the expression of which is coded by about 1000 genes; they form the basis of the organisms' antigen variation (see below).

The trypanosomes taken up by *Glossina* (tsetse flies) when they suck blood from an infected host go through a complex developmental and reproductive cycle in the insects lasting 15–35 days (Fig. 9.**6**). The resulting (metacyclic) stages can then be inoculated into the skin of a host with the fly's saliva. Infected *Glossina* can transmit the trypanosomes throughout their entire lifespan (up to six months).

Trypanosoma brucei rhodesiense

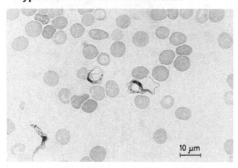

Fig. 9.**5** Giemsa staining of a blood smear preparation.

10 µm

Trypanosoma gambiense and rhodesiense: Life Cycle

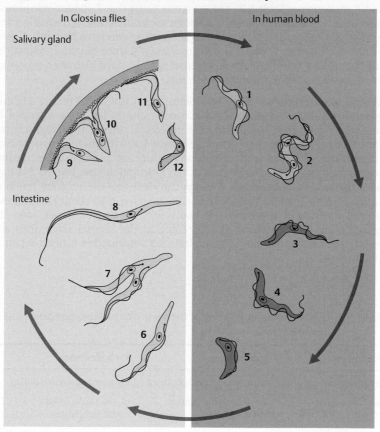

Fig. 9.**6** **Human blood:** **1** trypomastigote, slender form with variant specific surface antigen (VSSA); **2** binary fission form; **3, 4** slender forms with other VSSA type; 5 short ("stumpy") form.

***Glossina* intestine:** **6–8** procyclic forms without VSSA (reproduction by longitudinal fission).

Salivary gland of *Glossina*: **9, 10** epimastigote forms on epithelium; **11** trypomastigote form without VSSA; **12** trypomastigote form with VSSA (metacyclic form). (According to Vickerman K, Barry JE, in Kreier JP, Baker JR, eds. *Parasitic Protozoa*, Vol. 2, San Diego: Academic Press; 1992: 94.)

9

Epidemiology. There are epidemiological differences between *T. gambiense* and *T. rhodesiense* (Table 9.**2**), the main one being that *T. rhodesiense* persists in a latent enzootic cycle in wild and domestic animals and is normally transmitted by *Glossina* from animal to animal, more rarely to humans. *T. gambiense*, on the other hand, is transmitted mainly from human to human by the tsetse flies, although various animal species have also been identified as reservoir hosts for *T. gambiense* strains.

Clinical manifestations. Sleeping sickness is, in the initial phase, a febrile, generalized disease with lymphadenopathy and is later characterized by meningoencephalitic symptoms. The infection runs a two-stage course: the febrile-glandular or hemolymphatic stage 1 and the meningoencephalitic stage 2. The difference is therapeutically significant. In stage 1, the trypanosomes multiply in the tissue fluid at the inoculation site. Within 2–4 days an inflammatory, edematous swelling can develop—the primary lesion or "trypanosome chancre," which then disappears within about three weeks. Within a period of approximately two weeks the trypanosomes enter the bloodstream and lymphatic system. Later, in the second stage, they also invade the central nervous system. Table 9.**3** summarizes further details of the disease.

Table 9.**2** Epidemiological Differences between *Trypanosoma gambiense* and *T. rhodesiense*

Parameter	*T. gambiense*	*T. rhodesiense*
Distribution:	Western and central Africa	Eastern and central Africa
Vector:	*Glossina palpalis* group: Moist biotopes	*G. morsitans* group: Savanna biotopes
Sites of transmission:		
■ Frequently focal:	At rivers, lakes, watering holes, etc.	–
■ Less localized:	In moist forest areas	Savannas
Dominant cycle:	Human → human	Wild and domestic ruminants, other wild animals → humans
Reservoir hosts (for certain *Trypanosoma* strains)	Pigs, cattle, sheep, dogs, a small number of antelope species	Antelope species, cattle, sheep, goats, warthogs, lions, hyenas, dogs, etc.

Table 9.**3** Infection Course and Clinical Manifestations of Sleeping Sickness

Stage, course and symptoms	*T. gambiense*	*T. rhodesiense*
1st stage: Febrile-glandular or hemolymphatic phase		
▧ Trypanosome chancre	In Africans: <5% In Europeans: approximately 20%	Approximately 50%
▧ Onset of parasitemia:	2–3 weeks p.i.	1–2 weeks p.i.
▧ Type of parasitemia:	Low-level, intermittent	High-level, often persistent
▧ Parasitemia-associated symptoms:	Fever, chills, headache, joint and muscle pain, transitory edemas, weight loss, generalized lymphadenopathy (swelling of lymph nodes in neck = Winterbottom's sign); cardiac dysfunction (especially in *T. rhodesiense* infections), anemia, thrombocytopenia, raised serum IgM	
Course:	Chronic (also acute in persons without immunity)	
2nd stage: Meningoencephalitic phase		
▧ Penetration of trypanosomes into CNS:	4–6 months p.i. or later	Frequently after only a few weeks
▧ Symptoms:	Signs of progressive meningoencephalitis, epileptiform convulsions, later somnolence, apathy, coma. Pleocytosis in cerebrospinal fluid, raised total protein and IgM levels.	
Duration of disease, both stages	Months to >6 years	Rarely >3–7 months

9

Pathogenesis and immunology. The course of the infection is characterized by successive waves of parasitemia caused by antigenic variation in successive trypanosome populations (see above). Parallel to an increasing parasitemia, IgM antibodies are produced that are directed against a certain variant specific surface antigen (VSSA) of the trypanosomes, whereupon they eliminate the segment of the parasite population bearing this VSSA. The parasitemia then declines, but the trypanosomes with a different VSSA multiply, whereupon specific antibodies are once again produced. Antigen variation is one of a number of strategies to circumvent host defenses (immunoevasion). About the time when one VSSA variant of trypanosomes is being eliminated from the body, the concentrations of IgG antibodies rise and immune complexes form.

Many factors contribute to the pathogenesis of sleeping sickness, among them the activation of kallikrein, kinin, complement, and the coagulation system by circulating immune complexes (resulting in increased vascular permeability, edema, hemostasis, tissue hypoxia, tissue damage, disseminated intravasal coagulation), in addition anemia, deposition of immune complexes in the kidneys and other organs, immunosuppression, endocrinal disturbances, and CNS damage. The trypanosomes cause CD8+ T cells and macrophages to produce IFNγ and TNF. IFNγ stimulates trypanosomes to multiply. TNF contributes to immunosuppression and may initiate tissue damage.

Diagnosis. Important diagnostic tools include direct detection of the trypanosomes in the blood, lymph node aspirate and, in cerebral forms, in the cerebrospinal fluid (Fig. 9.**5**). Trypanosomes can be detected in native blood preparations, in Giemsa-stained thin smears or in thick blood films (p. 622). Since low-level parasitemias are often present, concentration methods may be required, e.g., microhematocrit centrifugation, anion exchange chromatography, or the QBC technique (p. 531). Other methods are cultivation and mouse inoculation tests (suitable for *T. rhodesiense*). Analysis of lymph node aspirate has a high diagnostic value in infections with *T. gambiense*. To confirm or exclude CNS infections obtain a cerebrospinal fluid sample, centrifuge it, and examine the sediment for trypanosomes. Antibodies in the bloodstream can be detected using various techniques (p. 625). The card agglutination trypanosomosis test (CATT) has proved valuable in epidemiological surveys. Indicators of a stage 2 infection include presence of trypanosomes and/or raised leukocyte numbers and elevated concentrations of protein and IgM in cerebrospinal fluid.

Therapy. Medical treatment of sleeping sickness is highly problematical, since only a small number of effective drugs are available, serious side effects are fairly frequent and drug-resistant trypanosomes are to be expected. In stage 1, *T. gambiense* infections are mainly treated with pentamidine, whereas *T. rhodesiense* infections are treated with suramin. These drugs are not effective in the second stage (cerebrospinal fluid-positive cases), so that the arsenic compound melarsoprol, a relatively toxic substance, must be used in these cases. The worst side effect of this substance is a potentially lethal encephalopathy observed in 1–10% of patients treated with melarsoprol. Eflornithine is used for treating the late stage of the *T. gamibiense* infection. Treatment of sleeping sickness victims should be entrusted to specialists if possible.

Prevention and control. Use individual prophylactic measures to protect against the diurnally active (!) *Glossina* flies. It is very important that tourists wear clothing that covers the skin as much as possible and treat uncovered skin with repellents (see Malaria, p. 535). They should also inspect the interior of cars for tsetse flies and spray with insecticides. *Glossina* flies are targeted by insecticide sprayings in preventive programs. More recently, the flies are also being caught in insecticide-charged traps using attractant colors and odors.

Trypanosoma cruzi
Causative agent of American trypanosomosis (Chagas disease)

Occurrence. Human Chagas disease is endemic in Central and South America and is caused by *Trypanosoma cruzi* (discovered in 1908 by Chagas). This parasite circulates in endemic sylvatic foci between vertebrates and insects (reduviid bugs), the latter transmitting it to humans. Until a few years ago, the endemic area of Chagas disease extended from Mexico to southern Argentina. In recent years parasite transmission to humans has been reduced or prevented in some countries (Argentina, Brazil, Chile, Paraguay, Uruguay) by control measures. The number of infected persons is currently estimated to be 16–18 million (WHO, 2000).

Causative agent and life cycle. In the natural cycle, the reduviid bugs ingest trypomastigote forms of *T. cruzi* in bloodmeals from infected hosts (vertebrate animals, humans). In the intestine of the vector, the parasites convert into intensively multiplying epimastigote stages, and later into trypomastigote forms that are excreted in feces after six to seven days. At subsequent bloodmeals, infected reduviids excrete droppings from which the trypomastigotes infect the host through skin lesions (e.g., lesions of bug bites) or the mucosa (e.g., conjunctiva).

Once in the human body, the parasites are phagocytosed by macrophages or invade other cells, mainly muscle cells (heart, skeletal, or smooth musculature) as well as neuroglial cells. Within the cells, they transform into amastigote forms (1.5–4.0 μm) and multiply by binary fission. Cells filled with up to 500 parasites are called "pseudocysts." After about five days the parasites develop into to the epimastigote form and then the trypomastigote form and return to the bloodstream, whereupon the cell infection cycle is repeated.

The *T. cruzi* organism in the blood of infected hosts (vertebrate animals, humans) is 16–22 μm long. It has a pointed posterior end and a large kinetoplast. Multiplication does not take place in the blood.

Epidemiology. The bloodsucking bugs of the family Reduviidae find a hiding place for the day and quest for food at night. The natural habitats of these insects are nests, animal dens, and other places frequented by vertebrate animals whose blood provides their sustenance. Some species of reduviids (e.g., *Triatoma infestans*, *Rhodnius prolixus*, *Panstrongylus megistus*) have invaded domestic habitats (also in urban areas!) and are typically found in simple human domiciles. Potential carriers of *T. cruzi* include over 150 species of wild

9

and domestic mammals. The most important in epidemiological terms are dogs, cats, rodents, chickens, opossums, and armadillos. Aside from the reduviid vector, *T. cruzi* can be transmitted between humans by blood transfusions, diaplacental infection, or organ transplants.

Clinical manifestations and pathogenesis. Some infected persons react to entry of the parasite into the skin or conjunctiva with a local, inflammatory dermal reaction (chagoma) or conjunctivitis with eyelid edema (Romaña sign). The following symptoms are observed in the acute phase, which follows an incubation period of seven to 30 days: fever, edema, lymph node swelling, hepatomegaly, splenomegaly, myocarditis, and, less frequently, meningoencephalitis. Beginning about eight to 10 weeks after the acute phase the infection turns to an inapparent phase: serum antibodies are detectable, as are parasites in 20–60% of cases (by means of xenodiagnosis). Clinical manifestations of the chronic phase, often starting 10–20 years after the acute phase, are cardiopathy (cardiomegaly, 30% of cases), digestive tract damage (megaesophagus, megacolon, etc., 6%), and neuropathies (3%).

The important pathogenic processes include immunologically induced destruction of ganglial cells in the autonomic nervous system that have adsorbed *T. cruzi* antigen (resulting in dysfunction and organomegaly in various organs) and inflammatory processes, especially in the myocardial tissues, probably the result of autoimmune reactions. Inapparent *T. cruzi* infections can be reactivated by AIDS.

Diagnosis. In the acute phase, trypanosomes are detectable in peripheral blood at the earliest one to two weeks after infection (thick blood films, centrifugation in hematocrit tubes, blood cultures; sensitivity 60–100%). In the chronic phase, detection of the parasites by conventional means is no longer reliable (sensitivity <10%). Tools for detection of low-level parasitemias include xenodiagnosis (from *xenos*, foreign: reduviids free of trypanosomes are allowed to suck the blood of persons in whom an infection is suspected or suck patient blood through a membrane; after a few weeks, the reduviids are examined for trypanosomes) or specific DNA detection by PCR. The apathogenic species *Trypanosoma rangeli* must be taken into consideration in differential diagnosis. Serological methods are also available that can be diagnostically useful in the chronic phase in particular (Table 11.**5**, p. 625).

Therapy and prevention. In the early phase of an infection, cure rates of 80% have been achieved with nifurtimox and benznidazole. Both of these preparations frequently cause side effects. Preventive measures concentrate mainly on vector eradication with insecticides, improvement of living conditions, individual protection from reduviid bites with mosquito nets (see Malaria, p. 535), and measures to prevent transfusion and transplantation infections.

Leishmania

Causative agent of leishmanioses

■ Leishmanias are transmitted by sandflies (Phlebotomidal) and cause the following main forms of leishmanioses in warm regions: visceral leishmanioses (VL), cutaneous leishmanioses (oriental sore) (CL), and mucocutaneous leishmanioses (MCL). In Central Europe, leishmaniosis is of significance as an imported disease and as an HIV-associated infection.   ■

Distribution of Leishmanioses

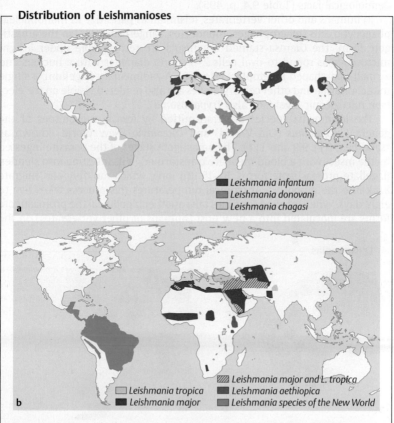

Fig. 9.**7**   **a** Visceral leishmaniosis, **b** cutaneous and mucocutaneous leishmanioses (according to Bryceson ADM, in Cook GC, ed. *Manson's Tropical Diseases*. 20th ed., London: Saunders; 1996: 1217–1219).

Occurrence. Various forms of leishmanioses occur in the warmer regions of 88 countries in Asia, Africa, Europe (Mediterranean countries!), and Latin America (Fig. 9.**7**). The annual number of new cases is estimated at 1.5–2 million (0.5 million VL, 1–1.5 million CL and MCL). Both geographic distribution and case numbers are reported to be on the increase (WHO, 2000).

Parasites and life cycle. The many (about 15) species of the genus *Leishmania* pathogenic to humans do not show morphological differences. They can be differentiated on the basis of biological criteria, laboratory analyzes (mainly isoenzyme patterns and DNA analysis), the different clinical pictures, and epidemiological facts (Table 9.**4**, p. 495).

In humans and other vertebrates, leishmanias parasitize in mononuclear phagocytic cells (macrophages, monocytes, Langerhans cells) in the amastigote form. The Giemsa-stained organisms are recognizable under a light microscope as round-to-oval cells 2–5 μm in diameter with a nucleus and a small, rod-shaped kinetoplast (Fig. 9.**8**). A rudimentary flagellum, a single mitochondrion and other cell organelles are also rendered visible on the electron microscopic level (see also *Trypanosoma*).

The leishmania species are transmitted by female mosquitoes of the genera *Phlebotomus* (Old World) and *Lutzomyia* (New World) known as "sandflies" (Fig. 9.**9** and 11.**1**). The amastigote stages of the parasite ingested by the insect with a blood meal are transformed in its intestine into slender, flagellate promastigote forms 10–15 μm long, which multiply and migrate back into the proboscis. At tropical temperatures this process takes five to eight days. When infected sandflies take another bloodmeal the promastigote forms are inoculated into a new host (humans or other vertebrates). In the

Leishmanias

Fig. 9.**8** **a** Leishmanias in a macrophage. **b** *Leishmania infantum* in a bursting macrophage; Giemsa staining of a bone marrow smear.

Table **9.4**   Selected Forms of Leishmanioses in Humans
(L.: subgenus *Leishmania*, V.: subgenus *Viannia*)

Visceral leishmanioses [1]

Main localization:	Internal organs, less often skin.
Incubation:	In most cases 3–6 months, also: several weeks to years
Primary symptoms:	Fever, splenomegaly, hypergammaglobulinemia, progressive anemia, leucopenia etc.

■ *L. (L.) donovani:*   Asia: India, Bangladesh, southern Nepal. Mainly in adults. Reservoir hosts[2]: humans. Vectors: *Phlebotomus* species.

■ *L. (L.) donovani:*   Africa: Mainly Sudan, Ethiopia, Kenya. Reservoir hosts: humans, dogs (*Felidae*, rodents?)[2]. Vectors: *Phlebotomus* species.

■ *L. (L.) infantum:*   Mediterranean region (Iberian Peninsula to Turkey, northern Africa), Middle East and central Asia, China. In children and adults; in adults cutaneous manifestations as well: Reservoir hosts: humans, dogs, wild *Canidae*. Vectors: *Phlebotomus* species.

■ *L. (L.) chagasi[3]:*   Central and northern South America. Mainly in youths. Reservoir hosts: humans, dogs, fox species, (opossum?). Vectors: *Lutzomyia* species.

Cutaneous leishmanioses (oriental sore)

Main localization:	Skin.
Incubation:	Weeks to months.
Primary symptoms:	On skin accessible by *Phlebotomus* species, development of solitary or multiple, dry, later possibly ulcerating papules; rarely spread to lymph vessels and nodes. Healing with scarification. Solid immunity is conferred by infections with *L. major* and *L. tropica*.

■ *L. (L.) major:*   Northern Africa, Middle East, Sahel Zone, western Asia. Incubation: up to 2 months. "Moist," (= "rural," or "zoonotic") form. Rapid growth of cutaneous lesion, later ulceration and healing within 6 months. Reservoir hosts: rodents. Vectors: *Phlebotomus* species.

■ *L. (L.) tropica:*   Mediterranean region, southwestern Asia to India. Incubation: 2–24 months. "Dry," (= "urban," or "anthroponotic") form. Development of lesions and persistence longer than with *L. major*. Reservoir hosts: humans. Vectors: *Phlebotomus* species.

9

Table **9.4** *Continued: Selected Forms of Leishmanioses in Humans*

■ *L. (L.) aethiopica:*	Ethiopia, Kenya. Cutaneous leishmaniosis. Reservoir hosts: rock hyrax and bush hyrax. Vectors: *Phlebotomus* species.

American cutaneous and mucocutaneous leishmanioses

Main localization:	Skin, mucosa.
Primary symptoms:	Skin changes similar to oriental sore. Some forms tend to spread to mucosa and cause severe tissue destruction.
■ *L. (L.) mexicana-* complex:	Southern US (Texas), parts of Central America and northern South America. Various *Leishmania* subspecies. Destructive cutaneous form. Reservoir hosts: woodland rodents. Vectors: *Lutzomyia* species.
■ *L. (V.) braziliensis* complex:	Parts of Central and South America. Various *Leishmania* subspecies. Mucocutaneous form ("espundia"). Reservoir hosts: woodland rodents, sloth, opossum. Vectors: *Lutzomyia* species.
■ *L. (V.) peruviana:*	Peru (Andes). Cutaneous form ("uta"). Reservoir hosts: dogs. Vectors: *Lutzomyia*

[1] Kala (Hindi) azar (Persian) = black disease (due to hyperpigmentation of skin caused by the infection) is the name given in India to the infection caused by *L. (L.) donovani*.
[2] Reservoir hosts: Epidemiologically significant hosts from which vectors can transmit parasites to humans. In parentheses with question mark: significance questionable.
[3] *L. chagasi* and *L. infantum* have many similarities. It is therefore assumed that *L. infantum* was imported to South America in dogs from Europe.

host, they bind host components to their surface (IgM, complement, erythrocyte receptor) and, thus equipped, couple to macrophage receptors. They are then phagocytosed and enclosed in a phagolysosome, where they are protected from the effects of lysosomal enzymes inter alia by substances in their cell membrane. The promastigotes quickly (within 12–14 hours) transform into amastigote stages, which are finally surrounded by a parasitophorous vacuole within the phagolysosome and reproduce by binary fission. The amastigote forms are then released in a process resembling exocytosis and can infect new cells.

Clinical manifestations and immunology. The most important human forms of leishmanioses are summarized in Table 9.**4**. It is important to note that in CL and MCL the parasites generally remain restricted to the skin or skin and mucosa. CL lesions may persist for long periods, but tend to heal spontaneously, whereas a greater tendency to destructive changes is seen in MCL infections. By contrast, in VL the leishmania organisms can invade the entire

Leishmania infantum: **Life Cycle**

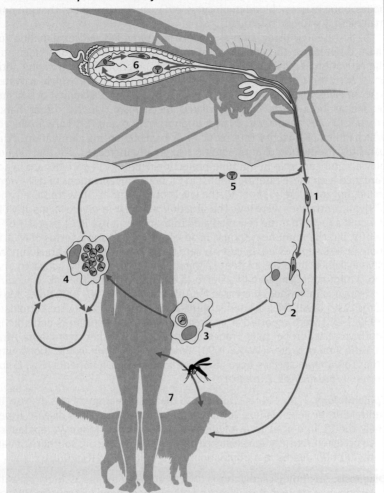

Fig. 9.**9** **1** Inoculation of promastigote stages by sandfly; **2** ingestion of parasites by phagocytes (Langerhans cells, dendritic cells, macrophages); **3** amastigote form in parasitophorous vacuole of a macrophage; **4** reproduction of amastigote forms in a macrophage; **5** ingestion of amastigote forms by sandfly with blood meal; **6** transformation into promastigote form and multiplication in insect; **7** dog as reservoir host.

mononuclear phagocytic system in various organs (spleen, liver, lymph nodes, bone marrow, blood monocytes, etc.), causing infections that are normally lethal without treatment.

Basic research using animal models has provided and explanation for these differences: the course of an infection is apparently dependent on the activation of various T lymphocyte subpopulations by *Leishmania* antigens. Activation of TH1 cells involves production of IFNγ, which activates macrophages that exert a protective effect by killing *Leishmania* organisms by means of a nitric oxide-mediated mechanism. On the other hand, when TH2 cells are activated large amounts of IL-4 and IL-10 are produced, which inhibit NO activity, thus reducing or even preventing elimination of the parasites. Production of antibodies is also greatly increased, but they do not play a significant role in immune protection. Findings in patients are in accordance with these interpretations: in CL, high concentrations of IFNγ were found, but in severe cases of VL the levels of IL-4 and IL-10 were raised and IFNγ concentrations were low. The situation is similar in severe forms of MCL. It would appear that the cell-mediated immune response in CL protects efficiently, but the immune response in advanced VL and some forms of MCL is more or less suppressed. In cases where the immune defenses are additionally weakened by AIDS, a latent *Leishmania* infection may be activated and take a fulminant symptomatic course. In endemic regions, the risk to acquire a *Leishmania* infection is increased for AIDS patients by 100–1000 times. Most of the cases of AIDS-associated leishmaniosis (about 50%) registered to date (1990–1998) were reported from areas in which *L. infantum* is endemic in southwestern Europe (Italy, France, Spain, Portugal) (others from India, Africa, Latin America, etc.) (WHO, 1999). Besides *L. infantum*, coinfections with other *Leishmania* species have also been found in AIDS patients (e.g., *L. donovani*, *L. braziliensis*, *L. tropica*).

Epidemiology. Table 9.**4** refers briefly to the epidemiology of this disease. In central Europe, leishmaniosis deserves attention as a travelers' disease, especially the VL imported from Mediterranean countries. Major VL epidemics have occurred recently in various parts of the world, e.g., in southern Sudan with 100 000 deaths in a population of <1 million (WHO, 2000).

Diagnosis. An etiological diagnosis of VL is made by means of direct parasite detection in aspirate material from lymph nodes or bone marrow (in HIV patients also in the enriched blood leukocyte fraction) in Giemsa-stained smears (uncertain!), in cultures (in which promastigotes develop) or using PCR. Cultivation and PCR have about the same high level of sensitivity. Antibodies are detectable in nearly all immunocompetent patients (around 99%), but 40–50% of HIV-coinfected patients are seronegative (Table 11.**5**, p. 625).

Diagnosis of a cutaneous leishmaniosis is usually based on clinical evidence. Etiological verification requires direct parasite detection (see above) in smears or excised specimens from the edges of the skin lesions. More reliably, the parasites can be detected by cultivation or PCR. Serological antibody tests are positive in only a small proportion of cases.

Therapy and prevention. Treatment of VL is usually done with pentavalent antimonials (meglumine antimonate, sodium stibogluconate) pentamidine, or amphotericin B. The recurrence rate is relatively high, especially in HIV patients. Miltefosine, a newly developed and well tolerated antitumor alkylphospholipid for oral application, has proved effective against VL. Various forms of CL (for instance *L. major* and *L. tropica*) can be influenced by injecting antimonial preparations into the lesions; mucocutaneous leishmaniosis (*L. braziliensis*) is treated systemically with antimonials (see above, amphotericin B, or pentamidine). An effective chemoprophylaxis has not yet been developed. It is therefore important to prevent Phlebotome bites with fine-meshed, insecticide-impregnated "mosquito nets" (p. 535). Control of the vectors involves use of insecticides and elimination of breeding places.

Entamoeba histolytica and Other Intestinal Amebas

Causative agents of amebosis (entamebosis, amebiasis)

■ Of the various amebic species that parasitize the human intestinal tract, *Entamoeba histolytica* is significant as the causative agent of the worldwide occurring entamebosis, a disease particularly prevalent in warmer countries. The vegetative stages (trophozoites) of *E. histolytica* live in the large intestine and form encysted stages (cysts) that are excreted with feces. The infection is transmitted by cysts from one human to another. The trophozoites of *E. histolytica* can penetrate into the intestinal wall and invade the liver and other organs hematogenously to produce clinical forms of amebosis, most frequently intestinal ameboses (amebic dysentery) and hepatic amebosis ("amebic liver abscess"). Diagnosis of an intestinal infection is primarily confirmed by detection of the parasites in stool. If an invasive, intestinal or extraintestinal infection with *E. histolytica* is suspected, a serological antibody test can also provide valuable information. Morphologically, *E. histolytica* is indistinguishable from the apathogenic *Entamoeba dispar* (collective term for both species: *E. histolytica/E. dispar* complex). ■

Occurrence. In endemic areas in Africa, Asia, and Central and South America up to 70–90 % of the population can be are carriers of *E. histolytica/E. dispar*, in the USA and Europe about 1–4 %. Worldwide the annual number of new cases is estimated at 48 million, with about 70 000 lethal outcomes (WHO, 1998).

Parasites. The causative agent of amebosis is the pathogenic *E. histolytica*. This species is morphologically identical with the apathogenic *E. dispar*. They can be differentiated by means of zymodeme and DNA analysis and with monoclonal antibodies. The two species occur in the form of trophozoites (vegetative stages) and cysts (Figs. 9.**10** and 9.**11c**).

■ The **trophozoites** of *E. histolytica* are cells of variable shape and size (10–60 μm) that usually form a single, broad pseudopod (protrusion of cell membrane and cytoplasm) that is often quickly extended in the direction of movement. Stained preparations of the genus *Entamoeba* show a characteristic ring-shaped nucleus with a central nucleolus and chromatin granula on the nuclear membrane. Trophozoites that have penetrated into tissues often contain phagocytosed erythrocytes.

■ The spherical, nonmotile **cysts** (10–16 μm) have a resistant cyst wall. At first each cyst contains a uninucleate ameba, with glycogen in vacuoles and the so-called chromidial bodies, which are cigar-shaped. The nucleus divides once to produce the binuclear form and later once again to produce the infective tetranuclear cyst (Fig. 9.**11c**). The cysts are eliminated in the stool of infected persons, either alone or together with trophozoites.

Life cycle and pathogenesis. The cycle of *E. histolytica* is shown in Fig. 9.**10**.

■ **Symptomatic intestinal amebosis.** Following peroral ingestion of a mature *E. histolytica* cyst, the tetranuclear ameba is released, divides to produce four or eight uninucleate trophozoites, which then continue to multiply and encyst (Fig. 9.**10**). The trophozoites colonize the large intestine mucosa or lumen. Their potential for invading and destroying tissue is high and is based on the following characteristics and processes: adhesion of trophozoites to intestinal cells by means of surface lectins, killing of cells with pore-forming peptides (amebapore, types A–C) and dissolution of the extracellular matrix by cysteine proteases. This enables the amebas to penetrate into the intestinal wall, where they multiply and cause pathological changes (necrotic foci, ulcers, inflammatory reactions) (see below).

■ **Asymptomatic intestinal amebosis.** This condition is usually caused by *E. dispar*, less frequently by *E. histolytica*. Characterizing *E. dispar* as "apathogenic" is not entirely accurate, since these organisms can cause slight intest-

Fig. 9.**10** **1** Cyst of *E. histolytica*, following peroral ingestion, in stomach; **2** ameba emerging from a cyst; **3** dividing stage of ameba; **4** uninucleate trophozoites result from division; **4a** invasive stage with phagocytosed erythrocytes, extraintestinal; **4b** lesions in the intestinal wall; **5** the amebas encyst; **6** cysts excreted with feces and different transmission routes; **7** peroral ingestion of cysts. ▶

Entamoeba histolytica: Life Cycle

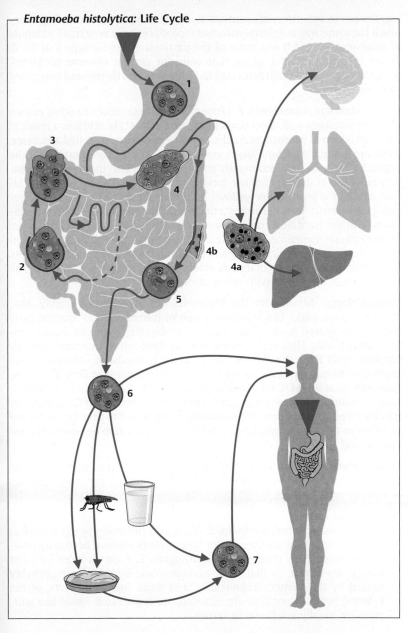

9

inal lesions in experimental animals. *E. dispar* adheres to host cells in very much the same way as *E. histolytica*, but it produces only very small amounts of amebapore A and B and none of the particularly potent type C at all. *E. dispar* is lacking several genes that code for certain cysteine proteases. Also, the activity of certain proteases in *E. dispar* is greatly reduced compared to *E. histolytica*.

■ **Extraintestinal amebosis.** *E. histolytica* can disseminate to other organs from the intestinal wall, most particularly to the liver (Fig. 9.**10**). As a result of the destruction of parenchymal cells, small necrotic foci, so-called abscesses, form and gradually become larger and can even affect major portions of the organ. Bacteria are involved in only about 5% of cases, so that the inflammatory reactions at the edges of the foci are usually mild. The decomposing lesion contains a brownish or yellowish, puslike liquid, in most cases bacteriologically sterile, later becoming a necrotic mass; amebas are often only detectable in the transition zone between the lesion and intact hepatic tissue. Liver abscesses sometimes perforate into the pleural space or lung; less often a hematogenous dissemination of amebas results in an invasion of the spleen, brain, and other organs. Cutaneous amebosis most frequently occurs in the perianal area, associated with rectal changes.

Epidemiology. Humans are the reservoirs for *E. histolytica* (rarely also: monkeys, dogs, cats). The infection is due to transmission of mature cysts with contaminated foods (fruit, vegetables), drinking water or fecally contaminated hands. Flies and cockroaches can function as intermediaries by carrying cysts from the feces of an excretor to foods. In contrast to the vegetative forms, the cysts are quite resistant in a moist environment (i.e., they survive at 28–34 °C for about eight days, at 10 °C for about one month); under conditions of desiccation and temperatures exceeding 55 °C they are quickly killed. The amounts of chlorine normally added to drinking water are insufficient to kill the cysts. Monkeys have been shown to be hosts of *E. histolytica* and *E. dispar*.

Clinical manifestations. Clinical symptoms can develop as early as two to four weeks after infection with *E. histolytica* or after asymptomatic periods of months or even years.

■ **Intestinal forms**
— **Asymptomatic intestinal form.** *E. histolytica* can colonize the intestinal mucosa, reproduce, and persist for long periods without becoming invasive or causing any changes. The apathogenic *E. dispar* is more frequent than *E. histolytica*, so that most asymptomatic infections are probably caused by the former. Trophozoites, and more frequently cysts, of the *E. histolytica*/*E. dispar* type are excreted, antibodies to *E. histolytica* antigens are usually not found in serum.

— The **invasive intestinal form** results from the invasion of the intestinal wall by the pathogenic *E. histolytica* and reflects large intestine disease. The intestinal parts affected (colon, cecum, rectum, sometimes terminal ileum) show either circumscribed or more expanded lesions of varying intensity, ranging from edematous swelling and reddening to pinhead-sized foci with central necrosis or larger, bottle-shaped ulcers extending deep into the intestinal wall with swollen edges and large decomposing foci. The ulcers sometimes perforate into the peritoneal cavity. Healing processes with scar formation may reduce the intestinal lumen; pronounced inflammatory processes can lead to a tumorlike thickening of the intestinal wall (ameboma). The **acute disease** usually begins with abdominal discomfort and episodes of diarrhea of varying duration, at first mushy then increasing mucoid, including blood-tinged, so-called "red currant jelly stools" in which amebas can be detected, including trophozoites containing erythrocytes. In such cases, antibodies are usually present in serum. The symptoms may abate spontaneously, but fairly often a recidivating **chronic colitis** develops that can last for months or even years.

■ **Extraintestinal forms**
— Extraintestinal forms develop because of hematogenous dissemination of *E. histolytica* originating in the intestine. The most frequent form is the so-called "**liver abscess**," which may develop in some infected persons. Only about 10% of patients with liver abscesses are also suffering from amebic colitis; coproscopic methods often do not reveal amebas in stool. The liver abscess causes remittent fever (sometimes high), upper abdominal pain, liver enlargement, elevation of the diaphragm, general weakness, and other symptoms. Large liver abscesses that are not treated in time are often lethal. Antibodies are detectable in most cases (around 95%) (see also Diagnosis). **Other forms** of extraintestinal amebosis are much rarer and include involvement of the lungs, brain, and skin.

Immunity. Reinfections are possible since sufficient immunity is not conferred in the course of an infection. Antibodies are usually detectable in serum in invasive intestinal and extraintestinal amebosis caused by *E. histolytica*.

Diagnosis

■ **Intestinal amebosis**
— **Coproscopic diagnosis.** For diagnosis of intestinal amebosis a body-warm stool specimen must be fixed without delay in SAF solution and examined microscopically following laboratory processing (p. 621). A single stool analysis has a statistical sensitivity of only 50–60%, but this can be raised to 95% by examining stool specimens from three consecutive days. Since *E. histolytica* and *E. dispar* are morphologically indistinguishable, a finding is classified as *E. histolytica/E. dispar* complex.

Differential Diagnosis of Intestinal Protozoa

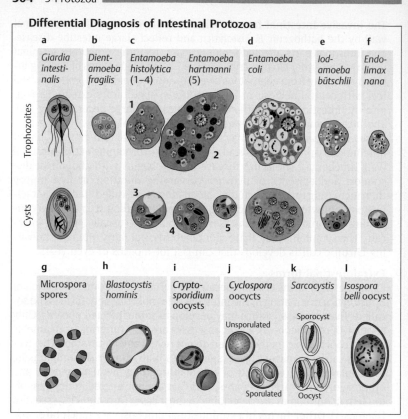

Trophozoites

Cysts

a — *Giardia intestinalis*
b — *Dientamoeba fragilis*
c — *Entamoeba histolytica (1–4)* / *Entamoeba hartmanni (5)*
d — *Entamoeba coli*
e — *Iodamoeba bütschlii*
f — *Endolimax nana*

g — Microspora spores
h — *Blastocystis hominis*
i — Cryptosporidium oocysts
j — Cyclospora oocysts — Unsporulated / Sporulated
k — Sarcocystis — Sporocyst / Oocyst
l — *Isospora belli* oocyst

9

— **Differential diagnosis.** It is important to differentiate the *E. histolytica*/*E. dispar* complex from intestinal epithelia, granulocytes, macrophages, and fungi as well as from other, apathogenic, intestinal protozoa (amebas: *Entamoeba coli*, *E. hartmanni*, *E. polecki*, *Iodamoeba bütschlii*, *Endolimax nana*; flagellates: *Dientamoeba fragilis*, *Enteromonas hominis*, *Chilomastix mesnili*, *Pentatrichomonas hominis* (Fig. 9.**11**). *D. fragilis* is classified by some authors as potentially pathogenic. *Blastocystis hominis* is frequently found in stool samples (Fig. 9.**11h**): this intestinal inhabitant is considered a fungus or a protozoon; some authors ascribe it a certain significance as causative agent of diarrhea. It is important to remember that a number of drugs reduce the excretion of intestinal protozoa.

◀ Fig. 9.**11**

a *Giardia intestinalis* (pathogenic):
trophozoites: 9–21 × 5–12 μm;
cysts: 8–14 × 8–10 μm (see also p. 478).

b *Dientamoeba fragilis* (apathogenic or facultatively pathogenic):
trophozoites: 5–15 μm, 3/4 of stages with two nuclei, the rest with one;
karyosome consisting of four to six granules;
cysts: none.

c *Entamoeba histolytica* (pathogenic):
trophozoites: small form (1) 10–20 μm, with *Entamoeba* nucleus and small number of vacuoles containing bacteria; larger form (2) 20–60 μm, with phagocytosed erythrocytes; (3) cysts: 10–16 μm, one to four nuclei. Here binuclear cyst with glycogen vacuole and cigarshaped chromidial bodies and (4) a tetranuclear cyst.

Entamoeba dispar (apathogenic): morphologically identical with *E. histolytica* (see text).

Entamoeba hartmanni (5) (apathogenic): similar to *E. histolytica*, but smaller. Trophozoites and cysts approximately 3–10 μm.

d *Entamoeba coli* (apathogenic):
trophozoites: with *Entamoeba* nucleus, 10–50 μm, in most cases numerous vacuoles containing bacteria and particles.Cysts: 15–25 μm, one to eight nuclei, chromidial bodies slender, splinter-shaped.

e *Iodamoeba bütschlii* (apathogenic):
trophozoites: 6–20 μm, nucleus with large karyosome, either centrally located or contiguous with the nuclear membrane.
Cysts: 5–18 μm, one nucleus, rarely two.

f *Endolimax nana* (apathogenic):
trophozoites: 6–15 μm, nucleus with karyosome.
cysts: usually oval, 8–12 μm long.

g *Microsporidia* (pathogenic):
spores: very small (!), 1–3.5 μm long depending on species, oval shape; spores often not stained homogeneously by chromotropic staining according to Weber (see also Fig. 9.**20c**, p. 539).

h *Blastocystis hominis* (facultatively pathogenic?):
single cells: 5–20 μm.

i *Cryptosporidium* species (pathogenic):
oocysts: 4–5 μm (see also Fig. 9.**14a**, p. 516).

j *Cyclospora cayetanensis* (pathogenic):
oocysts: 4–5 μm, spherical, unsporulated in fresh stool; after sporulation two sporocysts with two sporozoites each (see also Fig. 9.**14a**, p. 516).

k *Sarcocystis* species (pathogenic):
sporocyst: 14 × 9 μm; oocyst: 20 × 13 μm.

l *Isospora belli* (pathogenic):
oocyst: 20–33 × 10–19 μm.

9

- **Differentiation of** *E. histolytica* and *E. dispar*. A new type of PCR is now used in specialized laboratories that facilitates direct detection of these amebic species in stool specimens as well as a differential diagnosis.
- **Detection of coproantigen.** *E. histolytica* antigen can be detected in stool specimens using an ELISA based on monoclonal antibodies with high levels of sensitivity and specificity.
- **Serological antibody assay.** Antibodies can be detected serologically in 95–100% of patients with amebic liver abscess. This is also frequently the case in invasive intestinal amebosis caused by *E. histolytica*. On the other hand, antibodies are produced far less often in *E. dispar* infections. When stages of the *E. histolytica*/*E. dispar* complex are detected in stool, the presence or absence of serum antibodies can be used in differential diagnosis of invasive vs. noninvasive intestinal amebosis.

■ **Extraintestinal amebosis.** This type of amebosis is diagnosed with the help of clinical methods (ultrasound, computer tomography, etc.) and serological antibody detection (see above).

Therapy. Nitromidazole derivatives are effective against symptomatic intestinal and extraintestinal forms of amebosis. On the other hand, amebicides with only luminal activity are effective against asymptomatic intestinal amebosis (e.g., diloxanide furoate) (Table 9.**5**). A new drug against intestinal amebic infections is nitazoxandide. Besides chemotherapy, other measures may also be required, e.g., surgery and symptomatic treatment for liver abscesses.

Prevention. Travelers to endemic areas should decontaminate drinking water by boiling or filtering it (e.g., with Katadyn filters), not eat salads, eat only fruit they have peeled themselves and exercise caution when it comes to changing their diet. Chemoprophylactic dugs are not available.

9

Table 9.**5** Chemotherapy in Amebosis (examples)

Group of amoebicides*	Active substance	Indication
Luminal amebicides	Diloxanide furoate Paromomycin Nitazoxanide	Asymptomatic cyst excreters, follow-up treatment of invasive intestinal form
Systemic amebicides	Nitroimidazoles: Metronidazole Ornidazole Tinidazole	Invasive intestinal and extraintestinal forms

*Application per os

Naegleria, Acanthamoeba, and Balamuthia

Causative agents of naegleriosis, acanthamebosis, and balamuthiosis

Free-living ameba of the genera *Naegleria*, *Acanthamoeba*, and *Balamuthia* have the potential to infect vertebrates and to cause diseases in humans. The morphological characteristics of these amebas include: nucleus with large karyosome, lack of chromatin granules at the nuclear membrane (see *Entamoeba*). Trophozoites: *Naegleria fowleri* (15–30 µm) with wide pseudopods, produces flagellated stages in water; *Acanthamoeba* spp. (24–56 µm) with fingerlike protrusions ("filopods"); *Balamuthia mandrillaris* (12–60 µm) has irregularly branched pseudopods. All of these genera produce cysts.

Naegleria. The causative agent of primary amebic meningoencephalitis (PAM) is *Naegleria fowleri*. This species occurs worldwide in bodies of freshwater, especially warm water in swimming pools, storage containers or thermally polluted lakes and rivers, etc.

Infection of humans occurs by the nasal route with water containing trophozoites, i.e., during a swim or shower. The amebas migrate from the olfactory epithelium along the nerve tracts into the CNS and cause, after an incubation period of two to seven (rarely as long as 15) days a hyperacute to acute meningoencephalitis that usually has a lethal outcome. The infection occurs mainly in children and youths. Sporadic occurrence is reported from all continents. Treatment with amphotericin B has been successful in a small number of cases.

Acanthamoeba. Potential human pathogens in this genus include *Acanthamoeba culbertsoni* and several other species. These amebas occur worldwide in soil, sand, dust (also house dust), air, and water (also in tap water). The cysts can survive for several years in a dry state and disseminate with dust. Inhalation of cysts with dust is considered to be one of the main transmission routes. Acanthamebas are frequent colonizers of human nasal mucosa and have been isolated from the oral mucosa, skin lesions, and the cornea. From the portal of entry, they can spread hematogenously to the CNS and other organs.

Acanthamoeba infections in humans frequently take an asymptomatic course. Keratitis is observed occasionally, especially in contact lens wearers. Diagnosis: culturing of amebas from conjunctival and contact lens rinsing liquids. Prevention: use only sterile lens rinsing liquid. In rare cases of generalized infection, *Acanthamoeba* can cause granulomatous amebic encephalitis (GAE) as well as granulomatous lesions in the lungs and other organs, especially in immunodeficient patients. *Balamuthia mandrillaris* can also cause GAE.

9

Toxoplasma gondii

Causative agent of toxoplasmosis

■ *Toxoplasma gondii* is the causative agent of a zoonosis that occurs worldwide with high prevalences (up to 80% depending on region and age). Humans are infected by ingesting oocysts excreted by the definitive hosts (cats) or by eating unprocessed meat containing *Toxoplasma* cysts. If a women contracts toxoplasmosis for the first time during pregnancy, diaplacental transmission of the pathogen to the fetus is possible with potential severe consequences (for example malformations, eye damage, clinical symptoms during childhood). There is, however, no risk to the fetus from mothers who had been infected before their first pregnancy and have produced serum antibodies (about 35–45%). Latent infections can be activated by immunodeficiencies (e.g., in AIDS patients) and may result in cerebral or generalized symptomatic toxoplasmosis. Serological surveillance in pregnant women is important to prevent prenatal infections. ■

Occurrence. *T. gondii* occurs worldwide. The low level of host specificity of this organism explains its ready ability to infect a wide spectrum of warm-blooded vertebrate species (for example humans, sheep, pigs, cattle, horses, dogs, cats, wild mammals, bird species). It is estimated that approximately one-third of the world population is infected with *T. gondii*, although prevalences vary widely depending on age and region. According to a seroepidemiological study in Switzerland (published in 1995) of 4000 persons aged one to 70, an average of 52% was infected with seroprevalence rates in different age groups as follows: one to nine years: 24%, 20–39 years: 43%, and 40–70 years: 69%. Of 9000 pregnant women, 46% were infected. Women of childbearing age groups in other European countries showed either lower or higher seroprevalences. High prevalences were also observed in various animal species (see Epidemiology p. 514).

Parasite. Various strains of *T. gondii* differ in virulence and certain biological and genetic characteristics. The life cycle of *T. gondii* includes various stages:

■ **Tachyzoites** (endozoites) (Fig. 9.**12a, b**) are proliferative forms that reproduce rapidly within a parasitophorous vacuole in nucleate host cells by means of endodyogeny (endodyogeny: formation of two daughter cells from a mother cell by endogenous budding). The tachyzoites are sickleshaped (*toxon*: bow) cells about 4–7 µm long and 2–4 mm wide. An apical complex is located at the anterior pole, consisting of serveal components, including the conoid (a conical structure of spirally arranged microtubuli), a pole ring complex, the rhoptries, and micronemes (Fig. 9.**12b**). The apical complex

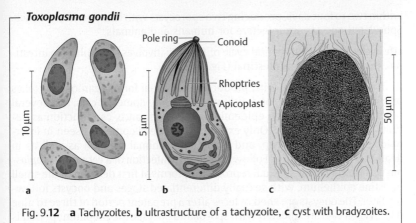

Toxoplasma gondii

Pole ring
Conoid
Rhoptries
Apicoplast
10 µm
5 µm
50 µm
a
b
c

Fig. 9.**12**   **a** Tachyzoites, **b** ultrastructure of a tachyzoite, **c** cyst with bradyzoites.

contributes to parasite penetration into host cells. The nucleus is located in the posterior half of the cell. More recent investigations have revealed that *Toxoplasma* and several other apicomplexan protozoa (e.g., *Plasmodium, Sarcocystis*) contain, in addition to the chromosomal and mitochondrial genomes, a further genome consisting of circular DNA (35 kb) localized in a special organelle called the apicoplast. This organelle, usually located anterior to the nucleus and close to the Golgi apparatus, is surrounded by several membranes and possesses outer and inner membrane complexes. There is evidence that the apicoplast has evolved from the plastids of endosymbiontic green or red algae. The function of the apicoplast remains uncertain but is indispensable for the host cell and may be a new and specific target for chemotherapy. Tachyzoites also multiply in experimental animals and cell cultures. This stage is highly labile outside of a host and usually does not survive the stomach passage following ingestion.

■ **Bradyzoites** (**cystozoites**) are stages produced by slow reproduction within the cysts (4–8 × 2–4 µm). The cysts develop intracellularly in various tissues (see below), have a relatively resistant wall, grow as large as 150 µm, and can contain up to several thousand bradyzoites (Fig. 9.**12c**). They have a long lifespan in the host. Humans and animals can be infected by peroral ingestion of meat containing cysts (Fig. 9.**13**).

■ **Oocysts** are rounded and encysted stages of the organism, surrounded by a resistant cyst wall, and are approx. 9 × 14 µm in size. They are the final product of a sexual reproductive cycle in the intestinal epithelia of *Felidae*. They contain a zygote and are shed in feces (Fig. 9.**13**). Sporulation takes place

9

within two to four days, producing two sporocysts with four sporozoites each. Sporulated oocysts are infective for humans and animals.

Life cycle. The developmental cycle of *T. gondii* involves three phases: intestinal, external, and extraintestinal (Fig. 9.**13**).

■ The intestinal **phase** with production of sexual forms (gamogony) takes only place in enterocytes of definitive hosts. Only domestic cats, and several other felid species of little epidemiological significance, can function as definitive hosts for *T. gondii*. Only extraintestinal development is seen in intermediate hosts (pigs, sheep, and many other animal species) as well as in dead-end hosts (humans). Following primary infection of a cat with *Toxoplasma* cysts in raw meat, asexual reproductive forms at first develop in the small intestine epithelium, with sexually differentiated stages and oocysts following later. The oocysts are shed in feces after a prepatent period of three to nine days. When cats are infected with sporulated oocysts, the prepatent period is extended to 20–35 days because in these cases the intestinal development of *Toxoplasma* is preceded by an extraintestinal asexual reproduction (see below). Oocyst shedding lasts for only a few days to a maximum of three weeks, but can be highly intensive (up to 600 million oocysts per eat during the patent period!).

■ **External phase.** Oocysts excreted in cat feces sporulate at room temperature within two to four days, rendering them infective. Kept moist, they remain infective for up to five years and are not killed by standard disinfectant agents. They die within a few minutes at temperatures exceeding 55 °C.

■ **Extraintestinal phase.** This phase follows a peroral infection with oocysts or cysts and is observed in intermediate hosts (dogs, sheep, pigs, other vertebrates, birds) and dead-end hosts (humans), as well as in the definitive hosts (cats). Starting from the intestine, the *Toxoplasma* organisms travel in blood or lymph to various organs and multiply in nucleate host cells, especially in the reticulohistiocytic system, in musculature, and in the CNS. Repeated endodyogenic cycles produce as many as 32 individual daughter cells in the expanding host cell before it bursts. The tachyzoites thus released attack neighboring cells.

These processes result in focal necroses and inflammatory reactions in affected tissues. Generalization of the infection can lead to colonization of the placenta and, about three to four weeks later, infection of the fetus. Cysts that elicit no inflammatory reactions in the near vicinity are produced early in the course of the infection. Such cysts (tissue cysts) are found above all in the CNS, in the skeletal and heart muscles as well as in the retina, the uterine wall, and other organs. They can remain viable for years without causing noticeable damage to the host.

Toxoplasma gondii: Life Cycle

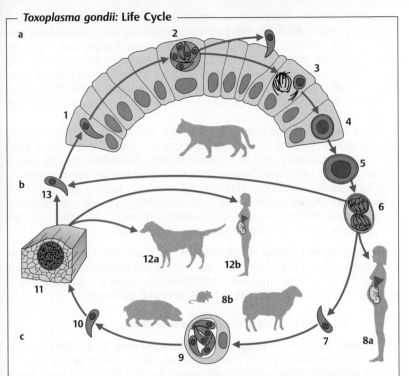

Fig. 9.**13** **a** Development in the definitive host (cat): intestinal phase with production of sexual forms: **1** *Toxoplasma* that has penetrated into a small intestine epithelial cell; **2** asexual reproductive stage with merozoites (can continue for several generations). The arrow indicates that an extraintestinal cycle precedes the enteral cycle when a cat is infected with oocysts; **3** production of sexual forms (gamogony) and formation of the zygote; **4** oocyst.
b External phase with sporogony: **5** unsporulated oocyst, shed in cat feces; **6** sporulated oocyst with two sporocysts each containing four sporozoites.
c Development in an intermediate host (mammals, birds, humans): extraintestinal phase with only asexual multiplication of parasites; **7** sporozoite released in organism following oral ingestion of oocysts; **8a** human infection; **8b** infection of various animal species; **9** asexual reproductive stages (tachyzoites) in a somatic cell; **10** free tachyzoite; **11** cyst with bradyzoites in musculature; **12a** infection of a dog with *Toxoplasma* cysts in animal meat; **12b** infection of a human with *Toxoplasma* cysts; **13** infection of cat with infective stages of cysts in meat or with oocysts.

9

Immunity. Various *Toxoplasma* antigens induce humoral and cellular immune responses which, following a primary infection, result in antibody production and inhibition of tachyzoite multiplication. Toxoplasmas then "escape" from the immune defense system by encysting (immunoevasion). This enables them to persist in a latent state for many years in immunocompetent hosts, at the same time maintaining an immune status that confers protection from new infections due to the continuous presentation of antigens.

The relevant immune defense mechanisms include mainly cellular mechanisms and production of IFNγ. Bradyzoites can also migrate out of cysts (without cyst rupture), are then, however, locally inactivated in immunocompetent persons, sometimes leading to formation of satellite cysts. In cases of cellular immune deficiency, this control system is lacking and the latent infection progresses to become an acute, manifest toxoplasmosis. Similarly, latent *Toxoplasma* infections in AIDS patients are usually activated and turn symptomatic when the CD4+ cell count falls below 200/μl.

Pathogenicity and clinical manifestations. Focal necrotic, inflammatory and immunopathological processes are the basis of the pathogenesis and varied clinical manifestations observed in toxoplasmosis. Cases are differentiated as to time of acquisition, i.e., postnatal and prenatal infections.

Forms of Postnatal Toxoplasma Infection

■ **Primary infection in immunocompetent persons.** This is the most frequent form without clinical manifestations, recognizable by the specific serum antibodies. The infection can persist for the life of the host, and it may exacerbate in response to immunosuppression. Subacute cervical lymphadenitis occurs in about 1% of infected persons.

■ **Primary infection during pregnancy.** This may cause prenatal infection of the fetus and thus become a significant threat (see prenatal toxoplasmosis p. 513).

■ **Primary infection in immunosuppressed persons.** In cases of immune deficiency (with significant disturbance of CD4+ and CD8+ cell functions) or immunosuppressant therapies (e.g., in organ transplantations) the infection gives rise to febrile generalized illness with maculopapulous exanthema, generalized lymphadenitis, necrotizing interstitial pneumonia, hepatosplenomegaly, mycocarditis, meningoencephalitis, eye damage, and other manifestations. There is a high rate of lethality if left untreated.

■ **Reactivation toxoplasmosis in cases of immune deficiency.** Local and generalized reactivation of a *Toxoplasma* infection originating from tissue cysts. Cerebral manifestations are the most frequent (up to 40% of patients in full-blown AIDS stage), for example, with multiple coagulative necroses, small-focus hemorrhages, and surrounding edema. Other organ systems are affected more rarely (in about 15% of cases), e.g., myocardium and lungs.

Prenatal Toxoplasmosis

Occurrence. The prenatal fetal infection occurs only in mothers who contract their *primary* (first!) infection with toxoplasmas during pregnancy! There is no risk of prenatal fetal infection in women having a latent infection with serum antibodies at conception.

Incidence. The rate of verified primary infections in pregnant women was estimated in Germany, Austria, and Switzerland in 1995 at 0.5–0.7%. A prenatal fetal infection is to be expected in some of these cases, whereby the infection risk for the fetus is lower in the first trimester than later in the pregnancy. The frequency of toxoplasmosis in newborns (prenatal toxoplasmosis) is between 0.1 and 0.3% in various European countries. The rate is lower in some countries, e.g., in Austria (0.01%), where monitoring examinations for pregnant women have been obligatory for a number of years (for details see Aspöck, 2000, p. 660).

Possible consequences of prenatal infection:

■ 10% clinically severe cases, 85% of these with brain damage (e.g., hydrocephalus, intracerebral calcifications), 15% perinatal deaths,

■ 15% milder symptoms (99% chorioretinitis, 1% brain damage),

■ 75% subclinical cases (15% no damage, 85% chorioretinitis).

Children in this last group appear to be clinically normal at birth, but signs of brain and eye damage, as well as other symptoms, may manifest later in infancy and early childhood.

Diagnosis. In **immunocompetent adults**, toxoplasmosis is normally diagnosed serologically by detection of parasite-specific IgG and IgM antibodies (Table 11.**5**, p. 625). IgM antibodies can be detected as early as one week after the primary infection, peak within two to four weeks, then drop to below the detection limit within a few weeks; in some cases persistence at low titers lasts longer. IgG antibodies appear somewhat later, peak after two to four months and persist for many years. A high or rising IgG titer with contemporal detection of IgM indicates an acute primary infection. The isolated cases of **ocular toxoplasmosis** normally cannot be diagnosed by serological methods.

Serological findings are often not reliable indicators in **immunodeficient patients** due to reduced antibody production. The cerebral form of the infection seen frequently in reactivated toxoplasmosis is therefore usually diagnosed by means of clinical imaging methods.

9

In **prenatal diagnostics**, PCR is seeing increasing use for direct detection of pathogens in the amniotic fluid. Detection of *Toxoplasma* DNA with this method is a reliable sign of fetal infection and demands a chemotherapeutic or other response accordingly. Diagnosis of **prenatal toxoplasmosis** in neonates is difficult, but highly important. Since IgG antibodies are transmitted from mother to child diaplacentally, detection of them in the child cannot serve as a definitive diagnostic indicator. IgM is only present in about 50% of prenatally infected children. In suspected cases, the blood or cerebrospinal fluid should by examined using the PCR.

Therapy. The following cases require treatment: acute or subacute, symptomatic infections in children and adults as well as symptomatic or asymptomatic primary infections in pregnant women. In an acute primary infection during pregnancy, the risk of infection for the developing fetus can be eliminated by starting chemotherapy immediately. Several different therapeutic schemes are recommended for this indication. For example, spiramycin daily for four weeks from diagnosis to the end of the 15th week of gravidity, and in the period beginning with the 16th week of gravidity pyrimethamine daily for four weeks together with sulfadiazine and folic acid. The recommendations also vary for treatment of toxoplasmosis in AIDS cases, e.g., pyrimethamine/sulfadiazine or pyrimethamine/clindamycin.

Epidemiology and prevention. Humans become infected by peroral ingestion of raw meat containing cysts or by uptake of sporulated oocysts. *T. gondii* is also transmitted diaplacentally and by transplantation of infected organs to uninfected recipients.

In Europe about 1–6% of domestic cats are oocyst excreters. Sheep and goats are frequently infected with toxoplasmas; infection prevalences of pigs have decreased significantly in pig farms with high hygienic standards as demonstrated in recent studies. Cattle have always been considered rare carriers, but recently in Switzerland *Toxoplasma* DNA was found using PCR in 1–6% of the animals examined ($n = 350$). The epidemiological significance of these findings has not yet been clarified. Certain wild animal species (e.g., wild boars) are relatively frequently infected, not so horses and chickens. Milk and eggs are not considered sources of infection.

Toxoplasma cysts remain viable and infectious in meat for up to three weeks at 4 °C. Deep-freezing to –20 °C kills bradyzoites within three days, heating to 70 °C is lethal to them within a few minutes. *Toxoplasma* oocysts show considerable environmental resistance, but can be killed rapidly by heat (70 °C).

Pregnant women should eat only meat that has been thoroughly heated or deep-frozen. Close contact with cats should be avoided. Cat litter boxes in the house should be cleaned out daily and flushed with boiling water (wear rubber gloves!). Cats can be fed canned (boiled) meat to protect them from infection. Of particular importance in prevention of prenatal toxoplasmosis is prophylactic serological monitoring, with one check per trimester as is obligatory in, for example, Austria (Aspöck, 2000 p. 660).

Isospora

Causative agent of isosporosis

The causative agent of human isosporiosis is *Isospora belli*. After peroral ingestion of sporulated oocysts and release of sporozoites, further development (schizogony, gamogony) takes place in the epithelium of the upper small intestine, leading finally to oocyst formation. In AIDS patients, encysted sporozoites have been found in various extraintestinal organs (lymph nodes, liver, gallbladder, spleen).

I. belli can cause severe clinical symptoms, especially in AIDS patients, for example persistent diarrhea, steatorrhea, cholecystitis, weight loss, and fever. Diagnosis is made by detection of unsporulated oocysts (20–30 μm long) in stool (Fig. 9.**11l**, p. 504) or of developmental stages in intestinal biopsies. High-dosed cotrimoxazole is the recommended therapy.

Cyclospora cayetanensis

Causative agent of cyclosporosis

Parasite and occurrence. *Cyclospora cayetanensis* was first identified as an apicomplexan parasite (family Eimeriidae) in 1994. The parasite occurs in various countries on all continents with generally low prevalences and with seasonal fluctuations, in children and adults, and also in AIDS patients.

Morphology and life cycle. Infection per os with sporulated oocysts in food or drinking water. Developmental stages in duodenal and jejunal enterocysts, probably two generations of schizonts; following gamogony formation of spherical oocysts 8–10 μm in size. Prepatency about one week; oocysts are shed unsporulated in feces, then sporulate outside of host within five to 12 days to become infective. The sporulated oocysts contain two sporocysts with two sporozoites each (Fig. 9.**11j**, p. 504).

Clinical manifestations. Villus atrophy, cryptic hyperplasia, and inflammatory changes in the intestinal mucosa. Incubation about one week, self-limiting diarrhea in immunocompetent persons (lasts for about two to three weeks) with loss of appetite, flatulence, and malaise, usually nonfebrile; the diarrhea may persist for months in immunodeficient patients.

Cyclospora and Cryptosporidium

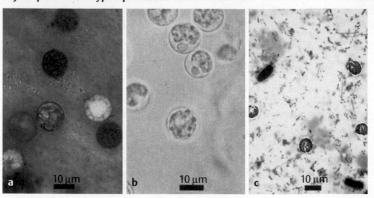

Fig. 9.**14 a** Oocysts of *Cyclospora cayetanensis* in stool smear, modified Ziehl-Neelsen staining. **b** Oocysts of *Cyclospora*, unstained, after isolation from stool. **c** Oocysts from *Cryptosporidium parvum* in stool smear. Staining as in **a**. (**b** and **c** from: *Bench Aids for the Diagnosis of Intestinal Parasites*. Geneva: WHO; 1995.)

Diagnosis and therapy. Detection of oocysts in stool specimens using concentration methods or in stained stool smears (for instance modified Ziehl-Neelsen staining or modified carbol-fuchsin staining). *Cyclospora* oocysts are easily confused with the oocysts of cryptosporidia (Fig. 9.**14**); they show autofluorescence in UV light and no reaction with monoclonal antibodies to *Cryptosporidium*. The drug of choice is cotrimoxazole.

Sarcocystis

Causative agent of sarcocystosis

Parasites, life cycle, and epidemiology. *Sarcocystis hominis* and *S. suihominis* are known as human intestinal parasites. Infection results from ingestion of raw or insufficiently heated meat from cattle or pigs, which frequently contains muscle cysts of these species. In the small intestine, bradyzoites are released from the muscle cysts. The bradyzoites undergo gamogony without an asexual reproductive phase in the lamina propria of the intestine. This process produces thin-walled oocysts that sporulate in the intestinal wall. Once the frail oocyst wall has burst, free sporocysts containing four sporozoites each are excreted with stool in most cases. The sporozoites are infectious for intermediate hosts. Prepatent periods of 14–18 and

11–13 days are reported for *S. hominis* and *S. suihominis*, respectively. Examination of large population groups in Germany (n = approx. 1500) and France (n = 3500) revealed 1.6% and 2% *Sarcocystis* excreters, respectively.

Clinical manifestations, diagnosis, therapy, and prevention. Both species can cause short-lived (six to 48 hours) symptoms within 24 hours of eating meat containing cysts, for example nausea, vomiting, and diarrhea as well as a mild fever. *S. suihominis* is more pathogenic than *S. hominis*.

An intestinal infection with *Sarcocystis* can be diagnosed by detection of sporocysts (14 × 9 µm), or more rarely oocysts (approx. 20 × 13 µm) (Fig. 9.**11k**, p. 504) in stool using the SAFC or the flotation method (p. 621). The two *Sarcocystis* species cannot be differentiated. An effective therapy has not yet been developed. Prevention consists in boiling or deep-freezing (–20 °C for three days) of pork and beef.

Cryptosporidium

Causative agent of cryptosporidiosis

■ Cryptosporidiosis in humans is predominantly caused by *Cryptosporidium hominis* (= human genotype of *C. parvum*) and the bovine genotype of *C. parvum*. Humans are infected by peroral ingestion of infective oocysts. In immunocompetent persons, the infection remains inapparent or manifests as a self-limiting diarrhea. Persistent, choleralike, life-threatening diarrheas are observed in AIDS patients. ■

Parasite species and occurrence. At least 10 species of the genus *Cryptosporidium* and several genotypes are currently known that occur mainly as parasites of the intestine (and rarely of other organs) in humans and numerous species of mammalian animals, birds, and reptiles. *Cryptosporidium hominis* is a parasite of humans and monkeys, the bovine genotype of *C. parvum* infects many species of mammalian animals (ruminants, dogs, cats, rabbits, rodents, etc.) and humans. Other species originating from animals have been found occasionally in AIDS patients, including *Cryptosporidium canis* (host: dog) *Cryptosporidium felis* (host: cat), *Cryptosporidium meleagridis* and *Cryptosporidium baileyi* (hosts: birds).

Cryptosporidiosis occurs worldwide. The mean prevalences in humans differ in developed and developing countries and are about 2% and 6% respectively for immunocompetent persons with diarrhea and 14% and 24% respectively in HIV-positive patients. Prevalences exceeding 50% are also known in the latter group. Among domesticated animals, particularly high prevalences are observed among young calves (often 20–100%).

Morphology and life cycle. *C. hominis* and *C. parvum* inhabit mainly the small intestine and produce oocysts 4–5 µm in diameter. Following peroral ingestion of infectious oocysts, each of which contains four sporozoites, the released sporozoites invade enterocytes where each stage resides within a parasitophorous vacuole just beneath the cell membrane in the microvillus region of the host cell. This localization is typical of cryptosporidia (Fig. 9.**15**). Following formation of type I meronts with eight merozoites, the latter can infect new cells. In the further course, type II meronts with four merozoites are produced that give rise to sexual forms (gamogony). The fertilized zygote encysts to produce about 80 % thick-walled and 20 % thin-walled oocysts. The oocysts sporulate while still intracellular in the intestine. Each sporulated oocyst contains four free sporozoites (i.e., not enclosed in a sporocyst). Thin-walled oocysts can burst within the host, releasing sporozoites that cause endogenous autoinfections. After a brief prepatent period (two to four, sometimes up to 12 days), thick-walled oocysts are shed with feces and can immediately infect new hosts. It is assumed that persistent infections in immunodeficient persons are due to endogenous autoinfections by sporozoites from thin-walled oocysts or by merozoites from type I meronts.

Epidemiology. *C. hominis* is transmitted within the human population. Humans may also acquire zoonotic infections with the bovine type of *C. parvum* (main source of infection: calves) or rarely with other species or genotypes of animal origin.

Transmission of the oocysts is by the direct fecal-oral route or in contaminated foods or drinking water. The oocysts of *C. parvum* remain viable in cool water for months. This explains the etiology of major epidemics due to fecal contamination and improper processing of drinking water such as occurred in Milwaukee in 1993 with 403 000 persons involved. Sewage contained up to 13 000 oocysts per liter, surface bodies of water up to 112 oocysts per liter. As few as 30–100 oocysts are sufficient to induce an infection in humans.

Clinical manifestations. Cryptosporidia inhabit mainly the small intestine, where they may cause destruction of microvilli, shortening, swelling, and fusion of the villi and cellular infiltration of the mucosa. The severity and course of an infection depends on the immune status of the infected person.

▪ **Immunocompetent persons.** Infections either take an inapparent course or result, after incubation periods of five to 28 days, in acute, self-limiting, in most cases mild illnesses lasting one to 26 days with diarrhea and various generalized symptoms.

▪ **Immunodeficient persons.** Chronic infections with severe diarrhea and long periods of oocyst excretion, e.g., in AIDS patients. The diarrhea is watery, voluminous, choleralike and often associated with other symptoms (abdominal pain, nausea, vomiting, mild fever, etc.). In HIV patients, cryptosporidia

Cryptosporidium: Life Cycle

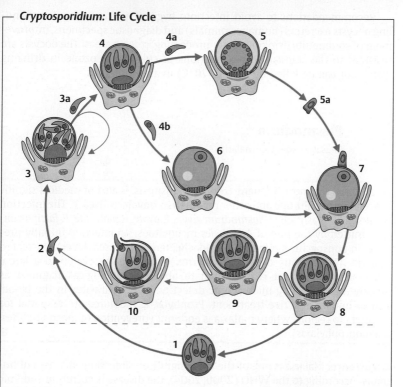

Fig. 9.**15** **1** Infective oocyst; **2** sporozoite before penetration into an enterocyte; **3** type I schizont with eight merozoites; **3a** free merozoite; **4** type II schizont with 4 merozoites; **4a, b** free merozoites; **5** microgamont; **5a** microgamete; **6** macrogamont; **7** macrogamete being fertilized by a microgamete; **8** thick-walled oocyst (shed with feces); **9, 10** thin-walled oocyst from which sporozoites are released in the host intestine (autoinfection).

are also found in other localizations (gallbladder, bile, and pancreatic ducts, esophagus, stomach, large intestine, respiratory tract).

Diagnosis, therapy, and prevention. *Cryptosporidium* oocysts can be diagnosed in stool smears after staining (e.g., modified Ziehl-Neelsen stain) (Fig. 9.**11i**, p. 504, Fig. 9.**14c**, p. 516), or visualization by immunofluorescence using monoclonal antibodies. In addition, coproantigens are detectable by ELISA. The only drug with efficacy against *Cryptosporidium* is nitazoxanide (see also *Giardia*).

9

Recommendations to avoid infection: hygienic precautions when handling oocysts excreters (humans, animals) and diagnostic specimens, improvement of community drinking water processing in some areas. The oocysts are resistant to the standard concentrations of chlorine or ozone in drinking water, but can be killed by heat ($>70\,°C$) in a few minutes.

Plasmodium

Causative agent of malaria

■ Malaria, the most frequent tropical parasitosis, is also of medical significance in central Europe and other regions as a travelers' disease. The infection is caused by plasmodia (*Plasmodium vivax*, *P. ovale*, *P. malariae*, *P. falciparum*) transmitted by the bite of *Anopheles* mosquitoes. An infection initially presents in nonspecific symptoms (headache, fatigue, nausea, fever). Untreated malaria tropica (caused by *P. falciparum*) can quickly develop to a lethal outcome. Therefore, it is important to obtain an etiological diagnosis as quickly as possible by microscopic detection of the parasites in the blood, and to initiate effective treatment. Prophylactic measures are essential for travelers to regions where malaria is endemic (prevention of mosquito bites, chemoprophylaxis). ■

Occurrence. Malaria is one of the most significant infectious diseases of humans. According to the WHO (2000, 2004), the disease is currently endemic in more than 100 countries or territories, mainly in sub-Saharan Africa, Asia, Oceania, Central and South America, and in the Caribbean. About 2.4 billion people (40% of the world's population) live in malarious regions. Fig. 9.**16** shows the geographic distribution of malaria (WHO, 2000). The annual incidence of malaria worldwide is estimated to be 300–500 million clinical cases, with about 90% of these occurring in sub-Saharan Africa (mostly caused by *P. falciparum*). Malaria alone or in combination with other diseases kills approximately 1.1–2.7 million people each year, including 1 million children under the age of five years in tropical Africa. About 7000 cases of imported malaria were reported in Europe in the period from 1985 to 1995, whereby the data are incomplete.

Parasites. Four *Plasmodium* species infect humans and cause different types of malaria:

■ *Plasmodium vivax*: tertian malaria (*malaria tertiana*),

■ *Plasmodium ovale*: tertian malaria (*malaria tertiana*),

Distribution of Malaria

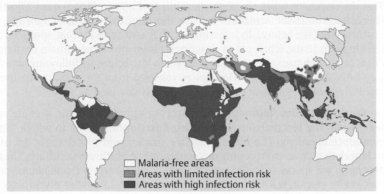

Malaria-free areas
Areas with limited infection risk
Areas with high infection risk

Fig. 9.**16**   Status: 1999. (From: *International Travel and Health*, Geneva. World Health Organization, 2000.)

■ *Plasmodium malariae*: quartan malaria (*malaria quartana*),

■ *Plasmodium falciparum*: malignant tertian malaria (*malaria tropica*).

These *Plasmodium* species can be identified and differentiated from each other by light microscopy in stained blood smears during the erythrocytic phase of the infection in humans (Fig. 9.**18**, p. 524). A reduced apical complex and other characteristics of apicomplexan protozoa are recognizable in various stages of the organism (sporozoite, merozoite, ookinete) on the electron microscopic level (see *Toxoplasma*, p. 509).

Life cycle. The life cycle of malaria plasmodia includes phases of asexual multiplication in the human host and sexual reproduction and formation of sporozoites in the vector, a female *Anopheles* mosquito (Fig. 9.**17**). The developmental cycle within the human host is as follows:

■ **Infection and exoerythrocytic development.** Humans are infected through the bite of an infected female *Anopheles* mosquito that inoculates spindleshaped sporozoites (see below) into the bloodstream or deep corium. Only a small number of sporozoites are needed to cause an infection in humans (about 10 *P. falciparum*). Within about 15–45 minutes of inoculation, the sporozoites of all *Plasmodium* species reach the liver in the bloodstream and infect hepatocytes, in which asexual multiplication takes place. In this process, the sporozoite develops into a multinuclear, large (30–70 μm) schizont (meront) described as a tissue schizont. Following cytoplasmic divi-

9

sion 2000 (*P. malariae*) to 30 000 (*P. falciparum*) merozoites are produced. This development takes six (*P. falciparum*) to 15 (*P. malariae*) days. Shortly thereafter, the tissue schizonts release the merozoites, which then infect erythrocytes (see below). In infections with *P. vivax* and *P. ovale*, sporozoites develop into tissue schizonts as described above, but some remain dormant as so-called hypnozoites, which may develop into schizonts following activation after months or years. Merozoites released from these schizonts then infect erythrocytes, causing relapses of the disease (see p. 527).

■ **Erythrocytic development.** The merozoites produced in the liver are released into the bloodstream where they infect erythrocytes, in which they reproduce asexually. The merozoites are small, ovoid forms about 1.5 µm in length that attach to receptor molecules on the erythrocyte surface. These receptors are species-specific, which explains why certain *Plasmodium* species prefer certain cell types: *P. malariae* infects mainly older erythrocytes, *P. vivax* and *P. ovale* prefer reticulocytes, and *P. falciparum* infects younger and older erythrocytes. Following receptor attachment, merozoites penetrate into the erythrocyte, where they are enclosed in a parasitophorous vacuole.

A *Plasmodium* that has recently infected an erythrocyte (<12 hours) appears ring-shaped with a thin cytoplasmic rim in a Giemsa-stained blood smear. Also visible are a central food vacuole and the dark-stained nucleus located at the periphery of the parasite. This stage is very similar in all four *Plasmodium* species (Fig. 9.**18**, p. 524). The ring forms develop into schizonts, which feed on glucose and hemoglobin. The latter is broken down to a brownish-black pigment (hemozoin)—after the amino acids used by the plasmodia are split off—and deposited in the parasite's food vacuole as "malaria pigment." The schizont undergoes multiple divisions to produce merozoites, in different numbers depending on the *Plasmodium* species (6–36). The merozoites enter

9

Fig. 9.**17 a** In humans: 1 sporozoite from infected *Anopheles* mosquito; **2** development in the liver; **2a** primary tissue schizonts and schizogony in hepatocytes (all *Plasmodium* species); **2b** hypnozoites and delayed schizogony in hepatocytes (*P. vivax* and *P. ovale* only); **3** further schizogenic development in erythrocytes; **3a** development of sexually differentiated plasmodia (female macrogametocytes and male microgametocytes).
b in the *Anopheles* mosquito: **4** macrogametocytes and microgametocytes taken up by bloodsucking mosquito; **5** fertilization of macrogametes (round) by microgametes (long); **6** fertilized macrogamete (ookinete) in intestinal wall of mosquito; **7** oocyst with sporozoites in intestinal wall; **8** infective sporozoites in salivary gland (according to Peters W. *Chemotherapy and Drug Resistance in Malaria*. Vol. 1, London: Academic Press; 1987:16). ▶

Malarial Plasmodia: Life Cycle

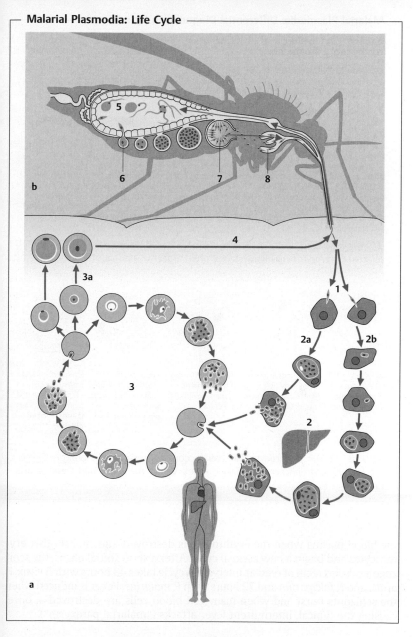

Malarial Plasmodia: Differential Diagnosis in Blood Smears

A: Young trophozoite	B: Older trophozoite	C: Schizont	D: Macro-gametocyte	E: Micro-gametocyte

Plasmodium falciparum
Infected erythrocyte: size and form normal, multiple infection more frequent than with other *Plasmodium species*, rarely: Maurer's clefts

Small rings; 1/3 to 1/5 of EDM, binuclear form frequent, narrow plasmic fringe, vacuole small	Vacuoles small or lacking, pigment dispersed or in clumps	8–24 merozoites, sometimes more, pigment usually peripheral	Sickle-shaped, nucleus compact and central, pigment arranged around nucleus	Sickle-shaped, plumper than D, nucleus larger and less compact

Plasmodium vivax
Infected erythrocyte beginning at stage B: often larger than normal, often with red Schüffner's dots

Rings 1/3 to 1/2 EDM, vacuole large, plasmic fringe narrow	Large rings or irregularly cleft form with diffuse pigment dispersal	12–24 merozoites, 1 to 2 pigment clumps, peripheral or central	Rounded, larger than EDM, nucleus small and excentric, with diffuse pigment dispersal	Rounded, nucleus larger than D, central or excentric, pigment finer than D and dispersed diffusely

Fig. 9.**18** EDM = erythrocyte diameter (according to Geigy R, Herbig A. *Erreger und Überträger tropischer Krankheiten*. Basel: Verlag für Recht und Gesellschaft; 1995).

the blood plasma when the erythrocyte is destroyed, they infect other erythrocytes and begin a new asexual cycle. After a short initial phase, the schizogonic cycles recur at regular intervals. A cycle takes 48 hours with *P. vivax, P. ovale*, and *P. falciparum* and 72 hours with *P. malariae*. Fever is induced when the schizonts burst and when many red blood cells are destroyed at once, causing the typical, intermittent fever attacks ("malarial paroxysm").

Malarial Plasmodia: Differential Diagnosis in Blood Smears

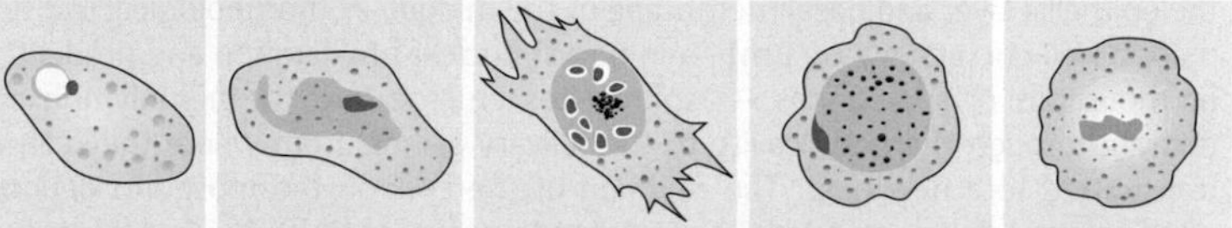

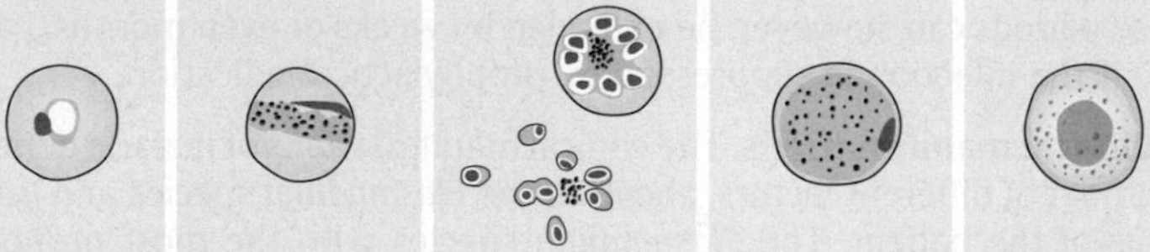

A: Young trophozoite	B: Older trophozoite	C: Schizont	D: Macro-gametocyte	E: Micro-gametocyte

Plasmodium ovale
Infected erythrocyte beginning at stage A: somewhat enlarged, often oval with ragged edges, Schüffner's dots more pronounced than in *Plasmodium vivax*

Rings similar to *Plasmodium vivax*	Rounded or cleft, pigment not very prominent	8 merozoites, pigment central	Similar to *Plasmodium vivax*, rare in oval erythrocytes	Similar to *Plasmodium vivax*, rare in oval erythrocytes

Plasmodium malariae
Infected erythrocyte: size normal or somewhat smaller than usual, multiple infection rare

Plasma ring wide, vacuole midsized	Band or rounded form, vacuoles lacking or small, pigment dark brown	6–12 merozoites, often in rosette form, pigment usually central	Similar to *P. vivax*, but smaller	Similar to *P. vivax*, but smaller

Fig. 9.**18**   *Continued*

9

■ After one or more schizogonic generations, some of the plasmodia in each generation develop into sexual forms, the male microgamonts (microgametocytes), and female macrogamonts (macrogametocytes). These sexual forms (gametocytes) persist for a certain period in the blood (*P. vivax* one day, *P. falciparum* up to 22 days), after which those not taken up by bloodsucking *Anopheles* females die.

Development in the Mosquito (Sexual Development and Sporogony)

This developmental stage is shown in detail in Fig. 9.**17b** and will only be described briefly here. In the mosquito midgut, each microgamont develops into (in most cases) eight uninucleate, flagellate microgametes and the macrogamont is transformed into a macrogamete → fusion of a microgamete and macrogamete to form a motile zygote (ookinete) → the ookinetes occupy the space between the epithelial layer and basal membrane of the midgut → morphological transformation into oocysts (40–60 µm) → in oocyst nuclear proliferation and production of thousands of sporozoites → sporozoites emerge into the hemolymph and migrate through the body cavity to the salivary glands, from where they can be transmitted to a new host. The duration of the cycle in the mosquito depends on the plasmodial species and the ambient temperature; at 20–28 °C, it takes eight to 14 days.

Clinical manifestations

Incubation periods. The clinical manifestations of malaria are caused by the asexual erythrocytic stages of the plasmodia and therefore commence shortly after parasitemia at the earliest. The incubation periods vary, depending on the *Plasmodium* species involved, from seven to 35 days after infection. These periods can, however, be extended by weeks or even months, particularly if the infection is suppressed by prophylactic medication.

Clinical manifestations. The clinical manifestations of malaria depend on a number of different factors, above all the *Plasmodium* species and immune status of the patient. The *Plasmodium* species with the most pronounced pathogenicity is *Plasmodium falciparum*, which causes "malignant tertian malaria" (malaria tropica), whereas the other *Plasmodium* species cause milder forms ("benign malaria"). Children and nonimmune adults from nonmalarious areas (e.g., European and US tourists), as well as children in endemic regions aged six months to three years, are most susceptible to infection.

Onset symptoms. Malaria begins with nonspecific initial symptoms that last several days, including for instance headache, pain in limbs, general fatigue, chills, and occasionally nausea as well as intermittent fever, either continuous or at irregular intervals. These symptoms can easily be mistaken for signs of influenza!

Febrile patterns. Several days to a week after onset of parasitemia, the schizogonic cycle synchronizes: in infections with *P. vivax*, *P. ovale*, and *P. falciparum*, a cycle is completed within 48 hours, in infections with *P. malariae* within 72 hours. Bouts of fever occur at the same intervals, i.e., on day 1, then 48 hours later on day 3 (hence "malaria tertiana") or on day 1 and then again after 72 hours on day 4 (hence "malaria quartana"). It is important to note that the malignant tertian malaria (malaria tropica) often does not show this typical periodicity.

■ **Classic malarial paroxysm.** After an initial rise in temperature to about 39 °C, peripheral vasoconstriction causes a period of chills (lasting for about 10 minutes to one hour), then the temperature once again rises to 40–41 °C (febrile stage two to six hours), whereupon peripheral vasodilatation and an outbreak of sweating follow. These bouts occur mainly in the afternoon and evening hours. Once the paroxysm has abated and the fever has fallen, the patient feels well again until the next one begins. In severe malaria tropica, however, circulatory disturbances, collapse, or delirium may occur without fever (algid malaria).

■ **Course of infection and recurrence.** The malarial paroxysms are repeated at intervals until parasite multiplication in the erythrocytes is suppressed by chemotherapy or the host immune response. Parasites that persist in the host can cause relapses for months or even years after the initial infection. Recurrence results either from persistence of erythrocytic forms (recrudescence) or reactivation of hypnozoites (p. 522) (relapse).

Types of malaria

■ **Tertian malaria** (*malaria tertiana*), caused by *P. vivax* or *P. ovale*:

Incubation period: nine to 20 days, also several weeks or months.
Parasitemia: generally low level, up to a maximum of 1–2%.
Course: usually benign ("benign malaria"). Febrile stage three to four hours, again 48 hours later. If untreated, disease lasts three to eight weeks or longer.
Recurrence: frequent relapses, after months and for up to five years; important: misdiagnosis is frequent!
Special characteristics: "tertiana quotidiana" is characterized by daily bouts of fever and results when two parasite populations overlap.

■ **Quartan malaria** (*malaria quartana*), caused by *P. malariae*:

Incubation period: 15–40 days (usually longer than with other species).
Parasitemia: generally low level, up to a maximum of 1%.
Course: usually benign. Febrile stage four to five hours, again 72 hours later. If untreated, disease lasts three to 24 weeks or longer.
Recurrence: frequent recrudescences, after months and even decades (30 years). Important: misdiagnosis is frequent!
Special characteristics: nephrotic syndrome, especially in African children.

■ **Malignant tertian malaria** (*malaria tropica*), caused by *P. falciparum*:

Incubation period:	seven to 15 days or longer.
Parasitemia:	often at very high level, up to 20 % or more!
Course:	initial symptoms often more pronounced than in other types. Rapid, severe course in nonimmune persons. High lethality rate if untreated (50–60 % in persons from central Europe).
	After short initial phase fever high, continuous or with <48 hour rhythm. If untreated, disease lasts two to three weeks.
Recurrence:	recrudescence is rare, usually within one year.
Special characteristics:	**severe complications are possible**, especially cerebral malaria (e.g., with convulsions, disturbed vision and coordination, altered states of consciousness, coma); severe normocytic anemia; pulmonary edema and respiratory insufficiency; renal insufficiency; gastrointestinal disturbances; circulatory collapse; hypoglycemia; liquid/electrolyte unbalance, spontaneous hemorrhaging; disseminated intravasal coagulation; hyperpyrexia (39.5–42 °C); hemoglobinuria ("blackwater fever"); hyperparasitemia.

■ **Mixed infections**

Mixed infections with two *Plasmodium* species are observed in about 3–4 % of all cases and may alter the course of the disease.

Pathogenesis and pathology. The clinical manifestations of malaria are caused by the erythrocytic stages ("blood stages") of the plasmodia and reflect multifactorial pathogenic process affecting many different organs. Only an outline of these processes can be drawn here, especially with regard to *falciparum* (tropical) malaria.

■ **The role of cytokines.** As a result of erythrocytic schizogony and the attendant rupture of erythrocytes (red blood cells = RBCs), malarial antigens (phospholipids and glycolipids) are released that stimulate macrophages and monocytes to produce tumor necrosis factor alpha (TNFα) and other cytokines (IL-1, IL-6, IL-8, etc.). Also associated with this process are bouts of fever, to which hemozoin presumably contributes as well. Cytokine production is also initiated by IFNγ produced in the immunological TH1 response. TNFα plays a special role in pathogenicity, since the concentration of this cytokine in the blood correlates with the severity of a *P. falciparum* infection. This substance also, at higher concentrations, induces fever, inhibits erythropoiesis, stimulates erythrophagocytosis, and causes various nonspecific symptoms such as nausea, vomiting, and diarrhea. At lower concentrations, TNFα can contribute to the killing of the intracellular parasites. Various other cytokines (see above) either synergize with TNFα or induce different reactions.

■ **Anemia.** An important factor in malarial pathogenesis, especially in malaria tropica, is anemia, caused by destruction of RBCs in schizogony, increased elimination of both infected and noninfected RBCs in the spleen, inhibition of erythropoiesis by TNFα, and other factors.

■ **Cytoadherence and rosette formation.** RBCs infected with maturing *P. falciparum* schizonts adhere to the endothelium of blood vessels in various organs, especially in postcapillary venules. This phenomenon is due to an interaction between strain-specific ligands of the parasite with host receptors. During the development of *P. falciparum* from the ring form to the maturing schizont, buttonlike protrusions of the erythrocytic membrane develop, under which high-molecular (200–300 kDa) proteins are enriched, then presented at the cell surface. These so-called *P. falciparum* erythrocyte membrane proteins (PfEMP) bind to a variety of endothelial receptors, for instance to the intercellular adhesion molecule (ICAM), thrombospondin, E-selectin (ELAM), and the CD36 molecule. ICAM-1 and ELAM-1 are thought to be mainly responsible for cytoadherence in the brain. These substances are produced in significant amounts there and are inducible by TNFα and other cytokines. Outside of the brain the receptor CD36 is apparently the most important recognition protein. The PfEMP antigens, coded for by about 150 genes, are variable and play a role in parasite immunoevasion. The advantage of cytoadherence for the plasmodia is that part of their population thus avoids elimination in the spleen. For the host, however, cytoadherence has pathological consequences: it hinders local microcirculation as well as gas and substance exchange processes, the resulting anemia exacerbates tissue hypoxia and, finally, it causes cell and organ damage with grave sequelae in the brain in particular. Rosette formation refers to clumping of RBCs infected by *P. falciparum* with other noninfected ones caused by mechanisms similar to cytoadherence.

■ **Other processes (a selection).** Due to the destruction of RBCs and parasites and resulting production of TNFα, phagocytosing cells of the reticuloendothelial system are activated. Signs of this include splenic swelling in the course of the infection and increased elimination of erythrocytes in the spleen (see anemia). Renal damage in acute malaria tropica is caused by capillary cytoadherence and tubular necrosis. In malaria quartana, such damage is due to deposition of immune complexes in the renal capillaries.

■ **Pathological changes.** Such changes are known from cases of malaria tropica in particular. Brain capillaries are clogged with infected RBCs (the pigment in the plasmodia is especially noticeable), hemorrhages, necrotic foci on obturated vessels surrounded by inflammatory reactions (Dürck granulomas). Further changes can be found in the spleen and liver (for instance swelling, hyperplasia of phagocytosing cells containing plasmodia and pigment), heart, lungs, kidneys, and other organs.

Resistance and immunity. Certain properties of blood are responsible for increased natural resistance to malarial infection. For instance, the intraerythrocytic development of *P. falciparum* is inhibited in persons with various hemoglobinopathies (HbS, HbE, HbF, HbC), in glucose-6-phosphate dehydrogenase deficiency (G6PDD) and β-thalassemia. On the other hand, persons with G6PDD are more sensitive to certain antimalarials (quinine, 8-aminoquinoline). Persons lacking the Duffy blood group antigen are resistant to *P. vivax*, but susceptible to *P. ovale*. A milk diet partially inhibits the development of malarial parasites in the RBCs because of a resulting reduced supply of p-aminobenzoic acid (vitamin H_1). This results in a milder malarial course, e.g., in infants.

In the course of a malaria infection, a host immune response develops, which, however, does not confer complete protection, but rather merely raises the level of resistance to future infections. Accordingly, the course of malaria infections is less dramatic in populations of endemic areas than in persons exposed to the parasites less frequently or for the first time. In these malarious areas, children are the main victims of the disease, which is less frequent and takes a milder course in older persons. Infants of mothers who have overcome malaria usually do not become ill in the first months of life due to diaplacental antibody transmission and a certain level of protection from the milk diet. On the other hand, children without maternal antibodies can become severely ill if they contract malaria, since their own immune defenses are developing gradually. Nonimmune travelers from nonmalarious regions are at special risk of infection.

The immunity conferred in humans by exposure to plasmodia develops gradually and is specific to the strains and stages that are capable of antigen variation. A particularly important part of the generalized immune response appears to be the component induced by asexual blood forms, which confers a protective effect against new infections. The specialist literature should be consulted for more details on this aspect. Despite many years of intensive effort, a decisive breakthrough in the development of malaria vaccines has not yet been achieved.

Epidemiology. Constant minimum temperatures of 16–18 °C (optimum: 20–30 °C) and high humidity for several weeks are preconditions for vectoral transmission of malaria. Further requirements for the plasmodial cycle are an epidemiologically relevant parasite reservoir in the population and the presence of suitable vectors.

Malarial parasites can be transmitted by female mosquitoes of about 80 species of the genus *Anopheles* (*Anopheles gambiae* complex, etc.). The larval and pupal stages of these mosquitoes develop in standing bodies of water, often near human dwellings. Anopheline mosquitoes are active from dusk to dawn. The females bite both in the outside and within buildings. Malaria often accompanies the rainy season, which provides the bodies of water the mosquitoes need. Occurrence is usually endemic, but epidemics do sometimes develop. The incidence of infections varies widely and the immune status of the population is a major factor (see immunity p. 530).

Alternative transmission routes for malarial plasmodia include diaplacental infection, blood transfusions (plasmodia survive in stored blood for five days, rarely longer), and contaminated needles used by drug addicts.

Diagnosis. Etiological confirmation of a clinical diagnosis is obtained by detecting malarial parasites in the blood (Fig. 9.**18**). Capillary blood is sampled before chemotherapy is started, if possible before the onset of fever, and examined microscopically in both thick and thin blood smears following Giemsa staining (p. 622). Stages of *P. falciparum*, *P. vivax*, and *P. ovale* can be found in blood five to eight days after the infection at the earliest, *P. malariae* not until after 13–16 days. The QBC (quantitative buffy coat) method can be used to concentrate the plasmodia. Rapid tests (ParaSight, MalaQuick) have also been available for some years to diagnose *P. falciparum* infections. Using a monoclonal antibody, these tests can detect a specific *Plasmodium* antigen (HRP2) in whole blood with a very high level of sensitivity and specificity. Another rapid test (OptiMAL) for diagnosis of all *Plasmodium* species is based on detection of specific lactate dehydrogenase.

Detection of specific antibodies in the serum of persons infected with plasmodia for the first time is not possible until six to 10 days after inoculation (Table 11.**5**, p. 625). In such cases, a serological antibody assay is not a suitable tool to confirm a diagnosis in an acute attack of malaria, although this method does provide valuable help in confirming older infections and screening out blood donors infected with plasmodia. DNA detection by means of PCR can be used to identify the different *Plasmodium* species for research purposes.

Therapy. Patients infected for the first time (e.g., travelers from the northern hemisphere returning from a stay in the tropics) may suffer highly acute and severe courses of malaria. Therapy and intensive clinical monitoring must therefore begin immediately, especially in acute malignant tertian malaria (malaria tropica) (medical emergency!). Table 9.**6** summarizes a number of antimalarials and their spectra of action. The best that can be offered here by way of a description of the highly complex field of malaria treatment is a brief sketch of the main principles involved.

Table 9.**6** Antimalarial Agents (a selection)

Chemical group and drug (P): used for prophylaxis	Spectrum of efficacy			
	Asexual blood stages	Game-tocytes	Liver schizonts	Hypnozoites of *P.vivax*, *P. ovale*
Arylaminoalcohls				
Quinine	+	VOM	–	–
Lumefantrine	+	VOM	–	–
Mefloquine (P)	+	VOM	–	–
4-Aminoquinolines	+	VOM	–	–
Chloroquine (P)	+	VOM	–	–
Amodiaquine	+	VOM	–	–
8-Aminoquinolines				
Primaquine	+/–	+	+	+
Naphtoquinones				
Atovaquone	+	VOM	+	–
Phenanthrene methanoles				
Halofantrine	+	–	–	–
Sesquiterpene lactones				
Artemisinin	+	+	–	–
Artemether	+	ni	ni	ni
Artesunates	+	ni	ni	ni
Sulfones/Sulfonamides				
Dapsone	+	–	F	–
Sulfadoxine (P)	F	–	F	–
Biguanides				
Proguanil (P)	+/–	?	+	–
Diaminopyrimidines				
Pyrimethamine (P)	+	–	–	v
Antibiotics (Tetracyclines)				
Doxycycline (P)	+	–	F	–

Table 9.**6** *Continued: Antimalarial Agents (a selection)*

Chemical group and drug (P): used for prophylaxis	Spectrum of efficacy			
	Asexual blood stages	Game-tocytes	Liver schizonts	Hypnozoites of *P.vivax*, *P. ovale*
Drug combinations				
Atovaquone + proguanil (P)	+	VOM	+	–
Artemether + lumefantrine	+	+	ni	–
Chloroquine + proguanil (P)	+	VOM	F	–
Sulfadoxine[2] + pyrimethamine[3]	+	VOM	–	–
Sulfadoxine[2] + pyrimethamine[3] + mefloquine	+	VOM	–	–

[1] Effectiveness: +: effective; +/–: moderately effective; ?: questionably effective; –: ineffective.

F: effective against *P. falciparum*; VOM: effective against *P. vivax, P. ovale, P. malariae*; ni: no information

[2] Dihydropteroate synthetase inhibitors (= sulfonamides and sulfones)

[3] Dihydrofolate reductase inhibitors (= antifolates)

■ **Treatment of acute disease.** The clinical symptoms of malaria are caused by the asexual forms in the erythrocytic schizogonic cycle. A clinical cure is thus achieved by eliminating these forms or stages with so-called schizonti-cides (Table 9.**6**). The antimalarials preferred in this indication are fast-acting schizonticides such as quinine, mefloquine, and halofantrine (in some countries artemisinin derivatives as well) as well as quinine combined with doxy-cycline (especially in complicated tropical malaria) and various combined preparations (Table 9.**6**). Some of the above substances are also effective against chloroquine-resistant and multiresistant *Plasmodium* strains. Chloro-quine, a former mainstay of malaria therapy, has now lost some of its importance due to widespread drug resistance of plasmodia.

■ **Prevention of relapses (radical cure).** Agents effective against blood schizonts do not eliminate the latent tissue forms (hypnozoites) of *Plasmo-dium vivax* and *Plasmodium ovale* in the liver. To prevent relapses, tissue forms can be eliminated with primaquine after the acute therapy is completed (Table 9.**6**). This therapy is not required for infections by *P. falciparum* and *P. malariae* since they do not produce hypnozoites.

9

Drug resistance. The resistance of malaria plasmodia to certain antimalarial drugs is a growing problem. Resistance is classified from RI (low grade) to RIII (high grade) and applies particularly to malaria tropica. Table 9.**7** and Fig. 9.**19** provide information on regions in which resistant *P. falciparum* strains have developed. Selection of drugs and their dosage in therapy and prevention must take this problem into account. In-vitro methods are available for resistance testing.

Prevention. Travelers to malarious areas should be informed well ahead of time concerning the risk of infection at their destination and the necessary prophylactic measures. This information is available from specialists and institutions in the field of tropical medicine, health offices, etc., as well as on the internet (WHO: www.who.int; Austria: www.reisemed.at; Germany: www.dtg.mwn.de; Switzerland: www.safetravel.ch). **It is important to remember that updated information is required because recommended malaria prevention measures vary from country to country and are subject to sudden changes.**

Prophylactic measures are necessary for travelers to malarious areas in **Africa**, **Central** and **South America**, and **Asia**. **Sub-Saharan Africa** in particular must be considered a high-risk area. Within a malarious area, the risk of infection may vary widely depending on the season, locality, and length of stay. Prophylactic measures must take this variation into consideration.

The following methods can be used to **prevent a malaria infection**:
— mosquito bite prevention,
— chemoprophylaxis,
— emergency stand-by therapy.

Malaria Prophylaxis by Areas

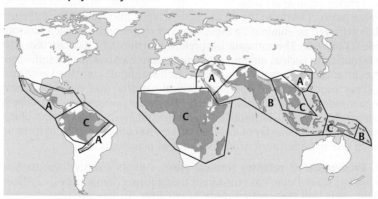

Fig. 9.**19** See Table 9.**7** for explanation (according to: *International Travel and Health*. Geneva: World Health Organization; 2000).

Table **9.7** Examples of Chemoprophylactic Regimens and Standby Medications by Areas[1]

Area	Characteristics of areas[2]	Prophylactic drugs	Standby drugs
A	Areas without chloroquine resistance or without *P. falciparum*	Chloroquine	None
		None	Chloroquine
B	Areas with chloroquine resistance	Chloroquine + proguanil or mefloquine	None
		None	Mefloquine or Atovaquone + proguanil
C	Areas with high chloroquine resistance or multiresistance	Mefloquine (doxycycline)[3]	None
		Doxycycline	Mefloquine or atovaquone + proguanil
		Chloroquine + proguanil	Mefloquine or atovaquone + proguanil

[1] Modified and supplemented according to: *International Travel and Health*. Geneva: World Health Organization; 2000 and other sources.
Note: Actual updates with detailed information on infection risk by country, region, and season can be obtained from the internet, for example: www.dtg.mwn.de.
[2] The data on resistance do not indicate the actual infection risk.
[3] In certain parts of Southeast Asia (border region Cambodia, Myanmar, Thailand).

The main aim of these measures is prevention of the life-threatening malignant tertian malaria (*malaria tropica*) caused by *P. falciparum.*

■ **Mosquito bite prevention (prevention of exposure):** in view of widespread drug resistance in plasmodia, it is very important to prevent mosquito bites in addition to chemoprophylactic measures. Remember, ***Anopheles* mosquitoes are active from dusk to dawn** and bites are possible both outside and inside buildings (although this is unusual in air-conditioned rooms). In general, the risk of being bitten by an *Anopheles* mosquito is lower in urban areas than in rural areas and may even be negligible in a city (exception: certain cities in tropical Africa and India). The following protective measures are recommended:

— Always wear **clothing** in the dusk and at night (long sleeves, long trousers) that prevents mosquito bites as far as possible. Spray clothing with a fast-acting insecticide (pyrethrines).

— Apply an **insect repellent** to uncovered skin (spray or spread by hand) (products with 20% diethyl-m-toluamide are protective for three to five hours).

— **Screen off** rooms to keep mosquitoes out (close doors and windows, fit fine-meshed screens on doors and windows).

— Spray mosquito resting places in room with **insecticide**. Use insecticide dispenser with renewable insecticide pellet or pyrethroid smoke coils.

— Screen off beds with mosquito nets (very important to protect infants and small children!).

— Impregnating bed nets with an insecticide (pyrethroids: permethrin, deltamethrin) increases their effectiveness.

■ **Chemoprophylaxis and emergency treatment. Chemoprophylaxis** comprises regular intake of antimalarial drugs before, during, and for a defined period after a stay in a malarious area. Depending on the target a distinction between suppressive and causal prophylaxis can be made: suppressive drugs prevent clinical symptoms by affecting the asexual stages in the erythrocytes, whereas causal drugs act against the tissue schizonts of *P. falciparum* in the liver, thus preventing the erythrocytic cycle. Most of the agents currently in use have a suppressive effect (Table 9.**6**). For short stays in low-risk areas, it may under certain circumstances make sense to refrain from chemoprophylaxis and take along an **emergency stand-by drug.** Self-treatment can be initiated in response to malarious symptoms if a physician cannot be reached within 12 hours. Taking along a stand-by drug is also worth considering if there is a high risk of infection with *P. falciparum* (especially multiresistant strains) and it is unclear whether the planned chemoprophylaxis will provide sufficient protection. Always remember the following principles:

— There is at present no chemoprophylactic regimen that can guarantee 100% efficacy. Therefore, a physician must be consulted immediately if fever occurs during or after the chemoprophylactic regimen.

— Specific antimalarials recommended by specialists must be used for chemoprophylaxis and emergency treatment. These substances may cause side effects.

— Specific advisement of travelers adapted to their individual situation (general health status, pregnancy, age, small children, allergies, etc.) and the specific situation at their destination is very important.

— Begin with chemoprophylaxis at the latest *one to two weeks before traveling* to a malarious area. During this period, potential side effects can be recognized and countermeasures can be taken or the medication changed as necessary.

— Duration of chemoprophylaxis: *during and four weeks after the traveler's stay* in the malarious area (with atovaquone/proguanil only one week). This measure is intended to prevent malaria tropica and does not affect hypnozoites of *P. vivax* and *P. ovale* (treatment with 8-aminoquinolines as required to prevent relapse, see above).

— The drugs are swallowed with liquid after meals. The dosages, intervals between intake and any restrictions (e.g., for pregnant women) must be strictly complied with.

■ Examples of chemoprophylaxis and use of emergency stand-by drugs. The modified and supplemented WHO recommendations are used as examples here (Table 9.**7**). NB: recommendations in some countries may differ considerably from the information in the table! The necessary measures differ in the different risk zones (Fig. 9.**19**) and apply to brief stays in malarious areas of up to three months for nonimmune persons. For longer stays (more than three months), the prophylaxis should be started as for a shorter stay, then a physician in the endemic area should be consulted concerning long-term measures.

Disease control. The main methods applied are *Anopheles* control by spraying houses and stables with insecticides (indoor spraying), environmental sanitation measures to eliminate mosquito-breeding places, and the usage of insecticide-impregnated bed nets to reduce vector-human contacts. Further measures in endemic areas are early diagnosis and treatment of malaria cases as well as chemoprophylaxis in selected population groups. Antimalaria vaccines are not available yet.

9

Babesia

Causative agent of babesiosis

Babesia species are apicomplexan blood parasites of the order *Piroplasmida* that occur quite frequently in domestic and wild animals in countries on all continents and are transmitted by hard tick species. In vertebrate hosts, they parasitize in erythrocytes and are detectable in stained blood smears, usually in the form of small rings and single or double pearshaped organisms (about 2–2.5 µm long). In contrast to plasmodia they do not contain pigment (hemozoin). *Babesia* infections are infrequently observed in humans, primarily affecting splenectomized, elderly, and immunocompromised patients. The causative agents were identified as *Babesia microti* from rodents, *B. divergens* from cattle, and some previously unknown *Babesia* species or strains. Such infections can cause severe malarialike symptoms.

Microspora

Causative agents of microsporosis

■ The clinical significance of the microspora is based mainly on their role as "opportunistic parasites" in HIV patients. The most important species are *Enterocytozoon bieneusi* and *Encephalitozoon intestinalis*. Transmission is by characteristic spores. Little is known about the epidemiology of these organisms that are closely related to the fungi. ■

Parasites. The phylum Microspora includes about 140 genera and 1300 species. They are parasites with intracellular development and spore formation. The host spectrum ranges from numerous invertebrates (e.g., protozoa, insects) to many species in all classes of vertebrates. The lack of mitochondria, peroxisomes, and typical Golgi membranes as well as their prokaryotelike ribosomes were previously regarded as characteristics of most primitive eukaryotes. Recently, analyzes of a variety of genes and proteins have revealed a close relationship to fungi. Therefore, some authorities now consider the Microspora to be highly specialized fungi rather than primitive protozoa and place them as a superclass into the subphylum fungi. A notable characteristic of the microspora is the unique morphology of their spores (see below).

Microspora, known since the middle of the last century, have attained attention as human pathogens and opportunistic parasites in the course of the AIDS epidemic. Several genera and species have been identified in humans to date (Table 9.**1**, p. 477).

Morphology and life cyle. Microspora reproduce intracellularly by means of repeated, asexual binary or multiple fission (merogony), then form spores in a subsequent phase (sporogony) (and sexual stages as well in *Thelohania*). The developmental stages are located freely in the host cell cytoplasm (*Enterocytozoon, Nosema*) or they inhabit a parasitophorous vacuole (*Encephalitozoon*); in other genera (*Pleistophora, Trachipleistophora*) the intracellular stages are separated from the cytoplasm by an amorphous layer (pansporoblastic membrane). Sporogony begins with formation of sporonts, which are derived from merogonic cells and possess a thicker cell wall. The sporonts divide to form sporoblasts, followed by morphological differentiation into spores.

The fine structure of these spores is typical of Microspora (Fig. 9.**20a, b**). The two-layered spore wall (exospore and endospore) encloses the uninucleate (rarely: binucleate) infective parasite stage called a sporoplasm or "ameboid organism" and a complex expulsion apparatus consisting of a coiled polar tubule and the polaroplast, a membranous anchoring component. The size of the spores of Microspora species infecting humans varies between about 1 and 4 µm. The number and position of the polar tubule windings as seen on the electron microscopical level (Fig. 9.**20a, b**) are of diagnostic importance.

The spores are eliminated in feces, urine, or sputum and can remain viable for several weeks outside of the host. Following peroral ingestion by a suitable host, the polaroplast swells up, the internal pressure in the spore in-

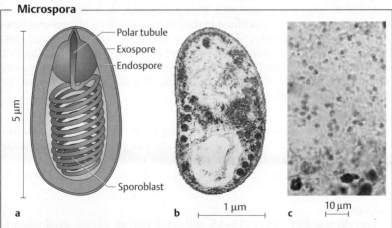

— **Microspora** —

Polar tubule
Exospore
Endospore

5 µm

Sporoblast

a

b   1 µm

c   10 µm

9

Fig. 9.**20**   **a** Spore (modified from Binford CH, Connor D, eds. *Pathology of Tropical and Extraordinary Diseases*. Vol. 1. Washington: Armed Forces Institute of Pathology; 1987: 336); **b** immature spore of *Encephalitozoon hellem* (TEM); **c** spores of *Enterocytozoon bieneusi* in stool smear, chromotropic stain according to Weber.

creases and the polar tubule, which is up to 100 µm long, is extruded rapidly. If the tip of the polar tubule penetrates the wall of an enterocyte, the sporoplasm migrates through the hollow tubule into the host cell. The Microspora then reproduce locally in intestinal cells or invade other organs from this site. Aerogenic infections appear probable in some genera. In animals, diaplacental transmission of *Encephalitozoon* has been confirmed.

It is not entirely clear by what mechanisms the Microspora are disseminated in the body. In cell cultures, the parasites are able to infect neighboring tissue cells by extruding their polar tubule and injecting the sporoplasm into them. In vitro, Microspora are phagocytosed by macrophages and other host cells (so-called nonprofessional phagocytes: epithelial and endothelial cells, mesenchymal cells). It is assumed that they may be transported within the body inside such cells.

Clinical manifestations. Microspora attain clinical significance almost exclusively in immunodeficient persons, in particular AIDS patients. The following list summarizes the diseases caused by the individual species together with some diagnostic information.

■ *Enterocytozoon bieneusi*

Occurrence:
Probably worldwide, found in 2–50% of HIV patients with chronic diarrhea, with prevalence showing a downward trend since the new type of antiretroviral therapy was introduced. Rarely diagnosed in immunocompetent persons. *E. bieneusi* was also found in the biliary epithelium of monkeys (macaques) and in fecal samples of animals, including pigs, cattle, dogs, and cats. The species *E. bieneusi* consists of number of various genotypes. Current knowledge suggests that humans acquire the infection predominantly from infected persons, whereas transmission of genotypes from animals to man—if it occurs at all—is a rare event.

Localization:
Mainly in the small intestine, in enterocytes at the tips of villi, less frequently in the colon as well, in the bile ducts and gallbladder. Intracellular localization in plasma without parasitophorous vacuole. Symptoms: chronic diarrhea, also with cholangiopathy; asymptomatic infections are known to occur.

Diagnosis:
Detection of tiny spores (1.1–1.6 × 0.7–0.9 µm) in stained stool smears. The spores have four to seven polar tubule windings in a double row (in other species: single row!).

■ *Encephalitozoon intestinalis* (formerly *Septata intestinalis*).

Occurrence:

In HIV patients, but less frequent than *Enterocytozoon bieneusi*; (in a German study this pathogen was found in 2% of 97 patients). There is unconfirmed evidence of animal reservoirs.

Localization:

Mainly in the small intestine, in enterocytes, lamina propria, fibroblasts, macrophages, and endothelial cells, also found disseminated, for instance in bile ducts, airways, and the kidneys. Within host cell located in "chambers," separated off by septa (hence the earlier name *Septata*).

Symptoms:

Chronic diarrhea as with *E. bieneusi*, other symptoms as per organ localization. Diagnosis: spore detection in urine or stool, spores somewhat larger than in *E. bieneusi* (1.5–2.0 × 1.0–1.2 μm); four to seven polar tubule windings.

■ *Encephalitozoon cuniculi*

Occurrence:

Worldwide; occur frequently in domestic and wild rabbits, also described in many other animal species (rodents, dogs, cats, foxes, monkeys); rarely found in HIV patients. Of the three known pathogenic strains, two (rabbit and dog strain) have also been found in humans (= zoonosis).

Localization and symptoms:

Intracellular development in parasitophorous vacuoles. In rabbits mainly in renal tubuli and CNS. In HIV patients with disseminated infection causing hepatitis, peritonitis, nephritis, pneumonia, sinusitis, and encephalitis.

Diagnosis:

Spore detection in urine and organ specimens. Spores 2.5–3.2 × 1.2–1.6 μm with four to six polar tubule windings, morphologically indistinguishable from *E. hellem* spores (see *E. hellem*).

■ *Encephalitozoon hellem*

Occurrence:

Rare, in HIV patients.

Localization and symptoms:

Keratoconjunctivitis, sinusitis, bronchitis, pneumonia, nephritis, urinary tract infection, disseminated infection.

Diagnosis:

Morphologically identical to *E. cuniculi*, differentiation possible based on immunology and molecular biology.

9

■ **Other species infecting humans**

Brachiola (formerly *Nosema*) *connori* (disseminated in internal organs), *Nosema ocularum* (cornea), *Microsporidium africanum*, *M. ceylonensis* (cornea), *Vittaforma corneae* (formerly *Nosema corneum*) (cornea), *Pleistophora* sp. (skeletal muscle), *Trachipleistophora hominis* (skeletal muscle, nasal mucosa), and *Trachipleistophora anthropophthera* (cardiac and skeletal muscle, liver, brain).

Epidemiology. Little is known about the epidemiology of the Microspora. Their spores can remain viable outside of a host for several weeks, are relatively heat-resistant, and are killed by 70% ethanol in 10 minutes. *E. cuniculi* has a reservoir in animals; isolates of this species from rabbits and humans are morphologically, immunologically, and genetically identical. Pigs, dogs, and cats can function as carriers and excreters of *E. bieneusi*, but the genotypes of animal origin are of little—if any—significance for humans.

Diagnosis. Direct detection of the Microspora and identification taking into account species-specific characteristics (see Figs. 9.**11g**, 9.**20c**). *Encephalitozoon* and *Nosema* species can be grown and concentrated in cultures in various cell types. Material obtained in this way can then be used to identify species or strains using antigen or DNA analysis. In vitro culturing of *Enterocytozoon* has not succeeded yet. Serological antibody assay methods are still being evaluated and do not currently play a significant role in diagnostic practice.

Therapy and prevention. According to case reports, treatment with albendazole is clinically and parasitologically beneficial in enteral and systemic infections with *Encephalitozoon* species; the substance is, however, less effective against *Enterocytozoon bieneusi*. Nitazoxanide was reported to be effective in single cases against this latter species.

9

Balantidium coli

Causative agent of balantidiosis

Balantidium coli is a worldwide distributed ciliate of highly variable size (30–150 μm long). It is frequently found as an inhabitant of the large intestine of monkeys, rats, and in particular pigs. It is also found, more rarely, in humans, in whom it occasionally causes intestinal necrosis and inflammation with ulceration. The disease is transmitted through spherical cysts (40–60 μm) from host to host on the fecal-oral route. Diagnosis involves detection of cysts or vegetative forms in fecal samples. Drugs recommended for treatment are tetracyclines and metronidazole.

10 Helminths

J. Eckert

Helminths (*helmins*: worm) are parasitic metazoans from the phyla Platy-helmintha (flatworms), Nematoda (roundworms), and Acanthocephala (thorny-headed worms). The organisms in this last phylum are of little significance as human parasites. Table 10.1, p. 545 provides a taxonomic overview of the groups covered in the text.

Eggs and Larvae of Important Helminths

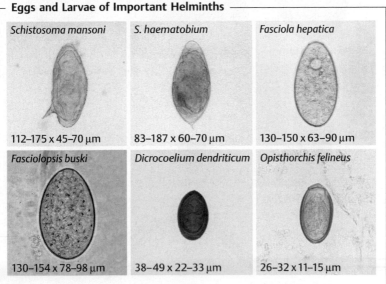

Schistosoma mansoni
112–175 x 45–70 μm

S. haematobium
83–187 x 60–70 μm

Fasciola hepatica
130–150 x 63–90 μm

Fasciolopsis buski
130–154 x 78–98 μm

Dicrocoelium dendriticum
38–49 x 22–33 μm

Opisthorchis felineus
26–32 x 11–15 μm

Fig. 10.1 Differential diagnosis of the eggs of important helminths (trematodes, cestodes, and nematodes) and of the larvae of *Strongyloides stercoralis*. Note: images are not to the same scale! (Images of *Hymenolepis* and *Enterobius*: H. Mehl-horn, Düsseldorf.)

Eggs and Larvae of Important Helminths

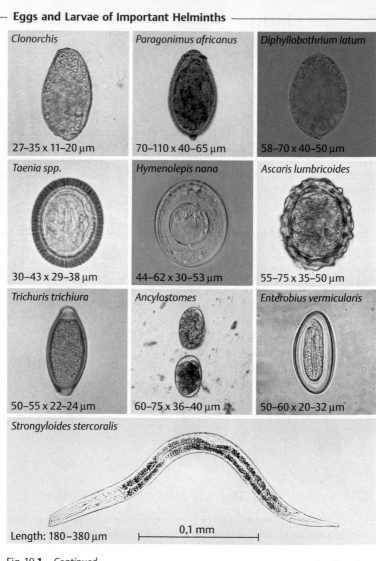

Clonorchis
27–35 x 11–20 µm

Paragonimus africanus
70–110 x 40–65 µm

Diphyllobothrium latum
58–70 x 40–50 µm

Taenia spp.
30–43 x 29–38 µm

Hymenolepis nana
44–62 x 30–53 µm

Ascaris lumbricoides
55–75 x 35–50 µm

Trichuris trichiura
50–55 x 22–24 µm

Ancylostomes
60–75 x 36–40 µm

Enterobius vermicularis
50–60 x 20–32 µm

Strongyloides stercoralis
Length: 180–380 µm
0,1 mm

Fig. 10.**1**   *Continued*

Table 10.1 Classification of Helminths Mentioned in the Text

Phylum ▪ Superclass*** ▪ Class** ▪ Subclass*	Order ▪ Superfamily	Genus
Platyhelmintha		
▪ Trematoda***	Strigeatida	*Schistosoma, Bilharziella, Trichobilharzia*
	Echinostomida	*Fasciola, Fasciolopsis, Echinostoma*
	Plagiorchiida	*Dicrocoelium, Paragonimus*
	Opisthorchiida	*Opisthorchis, Clonorchis, Heterophyes, Metagonimus*
▪ Cestoda**	Pseudophyllida	*Diphyllobothrium*
	Cyclophyllida	*Taenia, Echinococcus, Hymenolepis*
Nematoda		
▪ Secernentia*	Rhabditida	*Strongyloides*
	Strongylida	*Ancylsotsoma, Necator, Trichostrongylus, Angiostrongylus (= Parastrongylus)*
	Oxyurida	*Enterobius*
	Ascaridida	*Ascaris, Toxocara, Baylisascaris, Anisakis, Phocanema, Contracaecum*
	Spirurida	
	▪ Filarioidea	*Wuchereria, Brugia, Loa, Onchocerca, Mansonella, Dirofilaria*
	▪ Dracunculoidea	*Dracunculus*
▪ Adenophoria	Enoplida	*Trichuris, Trichinella*

Platyhelmintha (syn. Platyhelminthes)

Trematoda (Flukes)

General. Most of the trematode species that parasitize humans are dorsoventrally flattened with an oval to lancet shape, although others have different shapes such as the threadlike schistosomes. Suckers (*trema*: hole, opening) serve as attachment organs: an oral sucker around the mouth connected to the esophagus and the blind-ending intestine, and a ventral sucker. The body surface of adult trematodes is covered by a cellular tegument (composed of an outer annucleate, syncytial layer of cytoplasm connected by cytoplasmic strands to inner nucleated portions) through which substances can be absorbed from the environment. Most species are hermaphroditic, only the schistosomes have separate sexes. Snails are the first intermediate hosts; some species require arthropods or fish as second intermediate hosts.

Schistosoma (Blood Flukes)

Causative agents of schistosomosis or bilharziosis

■ Schistosomosis (bilharziosis) is one of the most frequent tropical diseases with about 200 million infected persons. The occurrence of schistosomosis depends on the presence of suitable intermediate hosts (freshwater snails). Human infections result from contact with standing or slow-moving bodies of water (freshwater) when *Schistosoma* cercariae penetrate the skin. *Schistosoma hematobium* causes urinary schistosomosis; *S. mansoni*, *S. japonicum*, *S. intercalatum*, and *S. mekongi* are the causative agents of intestinal schistosomosis and other forms of the disease. Diagnosis can be made by detection of either *Schistosoma* eggs in stool or urine or of specific antibodies in serum. ■

Parasite species and occurrence. Schistosomosis is also known as bilharziosis after the German physician Th. Bilharz, who discovered *Schistosoma hematobium* in human blood vessels in 1851. Schistosomosis occurs endemically in 74 tropical and subtropical countries of Africa, South America, and Asia (Fig. 10.**2**). The number of persons infected with schistosomes is estimated at 200 million (WHO, 2004).

The most important species pathogenic to humans are *Schistosoma hematobium* (Africa, the Near East, and questionable occurrence in India), *S. mansoni* (Africa, the Caribbean, the north-east of South America), and *S. japoni-*

Distribution of Schistosomes

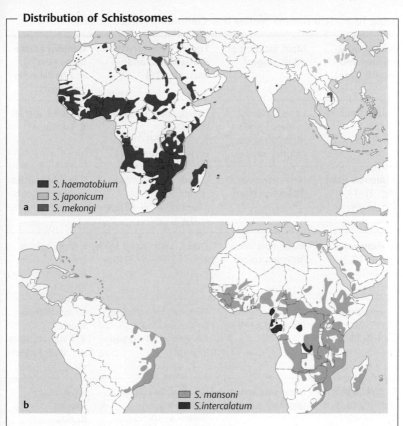

Fig. 10.**2** **a** *Schistosoma hematobium*, *S. japonicum*, and *S. mekongi*; **b** *S. mansoni* and *S. intercalatum* (according to *WHO Technical Report Series* No. 830. Geneva: World Health Organization; 1993).

10

cum (Southeast Asia and the western Pacific, especially China, Indonesia, the Philippines, but no longer in Japan). *S. intercalatum* occurs focally in central and western Africa, *S. mekongi* in Laos and Cambodia.

Morphology and life cycle. The various *Schistosoma* species can be differentiated morphologically (Table 10.**2**).

The relatively thick male forms a tegumental fold, the ventral groove (or canalis gynaecophorus) in which the threadlike female is enclosed. The male thus appears to be slit longitudinally (*schizein*: to split, *soma*: body) (Fig. 10.**3**).

Table 10.**2** Schistosoma Species that Commonly Infect Humans[1]

Schistosoma species and length (mm)	Main location of adult stages[2]	Eggs: characteristics, dimensions, and excretion (E)	I: Intermediate hosts (snails), R: Animal reservoir hosts[3]
S. haematobium ♂♂: 7–15 ♀♀: 9–20	Venous plexus in minor pelvis (draining urinary bladder, etc.)	Ovoid, with terminal spine, 83–187 × 60–70 μm E: urine, rarely stool	I: *Bulinus* species R: (Monkeys)
S. intercalatum ♂♂: 11–14 ♀♀: 13–24	Mesenteric veins (draining colon)	Ovoid, with terminal spine, 140–240 × 50–85 μm E: stool[3]	I: *Bulinus* species R: (sheep, goats)
S. mansoni ♂♂: 6–10 ♀♀: 7–15	Mesenteric veins (draining colon)	Ovoid, with lateral spine, 112–175 × 45–70 μm E: stool	I: *Biomphalaria* species. R: (monkeys, dog, rodents)
S. japonicum ♂♂: 7–20 ♀♀: 10–26	Mesenteric veins (draining intestine)	Elliptical, lateral spine tiny or lacking 70–100 × 50–65 μm E: stool	I: *Oncomelania* species. R: Cattle, buffalo, pig, dog, rodents, etc.
S. mekongi ♂♂: 10–18 ♀♀ : 14–20	Mesenteric veins (draining small intestine)	Elliptical, lateral spine tiny or lacking 50–65 × 30–55 μm E: stool	I: *Neotricula* species. R: dog

[1] Location not strictly specific; adult stages also found in vessels of liver, lungs, and, less frequently, in other organs.

[2] In parentheses: of secondary or local significance only.

[3] Stainable with Ziehl-Neelsen stain, in contrast to *S. hematobium*.

Schistosoma mansoni Pair

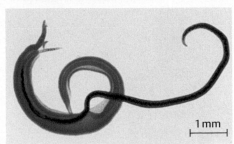

Fig. 10.**3** The threadlike female is enclosed in a groove in the body of the male.

1 mm

The adult parasites live in the lumen of veins. Table 10.**2** summarizes data on various *Schistosoma* species. Fig. 10.**4** (p. 550) shows their life cycle.

Sexually mature *Schistosoma* females lay about 100–3500 eggs a day, depending on the species, each containing an immature miracidium (= ciliate larva), which matures in the host within six to 10 days and remains viable for about three weeks (Fig. 10.**4**).

At the site of their deposition, the eggs lie in chainlike rows within small veins. Some penetrate through the vascular wall and surrounding tissue to reach the lumen of the urinary bladder or intestine (regarding the eggs that remain in the body see section on pathogenesis). Enzymes produced by the miracidium and secreted through micropores in the eggshell and granuloma formation (see below) contribute to the penetration process. The eggs are shed by the definitive host in stool or urine within a few weeks post infection (p.i.) (see below). If the eggs are deposited into freshwater, the miracidia hatch from the eggshell and begin their search for a suitable intermediate host (Fig. 10.**4**).

Various genera and species of freshwater snails serve as intermediate hosts (Table 10.**2**) in which the invading miracidia reproduce asexually, producing mother and daughter sporocysts, and finally numerous cercariae, which begin to swarm into the water three to six weeks p.i. at the earliest. A characteristic feature of the approximately 340–520 μm long cercariae is their forked tail. The cercariae swim freely about or cling to the surface of the water. Upon contact with a human host, enzyme secretion and vigorous movements enable them to penetrate the skin within a few minutes, or less frequently the mucosa when ingested with drinking water. During the infection process, the cercaria loses its tail, sheds the surface glycocalyx, forms a new tegument, and transforms into the schistosomulum.

10

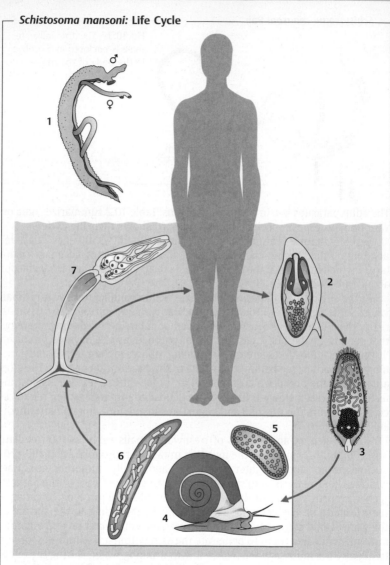

Schistosoma mansoni: **Life Cycle**

Fig. 10.**4** **1** Male and female; **2** egg with miracidium; **3** miracidium; **4** intermediate host (*Biomphalaria glabrata*); **5** sporocyst; **6** daughter sporocyst with cercariae; **7** fork-tailed cercaria (modified after Piekarski G, *Medizinische Parasitologie in Tafeln*. 2nd printing. Berlin: Springer; 1973).

Migration of Schistosomes in the Human Body

Infection → schistosomula penetrate subcutaneous tissues → find venous capillaries or lymph vessels → migrate through the venous circulatory system into the right ventricle of the heart and the lungs → travel hematogenously into the intrahepatic portal vein branches where development into adult worms takes place as wells as male-female pairing just prior to sexual maturity → retrograde migration of pairs into mesenteric veins or to the vesical plexus (Table 10.**2**).

Depending on the *Schistosoma* species involved, the prepatent period lasts about four to 10 weeks. Schistosomes remain in the definitive host for an average of two to five years, but in some cases for as long as 20–40 years.

Epidemiology. Schistosomosis occurs as an autochthonous infection in tropical and subtropical regions. Aquatic freshwater snails that prefer standing or slow-moving bodies of water are the intermediate hosts for *S. hematobium*, *S. mansoni*, *S. intercalatum*, and *S. mekongi* (Table 10.**2**). The intermediate hosts of *S. japonicum* are amphibious snails also found on moist ground and plants, e.g., in rice paddies.

Although the cycles of all *Schistosoma* species can include animals as hosts, humans are the most important parasite reservoirs (Table 10.**2**). However, animals contribute significantly to the dissemination of the eggs of *S. japonicum* and *S. mekongi*. Travelers to endemic tropical areas can acquire the infection by a single instance of contact with water containing cercariae.

Pathogenesis and clinical manifestations. The infection can be divided into the following phases:

■ **Penetration phase:** penetration of cercariae into the skin, either without reaction or—especially in cases of repeated exposure—with itching and skin lesions (erythema, papules), which disappear within a few days.

■ In the **acute phase**, about two to 10 weeks after a severe initial infection, the symptoms may include fever, headache, limb pains, urticaria, bronchitis, upper abdominal pain, swelling of the liver, spleen and lymph nodes, intestinal disturbances, and eosinophilia (= Katayama syndrome). Due to release of *Schistosoma* antigens, the serum antibody levels (IgM, IgG, IgA) rise rapidly and immune complexes are formed that can cause renal glomerulopathies. These symptoms persist for several days to several weeks. Normally, *Schistosoma* eggs are not yet excreted at the beginning of this phase (see prepatent periods). In low-level infections this phase is usually inapparent or subclinical.

■ **Chronic phase:** the most significant phase in pathogenic terms begins after an incubation period of about two months with oviposition by the *Schis-*

Schistosoma granuloma in the Liver

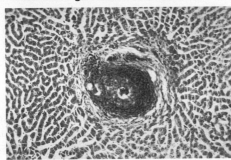

Fig. 10.**5** A section of an egg is visible in the center of the granuloma.

tosoma females. A large proportion (up to 50%) of the eggs laid remain in human body tissues, not only near the worms (urinary bladder, intestine), but also in more distant localizations due to hematogenous spreading (mainly to the liver and lungs, more rarely to the CNS, the skin, and other organs), where they lodge in small vessels.

The miracidia, which remain viable for about three weeks, produce antigens (proteins, glycoproteins), which are secreted through the eggshell into the tissue and are still present in the egg after the ciliated larva has died off. After antigenic stimulation of T lymphocytes secreted cytokines contribute to produce granulomatous reaction foci (so-called "pseudotubercles"): above all macrophages, neutrophilic and eosinophilic granulocytes, as well as fibroblasts, aggregate around single eggs or a number of centrally located eggs (Fig. 10.**5**). These foci may merge and form a starting point for larger, granulomatous proliferations that protrude into the lumen of the urinary bladder or intestine. The eggs in the tissues die off within about three weeks and are either broken down or they calcify. The granulomas are replaced by connective tissue, producing more and more fibrous changes and scarring.

The **main forms of schistosomosis** are differentiated according to the localization of the lesions:

■ **Urinary schistosomosis (urinary bilharziosis).** Causative agent: *S. hematobium.* Incubation 10–12 weeks or longer, morbidity rate as high as 50–70%. Hematuria (mainly in the final portion of urine), micturition discomfort, hyperemia, increasing fibrosis, 1–2 mm nodules, necroses, ulcers and calcification of the bladder wall, pyelonephrosis and hydronephrosis, urethral strictures, lesions in the sexual organs. In some endemic areas, an increased incidence of urinary bladder cancer has been associated with the *S. hematobium* infection.

■ **Intestinal schistosomosis (intestinal bilharziosis).** Causative agents: mainly *S. mansoni* and *S. japonicum*, also *S. mekongi* (rare: rectal lesions caused by *S. hematobium*). Incubation four to 13 weeks (acute phase), months to years (chronic phase). The course of an initial infection is only rarely symptomatic (see above: Katayama syndrome), inapparent and subclinical courses being the rule. Manifestations in the chronic phase are restricted almost entirely to large intestine with hyperemia, granulomatous nodules, papillomas ("bilharziomas"), ulcerations, hemorrhages, and increasing fibrosis, abdominal pain and bloody diarrhea.

■ **Other forms:** the causative agents of the **hepatosplenic form** are mainly *S. japonicum*, less frequently *S. mansoni*. This fibrotic form is caused by eggs deposited around the branches of the portal vein in the liver ("pipestem" fibrosis according to Symmers) and results in circulatory anomalies, portal hypertension, splenomegaly, ascites, hemorrhages in the digestive tract, and other symptoms. **Pulmonary schistosomosis** is observed mainly in severe *S. mansoni* infections, more rarely in infections with other species (including *S. hematobium*). **Cerebral schistosomosis** is relatively frequent in *S. japonicum* infections (2–4%).

■ **Cercarial dermatitis.** Cutaneous lesions (itching, erythema, urticaria, papules) in humans, caused by (repeated) skin penetration of schistosomatid cercariae parasitizing birds (e.g., *Bilharziella*, *Trichobilharzia*) or mammals (e.g., *Schistosoma spindale*). The infection occurs worldwide in freshwater or brackish water and is known as "swimmer's itch." The symptoms generally abate after a few days. The cercariae of schistosomes from humans can cause similar, although usually milder, symptoms.

Immunity. The prevalence and intensity of *Schistosoma* infections rise in endemic regions in children until the age of about 14, followed by a decline usually also accompanied by reduced egg excretion. This acquired immune status, known as "concomitant immunity," is characterized by total or partial protection against cercarial infection. However, the schistosomes already established in the body are not eliminated and may persist for years or even decades.

The immune defense is directed against schistosomula that have penetrated the skin, are a few hours old, and present their own antigens on their surface. Young schistosomula can be killed mainly by eosinophils and macrophages assisted by specific antibodies to these antigens and/or by complement. By the time the schistosomula reach the lungs they are resistant to such cytotoxic attacks. The explanation for this phenomenon is that the older schistosomula are able to acquire host antigens (e.g., blood group or histocompatibility antigens) and to synthesize hostlike macromolecules, thus "masking" their surfaces (= molecular mimicry) to circumvent the immune

10

response (= immunoevasion). Additional immunoevasive mechanisms have also been described, e.g., shedding part of the tegument and secretion of immunosuppressive substances.

The current immune status of persons infected with *Schistosoma* is apparently also determined by the balance of those antibodies which enhance the above-mentioned immune response (IgE and perhaps IgA) and others that inhibit it (IgM, IgG$_2$, or IgG$_4$).

Diagnosis. Following the prepatent period, i.e., four to 10 weeks p.i. at the earliest, the eggs can be detected in stool specimens or in urine sediment (Fig. 10.**1**, p. 545, Table 10.**2**, p. 547). The eggs can also be found in intestinal or urinary bladder wall biopsies. Immunodiagnostic methods (Table 11.**5**, p. 625) are particularly useful for detecting infections before egg excretion begins (important for travelers returning from tropical regions!). Detection of microhematuria with test strips is an important diagnostic tool in bladder schistosomosis. Clinical examination with portable ultrasonic imaging equipment has proved to be a highly sensitive method of detecting lesions in the liver and urogenital tract in epidemiological studies.

Therapy. The drug of choice for treatment of schistosomosis is praziquantel, which is highly effective against all *Schistosoma* species and is well tolerated. Oxamniquine is effective against *S. mansoni*.

Control and prevention. Current schistosomosis control strategies are based mainly on regular drug therapy of specific population groups. Morbidity, mortality, and egg excretion rates are clearly reduced by such programs. Hygienic and organizational measures (construction of latrines, improvement of water supply quality, etc.) aim to reduce *Schistosoma* egg dissemination and contact with contaminated bodies of water. Individual preventive measures in *Schistosoma*-contaminated areas include avoidance of skin contact with natural or artificial bodies of water (freshwater). Drinking water that could be contaminated with cercariae must be decontaminated before use by boiling, chlorination, or filtration.

10

Fasciola species

Fasciola hepatica (Common Liver Fluke) and F. gigantica (Large or Giant Liver Fluke)
Causative agents of fasciolosis

■ *Fasciola hepatica* and *F. gigantica* are frequent bile duct parasites of domestic ruminants. In their life cycle freshwater snails act as intermediate hosts. Humans become accidentally infected when they eat plants (e.g., watercress) to which infectious parasite stages (metacercariae) adhere. ■

Occurrence. *Fasciola hepatica* occurs worldwide as an important parasite in domestic ruminants that can also infect other animal species. Sporadic or endemic *F. hepatica* infections in humans have been reported from about 50 countries or regions on all continents (WHO, 1999). In Asia and Africa, human infections with the 7.5 cm long giant liver fluke (*F. gigantica*) are also reported. The number of persons infected with either *F. hepatica* or *F. gigantica* is estimated at 2.4 million (WHO, 1995).

Parasites, life cycle, and epidemiology. *F. hepatica* is a flattened, leaf-shaped parasite about 2–5 cm long and at most 1 cm wide. The cephalic cone with the oral sucker is somewhat demarcated from the rest of the body. A further characteristic feature is the pronounced branching of various inner organs (Fig. 10.**6a**).

Adult liver flukes parasitize in the bile ducts. They produce large (approx. 130 × 85 µm), golden-brown, operculated eggs (Fig. 10.**1**, p. 543) that are shed by the bile duct-intestinal tract route. Under favorable conditions, a ciliate larva, the miracidium, develops in the egg within a few weeks. The miracidia then hatch and penetrate into freshwater snails (*Lymnaea truncatula* in Central Europe), where they transform into sporocysts. After formation of further asexual reproductive stages (rediae), tailed cercariae develop and swarm out of the snails into the open water. They soon attach to plants and encyst, i.e., transform into infective metacercariae, which are then ingested with vegetable food of their definitive hosts. Eating watercress contaminated with metacercariae is one of the sources of infection for humans.

The juvenile liver flukes hatch from the cyst in the small intestine, penetrate the intestinal wall, and migrate through the peritoneal cavity to the liver. After migrating through the hepatic parenchyma for about six to seven weeks, the parasites finally reach the bile ducts, in which they develop to sexual maturity. Egg excretion begins two to three months p.i. at the earliest.

10

Liver Flukes

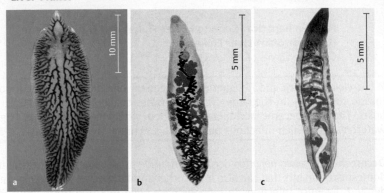

Fig. 10.**6** **a** *Fasciola hepatica*, adult stage with blood-filled intestinal branches; **b** *Dicrocoelium dendriticum*, adult stage; **c** *Opisthorchis felineus*, adult stage (Fig. a: K. Wolff, Zurich; c: V. Kumar, Antwerp).

Clinical manifestations. The infection may run an inapparent course or, after an incubation period of four to six weeks, become symptomatic with abdominal pain, hepatomegaly, fever, leukocytosis and eosinophilia (acute phase), or hepatocholangitic symptoms (chronic phase) and anemia. Occasionally, the parasites also migrate into other organs than the liver.

Diagnosis. The manifestations to be expected during the migration phase of the liver fluke include mainly leukocytosis, eosinophilia, and a rise in liver-specific serum enzymes. Detection of eggs (Fig. 10.1, p. 543) in stool or duodenal fluid is not possible until at least two to three months p.i. In patients from Asia, differential diagnosis of the eggs of the small intestinal parasites *Echinostoma* and *Fasciolopsis* (Fig. 10.1), which are very similar to those of *Fasciola*, must be kept in mind. Other diagnostic tools include detection of serum antibodies (Table 11.5, p. 625) and of coproantigen in stool.

Therapy and prevention. The drug of choice is triclabendazole, originally developed as a veterinary drug, is now registered ad usum humanum in several countries and is recommended by the WHO. The infection can be avoided by not eating raw watercress and other plants that may be contaminated with metacercariae.

Dicrocoelium

Dicrocoelium dendriticum (Lancet Liver Fluke)
Causative agent of dicrocoeliosis

The lancet liver fluke (0.5–1.0 × 0.2 cm) (Fig. 10.**6b**), a bile duct parasite in sheep, cattle, and other herbivores, occurs frequently in regional foci in the northern hemisphere (for instance southern Germany, Austria, Switzerland, North America). Its life cycle includes two intermediate hosts (terrestrial snails and ants). Humans become infected accidentally when they ingest ants containing infective metacercariae of the lancet liver fluke. Such infections are rare and either run an asymptomatic course or manifest in mild abdominal and hepatic symptoms. Diagnosis is based on detection of eggs in stool (about 40 × 25 µm, oval, dark brown, containing a miracidium with two rounded germinal cells) (Fig. 10.**1**. p. 543). Ingestion of contaminated beef or mutton liver can result in egg excretion in stool without infection (intestinal passage). The eggs of *Opisthorchis* and *Clonorchis* must be taken into consideration for a differential diagnosis (Fig. 10.**1**). Praziquantel has been shown to be effective against *Dicrocoelium* in animals (see also opisthorchiosis).

Opisthorchis and Clonorchis
(Cat Liver Fluke and Chinese Liver Fluke)
Causative agents of opisthorchiosis and clonorchiosis

■ Liver flukes of the genera *Opisthorchis* and *Clonorchis* occur mainly in river and lake regions of Asia and Eastern Europe; *Opisthorchis* is also found further westward as far as northern Germany. The life cycle of these organisms includes two intermediate hosts (aquatic snail, fish). Infections are contracted via raw fish containing infective stages (metacercariae). Diagnosis is based mainly on detection of eggs in stool or duodenal aspirate. ■

Parasites and occurrence. The members of these genera resemble the lancet liver fluke (*Dicrocoelium dendriticum*) in size (length 1–2 cm) and form. The position and structure of the testicles (*ophisten*: posterior; *orchis*: testicle; *clon*: branch) allow the discrimination of genera (Fig. 10.**6c**).

Opisthorchis and *Clonorchis* occur endemically in river and lake regions: *Opisthorchis felineus* in Eurasia (Russia, Kazakhstan, Ukraine; other endemic foci in the Baltic countries, northern Poland, and northern Germany), *Opisthorchis viverrini* in Thailand and Laos, *Clonorchis sinensis* in far-eastern Russia and other Asian areas (including China, Taiwan, Vietnam and Korea).

10

The number of persons infected with *Opisthorchis* and *Clonorchis* is estimated at 17 million, with about 350 million persons at risk for infection (WHO, 1995).

Life cycle and epidemiology. The definitive hosts of *Opisthorchis* and *Clonorchis* species are fish-eating mammals (cats, dogs, pigs, etc.) and humans, in which these trematodes colonize the bile ducts. The life cycle of these organisms involves various species of aquatic snails (*Bithynia*, etc.) as the first intermediate hosts and freshwater fish species as the second intermediate hosts. The infective metacercariae are localized in the musculature of the fish and, when raw fish is ingested, enter the intestinal tract of the definitive host, from where they migrate through the common bile duct (ductus choledochus) into the intrahepatic bile ducts. The prepatent period is four weeks.

Pathogenesis and clinical manifestations. *Opisthorchis* and *Clonorchis* infections cause proliferations of the bile duct epithelium, cystlike dilatation, inflammation, and fibrosis of the bile duct walls as well as connective tissue proliferation in the hepatic parenchyma. A high incidence of bile duct carcinomas has been reported from areas in which *C. sinensis and O. viverrini* are endemic. Clinical symptoms of more severe infections include variable fever, hepatocholangitic symptoms with hepatomegaly, leukocytosis, upper abdominal pains, and diarrhea.

Diagnosis, therapy, and prevention. Diagnosis is made by detection of eggs (26–32 μm long) in stool or duodenal fluid (Fig. 10.1, p. 543). Differential diagnosis must also consider the eggs of *Heterophyes heterophyes*, *Metagonimus yokogawai*, and other trematode species. Serum antibodies are found in some infected persons. The drug of choice is praziquantel; albendazole can also be used. Reliable preventive measures include boiling or frying fish to kill the metacercariae, which die at temperatures as low as 70 °C, and freezing to –10 °C for five days (WHO, 1995).

Paragonimus (Lung Flukes)

Causative agents of paragonimosis

■ Lung flukes of the genus *Paragonimus*, endemic in parts of Asia, Africa, and America, parasitize in pulmonary cysts and cause a tuberculosis-like clinical picture. Following development in two intermediate hosts (freshwater snails and crabs or crayfish), infective stages (metacercariae) can be transmitted to humans by eating the crabs or crayfish uncooked. Parasite eggs are detectable in sputum or stool. ■

Occurrence. At least nine *Paragonimus* species are known to be parasites of humans. They are found in East and Southeast Asia (*Paragonimus westermani, Paragonimus heterotremus,* and *Paragonimus uterobilateralis*), in North America (*Paragonimus kellicotti*), and in Central and South America (*Paragonimus mexicanus,* etc.). The number of infected persons is estimated at about 21 million (WHO, 1995).

Parasites, life cycle, and epidemiology. The plump, approx. 7–15 mm long, coffee bean-like *Paragonimus* species differ in appearance from other trematodes. The sexually mature parasites live in cystlike dilatations in the lungs, usually in connection with the bronchial tree. The yellow-brown, operculated eggs (about $80 \times 50\,\mu m$) laid by the adult worms are shed either in sputum or stool (Fig. 10.**1**, p. 544). The life cycle then continues in water, where a miracidium develops in each egg, hatches and invades an intermediate host. Egg-shaped cercariae with short tails develop in the first intermediate host, a freshwater snail (*Semisulcospira* and numerous other genera). The cercariae encyst in the second intermediate host (*Crustaceae*: crayfish or crabs) to form the infective metacercariae. When a suitable definitive host ingests the crustaceans uncooked, the young trematodes hatch in the small intestine, migrate through the peritoneal cavity to the diaphragm and finally into the lungs. The prepatent period is two to three months. Parasites that deviate from the normal migration route may enter other organs (e.g., the brain or the skin). Eggs distributed in the blood stream induce inflammatory granulomas in various organs.

Besides humans, crustacean eating mammals (Felidae, Canidae, pigs, etc.) play a significant epidemiological role as reservoir hosts.

Young lung flukes can be localized in the musculature of pigs and other "transport hosts" and be transmitted to humans who ingest the raw meat of these animals.

Clinical manifestations. Typical cases are clinically characterized by pulmonary symptoms (chronic cough, bloody expectoration, thoracic pain). Parasites following the normal or deviant migration routes can also cause abdominal, hepatic, pancreatic or CNS symptoms, or skin lesions (swelling, nodules).

Diagnosis, therapy, and prevention. An etiological diagnosis is based on detection of eggs in sputum or stool (Fig. 10.**1**, p. 544) and of serum antibodies (Table 11.**5**, p. 625). Regarding the differential diagnosis especially tuberculosis must be kept in mind. The drug of choice is praziquantel, but triclabendazole can also be used (see *Fasciola*, p. 556). Cooking crustaceans before eating them is a reliable preventive measure.

10

Cestoda (Tapeworms)

General. Various tapeworm species can parasitize in the small intestine of humans, including species from the "lower" (Pseudophyllida) and "higher" (Cyclophyllida) cestodes (from *kestos* = ribbon). These cestode species are hermaphrodites and consist of the head (scolex or "holdfast"), followed by an unsegmented germinative section (neck) and a posterior chain of segments (proglottids). There are no digestive organs, so nutrients are taken up through the absorptive integument. The life cycle of cestodes include one or two intermediate hosts.

Humans can also be infected by larval stages of various tapeworm species (cysticerci, metacestodes). These stages develop in body tissues and generally cause considerably greater pathological damage than the intestinal cestode stages.

Taenia species

Causative agents of taeniosis and cysticercosis

■ Taeniosis is a small intestine infection of humans caused by *Taenia* species. In the case of *T. saginata*, the intermediate hosts are cattle, in the musculature of which metacestodes (cysticerci) develop and can be ingested by humans who eat raw beef. The infection runs an inapparent course or is associated with mild intestinal symptoms. The metacestodes of *T. solium* develop in the musculature of pigs, or through accidental infection in humans as well (CNS, eyes, musculature, skin), causing cysticercosis. *T. saginata asiatica* is closely related to *T. saginata*, but its metacestodes parasitize mainly in the livers of pigs and ruminants. ■

Taenia saginata (Beef Tapeworm)
Causative agent of *T. saginata* taeniosis

10

Occurrence. This species occurs worldwide; the number of infected humans is estimated to be between 40 and 60 million. One indicator of infection frequency is the prevalence of *T. saginata*-cysticercosis in cattle (average prevalence in Europe approx. 0.3–6%, in some non-European regions more than 50%).

Parasites, life cycle, and epidemiology (see Fig. 10.**8**, p. 563). *T. saginata* (*taenia*: ribbon; *saginatus*: fattened) grows as long as 10 m and has a scolex with four suckers but a rostellum and hooks are lacking (see *T. solium*). The proglottids at the posterior end of the chain are longer than wide and each contains a treelike branched uterus containing 80 000–100 000 eggs (= gravid segments) (Fig. 10.**7c, d**). The eggs are released when a proglottid detaches from the tapeworm in the intestinal lumen or when a segment disintegrates outside the host. The eggs are small (diameter approx. 30–40 µm) and round (Fig. 10.**1**, p. 544). The outer shell forms a thick, brownish, radially striped embryophore enclosing an oncosphere with three pairs of hooks. The eggs are highly resistant and can remain infective in a moist environment for weeks or months (however, susceptible to desiccation!). Carried by feces of humans infected with *Taenia*, they contaminate pastures or feed either directly or via sewage. When cattle (or buffalo) ingest the eggs, the oncospheres hatch in the small intestine, migrate into the intestinal wall, and are transported with the bloodstream into the striated musculature, in which they develop into the infective metacestodes or cysticerci (= Cysticercus bovis) within three to four months. Each cysticercus is a pea-sized, fluid-filled cyst containing a single invaginated scolex (Fig. 10.**7e**).

Humans are infected by ingesting raw or undercooked beef containing cysticerci. In the small intestine, the cysticercus evaginates the scolex, at-

---

Cestodes

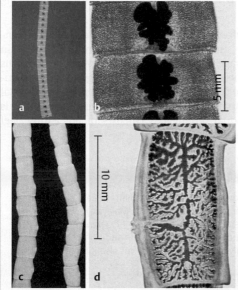

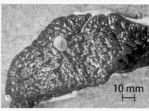

Fig. 10.**7 a** Chain of proglottids (strobila) of *Diphyllobothrium* sp., unstained; **b** strobila of *Diphyllobothrium latum*, stained; **c** strobila of *Taenia saginata*, unstained; **d** gravid proglottid of *T. saginata*, stained; **e** metacestode of *T. saginata* in bovine musculature (Fig. e: *Institut für Parasitologie der Tierärztlichen Hochschule Hannover*).

10

taches to the mucosa of the upper small intestine, and develops into an adult tapeworm, which can live for years or even decades. About two to three months after the infection, the first gravid segments detach from the strobila and then appear in feces or they can migrate out of the intestine without defecation. The segments remain motile for some time and frequently leave the stools.

Pathogenesis and clinical manifestations. In some infected persons, *T. saginata* causes morphological changes (villus deformation, enterocyte proliferation, cellular mucosal infiltration, etc.) and functional disturbances. Blood eosinophilia may occur sometimes. The infection takes an asymptomatic course in about 25 % of cases. Symptoms of infection include nausea, vomiting, upper abdominal pains, diarrhea or constipation and increased or decreased appetite. Infection does not confer levels of immunity sufficient to prevent reinfection.

Diagnosis. A *Taenia* infection is easy to diagnose if the 1.5–2 cm long and 0.7 cm wide segments are eliminated in stool (Fig. 10.**7c, d**). Morphological species differentiation (*T.saginata* vs. *T. solium*) is often not possible based on the gravid proglottids, but can be done by DNA–analysis (PCR). *T. saginata* eggs are shed irregularly in stool and cannot be differentiated morphologically from *T. solium* eggs (Fig. 10.**1**, p. 544). Using an ELISA, coproantigens are detectable in stool fluid even when neither proglottids nor eggs are being excreted.

Therapy and prevention. The drug of choice is the highly effective praziquantel. Albendazole, mebendazole, and paromomycin are less reliable. The main prophylactic measures are sewage treatment and the detection of cysticercus carriers at inspection of slaughter animals. Meat containing numerous cysticerci ("measly meat") has to be confiscated, but meat with small numbers of cysticerci can be used for human consumption after deep-freezing that is lethal to the parasites. Individual prophylaxis consists of not eating beef that is raw or has not been deep-frozen.

■ *Taenia saginata asiatica* ■

Causative agent of Asian taeniosis

This form of *Taenia* occurs in the small intestine of humans in East and Southeast Asia (Korea, Taiwan, the Philippines, Thailand, Indonesia, Malaysia). Genetic analysis has revealed a close subspecies-relation to *T. saginata* (= *T. saginata asiatica*). The two forms differ in a number of morphological features; in addition, the cysticerci of *T. saginata asiatica* develop mainly in the livers of pigs, but also infect cattle, goats, and monkey species.

Taenia saginata and *T. solium*: Life Cycles

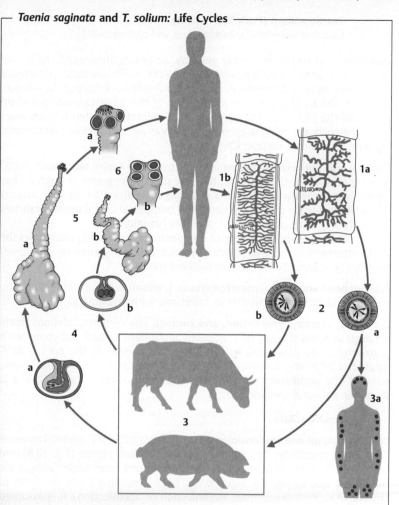

Fig. 10.8 **1a, b** Gravid segment containing eggs of *T. solium* (**a**) and of *T. saginata* (**b**); **2** free *Taenia* eggs; **3** natural intermediate hosts of *T. saginata* (cattle) and *T. solium* (pigs); **3a** human as accidental host of *T. solium*; **4a, b** infective metacestodes of *T. solium* (**a**) and of *T. saginata* (**b**); **5a, b** the same metacestodes with protoscoleces evaginated; **6a, b** "armed" head of *T. solium* (**a**) and "unarmed" head of *T. saginata* (**b**) from human small intestine (modified after Piekarski, G., *Medizinische Parasitologie in Tafeln*. 2nd ed., Berlin: Springer; 1973). Red dots in human host: possible location of *T. solium* metacestodes.

10

Taenia solium (Pork Tapeworm)

Causative agent of *T. solium* taeniosis and cysticercosis

Occurrence. *T. solium* is mainly endemic in poorly developed regions of Central and South America, Africa, and Asia, with sporadic occurrence in the USA as well as western, eastern, and southern Europe. In Mexico, 0.1–7% of the rural population are carriers of the adult tapeworm and up to 25% of the pigs carry the cysticerci of *T. solium*. Imported human cases of cysticercosis are being diagnosed in increasing numbers in nonendemic regions (e.g., central Europe, USA).

Parasite and life cycle. *T. solium* (*solium*: from the Arabic word *sosl*: chain) is 3–4 m long and is thus smaller than *T. saginata*. The scolex of *T. solium* has a rostellum armed with two rows of hooks in addition to the four suckers (Fig. 10.**8**). Inside the gravid segments, the number of lateral uterus branches is usually 7–13, i.e., less than in *T. saginata* (usually >15).

The life cycle is similar to that of *T. saginata*, except that *T. solium* uses the pig as intermediate host, in which the metacestode (Cysticercus cellulosae) develops to infectivity within two to three months.

Pathogenesis and clinical manifestations. *T. solium* in the intestine causes no or only mild symptoms, similar to infections with *T. saginata*.

Diagnosis, therapy, prevention, and control. The recommendations made for diagnosis and therapy of *T. saginata* apply here as well. Infections with *T. solium* can be prevented by cooking or deep-freezing the pork (–20 °C for at least 24 hours). Control measures in endemic areas include mass treatment of the population with praziquantel, improvement of hygiene and slaughter animal inspection.

Cysticercosis

Causative agent and epidemiology. The metacestodes of *T. solium*, known as Cysticercus cellulosae, can colonize various human organs (Fig. 10.**8**) and cause the clinical picture of cysticercosis. Infections occur under unhygienic conditions due to peroral ingestion of eggs stemming from the feces of tapeworm carriers (exogenous autoinfection or alloinfection). It is assumed that oncospheres hatching from eggs released from gravid proglottids in the human digestive tract may also cause an infection (endogenous auto-infection). In some countries of Latin America, Asia, and Africa, human cysticercosis is a public health problem. In Latin American countries, seroprevalences up to 10% and above have been found, and cysticerci were detected in 0.1–6% of the autopsy cases.

Clinical manifestations. Cysticercosis of the central nervous system (neurocysticercosis) or of the eye (ocular cysticercosis) is among the more severe forms of the infection. In the CNS, the metacestodes are usually localized in the cerebrum (ventricle, subarachnoidal space), more rarely in the spinal cord; they can cause epileptiform convulsions, raised intracranial pressure, and other neurological symptoms. The cysticerci can also develop in subcutaneous tissues, in the heart, and in the skeletal musculature.

Diagnosis. If metacestodes are localized in the subcutis, palpation of subdermal nodules may supply initial evidence of cysticercosis. Tools useful in diagnosing internal organ infections include imaging procedures and immunodiagnostic methods (Table 11.**5**, p. 625). In over 90 % of cases of cerebral cysticercosis, the use of purified glycoprotein antigens from *T. solium* metacestodes in a Western blot assay reveals serum antibodies.

Therapy. Praziquantel in combination with corticosteroids has proved effective in a large percentage of cases treated (including neurocysticercosis) in which the metacestodes were not yet calcified. Close patient monitoring is required for this therapy. Albendazole is also used in treatment of human cysticercosis.

Echinococcus
Causative agent of echinococcosis

■ The most important species of the genus *Echinococcus* are *Echinococcus granulosus* (intestinal parasite of Canidae) and *E. multilocularis* (intestinal parasite of fox species, dogs, cats, and other carnivores). Both species occur in Europe. Their metacestodes can cause cystic echinococcosis (CE, hydatid disease) or alveolar echinococcosis (AE) in humans. Humans are infected by peroral ingestion of *Echinococcus* eggs, from which in CE, liquid-filled cystic metacestodes (the hydatids) develop, particularly in the liver and lungs. In AE the metacestodes primarily parasitize the liver, where the metacestodes proliferate like a tumor and form conglomerates of small cysts; secondary metastatic spread to other organs is possible. Clinical imaging and immunodiagnostic methods are used for diagnosis. Treatment involves surgery and/or chemotherapy. ■

10

Parasite species. *Echinococcus* species are small tapeworms that parasitize the small intestine of carnivores and produce eggs that are shed to the environment by the host. Pathogenic larval stages (metacestodes) develop following peroral ingestion of such eggs by the natural intermediate hosts (various mammalian species), as well as in humans and other accidental hosts (which do not play a role in the life cycle). Four *Echinococcus* species are currently known, all of them pathogenic for humans (*Echinococcus granulosus*, *E. multilocularis*, *E. vogeli*, and *E. oligarthrus*).

Echinococcus granulosus (Dwarf Dog Tapeworm)
Causative agent of cystic echinococcosis (CE)

Occurrence. *E. granulosus* occurs worldwide, with relative high prevalences in eastern and southeastern Europe, the Mediterranean countries, the Near East, northern and eastern Africa, South America, and various parts of Asia and Australia. The parasite has become rare in northern and central Europe; most of the human cases of CE diagnosed in these areas are imported, in particular from Mediterranean countries. *E. granulosus* and *E. multilocularis* occur together in some areas.

Morphology and development

■ **Adult stage.** *E. granulosus* is a 4–7 mm long tapeworm with a scolex (bearing rostellar hooks) and normally three (two to six) proglottids. A notable characteristic is the uterus with its lateral sacculations, containing up to 1500 eggs (Fig. 10.**10a** p. 569).

■ **Definitive (final) and intermediate hosts.** The most important definitive host for *E. granulosus* is the dog, whereby other Canidae (jackal, dingo, and other wild canids) are involved in certain regions. Herbivorous and omnivorous vertebrates function as intermediate hosts, in particular domestic animals (ruminants, pigs, horses, camels) and in some areas wild animals as well.

■ **Life cycle** (Fig. 10.**9**). The adult tapeworms live in the small intestine of the definitive host for about six months, a few for up to two years (Fig. 10.**10c**). Eggs are either released from gravid proglottids in the intestine and shed with feces or pass out of the host still enclosed in the tapeworm segments. The eggs (diameter approx. 30–40 μm) are nearly spherical, contain an oncosphere and feature a radially striped shell. They cannot be morphologically differentiated from the eggs of other *Echinococcus* or *Taenia* species (see Fig. 10.**1**, p. 544). Infection of the intermediate hosts, humans, and other accidental hosts is by peroral ingestion of eggs, from which the oncospheres are released in the small intestine, penetrate into its wall and migrate hematogenously into the liver, as well as sometimes into the lungs and other organs. At first, the oncospheres develop into little vesicles, then gradually into metacestodes.

■ The metacestode of *E. granulosus* (also known as hydatid cysts, from *hydatis* = water bladder) is normally a fluid-filled cyst with one or multiple chambers, the wall of which is made up of an inner, cellular, germinative layer and an outer, acellular, laminated layer (cuticular layer), enclosed by a layer of host connective tissue (Fig. 10.**10d, f**). Brood capsules develop five to six months or later p.i. on the germinative layer, each containing up to 20 or

Echinococcus granulosus and *E. multilocularis*: Life Cycles

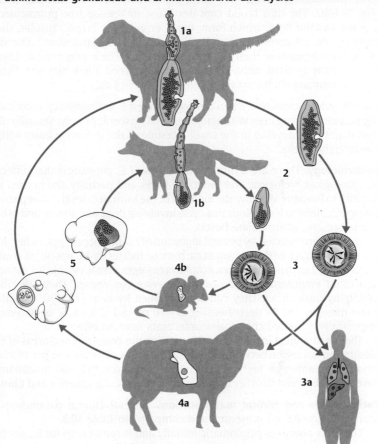

Fig. 10.**9** **1a, b** Adult parasites in final hosts: *E. granulosus* in dogs, *E. multilocularis* in red foxes (also: dogs, cats, and other carnivores); **2** gravid proglottids containing eggs; **3** *Echinococcus* eggs, infection of natural intermediate host or humans (accidental host) (**3a**); **4** natural intermediate hosts: of *E. granulosus*: sheep, cattle, horses, and other ungulates (**4a**); of *E. multilocularis*: rodents (**4b**); **5** metacestodes in the livers of intermediate hosts.

Red dots in human host: most frequent location of metacestodes (see text).

10

more protoscoleces with four suckers and tow rows of rostellar hooks (Fig. 10.**10h**). The thin brood capsules burst to release free protoscoleces into the hydatid fluid, which form, together with the brood capsules, their remains and calcareous corpuscles the so-called "hydatid sand." The size of the cysts depends on their age and other factors. The average cyst diameter in humans is 1–15 cm, although it can vary between a few mm and 20 cm. Cysts in humans often contain smaller daughter cysts.

The life cycle is completed when carnivores ingest *E. granulosus* cysts containing mature protoscoleces with slaughter offal (viscera) or prey. Sexually mature stages then develop in the small intestine of the definitive hosts within five to eight weeks.

Epidemiology. There are a number of strains of *E. granulosus* that differ in morphological, biological, and genetic features and partially also in their infectivity to humans. Worldwide, for most of the human cases the sheep strain is responsible which develops in a cycle involving dogs and sheep (and other, less important, intermediate hosts).

Humans are infected by peroral ingestion of *Echinococcus* eggs, either during direct contact with tapeworm carriers or indirectly by uptake of contaminated food or drinking water. *Echinococcus* eggs remain viable for months in a moist environment and can also survive the winter. They are killed rapidly by desiccation. They can also be killed by heat (75–100 °C) within a few minutes and by deep-freezing at –70 or –80 °C for four or two days, respectively. Standard chemical disinfectants have no effect.

The mean annual incidence of CE varies in the countries and areas of the Mediterranean region between about one to 10 new clinical cases per 100 000 inhabitants, although higher incidences (>40 cases/100 000 inhabitants) have been observed in other endemic areas (e.g., South America and China).

Pathogenesis and clinical manifestations. Several clinical parameters of human CE and AE are presented and compared in Table 10.**3**.

The CE is always asymptomatic initially and it remains so for longer periods in a proportion of cases (up to 30%), especially when only small, well-

10

Fig. 10.**10** **a** *Echinococcus granulosus*, adult; **b** *E. multilocularis*, adult; **c** dog intestine with *E. granulosus*; **d** cystic echinococcosis in human liver: mother cyst of *E. granulosus* with daughter cysts; **e** alveolar echinococcosis in liver; **f** cyst of *E. granulosus*: histological section through cyst wall; **g** section through *E. multilocularis* in human liver; **h** isolated protoscoleces of *E. granulosus*; **i** section through metacestodes of *E. multilocularis* with protoscoleces, from rodent. (d: A. Akovbiantz, Waidspital, Zurich.) ▶

Echinococcus granulosus and *E. multilocularis*

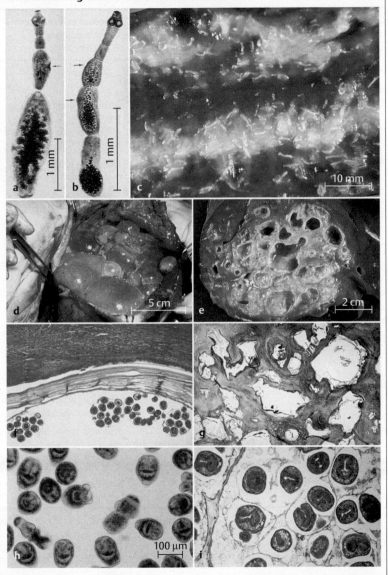

Table 10.**3**   Clinical Parameters of Human Cystic and Alveolar Echinococcosis[1]

Clinical parameters	Cystic echinococcosis Causative agent: E. granulosus	Alveolar echinococcosis Causative agent: E. multilocularis
Incubation period:	Months to several years	>5–15 years
Metacestode: ■ Typical form:	Cysts (see text)	Alveolar conglomerates (see text)
■ Growth:	Expansive	Infiltrative, like malignant tumor
Primary target organs:	Liver (60–70%), lungs (15–25%), less frequently spleen, kidneys, musculature, CNS, etc. Approx. 70% of patients have solitary cysts	Liver (98–100%)
Complications:	Secondary echinococcosis[2], mainly in peritoneal and pleural cavities	Metastasis to abdominal organs, lungs, brain, bones, etc.
Manifestations of disease in age groups: mean and (extremes[3])	38 years (3–86)	>54 years (20–84)
Symptoms:	Depends on localization, size, and number of cysts	Depends on extent of changes in liver and other organs
■ Liver:	Upper abdominal pains, hepatomegaly, cholestasis, jaundice, etc.	Upper abdominal pains, jaundice, weight loss, also fever and anemia
■ Lungs:	Thoracic pains, cough, expectoration, dyspnea, etc.	Thoracic pains, etc.
■ CNS:	Neurological symptoms	Neurological symptoms
Lethality in untreated patients:	Exact data unavailable	Very high: >94–100%

[1] For further information see Amman and Eckert: *Gastroenterological Clinic N. Amer.* 1996: 25: 655–689.
[2] See text for explanation.
[3] According to a study conducted in Switzerland.

encapsulated or calcified cysts are present. Symptoms may appear after months or years when one or more cysts begin to disrupt organ functions due to their size, expansive growth, or localization (Table 10.**3**). Acute symptoms may appear following spontaneous, traumatic, or intraoperative cyst ruptures, whereby the release of antigen containing hydatid fluid can cause symptoms of anaphylactic shock. There is also a risk that protoscoleces will be released and develop into new cysts in the human host (secondary CE). On the other hand, cyst rupture can also result in spontaneous cure.

Diagnosis is based on detection of cysts using imaging techniques (ultrasonography, computer tomography, thoracic radiography, etc.) in connection with serological antibody detection (Table 11.**5**, p. 625). Specific antibodies occur in about 90–100% of patients with cystic hepatic echinococcosis, but in only about 60–80% of cases with pulmonary echinococcosis. Diagnostic cyst puncture is generally not advisable due to the risks described above (secondary echinococcosis, anaphylactic reactions).

Therapy. The disease can be cured by removing the *Echinococcus* cysts surgically. Inoperable patients (e.g., with multiple cysts in lungs and liver) can be treated during several months with albendazole or mebendazole. Chemotherapy results in cure in about 30% of cases and in improvement in a further 30–50% (WHO, 1996). PAIR (**p**uncture **a**spiration **i**njection **r**easpiration) therapy is a new technique still under evaluation: after puncturing the cysts (not all cysts are suitable, e.g., pulmonary cysts!) under ultrasonic guidance, most of the hydatid fluid is aspirated, after which an adequate amount of 95% ethanol is injected into the cyst, left in it for 15 minutes and removed (reaspirated). If effective, the PAIR procedure often succeeds in killing the germinative layer and protoscoleces by ethanol. Since long-term experience with this method is lacking, it is recommended that the procedure be accompanied by a short-term drug regimen (WHO, 1996).

Control and prevention. Control of CE in humans includes regular mass treatment of dogs to eliminate *E. granulosus*, preventing access of dogs to viscera of domestic or wild animals, and dog population control. Special hygienic principles must be observed when handling dogs in endemic areas.

10

Echinococcus multilocularis (Dwarf Fox Tapeworm)
Causative agent of alveolar echinococcosis (AE)

E. multilocularis is widespread in the northern hemisphere with endemic regions in Europe, Asia (Turkey, Iran, Russia, and bordering countries all the way to Japan), and North America (Alaska, Canada, northern and central US states) (Fig. 10.**11**). In Central Europe, the parasite is widely distributed with prevalence levels in foxes exceeding 50% in some areas.

Distribution of *Echinococcus multilocularis*

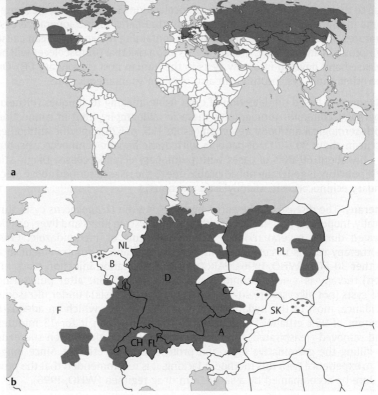

Fig. 10.**11** **a** Approximate global distribution (status: 1999); **b** approximate distribution in Central Europe (status: 1999) (© Institut für Parasitologie, Universität Zürich, J. Eckert, F. Grimm, and H. Bucklar). A: Austria, B: Belgium, CH: Switzerland, CZ: Czech Republic, D: Germany, F: France, FL: Liechtenstein, L: Luxembourg, NL: the Netherlands, PL: Poland, SK: Slovak Republic. Foci have been located in Denmark and on the Norwegian Svalbard Islands in the Arctic Ocean.

Morphology and development

■ **Adult stage.** *E. multilocularis* is only 2–4 mm long. Typically, the adult cestode has five (two to six) proglottids and is characterized by a sac-shaped uterus containing up to 200 eggs (Fig. 10.**10b**).

■ **Definitive hosts, intermediate hosts, and accidental hosts.** The most important definitive hosts for *E. multilocularis* are red and polar foxes, although other wild carnivores (e.g., coyotes, raccoons, wolves) as well as dogs and cats can also carry this tapeworm species. The intermediate hosts are usually rodents (field mice, voles, muskrats, etc.). Accidental hosts include humans and various mammalian animals such as monkey species, domestic and wild pigs, horses, and even dogs.

■ **Life cycle.** The *E. multilocularis* cycle is similar to that of *E. granulosus* (Fig. 10.**9**). In natural intermediate hosts, protoscoleces develop in the metacestode (see description below) within 40–60 days. Ingestion of metacestodes containing protoscoleces by a definitive host results in development of a new generation of tapeworms in its small intestine with infective eggs produced as early as 26–28 days p.i.

■ The **metacestode** of *E. multilocularis* is a conglomerate with an alveolar structure comprised of small cysts (microscopical to 3 cm in diameter) surrounded by granulomatous or connective tissue. Each cyst is structured as in *E. granulosus*, but contains a gelatinous mass. *E. multilocularis* rarely produce (small numbers of) protoscoleces in humans (max. 10% of cases) (Fig. 10.**10e, g, i**).

A pathologically significant aspect is that the individual cysts proliferate by exogenous budding and that thin cellular, rootlike extensions of the germinative layer can infiltrate into surrounding tissues. Presumably, cell groups released by these structures or very small vesicles spread hematogenously to cause distant metastases, e.g., in the brain or bones. Therefore the metacestode behaves like a malignant tumor. Metacestode conglomerates can grow to 20 cm in diameter in humans and may develop central necrosis and cavitation.

Epidemiology. In Europe, *E. multilocularis* develops mainly in a sylvatic cycle with the red fox as the definitive host and main source of human infections. Dogs and cats can become carriers of *E. multilocularis* by eating small mammals containing metacestodes. In the environment, the eggs of *E. multilocularis* show resistance similar to that of *E. granulosus*. The eggs are transmitted to humans by various routes, but it is not yet clear which are the most important:

10

■ Contamination of hands with eggs of *E. multilocularis* by touching definitive hosts (fox, dog, cat) having such eggs adhering to their fur or from working with soil or plants contaminated by the feces of definitive hosts.

■ Ingestion of contaminated food (wild berries, vegetables, windfall fruit, etc.) or drinking water.

Despite the frequent and widespread occurrence of *E. multilocularis* in foxes, the incidence of AE in humans is currently low. Statistics on national or regional incidences recorded in recent years in France, Germany, Austria, and Switzerland varied between 0.02 and 1.4 new cases per 100 000 inhabitants per year. It is possible that the growing fox population and increasing invasion of cities by foxes, combined with other factors, may raise levels of incidence in the future. In a highly endemic focus in China 4% of several thousand persons had documented AE.

Pathogenesis and clinical manifestations. The initial phase of an infection is always asymptomatic. Following a long incubation period, usually 10–15 years, the infection of the liver may present with symptoms resembling those of a malignant tumor (Table 10.**3**). The infection runs a slowly progressing, chronic course, lasting several weeks to several years. The lethality rate can exceed 94% in untreated patients. Spontaneous cure is possible, although no reliable statistics are available.

Diagnosis. The diagnostic procedure for AE is the same as for CE. Sensitive and specific methods are available for serological antibody detection (ELISA, Western blot) (Table 11.**5**, p. 625).

Therapy. Radical surgical removal of the parasites is potentially curative, but not always a feasible option (in only 20–40% of clinically manifest cases). During to the infiltrative mode of growth of *E. multilocularis* metacestodes it is impossible to be certain that all parts of the parasite have been removed, so that chemotherapy with mebendazole or albendazole must be carried out following such surgery for at least two years with patient monitoring continued for up to 10 years. Chemotherapy lasting years, or even for the life of the patient, is required in inoperable cases (WHO, 1996). Long-term studies have revealed that chemotherapy combined with other medical measures significantly increases life expectancy and quality of life in the majority of patients.

Control and prevention. Trials are currently in progress to evaluate drug-based control of *E. multilocularis* in fox populations, but an established and effective control program is not yet available. Personal prophylaxis in endemic areas should include special precautions when handling potentially infected foxes and other definitive hosts. Thorough washing, and better yet cooking, of low-growing cultivated and wild plants and windfall fruit before eating them and washing the hands after working with soil are further basic preventive measures. Persons known to have had contact with definitive hosts that are confirmed or potentially infected carriers, or who are in frequent contact with foxes or are exposed to other concrete infection risks can have their blood tested for antibodies to *E. multilocularis*, the objective being exclusion or early recognition of an infection.

Echinococcus vogeli and E. oligarthrus

Causative agents of polycystic echinococcosis

These two species, endemic in Central and South America, develop in wild animal cycles (bush dog/*paca* and wild felids/agoutis, paca etc., respectively). In humans, these organisms cause the rare polycystic echinococcosis, which affects the liver, lungs, and other organs.

Hymenolepis

Hymenolepis nana (Dwarf Tapeworm)
Causative agent of hymenolepiosis

Occurrence, morphology, and life cycle. *Hymenolepis nana*, 1–4 cm long (rarely 9 cm) and 1 mm wide, is a small intestinal parasite that occurs worldwide, the highest prevalences being found in warm countries and in children. The final hosts are rodents and humans. Infection results from peroral ingestion of eggs, from which oncospheres hatch in the small intestine, penetrate into the villi, and develop there into larvae (cysticercoids). The larvae then return to the intestinal lumen, where they develop into adult tapeworms within two to three weeks. Alternatively, *H. nana* develops in a cycle with an intermediate host (insects: fleas, grain beetles, etc.). The closely related species *Hymenolepis diminuta* (10–60 mm) is not as frequent in humans. The developmental cycle of this species always involves intermediate hosts (fleas, beetles, cockroaches, etc.).

Clinical manifestations and diagnosis. Infections are often latent, but sometimes cause indeterminate gastrointestinal distress. The eggs (elliptical, about 60×50 μm, Fig. 10.**1**, p. 544) are released from the cestode in the intestine and are found by normal stool examination procedures.

Therapy and prevention. Praziquantel or albendazole are the drugs of choice. Preventive measures include general hygiene and treatment of infected persons.

10

Diphyllobothrium

Diphyllobothrium latum (Broad Tapeworm, Fish Tapeworm)
Causative agent of diphyllobothriosis

Occurrence, morphology, and life cycle. This tapeworm is endemic in lake regions in Europe (above all in Russia, less frequently in Scandinavia, Germany, Switzerland, Italy, etc.), Asia, and America and parasitizes in the small intestine of humans and fish-eating mammals such as pigs, dogs, and cats. The parasite has two elongated grooves (bothria) on its head, it is 2–15 m long with numerous (up to 4000) proglottids (Fig. 10.**7a, b**, p. 561). The oval, yellow-brown, operculated eggs (approx. 70 × 50 μm) are similar to those of trematodes (Fig. 10.**1**, p. 544). The life cycle includes copepods as primary and freshwater fish as secondary intermediate hosts. Humans acquire the infection when eating raw or undercooked fish containing infective stages (plerocercoids) of the tapeworm. Development of a sexually mature tapeworm can be completed within 18 days.

Clinical manifestations The course of a *Diphyllobothrium* infection is often devoid of clinical symptoms, with only mild gastrointestinal distress in some cases. Anemia and other symptoms due to vitamin B12 uptake by the parasite is observed in about 2% of tapeworm carriers.

Diagnosis, therapy, and prevention. Diagnosis is made by detection of eggs in stool, sometimes proglottids are excreted. Praziquantel is a suitable drug for therapy. Preventive measures include wastewater hygiene and not eating undercooked fish. The plerocercoids can be killed by boiling or deep-freezing (24 hours at −18 °C or 72 hours at −10 °C).

Nematoda (Roundworms)

General. The nematodes (*nema*: thread) are threadlike, nonsegmented parasites, a few mm to 1 m in length, with separated sexes. They possess a complex tegument and a digestive tract. The males are usually smaller than the females and are equipped with copulatory organs that often show features specific to each species. Development from the egg includes four larval stages and four moltings before the adult stage is reached. Some species require an intermediate host to complete development.

Intestinal Nematodes

■ *Ascaris lumbricoides* (large roundworm), hookworms (*Ancylostoma* species and *Necator americanus*), and *Strongyloides stercoralis* (dwarf threadworm) parasitize in the small intestine of humans; *Trichuris trichiura* (whipworm) and *Enterobius vermicularis* (pinworm) live in the large intestine. The transmission routes and life cycles of these parasites differ. *S. stercoralis* infections acquired in warm countries may persist in a latent state for many years and can be activated in response to immunodeficiency and develop into life-threatening systemic infections. Careful diagnostic examinations are therefore necessary if a *Strongyloides* infection is suspected. ■

Ascaris lumbricoides (Large Roundworm)
Causative agent of ascariosis

Occurrence. The human large roundworm occurs worldwide. The number of infected persons is estimated at 1.38 billion (WHO, 1998). The main endemic regions, with prevalence rates of approx. 10–90%, include countries in Southeast Asia, Africa, and Latin America. Autochthonous infections are rare in central Europe.

Parasite and life cycle. The adult ascarids living in the small intestine (*ascaris*: worm) are 15–40 cm in length, about as thick as a pencil and of a yellowish pink color (Fig. 10.**12**). The sexually mature females produce as many as 200 000 eggs per day, which are shed with feces in the unembryonated state. The round-to-oval eggs are about 60×45 µm in size, have a thick, brownish shell and an uneven surface (Fig. 10.**13**). At optimum temperatures of 20–25 °C with sufficient moisture and oxygen, an infective larva in the egg develops within about three to six weeks.

Human infections result from peroral ingestion of eggs containing larvae, which hatch in the upper small intestine and penetrate into the veins of the intestinal wall. They first migrate hematogenously into the liver and then, four to seven days p.i., into the lungs, where they leave the capillary network and migrate into the alveoli. Via tracheopharyngeal migration they finally reach the digestive tract, where they further differentiate into adults in the small intestine. The prepatent period lasts for seven to nine weeks. The lifespan of these parasites is 12–18 months.

— *Ascaris lumbricoides* —

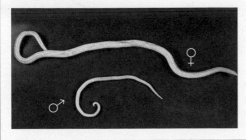

Fig. 10.**12** Male and female *Ascaris*.

10

Epidemiology. Reservoir hosts of the parasite are humans. The excreted eggs remain viable for years in a moist environment (soil), but are sensitive to desiccation. Infective *Ascaris* eggs can be ingested by humans with contaminated foods, soil (geophagia in children!) and, less frequently, in drinking water. In endemic areas, the prevalence and intensity of *A. lumbricoides* infections are highest in children.

Pathogenesis and clinical manifestations. Mild infections frequently remain inapparent. In more severe infections, **larval migration** in the lungs provoke hemorrhages and inflammatory infiltrations, which present as diffuse mot-

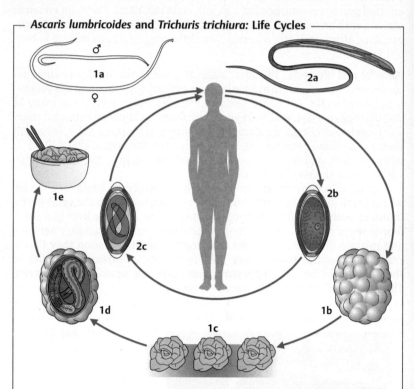

Ascaris lumbricoides and **Trichuris trichiura: Life Cycles**

Fig. 10.**13** **1a** Adult stages of *A. lumbricoides*; **1b** freshly shed egg, not yet infective; **1c** contamination of vegetables with eggs; **1d** infective egg with larva; **1e** ingestion of infective eggs with contaminated food. **2a** Adult stage of *T. trichiura*; **2b** freshly shed egg, not yet infective; **2c** infective egg with larva. (The transmission routes of *T. trichiura* are similar to those of *Ascaris*.)

10

tling and prominence of peribronchial regions in radiographs (Löffler syndrome). Blood eosinophilia is often concurrently observed. This syndrome may be accompanied by coughing, dyspnea, and mild fever. During the **intestinal phase** of the infection, only some patients develop distinct clinical symptoms: abdominal discomfort with nausea, vomiting, pains, and diarrhea. Ascarids sometimes also migrate into the stomach, the pancreatic duct or the bile ducts and cause symptoms accordingly. Infection or frequent contact with volatile *Ascaris* antigens (laboratory staff!) can cause allergies.

Diagnosis. An infection with sexually mature roundworms can be diagnosed by finding eggs in the stool (Figs 10.**1** and 10.**13**). Migrating *Ascaris* larvae can be indirectly detected by means of serological antibody detection (especially specific IgE), but this technique is seldom used in practice.

Therapy and control. Pyrantel, mebendazole, albendazole, and nitazoxanide are highly effective against the intestinal stages of *Ascaris*. Migratory stages are not affected by normal dosage levels. Due to the possibility of reinvasion of the intestine by larvae migrating in the body, the treatment should be repeated after two to three weeks. Preventive measures include sewage disposal, improvement of sanitation, good food hygiene practices (washing fruits and vegetables, cooking foods, etc.) and regular anthelminthic treatment of infected persons in endemic areas (see also filariosis, p. 593).

Trichuris trichiura (Whipworm)

Causative agent of trichuriosis

Occurrence. *Trichuris trichiura* occurs in humans and monkeys. Although this parasite has a worldwide distribution, it is found most frequently, like *Ascaris lumbricoides*, in moist, warm areas with low hygienic standards (prevalence around 2–90%). The number of infected persons worldwide is estimated at one billion (WHO, 1998).

Parasite, life cycle, and epidemiology (Fig. 10.13). The name whipworm characterizes the form of this 3–5 cm long nematode with a very thin anterior part reminiscent of a whiplash and a thicker posterior "handle." The adult nematodes live in the large intestine, mainly in the cecum. The females lay 2000–14 000 thick-shelled, yellow-brown eggs per day. The eggs are about 50–55 μm long and are readily identified by their lemonlike shape and hyaline polar plugs (Fig. 10.1, p. 544). An infective larva develops in the egg within a few weeks. In moist surroundings, *Trichuris* eggs remain viable for months or even years.

10

Following peroral ingestion of infective eggs, the larvae hatch in the digestive tract, migrate into the mucosa, and return to the intestinal lumen after a histotropic phase lasting about 10 days. There the adult stages develop and remain with their slender anterior ends anchored in the mucosa. The prepatent period is two and a half to three months, the parasite can live for several years.

A moist, warm climate and unhygienic practices favor infections, which are contracted as described for *Ascaris*.

Pathogenesis and clinical manifestations. The whipworms, with their thin anterior ends anchored in the mucosa, ingest blood. Mild infections are asymptomatic. More severe infections, with hundreds or several thousand whipworms, cause catarrhal or hemorrhagic inflammations of the large intestine.

Diagnosis, therapy, and control. A *Trichuris* infection is diagnosed by detecting eggs in stool (Fig. 10.**1**, p. 544). Effective drugs include albendazole, mebendazole, and oxantel. See ascariosis for appropriate prevention and control measures.

Ancylostoma and Necator (Hookworms)

Causative agents of ancylostomosis and necatorosis (hookworm infection)

Parasites. *Ancylostoma duodenale* and *Necator americanus* are common parasites of the human small intestine, causing enteritis and anemia. Infection is mainly by the percutaneous route. The dog parasite *Ancylostoma caninum* has been identified as the cause of eosinophilic enteritis in humans. Larvae of various hookworm species from dogs and other carnivores can penetrate into human skin, causing the clinical picture of "cutaneous larva migrans" (p. 602).

Occurrence. Human hookworm infections are most frequent in the subtropics and tropics (for instance in southern Europe, Africa, Asia, southern US, Central and South America). The number of persons infected worldwide is estimated at about 1.25 billion (WHO, 1998). In central Europe, hookworm infections are seen mainly in travelers returning from the tropics or in guest workers from southern countries.

Morphology, life cycle, and epidemiology (Fig. 10.**14**). The hookworms that parasitize humans are 0.7–1.8 cm long with the anterior end bent dorsally in a hooklike shape (*ankylos*: bent, *stoma*: mouth, *necator*: killer). The entrance to the large buccal capsule is armed with toothlike structures (*Ancylostoma*) or cutting plates (*Necator*). The thin-shelled, oval eggs (about 60 μm long) containing only a small number of blastomeres are shed with feces. In one to two days the first-stage larvae leave the eggshells, molt twice, and develop into infective third-stage larvae. Since the shed second-stage cuticle is not entirely removed, the third-stage larva is covered by a special "sheath." Larvae in this stage are sensitive to dryness. In moist soil or water they remain viable for about one month. Higher temperatures (optimum: 20–30 °C) and sufficient moisture favor the development of the parasite stages outside of a host.

Humans are infected mainly by the percutaneous route. Factors favoring infection include working in rice paddies, walking barefoot on contaminated

Life Cycles of Hookworms

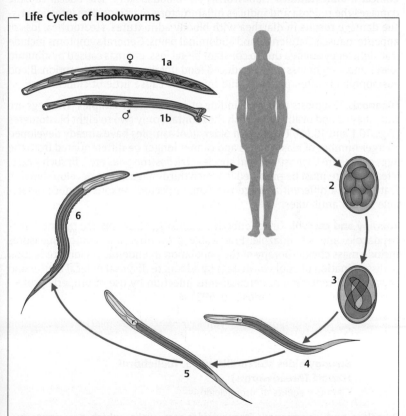

Fig. 10.**14   1** Female and male hookworms; **2** hookworm egg shed in stool with blastomeres; **3** development of first-stage larva (L1) in egg; **4** hatched L1 larva; **5** L2 larva; **6** L3 larva with sheath, infective stage.

10

soil, etc. While penetrating the skin the larvae shed their sheaths and migrate into lymphatic and blood vessels. Once in the bloodstream, they migrate via the right ventricle of the heart and by tracheal migration (conf. *Ascaris*) into the small intestine, where they develop to sexual maturity. The prepatent period lasts five to seven weeks or longer (reason: arrested larval development). Following oral infection, immediate development in the intestine is probably possible (i.e., without the otherwise necessary migration through various organs). The parasites can survive in the human gut for one to 15 years.

Clinical manifestations. Hookworms are bloodsuckers. The buccal capsule damages the mucosa and induces inflammatory reactions. The intestinal tissue damage results in diarrhea with bloody admixtures, steatorrhea, loss of appetite, nausea, flatulence, and abdominal pains. General symptoms include iron deficiency anemia due to constant blood loss, edemas caused by albumin losses and weight loss due to reduced food uptake and malabsorption. Blood eosinophilia is often present. Mild infections cause little of clinical note.

Diagnosis. Diagnosis relies on finding of eggs in stool samples. The eggs are thin-shelled and oval; when fresh they contain only two to eight blastomeres (Figs. 10.**1** and 10.**14**). The eggs in older stool samples have already developed a larger number of blastomeres and cannot longer be differentiated from the eggs of the rare trichostrongylid species (*Trichostrongylus* etc.). In such a case, a fecal culture must be prepared in which third-stage larvae develop showing features for a differential diagnosis. Some infected persons produce detectable serum antibodies.

Therapy and control. Drugs effective against hookworms are pyrantel, mebendazole, and albendazole. Practicable preventive and control measures include mass chemotherapy of the population in endemic regions, reduction of dissemination of hookworm eggs by adequate disposal of fecal matter and sewage, and reduction of percutaneous infection by use of properly protective footwear (see also filariosis, p. 593).

10

Strongyloides

Strongyloides stercoralis and S. fuelleborni (Dwarf Threadworms)
Causative agents of strongyloidosis

Parasites and occurrence. *Strongyloides stercoralis*, which parasitizes humans, dogs, and monkeys, occurs mainly in moist, warm climatic zones, and more rarely in temperate zones (e.g., southern and eastern Europe). About 50–100 million persons are infected worldwide (WHO, 1995). *Stron-*

gyloides fuelleborni is mainly a parasite of African monkeys, but is also found in humans.

Morphology, life cycle, and epidemiology (Fig. 10.**15**). Only *Strongyloides* females are parasitic. They are 2–3 mm long and live in the small intestine epithelium, where they produce their eggs by parthenogenesis. During the intestinal passage first-stage larvae (0.2–0.3 mm long) hatch from the eggs and are shed in stool (whereas eggs are shed in *S. fuelleborni* infections). Within a few days first-stage larvae develop into infective third-stage larvae.

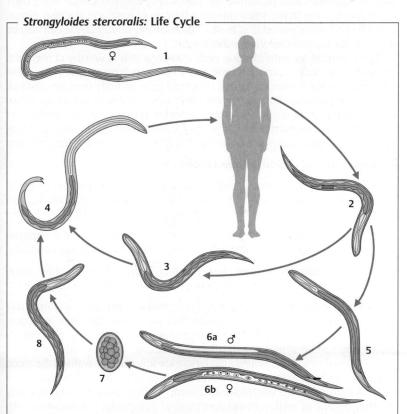

Strongyloides stercoralis: Life Cycle

Fig. 10.**15**   **1** Female *Strongyloides* from the small intestine; **2** first-stage larva (L1) shed in stool; **3** L2 larva; **4** infective L3 larva; **5** development of L1 larva to adult stages including four moltings (**6**); **6a** free-living male (not host-bound); **6b** free-living female; **7** egg of free-living generation; **8** larva hatched from egg, develops into infective larva including two moltings.

10

Given certain conditions, the first-stage larvae can develop into a free-living (nonparasitic) generation of males and females. The fertilized eggs laid by the females of this generation develop into infective third-stage larvae. This capacity for exogenous reproduction explains the enormous potential for contamination of a given environment with *Strongyloides* larvae. Third-stage larvae are highly sensitive to desiccation, but remain viable for two to three weeks in the presence of sufficient moisture.

The parasitic part of the life cycle is similar to that of the hookworms in that *Strongyloides* also penetrate the host's skin and the larvae reach their target localization in the small intestine by way of lung and tracheal migration. The prepatent period is at least 17 days. *Strongyloides* larvae can also be occasionally transmitted via mother's milk.

The potential for autoinfection with this organism is worthy of mention. The first-stage larvae can transform into infectious larvae during the intestinal passage or in the anal cleft and penetrate into the body through the large intestine or perianal skin. Continuous autoinfection can maintain an unnoticed infection in an immunocompetent person for many years (see below).

Humans are the main reservoir hosts of *S. stercoralis*; infections can also be transmitted from monkeys or dogs, but this route of infection is insignificant.

Pathogenesis and clinical manifestations

■ **Skin lesions** are observed when the larvae of *Strongyloides* species penetrate the skin, in particular in sensitized persons. Larvae of *Strongyloides* species from animals can cause "cutaneous larva migrans" (p. 602).

■ In the **lungs**, the migrating larvae provoke hemorrhages and inflammatory reactions that manifest clinically as pneumonic symptoms and coughing.

■ During the **intestinal phase**, heavy *Strongyloides* infections cause catarrhal, edematous, or ulcerative forms of enteritis as well as colitis.

■ **Systemic infection**. A *Strongyloides* infection can persist in a latent state for many years due to continuous autoinfection. If immune defense is compromised, for instance by AIDS or immunosuppressive therapy, parasite reproduction can be stimulated, resulting in massive systemic infections (hyperinfections) in which *Strongyloides* larvae are found in the walls of the colon and mesenteric vessels, in the bile ducts and in other organs. In such cases sexually mature female worms are also found in the lungs, and less frequently in other organs as well. A broad spectrum of symptoms is associated with systemic infection.

Diagnosis. Larvae (Fig. 10.1, p. 544) of *S. stercoralis* can be detected in fecal samples with the Baermann method and/or larval culture in about 60–70% of infected persons (egg detection with flotation technique for *S. fuelleborni*). Better results can be expected if duodenal fluid is examined.

Serum antibodies are present in about 85% of immunocompetent persons with *S. stercoralis* larvae in their stools (Table 11.5, p. 626). In infections with other helminths, especially filariae, cross-reactions occur that can be avoided by using recombinant proteins as antigens in the ELISA.

Therapy and prevention. The main drugs used for therapy are albendazole, mebendazole, and more recently ivermectin. Preventive measures resemble those taken to prevent hookworm infections. Travelers returning from tropical countries should be thoroughly examined for *Strongyloides* infections before any immunosuppressive measures are initiated (e.g., for a kidney transplantation).

Enterobius

Enterobius vermicularis (Pinworm)
Causative agent of enterobiosis (oxyuriosis)

Occurrence. The pinworm occurs in all parts of the world and is also a frequent parasite in temperate climate zones and developed countries. The age groups most frequently infected are five- to nine-year-old children and adults between 30 and 50 years of age.

Parasite, life cycle, and epidemiology. *Enterobius vermicularis* which belongs to the Oxyurida has a conspicuous white color. The males are 2–5 mm long, the females 8–13 mm. The long, pointed tail of the female gives the pinworm its name.

Sexually mature pinworms live on the mucosa of the large intestine and lower small intestine. Following copulation, the males soon die off. The females migrate to the anus, usually passing through the sphincter at night, then move about on the perianal skin, whereby each female lays about 10 000 eggs covered with a sticky proteinaceous layer enabling them to adhere to the skin. In severe infections, numerous living pinworms are often shed in stool and are easily recognizable as motile worms on the surface of the feces.

The eggs (about 50 × 30 µm in size) are slightly asymmetrical, ellipsoidal with thin shells (Fig. 10.1, p. 544). With their sticky surface they adhere to skin and other objects. Freshly laid eggs contain an embryo that develops into an infective first-stage larva at skin temperature in about two days. Eggs that become detached from the skin remain viable for two to three weeks in a moist environment.

Infection occurs mainly by peroral uptake of eggs (each containing an infective larva) that are transmitted to the mouth with the fingers from the anal region or from various objects. The sticky eggs adhere to toys and items of

10

everyday use or are disseminated with dust. In the intestinal tract, larvae hatch from the ingested eggs, molt repeatedly, and develop into sexually mature pinworms in five to six weeks. "Retroinfection" is also conceivable, whereby infective larvae would be released at the anus to migrate back into the intestine.

Pathogenesis and clinical manifestations. The pinworms living on the large intestine mucosa are fairly harmless. Occasionally, different stages of the pinworm penetrate into the wall of the large intestine and the appendix or migrate into the vagina, uterus, fallopian tubes, and the abdominal cavity, where they cause inflammatory reactions.

The females of *Enterobius* produce in particular a very strong pruritus that may result in nervous disorders, developmental retardation, loss of weight and appetite, and other nonspecific symptoms. Scratch lesions and eczematous changes are produced in the anal area and can even spread to cover the entire skin.

Diagnosis. A tentative diagnosis based on clinical symptoms can be confirmed by detection of pinworms spontaneously excreted with feces and eggs adhering to the perianal skin (Fig. 10.1). Standard stool examination techniques are not sufficient to find the eggs. Egg detection by the "adhesive tape method" has proved most efficient (p. 622).

Therapy and prevention. The following drugs are effective: albendazole, mebendazole, and pyrantel. Reinfections are frequent, so that treatment usually should be repeated once or more times, extended to include all potential parasite carriers (e.g., family members, kindergarten members), and combined with measures, the purpose of which is to prevent egg dissemination: washing the perianal skin (especially in the morning), covering it with ointments, washing the hands, hot laundering of underwear, and cleaning contaminated objects with hot water.

10

Nematodal Infections of Tissues and the Vascular System

Filarial nematodes, the Medina worm, and *Trichinella* are discussed in this section along with infections caused by the larvae of various nematode species.

Filarioidea (Filariae)
Causative agents of filarioses

━━

■ The nematode genera of the superfamily Filarioidea (order Spirurida) will be subsumed here under the collective term filariae, and the diseases they cause are designated as filarioses. In the life cycle of filariae infecting humans, insects (mosquitoes, blackflies, flies etc.) function as intermediate hosts and vectors. Filarioses are endemic in subtropical and tropical regions; in other regions they are observed as occasional imported cases. The most important filariosis is onchocercosis, the causative agents of which, *Onchocerca volvulus*, is transmitted by blackflies. Microfilariae of this species can cause severe skin lesions and eye damage, even blindness. Diagnosis of onchocercosis is based on clinical symptoms, detection of microfilariae in the skin and eyes, as well as on serum antibody detection. Other forms of filarioses include lymphatic filariosis (causative agent: *Wuchereria bancrofti*, *Brugia* species) and loaosis (causative agent: *Loa loa*). *Dirofilaria* species from animals can cause lung and skin lesions in humans (see p. 605). ■

━━

General. Filariae are threadlike (*filum*: thread) nematodes. The length of the adult stages (= macrofilariae) of the species that infect humans varies between 2–50 cm, whereby the females are larger than the males. The females release embryonated eggs or larvae called microfilariae. These are about 0.2–0.3 mm long, snakelike stages still surrounded by an extended eggshell (sheathed microfilariae) or they hatch out of it (unsheathed microfilariae) (Fig. 10.**17** p. 592). They can be detected mainly in the skin or in blood (Table 10.**4**).

Based on the periodic appearance of microfilariae in peripheral blood, periodic filaria species are differentiated from the nonperiodic ones showing continuous presence. The periodic species produce maximum microfilaria densities either at night (nocturnal periodic) or during the day (diurnal periodic). Different insect species, active during the day or night, function as intermediate hosts accordingly to match these changing levels of microfilaremia.

10

■ **Life Cycle of Filariae** ▬▬▬▬▬▬▬▬▬▬▬▬▬▬▬▬▬▬▬▬▬▬▬▬▬

Insect: → Ingestion of microfilaria with a blood meal → development in thoracic musculature with two moltings to become infective larva → migration to mouth parts and tranmission into skin of a new host through puncture wound during the next blood meal.

Human: → Migration to definitive localizations and further development with two more moltings to reach sexual maturity.

Wuchereria bancrofti and Brugia species
Causative agents of lymphatic filariosis

Parasites and occurrence. About 120 million people in 80 countries suffer from lymphatic filariosis caused by *Wuchereria bancrofti* or *Brugia* species (one-third each in India and Africa, the rest in southern Asia, the Pacific region, and South America), and 1.1 billion people are at infection risk (WHO, 2000). (Table 10.**4**). Humans are the only natural final hosts of *W. bancrofti* and the most widely disseminated *Brugia* strains. There are, however, other *Brugia* strains using also animals as final hosts (cats, dogs, and monkeys).

Life cycle and epidemiology. The intermediate hosts of *W. bancrofti* and *B. malayi* are various diurnal or nocturnal mosquito genera (Table 10.**4**). The development of infective larvae in the insects is only possible at high environmental temperatures and humidity levels; in *Wuchereria bancrofti* the process takes about 12 days at 28 °C. Following a primary human infection, the filariae migrate into lymphatic vessels where they develop to sexual maturity. Microfilariae (Mf) do not appear in the blood until after three months at the earliest (*B. malayi, B. timori*) or after seven to eight months (*W. bancrofti*). Tables 10.**4** and Fig. 10.**17** show their specific characteristics. The adult parasites survive for several years.

Pathogenesis and clinical manifestations. The pathologies caused by *W. bancrofti* and *Brugia* species are very similar. The initial symptoms can appear as early as one month p.i. although in most cases the incubation period is five to 12 months or much longer. The different courses taken by such infections can be summarized as follows:

■ **Asymptomatic infection**, but with microfilaremia that can persist for years.

■ **Acute symptomatic infection:** inflammatory and allergic reactions in the lymphatic system caused by filariae → swelling of lymph nodes, lymphangitis, intermittent recurrent febrile episodes, general malaise, swellings on legs, arms, scrotum and mammae, funiculitis, orchitis.

10

Table 10.4 Filarial Species Commonly Infecting Humans

Species and length (cm)	Distribution	Vector	Localization of adults	Microfilariae: characteristics and periodicity	Pathology
Wuchereria bancrofti ♂♂: 2.4–4.0 ♀♀: 5.0–10.0	Southeast Asia, Pacific, trop. Africa, Caribbean, trop. South America	**Mosquitoes:** *Culex, Anopheles, Aedes*	Lymphatic system	244–296 μm, sheathed, in blood, nocturnal, diurnal or subperiodic[2]	Lymphangitis and lymphadenitis, elephantiasis
Brugia malayi ♂♂: 2.2–2.5 ♀♀: 4.3–6.0	South and East Asia	**Mosquitoes:** *Anopheles, Aedes, Mansonia*	Lymphatic system	177–230 μm, sheathed, in blood, nocturnal or subperiodic	Lymphangitis and lymphadenitis, elephantiasis
Brugia timori	Indonesia	**Mosquitoes:** *Anopheles*		Nocturnal periodic	
Loa loa ♂♂: 3.3–3.4 ♀♀: 5.0–7.0	Tropical Africa	**Flies:** *Chrysops*	Subcutaneous connective tissue	250–300 μm, sheathed, in blood, diurnal periodic	Skin swellings, infection of conjunctiva
Onchocerca volvulus ♂♂: 2.0–4.5 ♀♀: 23–50	Africa, Central and South America	**Black flies:** *Simulium*	Subcutaneous connective tissue	221–358 μm, unsheathed, in skin, not periodic	Skin nodules, dermatitis, eye lesions
Mansonella perstans ♂♂: 4.5 ♀♀: 7.0–8.0	Africa, South America	**Midges:** *Culicoides*	Peritoneal and pleural cavities	190–200 μm, unsheathed, in blood, nocturnal subperiodic	Normally apathogenic
Mansonella streptocerca ♂♂:[3] ♀[3]	Tropical Africa	**Midges:** *Culicoides*	Subcutaneous connective tissue	180–240 μm, unsheathed, in skin, not periodic	Skin edema, dermatitis
Mansonella ozzardi ♂♂:[3] ♀♀: 6.5–8.1	Central and South America	**Midges:** *Culicoides*	Peritoneal cavity	173–240 μm, unsheathed, in blood (not periodic)	Normally apathogenic

[1] See Fig. 10.1 for details on differentiation of microfilariae.
[2] Subperiodic: periodicity is not pronounced.
[3] No exact data are available.

10

■ **Chronic symptomatic infection:** chronic obstructive changes in the lymphatic system → hindrance or blockage of the flow of lymph and dilatation of the lymphatic vessels ("lymphatic varices") → indurated swellings caused by connective tissue proliferation in lymph nodes, extremities (especially the legs, "elephantiasis"), the scrotum, etc., thickened skin (Fig. 10.**16**). Lymphuria, chyluria, chylocele etc. when lymph vessels rupture. This clinical picture develops gradually in indigenous inhabitants over a period of 10–15 years after the acute phase, in immigrants usually faster.

■ **Tropical, pulmonary eosinophilia:** syndrome with coughing, asthmatic pulmonary symptoms, high-level blood eosinophilia, lymph node swelling and high concentrations of serum antibodies (including IgE) to filarial antigens. No microfilariae are detectable in blood, but sometimes in the lymph nodes and lungs. This is an allergic reaction to filarial antigens.

Diagnosis. A diagnosis can be based on clinical symptoms (frequent eosinophilia!) and finding of microfilariae in blood (blood sampling at night for nocturnal periodic species!). Microfilariae of the various species can be differentiated morphologically in stained blood smears (Table 10.**4**, Fig. 10.**17**) and by DNA analysis. Conglomerations of adult worms are detectable by ultrasonography, particularly in the male scrotal area. Detection of serum antibodies (group-specific antibodies, specific IgE and IgG subclasses) and circulating antigens are further diagnostic tools (Table 11.**5**, p. 625). The recent development of a specific ELISA and a simple quick test (the ICT filariosis card test) represents a genuine diagnostic progress due to the high levels of sensitivity and specificity with which circulating filarial antigens can now be detected, even in "occult" infections in which microfilariae are not found in the blood.

Therapy. Both albendazole and diethylcarbamazine have been shown to be at least partially effective against adult filarial stages. However, optimal treatment regimens still need to be defined. Adjunctive measures against bacterial and fungal superinfection can significantly reduce pathology and suffering.

Control and prevention. In 1997, the WHO initiated a program to eradicate lymphatic filariosis. The mainstay control measure is mass treatment of populations in endemic areas with microfilaricides. Concurrent single doses of two active substances (albendazole with either diethylcarbamazine or iver-

Fig. 10.**16**   **a** Infection with *Wuchereria bancrofti*: elephantiasis; **b** infection with *Loa loa*: eyelid swelling; **c** onchocercosis: cutaneous nodules caused by *Onchocerca volvulus*; **d** blindness caused by *O. volvulus*; **e** *Trichinella spiralis*; larvae in rat musculature; **f** larva migrans externa. (Images a, b, d: *Tropeninstitut Tübingen*, c: *Tropeninstitut Amsterdam*; f: *Dermatologische Klinik der Universität Zürich*.)   ▶

Nematode Infections

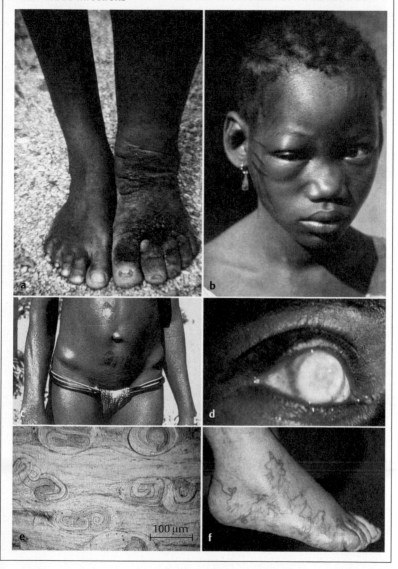

Microfilariae of Various Filarial Species

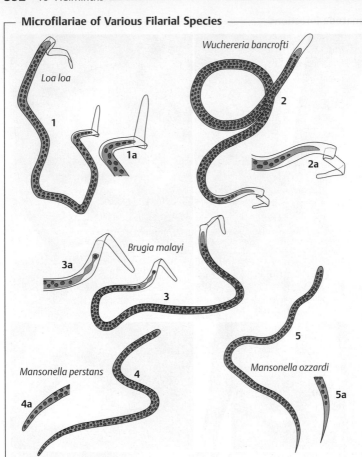

Fig. 10.**17** Differential diagnosis of microfilariae in human blood: sheathed, large: **1** *Loa loa*: tip of tail (**1a**) with several nuclei; **2** *Wuchereria bancrofti*: tip of tail (**2a**) without nuclei; **3** *Brugia malayi*: tip of tail (**3a**) with single nucleus. Unsheathed, smaller: **4** *Mansonella perstans*: tip of tail (**4a**) rounded with densely packed nuclei, often in several rows reaching nearly to the tip of the tail; **5** *Mansonella ozzardi*: tip of tail (**5a**) pointed, tip free of nuclei.

mectin) are 99% effective in removing microfilariae from the blood for one year after treatment. Mass-treatment with albendazole or ivermectin is also expected to have a controlling effect on intestinal nematodes (*Ascaris*, hookworms, *Strongyloides*, *Trichuris*). Measures to avoid mosquito bites are the same as for malaria.

Loa

Loa loa
Causative agent of loaosis (loiasis, *Loa loa* filariosis, African eyeworm)

Occurrence, life cycle, and epidemiology. Thirteen million people are infected with this filarial species in the tropical rainforest areas of Africa (western and central Africa, parts of Sudan) (WHO, 1995).

The adult and pre-adult parasites (Table 10.**4**) live in and migrate through the subcutaneous connective tissues. The microfilariae appear in a periodic pattern during the day in peripheral blood (Table 10.**4**, Fig. 10.**17**). Accordingly, the intermediate hosts are diurnally active horsefly species (Tabanidae: *Chrysops* species). The prepatent period is five to six months. In some cases, microfilariae do not appear in the blood even in older cases of infection. The adult filariae live for several years.

Pathogenesis and clinical manifestations. Clinical symptoms can occur two to 12 months after the infection. They are probably mainly allergic in nature. The filariae migrating through the connective tissues cause edematous swellings in the limbs, face, and body ("Calabar swellings") and itching nodules (Fig. 10.**16b**). The infection is often accompanied by blood eosinophilia. Migration of a parasite beneath the conjunctiva causes lacrimation, erythema, and other symptoms.

Diagnosis, therapy, and prevention. Diagnosis involves observation of typical symptoms, adult parasites in subcutis or conjunctiva and microfilariae in peripheral blood (in blood specimens sampled during the day!) (Table 10.**4**, Fig. 10.**17**). The drug of choice is diethylcarbamazine that kills microfilariae and damages macrofilariae after long-term therapy (N.B.: possible side effects).

10

Mansonella species

See Table 10.**4** and Fig. 10.**17** for *Mansonella* species that should be taken into account in differential diagnostic procedures.

Onchocerca

Onchocerca volvulus
Causative agent of onchocercosis

This filarial species causes onchocercosis, a disease that manifests mainly in the form of skin alterations, lymphadenopathy, and eye damage, which latter is the reason for the special importance of the disease.

Occurrence. *Onchocerca volvulus* is endemic in 30 countries in tropical Africa (from the Atlantic coast to the Red Sea) and southern Arabia (Yemen) as well as in six countries in Central and South America (Mexico, Guatemala, Columbia, Venezuela, Brazil, Ecuador). About 17.6 million persons are currently infected and 267 000 are blind due to onchocercosis (WHO, 1998, 2000). The WHO has been coordinating successful control programs in 11 African countries since 1974, and in six Latin American countries since 1991 (see below).

Life cycle. The adult *Onchocerca* live in the connective and fatty tissues, usually tightly coiled in connective tissue nodules in the subcutis or deeper tissue layers (Fig. 10.**16c**). Sexually mature parasites can live as long as 15 years.

Female *Onchocerca* produce microfilariae that live in the tissue within the nodules or skin. Starting from the site of the female worms, the microfilariae migrate through the deep corium of the dermis into other skin regions and can also affect the eyes—especially if the nodule is located on the head or upper body. Through the lymphatics, the microfilariae can penetrate into the bloodstream and also appear in urine, sputum, and cerebrospinal fluid. The relatively large microfilariae have no sheath (Table 10.**4**); their lifespan in human hosts is from six to 30 months.

Simuliidae (blackflies) are the intermediate hosts and vectors. The development of the infective larvae, transmitted by a blackfly to a human host, takes many months before the nematodes reach sexual maturity. Microfilariae are usually be detected in skin after 12–15 months (seven to 24 months) (prepatent period).

Epidemiology. Humans are the sole parasite reservoir of *O. volvulus*. Onchocercosis occurs in endemic foci along the rivers in which the larvae and pupae of the blackflies develop. Therefore, the blindness caused by onchocercosis is designated as "river blindness."

Pathogenesis and clinical manifestations. Pathological reactions are provoked by adult parasites and by microfilariae. These reactions are influenced by the immune status of infected individuals.

■ **Reactions to adult parasites:** enclosure of adult filariae in fibrous nodules (onchocercomas), usually 0.5–2 cm (sometimes up to 6 cm) in diameter in the subcutis along the iliac crest, ribs, scalp, etc., more rarely in deeper tissues. Nodulation occurs about one to two years after infection and is either asymptomatic or causes only mild symptoms (Fig. 10.**16c**).

■ **Reactions to microfilariae:** microfilariae appear in the skin about 12–15 (seven to 24 months p.i.). Initial symptoms occur after about 15–18 months: for example, pruritus, loss of skin elasticity with drooping skin folds, papules, depigmentation, and swelling of lymph nodes; blood eosinophilia may also be present.

■ **Eye changes:** "snowflake" corneal opacities, in later stage sclerosing keratitis, the main cause of blindness, chorioretinitis and ocular nerve atrophy; tendency toward bilateral damage (Fig. 10.**16d**).

Diagnosis

■ **Adult parasites.** Onchocercomas can be identified by palpation and ultrasonic imaging. Presence of the parasites can be confirmed by surgical removal and examination of the cutaneous nodules.

■ **Microfilariae** can be found in skin snips after the prepatent period. A PCR is now available for species-specific detection of *Onchocerca* DNA (Oncho-150 repeat sequence) in skin specimens. Living or dead microfilariae can be seen in the anterior chamber of the eye with the help of a slit lamp or an ophthalmoscope. Various techniques and antigens (e.g., recombinant antigens) can also be used to detect serum antibodies (Table 11.**5**, p. 625).

Therapy. *Onchocerca* nodules can be removed surgically. Suramin—a quite toxic substance effective against macrofilariae—is now no longer used. It was recently discovered that *O. volvulus*, *Wuchereria bancrofti*, *Brugia* species, and several other filarial species contain endosymbionts of the genus *Wolbachia* (order Rickettsiales) that are transovarially transmitted from females to the following generation. Studies in animals and humans have shown that prolonged therapy with doxycyclin damages both the endosymbionts and the filariae. These results could lead to a new therapeutic approach. Ivermectin in low doses is highly effective against microfilariae (see prevention), and has some effect on macrofilariae in repeated higher doses.

Prevention and control. Protective clothing and application of repellents to the skin can provide some degree of protection from blackfly bites (see Malaria). WHO programs involving repeated applications of insecticides to streams and rivers with the aim of selective eradication of the developmental stages of *Simuliidae* in western Africa have produced impressive regional results. Mass treatment of the population in endemic areas with low-dose iver-

10

mectin (0.15 mg/kg of body weight) administered once or twice a year has been practiced since 1987. This can drastically reduce the microfilarial density in human skin for up to 12 months. Microfilariae in the eyes are also influenced. These measures prevent disease and reduce, or even interrupt parasite transmission. Simultaneous application of vector control measures and mass therapy with ivermectin has eliminated the parasite reservoir in the populations of seven of the 11 African countries participating in the above-mentioned control program (WHO, 2000). The manufacturer of ivermectin is providing the drug at no cost for the WHO-coordinated program. In further disease control campaigns, the vector control measures are to be stopped, but mass treatments with ivermectin or other potent drugs are to be continued once a year over the longer term (WHO, 2000).

Dracunculus medinensis (Medina or Guinea Worm)

Causative agent of dracunculosis (Medina or Guinea worm infection)

Male *Dracunculus medinensis* worms are 1–4 cm long, the females measure 50–100 cm in body length. Humans contract the disease by ingesting drinking water contaminated with intermediate hosts ("water fleas": fresh water crustacea, *Cyclops*) containing infective *Dracunculus* larvae. From the intestine the parasites migrate through the body, females and males mate in the connective tissue, and after approximately 10–12 months p.i. mature females eventually move to the surface of the skin of the legs and feet in 90% of the cases. There, the female provokes an edema, a blister, and then an ulcer. Skin perforation is accompanied by pain, fever, and nausea; secondary bacterial infections occur in approx. 30% of cases. When the wound contacts water, the female extends the anterior end out of it and releases numerous larvae. The larvae are ingested by intermediate hosts and develop into infective stages.

Diagnosis is usually based on the clinical manifestations.

The WHO has been running a control program since the early 1980s based mainly on education of the population and filtration of drinking water using simple cloth or nylon filters. Annual infection incidences have been reduced from three and a half million cases in 1986 to about 75 000 in 2000 (WHO, 2004). Dracunculosis now still occurs in 14 sub-Saharan African countries, but has been officially declared eliminated in some formerly endemic countries (including India, Pakistan, and some African countries). Approximately 73% of all cases are currently reported from Sudan.

Trichinella
Causative agent of trichinellosis

■ Humans can acquire an infection with larvae of various *Trichinella* species by ingesting raw meat (from pigs, wild boars, horses, and other species). Adult stages develop from the larvae and inhabit the small intestine, where the females produce larvae that migrate through the lymphatics and bloodstream into skeletal musculature, penetrate into muscle cells and encyst (with the exception of *Trichinella pseudospiralis* and some other species which does not encyst). Clinical manifestations of trichinellosis are characterized by intestinal and muscular symptoms. Diagnosis requires muscle biopsies and serum antibody detection. ■

Parasite species and occurrence. Eight *Trichinella* species and several strains have been described to date based on typical enzyme patterns, DNA sequences, and biological characteristics. The areas of distribution are listed in Table 10.**5**; several *Trichinella* species occur sympatrically, i.e., in the same geographic region (Table 10.**5**).

The most widespread and most important species is *Trichinella spiralis*, which develops mainly in a synanthropic cycle. Despite the generally low prevalence of *Trichinella* in Europe, a number of outbreaks have occurred since 1975 (e.g., in Germany, France, Italy, Spain, England, and Poland) affecting groups of persons of various sizes (the largest about 650). Worldwide, the annual incidences per 100 000 inhabitants (1991–2000) have varied widely, for example between 0.01 in Germany and the USA, 5.1 in Lithuania, and 11.4 in Bulgaria.

Morphology and life cycle (Fig. 10.**18**). Male *Trichinella spiralis* are approximately 1–2 mm long, the females 2–4 mm. A characteristic feature is the subdivided esophagus with a muscular anterior portion and a posterior part consisting of glandular cells ("stichocytes"). The other *Trichinella* species are of about the same length and do not show morphological differences, except *T. pseudospiralis*, *T. papuae*, and *Trichinella zimbabwensis* the muscle larvae of which do not encyst.

The life cycle described here refers to *T. spiralis*. Infection of humans and other hosts results from ingestion of raw or undercooked meat containing encysted *Trichinella* larvae (Fig. 10.**16e**). The larvae are released following exposure to the digestive juices, whereupon they invade epithelial cells in the small intestine, reaching sexual maturity within a few days after four moltings. The males soon die after copulation, the females live for about four to six weeks. Each female produces about 200–1500 larvae (each around 100 μm long), which penetrate into the lamina propria. The larvae disperse

10

Trichinella spiralis: Life Cycle

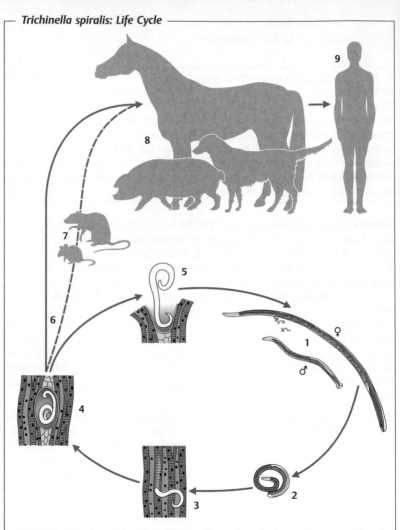

Fig. 10.**18** **1** Male and female in the small intestine of a host; **2** larvae produced by female; **3** larvae penetrating muscle cell; **4** larvae encapsulated in musculature; **5** release of larvae from capsule following peroral ingestion by host; **6** infection of hosts with muscle larvae; **7** rodent hosts; **8** domestic animal hosts; **9** transmission of parasites to humans with trichinellous meat.

10

into organs and body tissues by means of lymphogenous and hematogenous migration. Further development occurs only in striated muscle cells that they reach five to seven days p.i. at the earliest.

The larvae penetrate into muscle fibers, which are normally not destroyed in the process, but transformed into "nurse" cells providing a suitable environment for the parasite. The muscle cell begins to encapsulate the parasite about two weeks p.i. by depositing hyaline and fibrous material within the sarcolemma. Encapsulation is completed after four to six weeks. The capsules are about 0.2–0.9 mm long with an oval form resembling a lemon. Granulation tissue or fat cells form at the poles (Fig. 10.**16e**). The capsule may also gradually calcify beginning at the poles.

The *Trichinella* larvae at first lie stretched out straight within the muscle cell, but by the third week p.i. they roll up into a spiral form (not observed in *Trichinella pseudospiralis* and some other species, see Table 10.**5**). They differentiate further during this period to become infective. The encapsulated *Trichinella* remain viable for years in the host (demonstrated for up to 31 years in humans). The developmental cycle is completed when infectious muscle *Trichinella* are ingested by a new host.

Epidemiology. In many countries trichinellosis exists in natural foci with sylvatic cycles involving wild animals, in particular carnivores. Such cycles are known to occur in most of the *Trichinella* species but *T. spiralis* is predominantly perpetuated in a synanthropic cycle (Table 10.**5**). Humans can acquire the infection from sylvatic cycles by eating undercooked meat of wild boar, bear etc. containing infective *Trichinella* larvae. Sylvatic cycles may remain restricted to natural foci without spreading to domestic pigs or other domestic animals. This is apparently the case with *T. britovi* in Switzerland, for example. Human infections are most frequently derived from the synanthropic cycle of *T. spiralis*.

Encapsulated muscle larvae are very resistant. They remain infectious for at least four months in rotting meat. Cooled to 2–4 °C, they survive in musculature for 300 days. They are generally killed by deep-freezing to –25 °C within 10–20 days, although muscle larvae of the cold-resistant species *T. nativa* may remain infective for many months at –20 °C (Table 10.**5**). Heat is rapidly lethal, but the larvae can survive drying and pickling.

The sources of human infection are raw and insufficiently cooked or frozen meat products from domestic pigs and wild boars, horses, and less frequently from bears, dogs, and other animal species. Dried and pickled meat containing trichinellae can also be infective.

Clinical manifestations. The severity and duration of clinical manifestations depend on the infective dose and the rate of reproduction of the trichinellae. As few as 50–70 *T. spiralis* larvae can cause disease in humans. The pathogenicity of the other species is apparently lower. Infections run a two-phase course:

10

Table 10.5 *Trichinella* species

Trichinella species and distribution	Cycle[1] and important hosts (selection)	Characteristics of muscle larvae R: Resistance at −30 °C, 12 h
T. spiralis Worldwide	*Mainly synanthropic, also sylvatic.* Domestic pig, rat, horse, wild boar, camel, dog, red fox, bear, humans	With capsule R: low
T. britovi Temperate zone of the palaearctic region	*Mainly sylvatic, also synanthropic.* Red fox, wolf, jackal, raccoon dog, wildcat, bears, badger, marten, rodents, domestic pig, wild boar, horse, humans	With capsule R: moderate
T. murrelli Temperate zone in North America (US)	*Sylvatic, also synanthropic.* Bear, raccoon, red fox, coyote, bobcat (*Felis rufus*), horse, humans	With capsule R: low
T. nativa Arctic and subarctic regions (north of the −6 °C January isotherm)	*Mainly sylvatic, also synanthropic.* Polar fox, red fox, polar bear, wolf, raccoon dog, jackal, dog, wild boar, humans	With capsule R: high
T. nelsoni Sub-Saharan Africa, Asia (Kazakhstan)	*Sylvatic.* Hyena, warthog, wild boar, domestic pig, humans	With capsule R: none
T. pseudospiralis Australia, India, Caucasus, Kazakhstan, US	*Sylvatic.* Quoll (Dasyuridae), raccoon, korsak (steppe fox), rodents, bird species, (birds of prey and others), humans	Without capsule R: none
Trichinella papuae Papua New Guinea	*Sylvatic.* Wild boar, domestic pig, humans	Without capsule R: ?
Trichinella zimbabwensis Zimbabwe	*Cycle in farmed crocodiles* Experimental hosts: pig, rat, monkey	Without capsule R: ?

[1] Animals involved: synanthropic cycle: animals living in proximity to human dwellings (domestic animals, rats etc.); sylvatic cycle: wild animals.

■ **Intestinal phase:** incubation period of one to seven days. Symptoms: nausea, vomiting, gastrointestinal disorders with diarrhea, mild fever, and other symptoms. An inapparent course is also possible.

■ **Extraintestinal phase:** incubation period of seven or more days. Symptoms caused by invasion of body tissues by *Trichinella* larvae: myositis with muscle pain and stiffness, respiratory and swallowing difficulties, fever, edemas on eyelids and face, cutaneous exanthema. Feared complications include mycocarditis and meningoencephalitis. Further characteristic features are blood eosinophilia, raised activity of serum lactate dehydrogenase, myokinase and creatine phosphokinase, and creatinuria. This phase lasts about one to six weeks. It is frequently followed by recovery, but rheumatoid and other symptoms can also persist (e.g., cardiac muscle damage). Lethal outcome is rare.

Diagnosis. Diagnosis during the intestinal phase is difficult and only rarely trichinellae can be found in stool or duodenal fluid. During the extraintestinal phase, *Trichinella* larvae are detectable in muscle biopsies (either by microscopy in press preparations, histologically or by PCR-based DNA detection). Beginning in the third week p.i. serum antibodies appear (Table 11.**5**, p. 626). Clinical chemistry (see above) furnishes further diagnostic data.

Therapy and prevention. The recommended drugs for therapy are mebendazole or albendazole in combination with prednisolone (to alleviate allergic and inflammatory reactions) (WHO, 1995). Heat exceeding 80 °C kills trichinellae in meat. The safest methods are to boil or fry the meat sufficiently (deep-freezing may be unreliable, see above!). Important disease control measures include prophylactic inspection of domestic and wild animal meat for *Trichinella* infection and not feeding raw meat wastes to pig livestock and other susceptible domestic animals.

Infections Caused by Nematodal Larvae

■ *Larva migrans externa* and Larva migrans *interna* are diseases caused by migrating nematode larvae. The first (*externa*) is a skin disease, usually caused by zoonotic hookworms or *Strongyloides* species. In the second type (*interna*), nematode larvae migrate into inner organs, e.g., in toxocarosis. In toxocarosis the infection results from peroral ingestion of infective eggs of roundworms of the genus *Toxocara* that are released to the environment in the feces of dogs, foxes, and cats (infection risk for children on contaminated playgrounds!). In humans, migrating *Toxocara* larvae can cause damage to liver, lungs, CNS, and eyes. Additional diseases caused by nematode larvae include anisakiosis, angiostrongylosis, and dirofilariosis. ■

Larva Migrans Externa or
Cutaneous Larva Migrans (CLM)
("Creeping Eruption")

Parasites. CLM designates a syndrome caused by migration of larval parasites in the skin of accidental hosts. Hookworm species of dogs and cats (e.g., *Ancylostoma braziliense, Ancylostoma caninum*) and *Strongyloides* species of various hosts (mammalian animals, humans) are mainly responsible for human CLM. Other potential causative organisms include insect larvae (*Hypoderma, Gasterophilus*, etc.).

Clinical manifestations. The infective larvae of the above-mentioned hookworm species can penetrate human skin (feet, hands, other body regions) upon contact with contaminated soil (e.g., on bathing beaches) and migrate through the dermis. This results in papules, twisted and inflamed worm burrows, and pruritus (Fig. 10.**16f**). These larvae rarely penetrate further into the body and normally do not reach sexual maturity in the host (however, see also p. 580). The larvae persist in the skin for several weeks to months, and then they die (see p. 617 for causative insect larvae).

Diagnosis and therapy. The clinical presentation with many 1–2 mm wide and centimeter-long worm burrows usually suffices for a diagnosis. Recommended treatments include topical application of thiabendazole ointment (15%), wetting with ivermectin solution, spray-freezing with ethyl chloride and peroral therapy with albendazole or ivermectin.

Larva Migrans Interna or
Visceral Larva Migrans (VLM)

Parasites. The main causative agents of this disease are the larvae of various roundworm species from domestic and wild animals, for instance *Toxocara canis* from dogs and foxes, *T. mystax* from cats, *Baylisascaris procyonis* from raccoons as well as roundworm species (Anisakidae) from marine mammals. Toxocarosis and anisakiosis are discussed here as examples from this group. Angiostrongyliosis and dirofilariosis can also be included in this disease category.

Toxocara

Causative agent of toxocarosis

Distribution, life cycle, and epidemiology. Dogs, cats, and foxes all over the world, especially younger animals, are frequently infected with adult *Toxocara* roundworms. The parasites live in the small intestine and in most cases produce large numbers of eggs. An infective larva develops in an egg shed into the environment within two to three weeks. Humans are infected by accidental peroral ingestion of infective eggs (geophagia, contaminated foods). Small children run a particularly high risk. Fairly high levels of contamination of public parks and playgrounds with *Toxocara* eggs (sandboxes >1–50%) have been found in many cities in Europe and elsewhere. Mean antibody prevalence levels of about 1–8% were measured in healthy persons in Germany, Austria, and Switzerland in serological screening based on a specific ELISA, with figures as high as 30% in some population subgroups.

After infection, the *Toxocara* larvae hatch from the eggshells in the small intestine, penetrate the intestinal wall, and migrate hematogenously into the liver, lungs, CNS, eyes, musculature, and other organ systems. Larvae caught in the capillary filter leave the vascular system and begin to migrate through the organ involved. This results in hemorrhages and tissue destruction as well as inflammatory reactions and formation of granulomatous foci. Living larvae are encapsulated in connective tissue in all organs except the CNS, but they can also leave the capsules and continue migrating. The larvae can live for a number of years (at least 10 years in monkeys). Development of adult *Toxocara* stages in the human intestine is a very rare occurrence.

Clinical manifestations. VLM remains inapparent in most cases. Symptomatic cases are most frequently observed in children aged two to five years. The clinical symptoms depend on the localization and degree of pathological changes and include nonspecific and varied conditions such as eosinophilia, leukocytosis, hepatomegaly, brief febrile episodes, mild gastrointestinal disorders, asthmatic attacks, pneumonic symptoms, lymphadenopathy, urticarial skin changes, central nervous disorders with paralyses, or epileptiform convulsions. Eye infections are seen in all age groups and present as granulomatous chorioretinitis, clouding of the vitreous body and other changes. Ocular toxocariosis is often observed without signs of visceral infection.

Diagnosis. Persistent eosinophilia and the other symptoms described above justify a tentative diagnosis. Etiological confirmation requires serological testing for specific antibodies. Highly sensitive and specific techniques are available (ELISA, Western blot) (Table 11.**5**, p. 625). Positive seroreactions can be expected four weeks after infection.

Therapy and prevention. Chemotherapy with albendazole is only indicated in symptomatic cases. Prophylactic measures include control of *Toxocara* infections in cats and dogs, especially in young animals, and reduction or prevention of environmental contamination with feces of dogs, cats, and foxes especially on children's playgrounds.

Anisakis
Causative agent of anisakiosis

Anisakis and related roundworm genera (*Phocanema* [= *Pseudoterranova*], *Contracecum*), live in the intestines of marine mammals or birds. The larvae of these parasites, which are ingested by humans with raw sea fish, are known as the causative agents of eosinophilic granulomas in the gastrointestinal tract ("herring worm disease"). In recent years, most cases reported have occurred in Japan. Reliable prophylactic practices include heating or deep-freezing of fish (–20 °C for at least 12–24 hours).

Angiostrongylus
Causative agent angiostrongylosis

Angiostrongylus cantonensis (syn. *Parastrongylus cantonensis*) occurs in the southern Asian and Pacific area, where it inhabits the lungs of rats. This parasite has been identified as the cause of an eosinophilic meningoencephalitis in humans. Larval stages of the parasite have been found in the brain, spinal cord, and eyes of persons who had previously fallen ill. Infection results from ingestion of raw intermediate hosts (snails) and transport hosts (crustaceans) containing infective larvae of *A. cantonensis*.

Angiostrongylus costaricensis (syn. *Parastrongylus costaricensis*) occurs in the USA, Central and South America, and Africa, where it parasitizes in the mesenteric vessels of cotton rats and other vertebrates. Human infections are caused by accidental ingestion of intermediate hosts (snails) containing larvae, resulting in the invasion of mesenteric vessels by parasites and development of inflammatory intestinal wall granulomas. Larvae are not shed in stool because, although the parasites produce eggs, no larvae hatch out of them.

Dirofilaria

Causative agent of dirofilariosis

The larvae of *Dirofilaria immitis* and *Dirofilaria repens*, which in the adult stages are parasites of dogs, cats, and wild carnivores, are occasionally transmitted to humans by mosquitoes: immature stages of *D. immitis* usually invade the lungs and produce 1–4 cm round foci there, whereas the stages of *D. repens* are usually found in subcutaneous nodules. In Europe, the majority of autochthonous cases are reported from Italy, France, and Greece. Imported infections are reported from other countries as well (Germany, Austria, Switzerland, etc.).

11 Arthropods

J. Eckert

Parasitic arthropods are ectoparasites that have a temporary or permanent association with their hosts. Their considerable medical significance is due to their capability to cause nuisance or skin diseases in humans and to act

Table 11.1 Classification of Arthropods Mentioned in the Text

Subphylum ▪ Class	Order* ▪ Suborder	Genus
Amandibulata		
▪ **Arachnida**	Metastigmata[1] (ticks)	Family Ixodidae: *Ixodes, Dermacentor, Rhipicephalus, Haemaphysalis* etc.; family Argasidae: *Argas, Ornithodoros*
	Mesostigmata[2] (mites)	*Dermanyssus, Ornithonyssus*
	Prostigmata[3] (mites)	*Cheyletiella, Neotrombicula*
	Astigmata[4] (mites)	*Sarcoptes, Notoedres, Psoroptes, Tyrophagus, Tyroglyphus, Glyciphagus, Dermatophagoides*
Madibulata		
▪ **Insecta**	Anoplura (lice)	*Pediculus, Phthirus*
	Heteroptera (bugs)	*Cimex, Oeciacus, Triatoma, Rhodnius, Panstrongylus*
	Diptera	
	▪ Nematocera (mosquitoes, black flies etc.)	*Anopheles, Culex, Aedes, Simulium, Phlebotomus, Lutzomyia*
	▪ Brachycera (flies)	*Musca, Glossina, Calliphora, Cochliomyia, Cordylobia, Lucilia, Sarcophaga, Wohlfahrtia, Gasterophilus, Hypoderma, Cuterebra*
	Siphonaptera (fleas)	*Pulex, Ctenocephalides, Ceratophyllus, Archaeopsylla, Xenopsylla, Tunga,* etc.

*Syn. [1]Ixodida, [2]Gamasida, [3]Trombidiformes, [4] Sarcoptiformes.

as vectors of viruses, bacteria, protozoa, or helminths. Some species or stages of arthropods are capable of penetrating to deeper skin layers or into body openings or wounds, where their effect is similar to that of endoparasites. Only a small selection of medically important arthropods will be described in the following chapter (see Table 11.**1**), in particular those that are of significance in central Europe. The reader is referred to the literature for more detailed information (see p. 660).

Arachnida

Ticks (Ixodida)

General. The order Ixodida includes two important families, the Argasidae (soft ticks) and Ixodidae (hard ticks). The latter is the most significant group worldwide. We will only be considering the Ixodidae here.

Approximately 20 hard tick species are indigenous to western and central Europe, belonging to the genera *Ixodes*, *Rhipicephalus*, *Dermacentor*, and *Haemaphysalis*. The most important species is *Ixodes ricinus* that accounts for about 90% of the tick fauna in this region. For this reason, human tick bites in central Europe are in most cases caused by *I. ricinus* and only occasionally by other tick species.

Ixodes ricinus

Vector of the causative agents of Lyme borreliosis and tickborne encephalitis

---

■ *Ixodes ricinus*, (common sheep tick, castor bean tick) is the most frequent hard tick species in central Europe. The medical significance of this species is due to its role as vector of the causative agents of Lyme borreliosis, tickborne encephalitis (European tickborne encephalitis, "early summer meningoencephalitis," ESME), and other pathogens. Ticks that have attached to the skin should be mechanically removed as soon as possible to reduce the risk of infection. ■

Morphology. *Male*: about 2–3 mm long with a highly chitinized scutum covering the entire dorsal surface. *Female*: 3–4 mm, up to 12 mm when fully engorged after a blood meal; the scutum covers only the anterior portion of the body (Fig. 11.**1a**). Adults and nymphs (the latter about 1 mm long) have four pairs of legs, the smaller larvae (about 0.5 mm long) only three pairs. Ticks possess characteristic piercing mouthparts.

11

Arthropod Parasites of Man

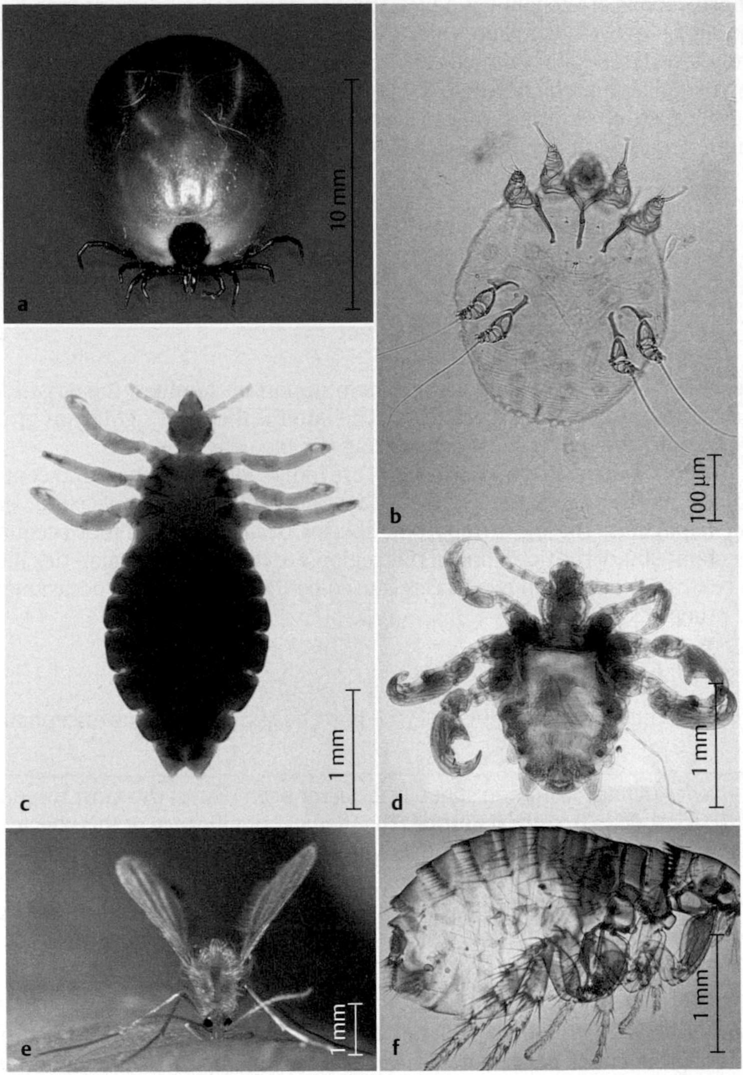

Fig. 11.**1** **a** *Ixodes ricinus*, female engorged with blood; **b** *Sarcoptes scabiei*, female; **c** body louse; **d** crab louse; **e** sandfly (*Phlebotomus papatasi*) feeding on human skin; **f** dog flea (*Ctenocephalides canis*). (Image e: H. M. Seitz, Institut für Medizinische Parasitologie, Bonn.)

Biology. The various stages of *I. ricinus* are dependent on blood meals from vertebrates throughout their developmental cycle. Having selected a suitable location on a host, a female tick inserts her piercing mouthparts into the skin within about 10 minutes. Using clawlike organs at the tip of stylettelike mouthparts, the chelicerae, the tick cuts a wound into which the unpaired, barbed, pinecone-shaped hypostome is then inserted to anchor the parasite in the skin. While sucking blood, ticks secrete large amounts of saliva, containing cytolytic, anticoagulative, and other types of substances. They ingest blood, tissue fluid and digested tissue components. The weight of the female increases considerably during a blood meal. When completely engorged, the tick resembles a ricinus seed. The epidemiologically important factor is the possible ingestion of pathogens with the blood meal, which can, at a following blood meal in the tick's next developmental stage, be inoculated into another vertebrate host (horizontal transmission). Female ticks even transmit certain pathogens by the transovarial route to the next generation of ticks (vertical transmission).

Table 11.**2** summarizes the life cycle of *I. ricinus*. The overall development period may be interrupted by periods of inactivity and starvation (maximum starvation capacity 13–37 months, depending on the stage) and can therefore take from one to three years.

Epidemiology. *I. ricinus* occurs widely in Europe, both in lowland and mountainous regions up to 800–1000 m above sea level, occasionally even higher. The habitats preferred by this species include coniferous, deciduous, and mixed forests with plentiful underbrush and a dense green belt. The different

Table 11.**2** Life Cycle of *Ixodes ricinus*

Developmental stages:	Egg →	Larva →	Nymph →	Imago
Host groups commonly used for blood feeding:	–	Rodents, birds, (humans)[1]	Birds, mammals[2], humans	Domestic and wild ruminants, dogs, cats, horses, and other animal species[2], humans
Duration of bloodsucking, in days:	–	2–6	3–7	5–14
Tick habitat when not attached to a host:	Humid soil, low vegetation, areas of woodland with underbrush, meadows with high grass, gardens etc.			

[1] Occasionally. [2] Many different host species; in Europe about 35.

11

stages of ticks inhabit grass, ferns, and branches in this low vegetation either quite close to the ground (mainly larvae and nymphs) or somewhat higher (up to about 80–100 cm, mainly adults) in questing for suitable hosts. When hosts approach, the ticks either let themselves drop onto them or cling to the skin on contact. *I. ricinus* becomes active at 7–10 °C. Maximum tick activity is registered in the periods May-June and August-October.

The great epidemiological significance of *I. ricinus* in central Europe is predominantly due to its function as vector of the causative agents of Lyme borreliosis (*Borrelia* spp., p. 324f.) and the European tickborne encephalitis (TBE) (virus of TBE, p. 443f.). In northern and eastern Europe the TBE virus is transmitted by *Ixodes persulcatus*; *Ixodes scapularis* (syn. *I. dammini*) is the vector of *Borrelia burgdorferi* in the USA.

Diagnosis. Identification of *I. ricinus* is either done macroscopically or with the help of a magnifying glass. Differential species identification requires the skills of a specialist. Skin reactions, in particular the erythema chronicum migrans resulting from a borreliosis infection, often provide indirect evidence of an earlier tick bite.

Tick bite prevention. Tick habitats with dense undergrowth, ferns, and high grasses should be avoided as far as possible. If this is unavoidable, proper clothing must be worn: shoes, long socks, long trousers (tuck legs of trousers into socks), long sleeves that fit closely around the wrists. Additional protection is provided by spraying the clothes with acaricides, especially pyrethroids, which have a certain repellent effect (e.g., flumethrin). The effect of repellents applied to the skin (see malaria) is in most cases insufficient to protect against ticks.

After staying in a tick habitat persons should search their entire body for ticks and remove any found attached to the skin as quickly as possible by mechanical means (do not apply oil or other substances to attached ticks!). Any bites should be watched during the following four weeks for signs of reddening (erythema), swelling, and inflammation. A "migrating," i.e., spreading rash (erythema migrans) is indicative for a *Borrelia* infection. On the other hand, this sign is not observed in all infected persons.

Mites

Sarcoptes scabiei
Causative agent of scabies ("the itch," "sarcoptic itch")

■ Infestation with *Sarcoptes scabiei* var. *hominis* causes human scabies, a condition characterized by pronounced pruritus, epidermal mite burrows, nodules, and pustules. Transmission is person to person. Various mite species that parasitize animals may also infest the human skin without reproducing, causing the symptoms of "pseudoscabies." ■

Occurrence. Scabies caused by *Sarcoptes scabiei* var. *hominis* does not occur frequently in Europe, although occasional outbreaks are seen in school classes, families, senior citizens' homes, and other groups.

Morphology and biology. *Sarcoptes scabiei*: mites about 0.2–0.5 mm long with ovoid bodies. The adults and nymphs have four pairs of legs (Fig. 11.**1b**), the larva has three pairs of legs. Following transmission to a human host the female mites penetrate into the epidermis and begin to tunnel. The resulting winding burrows are usually 4–5 mm and sometimes as long as 10 mm. Oviposition begins after only a few hours. Six-legged larvae hatch from the eggs after a few days. In further course of development involving moltings, the larvae transform into protonymphs (nymph I), then deutonymphs (nymph II), and finally adult males and females. The entire life cycle takes two to three weeks. The lifespan of the female mites is four to six weeks.

Epidemiology. Transmission is by close contact (sexual partners, family members, school children, healthcare staff) from person to person, whereby female mites translocate to the skin of a new host. Indirect transmission on clothes (underclothes), bed linens, etc. is not a primary route, but should be considered as a factor in control measures. Without a host, mites usually die off within a few days. Mite infections can also be acquired from animals to which humans have close skin contact.

Clinical manifestations. An early sign of an initial infestation with *Sarcoptes* mites is the **primary efflorescence** with mite tunnels up to 2–4 mm and sometimes 10 mm long—threadlike, irregularly winding burrows reminiscent of pencil markings. The female mite is found at the end of the burrow in a small swelling.

Following an inapparent period of about four to five weeks, during which time a hypersensitivity response to mite antigens develops, the **scabies exanthema** manifests in the form of local or generalized **pruritus**, which is particularly bothersome in the evening when body heat is retained under the bedcovers. The evolving skin lesions are papulous or papulovesicular exanthema and reactions due to scratching. In adults, these lesions are seen mainly in the interdigital spaces and on the sides of the fingers, on the wrists and ankles and in the genital region. Children also occasionally show facial lesions.

A special form of the infestation may develop in immunocompromised patients: **scabies crustosa** (formerly scabies norvegica). This type is characterized by pronounced crusted, flaking lesions, particularly in the head and neck region. Massive reproduction of the mites makes this condition highly contagious.

11

Diagnosis and control. Case history and clinical manifestations provide important diagnostic hints that require etiological confirmation by identification of the parasites (Fig. 11.**1b**). A papule is removed by tangential scalpel excision, whereupon the specimen is macerated in 10% potassium hydroxide (KOH), and then examined for mites under a microscope. Mites can also be isolated from skin tunnels after scarification with a needle or by pressing adhesive tape onto the skin. Therapy requires topical application of γ-hexachlorocyclohexane (lindane), permethrin or crotamiton in strict accordance with manufacturer's instructions. A recent development is peroral therapy with ivermectin. Underclothing and bed linens must be washed at a minimum temperature of 50 °C.

Other Mites

The preferred hosts of mites of the orders Astigmata (e.g., *Sarcoptes scabiei* var. *suis*, *S. scabiei* var. *canis*, *Notoedres cati*, *Psoroptes ovis*), Prostigmata (e.g., *Cheyletiella*, *Neotrombicula*), or Mesostigmata (e.g., *Dermanyssus*, *Ornithonyssus*) are vertebrate animals (usually domestic animals), with occasional human infestations. On human hosts the mites remain temporarily on or in the skin without reproducing, causing a variety of skin lesions involving pruritus, most of which abate spontaneously if reinfestation can be prevented. It is important to prevent such infestations by treating of mite-infested animals and—if needed—by decontaminating their surroundings.

Some groups of nonparasitic ("free-living") mites are known to induce allergies. The so-called forage or domestic mites (e.g., *Glyciphagus*, *Tyrophagus*, *Tyroglyphus*) develop mainly in vegetable substrates (grain, flour, etc.) and can cause rhinopathies, bronchial asthma, and dermal eczemas ("baker's itch," "grocer's itch") due to repeated skin contacts with or inhalation of dust containing mites. Widespread and frequent in human dwellings are several species of house-dust mites (above all *Dermatophagoides pteronyssinus*) that are an important cause of "house-dust allergy" (dermatitis, inhalation allergy).

Insects

Lice (Anoplura)

Causative agents of pediculosis and phthiriosis (louse infestations)

■ Head lice and crab lice occur more frequently in central Europe and elsewhere than is generally assumed and must therefore always be taken into consideration when diagnosing skin diseases. ■

Parasite species. Two species of lice infest humans, one of which is divided into two subspecies (Table 11.**3**).

General morphology and biology. Lice are dorsoventrally flattened insects, about 1.5–4 mm in length, wingless, with reduced eyes, short (five-segmented) antennae, piercing and sucking mouthparts, and strong claws designed to cling to hairs (Fig. 11.**1c**).

Lice develop from eggs (called nits) glued to hairs. The hatched louse grows and molts through three larval stages to become an adult. Lice remain on a host permanently; both males and females are hematophagous and require frequent blood meals. Lice are highly host-specific, so that animals cannot be a source of infestation for humans.

Medical significance. Among the various species of lice only the body louse is a vector of human diseases. It transmits typhus fever (caused by *Rickettsia prowazekii*), relapsing fever (caused by *Borrelia recurrentis*), and trench fever (caused by *Bartonella quintana*). In central Europe, the medical importance of lice is not due to their vector function, but rather to the direct damage caused by their bites (see below).

Pediculus humanus capitis (Head Louse)

Morphology and biology. Oval body, length 2.2–4.0 mm, morphology very similar to the body louse. Nits are 0.5–0.8 mm long. Localization is mainly in the **hair on the head,** occasionally also on other hairy areas of the head or upper body. The nits are glued to the base of the hair near the skin. Duration of development from nit to adult is 17 days. The lifespan of adults on human host about one month, survival off host at room temperature is for up to one week.

Occurrence and epidemiology. Occurs worldwide; in central Europe it is not frequent, but epidemic-like outbreaks of head louse infestation are observed regularly, especially in schools and kindergartens, homes, groups of neglected

Table 11.**3** Lice that Infest Humans

Species	Main localization of lice and sites of oviposition
Pediculus humanus capitis (head louse)	Hair on the head, rarely on beard hairs or hairy sites on upper body
Pediculus humanus corporis (body louse)	Stitching, seams, and folds in clothes, especially where it is in direct contact with the body
Phthirus pubis (crab louse)	Hair of pubic area, more rarely in the abdominal and axillary regions, beard, eyebrows, and eyelashes

11

persons, etc. Children and women are most frequently infested. About 60% of persons with lice show low levels of infestation with <10 adult lice, the others higher levels (up to >1000 lice). According to official statistics, head louse infestation in the UK increased between 1971 and 1991 about sevenfold; in 1997, about 18.7% of the schoolchildren in Bristol were infested with lice.

Transmission is in most cases by personal contact (mother-child contacts, children playing, etc.), but can also be mediated by such objects as combs, caps, pillows, head supports, stuffed animals, etc.

Clinical manifestations

■ Pruritus and excoriations in the scalp area, nits on hairs, especially in the retroauricular area.

■ In some cases scalp dermatitis, especially at the nuchal hair line: small papules, moist exanthema, and crusting.

■ Occasionally also generalized dermatitis on other parts of the body caused by allergic reactions to louse antigens.

■ Both objective and subjective symptoms may be lacking in up to 20% of cases.

Diagnosis. Determination of symptoms and detection (direct or with magnifier) of lice and/or nits, especially around the temples, ears, and neck.

It is important to clarify the epidemiological background regarding all possible sources of infestation (e.g., in schools). Some countries have introduced regulations on control of outbreaks of louse infestation in schools and other community institutions.

Therapy. In group outbreaks, all contact persons must be treated concurrently, e.g., entire school classes and the families of infested children. A variety of different insecticides are available for therapy, for instance pyrethrum, permethrin, malathion, and γ-hexachlorocyclohexane (γ-HCH, lindane). (Important: lice may show resistance to certain insecticides!) Follow the preparation application instructions and repeat application after seven to 10 days. Rinsing the hair with 5% vinegar in water followed by mechanical removal of the nits with a "louse comb" is a supportive measure.

Control. Clothing, pillows, etc. that have been in contact with lice must be decontaminated: wash laundry at 60 °C; keep clothes and other objects in plastic bags sealed with adhesive tape for four weeks or deep-freeze the bags for one day at –10 to –15 °C. Clean upholstered furniture, mattresses, etc. thoroughly with a vacuum cleaner and decontaminate as necessary (consult an expert for pest control).

11

Pediculus humanus corporis (Body Louse)

Occurrence, morphology, and biology. Very rare in central Europe. Oval body, length: 2.7–4.7 mm. Very difficult to distinguish from head louse (Fig. 11.**1c**). Localization mainly in clothing, where nits are deposited on fibers. These lice contact to the host only for blood meals. Duration of life cycle about three weeks, lifespan on host usually four to five weeks, rarely as long as two months; can survive without a host at 10–20 °C for about one week and at 0–10 °C for approximately 10 days.

Clinical manifestations, diagnosis, and control. Bite reactions on the body, especially around the underwear, are indicative of body louse infestation. To confirm diagnosis inspect clothing for nits and lice. Control: see head louse p. 614.

Phthirus pubis (Crab or Pubic Louse)

Occurrence, morphology, and biology. The crab louse occurs with some regularity in central Europe. Infestations are more frequent in adults than in children and in men more frequently than in women. This louse species can be readily differentiated from the head or body louse: small, length 1.3–1.6 mm, with trapezoid or crablike body form (Fig. 11.**1d**). The parasites are most often found on hair of the **pubic and perianal region**, more rarely on hairy areas of the abdominal region, hairs around the nipples, beard hairs, eyelashes, and eyebrows. The life cycle takes three to four weeks. Deprived of a host, crab lice die at room temperature within two days.

Epidemiology. Transmission of crab lice is almost solely by way of close body contact (sexual intercourse in adults or parent-child contact). Indirect transmission on commonly used beds, clothes, etc. is possible, but is not a major factor.

Clinical manifestations

■ Pruritus and scratches in the genital area and other infestation sites (see above).

■ In some patients typical slate-blue spots, a few mm to 1 cm in size (maculae coeruleae, macula = spot, coeruleus = blue, blackish).

Diagnosis, therapy, control. Detection of lice and nits in the pubic area and other possible localizations by means of inspection (magnifying glass!). Treatment with lindane, malathion, or other substances (see also head louse). It is important to identify contact persons and have them treated as necessary.

11

Bugs (Heteroptera)

Cimex lectularius (family *Cimicidae*), the bedbug, occurs worldwide. Now rare in central Europe, it is therefore often not considered when diagnosing skin lesions. Bedbugs live on human blood. Especially in repeated infestations, their bites induce hemorrhagic or urticarial-papulous reactions, often visible as lesions arranged in groups or rows. The bugs are about 3–4 mm long, with dorsoventrally flattened bodies, greatly reduced wings and a bloodsucking proboscis that can be folded back ventrally. Development from the egg through five larval stages to the adults takes about one and a half months under suitable conditions, but can be extended to as long as one year. Bedbugs require several blood meals during development and egg production. Their ability to starve for as long as a year means they can persist for long periods in rooms, hiding by day (under mattresses, behind furniture, in cracks in the walls, etc.) and emerging at night questing for a blood meal. Diagnosis: skin lesions and detection of bugs in the vicinity. Therapy: symptomatic. Control by means of room decontamination. Other bugs do at times bite humans, e.g., the swallow bug (*Oeciacus hirundinis*), which sometimes leave birds' nests to invade human dwellings. Bugs of the family *Reduviidae* (genera *Triatoma*, *Rhodnius*, etc.) transmit Chagas disease (see p. 491).

Mosquitoes and Flies
(Diptera: Nematocera and Brachycera)

■ Many dipteran species act as vectors of pathogens. Their bites also cause local reactions, and fly maggots may even penetrate into and colonize the skin, wounds, or natural orifices, thereby causing considerable tissue damage. ■

Role as vectors. Many species of Nematocera are significant vectors of pathogens, e.g., *Anopheles* mosquitoes transmitting the malaria parasites, *Aedes aegypti* which is the principal vector of the Dengue virus, or *Phlebotomus* sandflies (Fig. 11.**1e**) transmitting the causative agents of leishmanioses (see Chapter 9). Nematocera also transmit many other pathogens—not only in the tropics, but in central Europe as well.

The same applies to numerous fly species e.g., *Glossina* flies, the vectors of the sleeping sickness agents. Flies can also disseminate various pathogens mechanically (e.g., bacteria, parasites).

Bite reactions. The bites of Nematocera and flies can cause more or less pronounced primary dermal reactions (e.g., mosquitoes of the genus *Aedes* or blackflies of the family *Simuliidae*) or allergic skin reactions.

Table 11.**4** Important Forms of Myiasis in Humans

Form of myiasis	Type of infestation	Infesting flies (genera, selection)
Cutaneous myiasis		
■ Furuncular myiasis	Larvae form focal skin swellings with central small hole	*Dermatobia, Cordylobia, Cuterebra*
■ "Creeping eruption"	Larvae tunnel in epidermis and induce focal skin swellings	*Hypoderma, Gasterophilus*
■ Wound myiasis	Deposition of eggs or larvae in wounds	*Sarcophaga, Calliphora, Musca, Wohlfahrtia, Lucilia, Cochliomyia*
Other forms		
■ Nasopharyngeal, ocular, auricular, and urogenital myiasis	Deposition of eggs or larvae in nasal orifices, eyes, auricular orifices, vulva, etc.	*Sarcophaga, Calliphora, Musca, Wohlfahrtia, Lucilia*

Myiasis. Larvae (maggots) of various fly species can penetrate and colonize the skin, skin lesions, and body orifices, thereby causing the type of tissue damage known as myiasis. There are various forms of myiasis, the most important of which are summarized in Table 11.**4**. Cases of imported myiasis and autochthonous wound myiasis have increased in central Europe in recent years. Diagnosis: inspection and identification of the larvae. Therapy: mechanical removal of the parasites, control of secondary infections, if required oral therapy with ivermectin (extralabel drug use).

The maggots of certain fly species (*Lucilia* spp.) raised under sterile conditions are sometimes used for treating patients with necrotizing or nonhealing dermal lesions. In many cases, the maggots are able to clean such wounds in short order.

11

Fleas (Siphonatera)
Causative agents of flea infestation

■ The "human flea" (*Pulex irritans*) is rare, but humans are frequently attacked by flea species that normally parasitize animal species. Bite reactions can be identified on the human skin, but the parasites must be found and controlled on animals or in their environment. Travelers to tropical areas may become infested with sand fleas (*Tunga penetrans*).   ■

Species and occurrence. At least 2500 species of fleas have been described worldwide. About 100 of these occur in central Europe, of which the medically important species belong mainly to the families Pulicidae and Ceratophyllidae. Encounters with *Pulex irritans*, the so-called "human flea," are rare, but humans are often bitten by flea species normally found on animals, e.g., the dog flea (*Ctenocephalides canis*), cat flea (*Ctenocephalides felis felis*), hedgehog flea (*Archaeopsylla erinacei*), and European chicken flea (*Ceratophyllus gallinae*). All flea species show low levels of host specificity and therefore may infest various animal species as well as humans.

Due to their life cycle the sand fleas (family Tungidae) represent a special group of the fleas. *Tunga penetrans*, endemic in tropical Africa as well as Central and South America, is the most important species in this family from a medical point of view. Sand flea infestation is occasionally reported in travelers returning from tropical regions.

Fleas of the Families Pulicidae and Ceratophyllidae

Morphology. The fleas in this group are about 2–5 mm long, laterally flattened, wingless and have three pairs of legs, the hindmost of which are highly adapted for jumping. The mouthparts form a beaklike proboscis for bloodsucking, the antennae are short. Combs of spines (ctenidia) can adorn the head and first thoracic segment (Fig. 11.**1f**).

Life cycle. Fleas are ectoparasites in humans and vertebrate animal species. Frequent blood meals are needed during the one to three month egg-laying period. Most of the eggs fall off the host and continue to develop in cracks and crevices (e.g., between floorboards, under rugs, under dog or cat cushions or in birds' nests). The life cycle from egg to adult includes three larval stages and one pupal stage and takes three to four weeks under ideal conditions. This time period can also be extended by a matter of weeks depending on the environmental conditions. The lifespan of an adult flea varies from a few weeks to one year including longer starving periods as well as egg and pupa survival maxima of eight and five months, respectively. This explains why dog and cat flea populations can persist in human dwellings for months if control measures are not taken.

Epidemiology. The fleas in this group are periodic ectoparasites. The adult stages remain for the most part on the host while the larvae and pupae live in the vicinity of their hosts in the so-called "nest habitat." In certain regions, fleas serve as vectors for viruses, bacteria, rickettsiae, protozoa, and helminths. Fleas are best-known as the vectors of the causative agent of plague, *Yersinia pestis* (rodent-infesting fleas of the genus *Xenopsylla*, among others).

Clinical manifestations. Dermal reactions to fleabites go through several phases:

■ **Early reaction:** within five to 30 minutes after the bite, a dotlike hemorrhage (at the site of the bite) and a reddening (erythema) with or without a central blister are formed, accompanied by pruritus.

■ **Late reaction:** after 12–24 hours, itching papules form, surrounded by erythemas up to palm-size, some with a central blister or purulent pustule; this reaction persists for one to two weeks.

■ **Predilection sites for lesions:** extremities, neck, nape of neck, shoulders, less often the trunk. Reactions are usually in multiple groups, sometimes in rows.

Diagnosis and control. A diagnosis is reached based on the skin lesions and the case history. Fleas are rarely found on the human body. It is important to find the potential source of flea infestation on animal hosts (dog, cat, hedgehog, birds, etc.) or in their environment, and to identify the fleas found. Once the species is known, specific control measures can be carried out.

Fleas of the Family Tungidae (Sand Fleas)

Tunga penetrans
Causative agent of tungaosis (tungiasis)

Morphology and biology. *Tunga penetrans*, the chigoe, jigger, or sand flea, infest humans and animal species, for example dogs. The males, young females, and other stages live in sandy soil. Fertilized females are highly active in questing for a host. If they succeed, they penetrate the skin head first, then swell up within one to two weeks, sometimes reaching the size of a pea, from their original size of 1–2 mm in length. They lay eggs over a period of about two weeks, and then die while still under the skin.

11

Clinical manifestations

■ Lesions, mainly on the soles of the feet and between the toes, more rarely on other parts of the body.

■ Formation of reddened, pea-sized, painful nodules with a craterlike central depression. Inflammatory and sometimes purulent infiltration of the lesion.

Diagnosis, therapy, and prevention. The diagnosis is based on the characteristic skin lesions and can be confirmed by parasitological or histological examination of the material removed from the sores. Treatment consists of mechanical removal of the female flea under local anesthesia and control of the secondary infection. Topical application of ivermectin is also effective. Prevention demands that shoes that fit and close properly be worn.

Appendix to Chapters 9–11

Laboratory Diagnosis of Parasitoses

This section contains short instructions for sampling and shipment of specimens to diagnostic laboratories and describes current options of diagnosing parasitoses. Readers are referred to the specialized literature for more detailed information.

■ In addition to the usual patient data, a diagnostic laboratory requires in particular information on previous stays in foreign countries, especially travel to tropical or developing countries, as well as any clinical symptoms or previous treatments.

Shipment of Materials

Proper shipment of specimens is an important precondition to obtain reliable results! Request specific instructions from officially recognized (accredited) analytical laboratories. The following specimen types are suitable as test materials for the various parasites:

Stool

■ **Intestinal protozoa (*Entamoeba*, *Giardia*, *Cryptosporidium*, *Sarcocystis*, *Cyclospora*, Microspora):** stool specimen preserved in SAF solution. Add about 1 g of fresh (body-warm!) stool to 10 ml SAF solution (**s**odium aceta**t**e–**a**cetic acid–**f**ormalin), shake vigorously, and submit to laboratory. If the test result is negative and an infection is still suspected, repeat the test once or twice on different days. Request transport tubes and solution from the laboratory. Commercial test kits are also available for shipment and processing of stool specimens.

11

Important: treatment with certain drugs may reduce fecal excretion of intestinal protozoa!

■ **Helminth eggs (without *Enterobius*):** one to two specimens of SAF stool, or better yet 10–20 g fresh stool. With larger amounts of fresh stool, concentration methods can be used, thus improving the chances of parasite detection.

■ *Enterobius* **(oxyurid) eggs:** adhesive tape on slide.

In the morning, press the adhesive side of a piece of transparent adhesive tape about 4 cm long and 1 cm wide onto the perianal skin, then strip it off and press the adhesive side smoothly onto a slide. Submit to laboratory or examine under a microscope.

■ **Larvae of** *Strongyloides* or hookworms: about 10–20 g fresh stool (unrefrigerated) for examination using the Baermann technique and for preparing a larval culture.

■ **Coproantigens:** parasite antigens excreted in stool (coproantigens) can be detected using predominantly the ELISA. Laboratory procedures or commercial kits are now available for diagnosing various intestinal parasites, including *Giardia*, *Cryptosporidium*, *Entamoeba*, and *Taenia*.

Blood

■ **Malaria plasmodia**

Important: the blood specimen must be taken before commencement of malaria therapy, if possible at the onset of a febrile episode. Send the material to the laboratory by the fastest means available!

5–10 ml EDTA blood (to test for *Plasmodium falciparum* antigen, for blood smears and "thick film" preparations).

If possible, add two to four thin, air-dried blood smears (for Giemsa staining and detection/identification of *Plasmodium* species).

■ **Other blood protozoa** (trypanosomes, *Babesia*): 5–10 ml EDTA blood.

■ **Microfilariae:** 5–10 ml blood with EDTA. Important: take blood samples in accordance with periodicity of microfilariae (Table 10.**4**, p. 519), either at night or during the day.

11

Serum

■ **Antibodies to various parasites:** 2–5 ml serum or 5–10 ml of whole blood (both without additives) (see also Table 11.**5**, p. 625).

Cerebrospinal fluid

■ **Antibodies to** *Taenia solium* (suspected cysticercosis): 1–2 ml of cerebrospinal fluid, no additives.

■ **Trypanosomes:** 1–2 ml of cerebrospinal fluid, no additives.

Bronchial Specimens

■ **Microspora and** *Pneumocystis carinii*: induced sputum or 20 ml of bronchial lavage.

Urine

■ *Schistosoma* eggs and microsporidia: sediment (about 20 ml) from 24-hour urine.

Cultivation

■ **Visceral leishmaniosis:** sample obtained under aseptic conditions by puncture from lymph nodes or bone marrow must be transferred immediately to culture medium (order from laboratory).

■ **Cutaneous leishmaniosis:** take specimen tissue from the edges of the lesion (following surface disinfection) and transfer to culture medium.

■ **Acanthamoebas:** 1–2 ml of contact lens rinsing liquid or conjunctival lavage, no additives.

Material for Polymerase Chain Reaction (PCR)

The PCR (see p. 409) is now used to detect or identify species or strains of different parasites, including for example *Leishmania*, *Toxoplasma*, Microspora, *Echinococcus*, *Taenia*, and filarial worms. For analysis with this technique, the following materials can be sent to the laboratory, depending on the parasite species involved: biopsy or tissue specimens from hosts, blood (with EDTA or heparin added), sputum, fecal specimens or other materials in native condition, and parts of parasites (for example proglottids of *Taenia*). Some specimens can also be fixed in 70% ethanol (consult with the laboratory).

Tissue Specimens and Parasites

■ **Skin snip:** for detection of microfilariae in skin. Remove about a 5 mm^2 surface skin specimen using a scalpel and needle, without opening any blood vessels, at the pelvic crest, thigh or other suitable localization, transfer immediately to 0.9% NaCl solution and transport to laboratory immediately or send by express delivery.

■ **Surgical preparations and biopsies:** either by standard method fixed in 4% formalin or finished section preparations.

■ **Parasites:** place tapeworm parts, trematodes, and nematodes in liquid (physiological saline). Fix arthropods in hot 70% ethanol. Consult with laboratory on sending in other parasites.

Immunodiagnostic and Molecular Techniques

A number of parasitoses can be diagnosed by immunological techniques (detection of antibodies or circulating antigens in serum or of coproantigens in stool) and/or by DNA analysis using the PCR or another technique. Table 11.5 provides an overview of selected options.

11

Table 11.**5**   Immunological and Molecular Diagnosis of Parasitoses in Humans: A Selection of Techniques and Established Methods

Parasitosis	Methods Antibody assay[1]	Antigen assay	DNA analysis
African trypanosomosis (sleeping sickness)	IFAT, ELISA, HA		PCR (blood)
American trypanosomosis (Chagas disease)	IFAT, ELISA, HA		PCR (blood)
Leishmaniosis			
■ visceral	IFAT, ELISA		PCR (blood, lymph node aspirate)
■ cutaneous/mucocutaneous	(IFAT, ELISA)		PCR (biopsy)
Giardiosis		IFAT, ELISA (stool)	
Amebosis (Entamebosis)			
■ intestinal	ELISA, IFAT	ELISA (stool)	PCR (stool)
■ extraintestinal	ELISA, IFAT		
Toxoplasmosis	ELISA, IFAT, SFT, CFT, ISAGA, WB, IgG avidity test		PCR (amniotic fluid, placenta, etc.)
Cryptosporidiosis		ELISA, IFAT (stool)	
Malaria	IFAT	Rapid test (blood)[2]	PCR (blood)
Microsporosis			PCR (stool, urine, etc.)
Schistosomosis	IFAT, ELISA		
Fasciolosis	IFAT, ELISA	ELISA (stool)	
Opisthorchiosis	ELISA		
Paragonimosis	ELISA, HA		
Echinococcosis	ELISA, IFAT, WB		PCR (metacestodes)
Cysticercosis	WB, ELISA		
Taeniosis		ELISA (stool)	PCR (proglottids)
Toxocarosis	ELISA, WB		
Filariosis	ELISA, IFAT	ELISA (serum)	

11

Table 11.5 *Continued: Immunological and Molecular Diagnosis of Parasitoses in Humans*

Parasitosis	Methods Antibody assay[1]	Antigen assay	DNA analysis
Trichinellosis	ELISA, IFAT, WB		PCR (biopsy)
Strongyloidosis	ELISA, IFAT, WB		
Ascariosis	ELISA		
Anisakiosis	ELISA		

[1] In parentheses: techniques with low reliability.
[2] Rapid test to detect *Plasmodium*-specific antigens or lactate dehydrogenase.
Abbreviations: **ELISA**: enzyme-linked immunosorbent assay, **HA**: hemagglutination, **IFAT**: indirect immunofluorescent antibody test, **ISAGA**: immunosorbent agglutination assay, **CFT**: complement fixation test , **PCR**: polymerase chain reaction, **SFT**: Sabin-Feldman test, **WB**: Western blot (immunoblot).

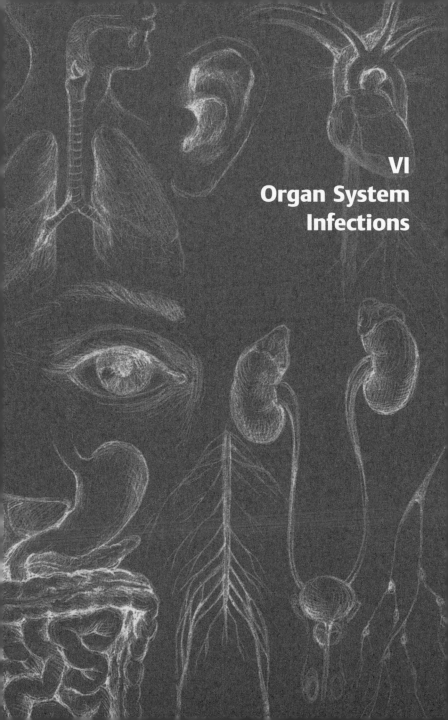

**VI
Organ System
Infections**

Medical microbiology explores how infectious diseases originate and develop. The focus of this branch of the life sciences is of course on infective pathogens, the causes of infections. This explains why the taxonomy of these microorganisms determines the structure of textbooks of medical microbiology, and this one is no exception. This approach does not, however, satisfy all the requirements of clinical practice. The practicing physician is confronted with a pathological problem affecting a specific organ or organ system, and therefore might well find good use for a brief reference tool covering the pathogenic agents that potentially affect specific organs and systems.

Medical microbiology must address two tasks: 1. describing the origins and development of an infection and 2. obtaining a laboratory diagnosis of the resulting disease that is of immediate clinical relevance to patient treatment. Chapter 12 of this book was written to help bridge the gap between basic microbiological science and the demands of medical practice. Concise information on etiology and laboratory diagnosis has been grouped in tabular form in 12 sections corresponding to the most important organs and organ systems. Infections that affect more than one organ system are listed with the system that is affected most severely and/or most frequently or in which the disease manifests most clearly. The pathogens in question are also listed with the other organ manifestations. In the tables, the most frequent causative pathogens in each case are printed in bold letters. Readers are referred to textbooks on internal medicine or specialist literature on infective diseases for exhaustive information on clinical aspects extending beyond etiology and laboratory diagnosis (see references at the end of the book). The descriptions of the diagnostic procedures used to clarify the different infections had to be kept concise in accordance with the tabular format. Since each laboratory offers its own specific set of testing techniques, a physician's choices are defined and limited by what is feasible and available in a given case. This applies in particular to the many different antibody assays now available (= serology). The most important serological tests are listed together with the relevant pathogens in the respective chapters.

12 Etiological and Laboratory Diagnostic Summaries in Tabular Form

FH Kayser, J Eckert, and KA Bienz

Table 12.**1** Upper Respiratory Tract

Infection	Most important pathogens*	Laboratory diagnosis
Rhinitis (common cold)	**Rhinoviruses** Coronaviruses Influenzaviruses Adenoviruses	Laboratory diagnosis not recommended
Sinusitis	*Streptococcus pneumoniae* *Haemophilus influenzae* *Staphylococcus aureus* *Moraxella catarrhalis* (children) *Streptococcus pyogenes* rarely: anaerobes	Microscopy and culturing from sinus secretion/pus (punctate) or sinus lavage
	Influenzaviruses Adenoviruses	Serology
	Rhinoviruses Coronaviruses	Laboratory diagnosis not recommended
Pharyngitis/tonsillitis/ gingivitis/stomatitis *Viruses*	**Adenoviruses** Influenzaviruses RS virus Rhinoviruses Coronaviruses	Isolation, if required, or direct detection in pharyngeal lavage or nasal secretion; serology
Herpangina	Coxsackie viruses, group A	Isolation if required
Gingivitis/stomatitis	Herpes simplex virus	Isolation Serology

12

Table 12.**1** *Continued: Upper Respiratory Tract*

Infection	Most important pathogens*	Laboratory diagnosis
Infectious mononucleosis	**Epstein-Barr virus (EBV)**	Serology
	Cytomegalovirus (CMV)	Culture from pharyngeal lavage and urine; serology
Bacteria	***Streptococcus pyogenes,*** rarely: streptococci of groups B, C, or G	Culture from swab; rapid antigen detection test for A-streptocci in swab material if required
Plaut-Vincent angina	***Treponema vincentii*** + mixed anaerobic flora	Microscopy from swab
Acute necrotic ulcerous gingivostomatitis	***Treponema vincentii*** + mixed anaerobic flora	Microscopy from swab
Diphtheria	***Corynebacterium diphtheriae***	Culture from swab
Laryngotracheobronchitis (croup)	**Parainfluenza viruses** **Influenza viruses** **Respiratory syncytial virus** **Adenoviruses** Enteroviruses	Isolation from pharyngeal lavage or bronchial secretion, combined with serology
	Rhinoviruses	Laboratory diagnosis not recommended
Epiglottitis	***Haemophilus influenzae*** (usually serovar "b") More rarely: *Streptococcus pneumoniae, Staphylococcus aureus, Streptococcus pyogenes*	Blood culture. Culture from swab (caution: respiratory arrest possible in taking the swab)

* The pathogens that occur most frequently are in bold type.

Table 12.**2** Lower Respiratory Tract

Infection	Most important pathogens	Laboratory diagnosis
Acute bronchitis. Acute bronchiolitis (small children)	**Respiratory syncytial virus** **Parainfluenza viruses** **Type A influenza viruses** Adenoviruses	Serology, combined with isolation from pharyngeal lavage or bronchial secretion
	Rhinoviruses	Not recommended
	Mycoplasma pneumoniae	Serology
	Chlamydia pneumoniae	Serology if required
Pertussis	*Bordetella pertussis*	Culture; special material sampling and transport requirements
		Direct immunofluorescence in smear
Acute exacerbation of "chronic obstructive pulmonary disease" (COPD)	***Streptococcus pneumoniae*** *Haemophilus influenzae* *Moraxella catarrhalis*	Culture from sputum or bronchial secretion
Tuberculosis	***Mycobacterium tuberculosis*** other mycobacteria	Microscopy and culture (time requirement: 3–6–8 weeks)
Pneumonia *Viruses* (15–20%) (usually community-acquired)	**Parainfluenza viruses** (children) **Respiratory syncytial virus** (children) **Influenza viruses** **Adenoviruses**	Serology, combined with isolation from pharyngeal lavage or bronchial secretion or antigen detection in nasal secretion
	Epstein-Barr virus (EBV)	Serology
	Cytomegalovirus (CMV) (in transplant patients) Measles virus	Serology, combined with isolation from pharyngeal lavage or bronchial secretion; cell culture if CMV pneumonia suspected. Antigen or DNA assay. Serology

Table 12.**2**   *Continued: Lower Respiratory Tract*

Infection	Most important pathogens	Laboratory diagnosis
	Pulmonary hantaviruses (USA)	Serology
	Enteroviruses	Isolation from pharyngeal lavage or bronchial secretion
	Rhinoviruses	Laboratory diagnosis not recommended
Bacteria (80–90%) "Community-acquired pneumonia"	*Streptococcus pneumoniae* (30%) *Haemophilus influenzae* (5%) *Staphylococcus aureus* (5%) *Klebsiella pneumoniae* *Legionella pneumophila* Mixed anaerobic flora (aspiration pneumonia)	Microscopy and culturing from expectorated sputum, or better yet from transtracheal or bronchial aspirate, from bronchoalveolar lavage or biopsy material. If anaerobes are suspected use special transport vessels
	Mycoplasma pneumoniae (10%)	Serology
	Coxiella burnetii *Chlamydia psittaci*	Serology Serology: CFT can detect only antibodies to genus. Microimmunofluorescence (MIF) species-specific
	Chlamydia pneumoniae	Serology: MIF
"Hospital-acquired pneumonia"	**Enterobacteriaceae** **Pseudomonas aeruginosa** **Staphylococcus aureus**	Laboratory procedures see above at "community-acquired pneumonia"
Fungi	*Aspergillus* spp. *Candida* spp. *Cryptococcus neoformans* *Histoplasma capsulatum* *Coccidioides immitis* *Blastomyces* spp. *Mucorales*	Microscopy and culture, preferably from transtracheal or bronchial aspirate, bronchoalveolar lavage or lung biopsy. Serology often possible (see Chapter 5)

Table 12.**2** *Continued: Lower Respiratory Tract*

Infection	Most important pathogens	Laboratory diagnosis
	Pneumocystis carinii (Pneumocystis carinii pneumonia (PCP) frequent in AIDS patients)	Pathogen detection in "induced" sputum or bronchial lavage by means of microscopy, immunofluorescence or DNA analysis
Protozoa	Microspora	As for *P. carinii*, DNA detection (PCR)
	Toxoplasma gondii	Serology
Helminths	*Echinococcus* spp.	Serology
	Schistosoma spp.	Serology; worm eggs in stool
	Toxocara canis (larvae)	Serology
	Ascaris lumbricoides (larvae)	Serology (specific IgE) (worm eggs in stool)
	Paragonimus spp.	Worm eggs in stool and sputum; serology
SARS (Severe Acute Respiratory Syndrome)	SARS Corona Virus	Reverse transcriptase PCR (RT-PCR) in respiratory tract specimens (swabs, lavage etc.). Serology (EIA).
Empyema	***Streptococcus pneumoniae Staphylococcus aureus Streptococcus pyogenes*** Numerous other bacteria are potential pathogens	Microscopy and culture from pleural pus specimen
Pulmonary abscess Necrotizing pneumonia	Usually endogenous infections with Gram-negative/Gram-positive mixed anaerobic flora Aerobes also possible	Microscopy and culture from transtracheal or bronchial aspirate, bronchoalveolar lavage or lung biopsy. Transport in medium for anaerobes
	Candida spp. *Aspergillus* spp. *Mucorales*	Microscopy and culture, serology as well if required

Table 12.**3** Urogenital Tract

Infection	Most important pathogens	Laboratory diagnosis
Urethrocystitis Pyelonephritis	*Escherichia coli* Other *Enterobacteriaceae* *Pseudomonas aeruginosa* Enterococci *Staphylococcus aureus* *Staphylococcus saprophyticus* (in women)	Microscopy and culture; test midstream urine for significant bacteriuria (p. 210)
Prostatitis	*Escherichia coli* Other *Enterobacteriaceae* *Pseudomonas aeruginosa* Enterococci *Staphylococcus aureus* *Neisseria gonorrhoeae* *Chlamydia trachomatis*	Microscopy and culture. Specimens: prostate secretion and urine. Quantitative urine bacteriology (p. 210) required for evaluation. To confirm *C. trachomatis*, antigen detection by direct IF or EIA or cell culture or PCR.
Nonspecific urethritis	*Chlamydia trachomatis*	Microscopy (direct IF) or antigen detection with EIA, or cell culture or PCR
	Mycoplasma hominis *Ureaplasma urealyticum*	Culture (special mediums)
Urethral syndrome (women)	*Chlamydia trachomatis* (30%) *Escherichia coli* (30%) *Staphylococcus saprophyticus* (5–10%) Unknown pathogens (20%)	See above: nonspecific urethritis Culture from urine. Bacteriuria often $\leq 10^4$/ml
Microsporosis of the genitourinary tract	*Encephalitozoon* spp.	Microscopy of urine sediment, DNA detection (PCR)
Nephropathia epidemica	Hantaviruses/Puumala virus	Serology
Tuberculosis of the urinary tract	*Mycobacterium tuberculosis*	Microscopy and culture Three separate morning urine specimens, 30–50 ml each

Table 12.**3** *Continued: Urogenital Tract*

Infection	Most important pathogens	Laboratory diagnosis
Listeriosis (pregnancy)	*Listeria monocytogenes*	Microscopy and culture from cervical and vaginal secretion, lochia. Blood culture if required
Schistosomosis of the urinary tract	*Schistosoma haematobium*	Microscopy of urine sediment; serology
Vulvovaginitis	Herpes simplex virus	Isolation or antigen detection in secretion
	Candida spp.	Microscopy, culture if required
	Trichomonas vaginalis	Microscopy (native). Submit two slides with air-dried secretion (for Giemsa staining or immunofluorescence), culture from vaginal secretion
Nonspecific vaginitis (vaginosis)	Several bacterial spp. often contribute to infection: *Gardnerella vaginalis* *Mycoplasma hominis* *Mobiluncus mulieri* *Mobiluncus curtisii* Gram-negative anaerobes	Attempt microscopy and culture of vaginal secretion. Look for "clue cells" in microscopy. Interpretation of many findings is problematic because the bacteria are part of the normal flora
Cervicitis Endometritis Oophoritis Salpingitis Pelveoperitonitis	***Neisseria gonorrheae*** ***Chlamydia trachomatis*** ***Mixed anaerobic flora*** Less frequently: *Enterobacteriaceae* *Streptococcus* spp. *Gardnerella vaginalis* *Mycoplasma hominis* *Mycobacterium tuberculosis*	Microscopy and culture from swab material. Use transport mediums. For detection of chlamydiae: direct IF microscopy, EIA antigen detection, cell culture or PCR. PCR kit available to detect gonococci simultaneously.

Table 12.**4** Genital Tract (venereal diseases)

Infection	Most important pathogens	Laboratory diagnosis
Gonorrhea	*Neisseria gonorrhoeae*	Microscopy (send two slides to the laboratory, for gram staining and IF); culture (swab in special transport medium); rapid antigen detection with antibodies in swab material; PCR (kit available to detect *C. trachomatis* simultaneously)
Syphilis (lues)	*Treponema pallidum* (ssp. *pallidum*)	Microscopy (dark field) of material from stage I and II lesions. **Serology** (see p. 321 for basic diagnostics)
Lymphogranuloma venereum	*Chlamydia trachomatis* (L serovars)	Microscopy (direct IF) of pus; cell culture or PCR
Ulcus molle (soft chancre)	*Haemophilus ducreyi*	Microscopy of pus. Culture (very difficult)
Granuloma inguinale	*Calymmatobacterium granulomatis*	Microscopy of scrapings or biopsy material (look for Donovan bodies); culture (embryonated hen's egg or special mediums)

Table 12.**5**   Gastrointestinal Tract

Infection	Most important pathogens	Laboratory diagnosis
Gastritis type B Gastric ulceration Duodenal ulceration Gastric adenocarcinoma Gastric lymphoma (MALT)	*Helicobacter pylori*	Direct fecal antigen detection Biopsy and histopathology Urea breath test Culture from biopsy Serology for screening
Gastroenteritis/enterocolitis		
Viruses	**Rotaviruses** Adenoviruses Rarely: enteroviruses, coronaviruses, astroviruses, caliciviruses, Norwalk virus	Direct virus detection with electron microscopy (reference laboratories) or direct detection with immunological methods (e.g., EIA)
Bacteria	*Staphylococcus aureus* intoxication (enterotoxins A-E)	Toxin detection (with antibodies) in food and stool
	Clostridium perfringens (foods)	Culture (quantitative) from food and stool
	Vibrio parahaemolyticus (food, marine animals)	Culture from stool
	E. coli (EPEC, ETEC, EIEC, EHEC, EAggEC)	No simple tests available; if necessary: culture from stool and identification of pathovars by means of DNA assay; serovar may provide evidence
	Campylobacter jejuni	Culture from stool
	Yersinia enterocolitica	Culture from stool
	Bacillus cereus	Culture from stool
Pseudomembranous colitis (often antibiotic-associated)	*Clostridium difficile*	Toxin detection (cell culture) in stool. DNA assay for toxin possible
Shigellosis (dysentery)	*Shigella* spp.	Culture from stool

Table 12.**5**   *Continued: Gastrointestinal Tract*

Infection	Most important pathogens	Laboratory diagnosis
Salmonellosis		
Enteric form	*Salmonella enterica* (enteric serovars)	Culture from stool
Typhoid form	*Salmonella enterica* (typhoid serovars) (or possibly enteric salmonellae in predisposed persons)	Culture from blood and stool; serology (Gruber-Widal results of limited significance)
Cholera	*Vibrio cholerae*	Culture from stool, possibly also from vomit
Whipple's disease	*Tropheryma whipplei*	Microscopy and DNA detection from small intestine biopsy. Culture not possible
Protozoa		
Amebosis	*Entamoeba histolytica*	Microscopy of stool, detection of coproantigen (or DNA); serology
Giardiosis	*Giardia intestinalis*	Microscopy of stool or duodenal fluid, coproantigen detection
Cryptosporidiosis	*Cryptosporidium* species	Microscopy of stool, coproantigen detection, DNA detection
Microsporosis	*Enterocytozoon bieneusi*	Microscopy of stool, DNA detection
Cyclosporosis	*Cyclospora cayetanensis*	Microscopy of stool
Sarcocystiosis	*Sarcocystis* spp.	Microscopy of stool
Isosporiosis	*Isospora belli*	Microscopy of stool
Blastocystosis	*Blastocystis hominis*	Microscopy of stool

12

Table 12.**5** *Continued: Gastrointestinal Tract*

Infection	Most important pathogens	Laboratory diagnosis
Helminths		
Trematode infections	*Schistosoma* spp.	Microscopical detection of worm eggs in stool; serology
	Fasciolopsis buski	Microscopical detection of worm eggs in stool
	Heterophyes heterophyes and others	Microscopical detection of worm eggs in stool
Cestode infections	*Taenia* spp. *Hymenolepis* spp. *Diphyllobothrium* spp.	Microscopical detection of worm eggs and/or proglottids in stool
Nematode infections	*Ascaris lumbricoides* *Trichuris trichiura* *Ancylostoma* and *Necator* spp.	Microscopical detection of worm eggs in stool
	Strongyloides stercoralis	Microscopy and culturing of larvae in stool (serology)
	Enterobius vermicularis	Microscopical detection of worm eggs (anal adhesive tape on slide) or worms in stool

Table 12.**6** Digestive Glands and Peritoneum

Infection	Most important pathogens	Laboratory diagnosis
Mumps (parotitis epidemica)	Mumps virus (paramyxovirus)	Serology
Infectious hepatitis	Hepatitis A virus	Serology (IgM)
	Hepatitis B and D virus	Antigen and antibody detection in blood, PCR
	Hepatitis C and G virus	Serology, PCR
	Hepatitis E virus	Serology (IgE, IgM), PCR
Yellow fever (liver)	Yellow fever virus (flavivirus)	Serology; isolation if required (use reference laboratory)
Cytomegalovirus infection (liver)	Cytomegalovirus (CMV)	Cell culture from saliva, urine and if required from biopsy material. Antigen assay or DNA test (PCR). Serology
Leptospirosis (liver)	*Leptospira interrogans* (serogroup ictero-haemorrhagiae)	Serology. Culture from urine and blood
Cholecystitis/Cholangitis	**E. coli** Other *Enterobacteriaceae* Gram-negative anaerobes	Culture from bile
	Fasciola hepatica	Worm eggs in stool; serology
	Opisthorchis *Clonorchis* *Dicrocoelium*	
Pancreatitis Pancreatic abscess	*Enterobacteriaceae* *Staphylococcus aureus* *Streptococcus* spp. *Pseudomonas* spp. Anaerobes	Microscopy and culture from pus (punctate or biopsy, if specimen sampling feasible)

Table 12.**6** *Continued: Digestive Glands and Peritoneum*

Infection	Most important pathogens	Laboratory diagnosis
Liver abscess	Usually mixed bacterial flora: *E. coli* Other *Enterobacteriaceae* Gram-negative anaerobes Gram-positive anaerobes *Staphylococcus aureus* *Streptococcus pyogenes* *Streptococcus milleri* *Entamoeba histolytica*	Microscopy and culture from pus if specimen sampling feasible (punctate, biopsy, surgical material) Serology
Splenic abscess	*Staphylococcus* spp. (in endocarditis) *Streptococcus* spp. (in endocarditis) *Enterobacteriaceae* Gram-negative and Gram-positive anaerobes	Microscopy and culture from pus if specimen sampling feasible; blood culture
Peritonitis Primary peritonitis (rare; usually the result of hematogenous dissemination)	*Streptococcus pneumoniae* *Streptococcus pyogenes* Gram-negative/-positive anaerobes; *Enterobacteriaceae;* enterococci; rarely *Staphylococcus aureus*	Microscopy and culture from pus; (specimen sampling during laparotomy, or puncture if necessary)
Secondary peritonitis (endogenous infection caused by enteric bacteria)	Usually mixed aerobic-anaerobic flora *Enterobacteriaceae* Gram-negative and Gram-positive anaerobes	Microscopy and culture from pus (specimen sampling during laparotomy, or puncture if necessary)

Table 12.**6** *Continued: Digestive Glands and Peritoneum*

Infection	Most important pathogens	Laboratory diagnosis
Peritonitis following peritoneal dialysis (CAPD)	Gram-positive bacteria (60–80%): *Staphylococcus* spp. *Streptococcus* spp. *Corynebacterium* spp. Gram-negative bacteria (15–30%): *Enterobacteriaceae* *Pseudomonas* spp. *Acinetobacter* spp. *Candida* spp. (rare)	Microscopy and culture from cloudy dialysis fluid. Concentration of fluid necessary (e.g., filtration or centrifugation)
Intraperitoneal abscesses	Usually mixed aerobic-anaerobic flora: *Enterobacteriaceae* *Staphylococcus aureus* Gram-negative/-positive anaerobes *Streptococcus milleri*	Microscopy and culture from pus (specimen sampling during laparotomy, or puncture if necessary)
Protozoan infections (liver) Visceral leishmaniasis	*Leishmania donovani* *Leishmania infantum*	Microscopy and culture from lymph node or bone marrow punctate; DNA detection; serology
Trematode infections (liver, bile ducts)		
Schistosomosis	*Schistosoma mansoni*	Microscopical detection of worm eggs in stool; serology
Fasciolosis	*Fasciola hepatica*	Microscopical detection of worm eggs in stool; serology
Opisthorchiosis Clonorchiosis Dicrocoeliosis	*Opisthorchis* spp. *Clonorchis sinensis* *Dicrocoelium dendriticum*	Microscopical detection of worm eggs in stool
Cestode infections Echinococcosis (liver, peritoneal cavity)	*Echinococcosus granulosus* *Echinococcosus multilocularis*	Serology

12

Table 12.**7**   Nervous System

Infection	Most important pathogens	Laboratory diagnosis
Meningitis		
Viruses	**Enteroviruses** **Herpes simplex virus** **Mumps virus**	Isolation from cerebrospinal fluid, stool, pharyngeal lavage; serology if herpes or mumps suspected PCR from cerebrospinal fluid
	Togaviruses Bunyaviruses Arenaviruses	In tropical viroses virus isolation from cerebrospinal fluid and blood and serology in reference laboratory
	Lymphocytic choriomeningitis virus Tickborne encephalitis virus (flavivirus)	Serology in blood, in cerebrospinal fluid if necessary
Bacteria	***Neisseria meningitidis*** (~20%) ***Streptococcus pneumoniae*** (~30%) ***Haemophilus influenzae b*** (Less frequent now due to vaccination in children) Rare: *Enterobacteriaceae* (senium) *Mycobacterium tuberculosis* *Leptospira interrogans* *Listeria monocytogenes* Neonates: *E. coli* Group B streptococci	Microscopy and culture from cerebrospinal fluid; antigen detection if required (rapid test)
Fungi	*Cryptococcus neoformans* *Candida* spp. *Coccidioides immitis*	Microscopy and culture from cerebrospinal fluid; antigen detection; serology

12

Table 12.**7** *Continued: Nervous System*

Infection	Most important pathogens	Laboratory diagnosis
Encephalomyelitis		
Viruses	**Measles virus** Epstein-Barr virus	Serology
	HIV-1, HIV-2 **Herpes simplex virus** Varicella zoster virus Cytomegalovirus	PCR and isolation in brain biopsy or cerebrospinal fluid if required
	Mumps virus	Additionally: isolation from pharyngeal lavage
	Enteroviruses	Additionally: isolation from stool
	Togaviruses Bunyaviruses Arenaviruses	In tropical viroses viral serology in reference laboratories
	Rabies virus (lyssa virus)	Direct Immunofluorescence with brain specimen (autopsy) and/or corneal epithelium Serology
	Tickborne encephalitis virus	Serology
Bacteria	*Rickettsia* spp. *Brucella* spp.	Serology
	Borrelia burgdorferi	Serology and PCR; culture in biopsy if required
	Leptospira interrogans	Serology and culture in biopsy if required
	Treponema pallidum	Syphilis serology
	Listeria monocytogenes	Try microscopy and culture from cerebrospinal fluid and blood
	Mycobacterium tuberculosis	Microscopy and culture from cerebrospinal fluid; DNA test if required
Fungi	*Cryptococcus neoformans* *Aspergillus* spp. *Mucorales*	Try microscopy and culture from cerebrospinal fluid and blood; *Cryptococcus* antigen can be detected in cerebrospinal fluid. Serology

12

Table 12.**7** *Continued: Nervous System*

Infection	Most important pathogens	Laboratory diagnosis
Protozoa	*Naegleria fowleri* *Acanthamoeba* spp.	Microscopy (cerebrospinal fluid), culture, DNA detection
	Toxoplasma gondii	Serology, microscopy, culture, DNA detection (cerebrospinal fluid)
	Trypanosoma brucei gambiense *Trypanosoma brucei rhodesiense*	Microscopy (cerebrospinal fluid); Serology
	Plasmodium falciparum	Microscopy (blood); Serology
Helminths	*Taenia solium* (cysticercosis of the CNS)	Serology
	Echinococcus granulosus *Echinococcus multilocularis*	Serology
	Toxocara canis *Toxocara mystax*	Serology
Cerebral abscess Epidural abscess Subdural empyema	*Streptococcus milleri* Gram-negative anaerobes *Enterobacteriaceae* *Staphylococcus aureus*	Microscopy and culture for bacteria from pus
	Mucorales *Aspergillus* spp. *Candida* spp.	Microscopy and culture for fungi from pus; serology
	Toxoplasma gondii	Serology. Microscopy; DNA test (in cerebrospinal fluid)
Tetanus	*Clostridium tetani*	Toxin (animal test, PCR) in material excised from wound. Try microscopy and culture from excised material
Botulism	*Clostridium botulinum*	Toxin detection in blood or food (animal test, PCR)
Leprosy (peripheral nerves)	*Mycobacterium leprae*	Microscopy of biopsy specimen or scrapings from nasal mucosa

Table 12.**8**   Cardiovascular system

Infection	Most Important Pathogens	Laboratory diagnosis
Endocarditis	*Streptococcus* spp. (60–80%) *Staphylococcus* spp. (20–35%) Gram-negative rods (2–13%) Numerous other bacterial spp. (5%) Fungi (2–4%) Culture negative (5–25%)	**Blood culture**, three sets from three different sites, within 1–2 h, before antimicrobials if possible. 10–20 ml venous blood into one aerobic and one anaerobic bottle, respectively.
Myocarditis/ pericarditis		
Viruses	**Enteroviruses** Adenoviruses Herpes virus group Influenzaviruses Parainfluenzaviruses	Serology, if necessary combined with isolation and PCR of punctate
Bacteria	***Staphylococcus aureus*** ***Streptococcus pneumoniae*** ***Enterobacteriaceae*** ***Mycobacterium tuberculosis***	Microscopy and culture from punctate DNA test from punctate if required
	Mycoplasma pneumoniae	Serology; culture from punctate
	Neisseria spp. Gram-negative anaerobes *Actinomyces* spp. *Nocardia* spp.	Microscopy and culture from punctate
	Rickettsia spp. *Chlamydia trachomatis*	Serology
Fungi	**Candida spp.** **Aspergillus spp.** *Cryptococcus neoformans*	Serology; microscopy (direct IF); cell culture or PCR if required
Protozoa	*Toxoplasma gondii* *Trypanosoma cruzi*	Serology, if necessary in combination with culture and microscopy from punctate
Helminths	*Trichinella spiralis*	Serology

12

Table 12.**9** Hematopoietic and Lymphoreticular System

Infection	Most important pathogens	Laboratory diagnosis
HIV infection (AIDS)	HIV-1; HIV-2	Serology: EIA and Western blot. Also p24 antigen assay for primary infection. Quantitative genome test with RT-PCR for therapeutic indication and course (viral load).
Infectious mononucleosis	**Epstein–Barr virus (EBV)** Cytomegalovirus (rare)	Serology Isolation from urine and saliva; serology
Brucellosis	*Brucella abortus* *Brucella melitensis* *Brucella suis*	Blood culture: three sets from three different sites, within 1–2 h, before antimicrobials if possible. 10–20 ml venous blood into one aerobic and one anaerobic bottle, respectively. Incubation for up to 4 weeks is necessary—inform laboratory of suspected *Brucella* infection. Serology
Tularemia	*Francisella tularensis*	Culture from lymph node biopsy, sputum and blood; serology
Plague	*Yersinia pestis*	Microscopy and culture from bubo pus, possibly from sputum (pulmonary plague)
Melioidosis	*Burkholderia pseudomallei*	Microscopy and culture from sputum, abscess pus or blood
Malleus (glanders)	*Burkholderia mallei*	Microscopy and culture from nasal secretion, abscess pus or blood
Rat-bite fever	*Streptobacillus moniliformis*	Culture from lesion specimen
Sodoku	*Spirillum minus*	Attempt microscopical detection in blood or wound secretion

Table 12.**9** *Continued: Hematopoietic and Lymphoreticular System*

Infection	Most important pathogens	Laboratory diagnosis
Oroya fever and verruga peruana	*Bartonella bacilliformis*	Blood culture (see above for brucellosis)
Relapsing fever	*Borrelia recurrentis* *Borrelia duttonii* Other borreliae	Microscopy (Giemsa staining) of blood while fever is rising
Bacillary angiomatosis (AIDS)	*Bartonella henselae*	Serology; microscopy and culture from lymph node biopsy as required
Cat scratch disease	*Bartonella henselae; Bartonella claridgeia Afipia felis* (rare)	Microscopy of puncture pus: Warthin-Starry silver stain. Culture on special medium (difficult)
Malaria	*Plasmodium* spp.	Microscopy (blood smear, thick film); antigen detection with ParaSight test. Serology (not in acute malaria)
Babesiosis	*Babesia* spp.	Microscopy of blood swabs
Toxoplasmosis	*Toxoplasma gondii*	Serology
Visceral leishmaniosis	*Leishmania donovani Leishmania infantum*	Serology; microscopy and culture of lymph node or bone marrow punctate, DNA detection
Filariosis (lymphatic)	*Wuchereria bancrofti Brugia malayi*	Microscopical detection of microfilaria in nocturnal blood; serology
Ehrlichiosis	*Ehrlichia* spp.	Isolation in cell culture. PCR. Serology (immunofluorescence)

12

Table 12.**10** Skin and Subcutaneous Connective Tissue (local or systemic infections with mainly cutaneous manifestation)

Infection	Most important pathogens	Laboratory diagnosis
a) Viruses		
Smallpox	Variola virus Parapox viruses (orf virus, milker's nodules virus)	Electron microscopy of vesicle/pustule content; isolation; serology; (use reference laboratory)
Herpes	Herpes simplex virus	Electron microscopy of vesicle content; cell culture
Varicella (chicken pox)	Varicella zoster virus	Serology (IgG, IgM); electron microscopy of vesicle content; direct IF, cell culture
Measles (morbilli, rubeola)	Measles virus (*Morbillivirus*)	Isolation from pharyngeal lavage and urine if required; serology
German measles (rubella)	Rubella virus (*Rubivirus*)	Serology
Hemorrhagic fever	Bunyaviruses (e.g., hantavirus) Arenaviruses Flaviviruses (e.g., Dengue viruses) Marburg virus Ebola virus	Serology; cell culture and PCR from blood or liver as required; animal test as required; laboratory diagnosis only possible in reference laboratories
Molluscum contagiosum	Molluscum contagiosum virus	Microscopy of skin lesions; molluscum bodies
Warts Papillomas	*Papillomavirus*	Genomic test with DNA probe or electron microscopy
Erythema infectiosum	*Parvovirus* B19	Serology
Exanthema subitum	Human herpes virus 6 (HHV 6)	Serology

Table 12.**10** *Continued: Skin and Subcutaneous Connective Tissue*

Infection	Most important pathogens	Laboratory diagnosis
b) Bacteria and fungi		
Furuncles Carbuncles Pemphigus Folliculitis Impetigo Erysipelas	***Staphylococcus aureus*** ***Streptococcus pyogenes***	Microscopy and culture from swab
Gangrenous cellulitis	**Often mixed flora:** *Clostridium* spp. Gram-negative anaerobes *Pseudomonas* spp. *Enterobacteriaceae*	Microscopy from swab or pus, use transport medium for anaerobes
Erysipeloid	*Erysipelothrix rhusiopathiae*	Microscopy and culture from skin lesion swab
Erythema migrans	*Borrelia burgdorferi*	Serology
Cutaneous anthrax	*Bacillus anthracis*	Microscopy and culture from skin lesion swab
Leprosy	*Mycobacterium leprae*	Microscopy (Ziehl-Neelsen stain) of material from skin lesions (biopsy) or scrapings from nasal mucosa
Rickettsioses (spotted fever and others)	*Rickettsia* spp.	Serology, culturing (embryo-nated hen's egg) or animal test if necessary
Nonvenereal treponema infections (endemic syphilis, pinta, yaws)	*Treponema pallidum* (subsp. *endemicum*) *Treponema pallidum* (subsp. *pertenue*) *Treponema carateum*	Try microscopy of material from skin lesions; serology (syphilis tests)

Table 12.**10**   *Continued: Skin and Subcutaneous Connective Tissue*

Infection	Most important pathogens	Laboratory diagnosis
Madura foot mycosis/mycetoma		
Bacteria	*Nocardia brasiliensis* *Actinomadura madurae* *Streptomyces somaliensis*	Microscopy and culture from lesion material
Fungi	*Madurella* spp. *Pseudoallescheria* spp. *Aspergillus* spp., and others	Microscopy and culture from lesion material
Dermatomycoses	Dermatophytes *Candida* spp.	Microscopy and culture from cutaneous scales
Sporotrichosis	*Sporothrix schenckii*	Microscopy and culture from lesion pus
Chromomycosis	Black molds (various types)	Microscopy and culture from lesion pus
c) Protozoa, helminths, and arthropods		
Cutaneous leishmaniosis (oriental sore)	*Leishmania tropica* *Leishmania major*	Microscopy and culture from lesion biopsy; DNA detection (PCR)
American cutaneous and mucocutaneous leishmaniosis	*Leishmania braziliensis* *Leishmania mexicana*	Microscopy and culture from skin and mucosal lesion biopsy; DNA detection (PCR)
Cercarial dermatitis	Cercariae from *Schistosoma* spp.	Serology
Cutaneous larva migrans ("creeping eruption")	Larvae of *Ancylostoma* spp. and *Strongyloides* species	Clinical diagnosis
Onchocercosis	*Onchocerca volvulus* (microfilariae)	Microscopical detection of microfilariae in "skin snips"; serology

Table 12.**10**   *Continued: Skin and Subcutaneous Connective Tissue*

Infection	Most important pathogens	Laboratory diagnosis
Loaosis	*Loa loa* (migrating filariae)	Microscopy of diurnal blood for microfilariae; serology
Cysticercosis	*Taenia solium*	Serology (radiology)
Dracunculosis	*Dracunculus* spp.	Clinical diagnosis
Tickbite	*Ixodes ricinus* and other tick species	Inspection of skin
Scabies	*Sarcoptes scabiei*	Microscopy
Louse infestation	*Pediculus* spp., *Phthirus pubis*	Inspection of hair, skin, and clothing (body lice) for lice and nits
Myiasis	Fly larvae (maggots)	Inspection
Flea infestation	Various flea species, in most cases from animals	Detection of fleas and flea fecal material on animals and in their surroundings
Sand flea bites	*Tunga penetrans*	Clinical diagnosis, histology if needed

Table 12.**11**   Bone, Joints, and Muscles

Infection	Most important pathogens	Laboratory diagnosis
Pleurodynia, epidemic myalgia (Bornholm disease)	**Coxsackie viruses group B** (possibly echoviruses)	Isolation from stool and pharyngeal lavage; serology
Clostridial infections 1. Gas gangrene (with myonecrosis) 2. Clostridial cellulitis (without myonecrosis)	***Clostridium perfringens*** Other clostridial spp.	Microscopy and culture from wound secretion. Transport materials in anaerobic system

12

Table 12.**11** Bone, Joints, and Muscles

Infection	Most important pathogens	Laboratory diagnosis
Necrotizing fasciitis Type 1 (syn. polymicrobial gangrene)	Often aerobic/anaerobic mixed flora: *Clostridium* spp., Gram-positive and Gram-negative anaerobes, *Staphylococcus aureus*, *Streptococcus bovis*, *Enterobacteriaceae*	Microscopy and culture from wound secretion. Transport materials in anaerobic system
Type 2 (syn. Streptococcal necrotizing myositis)	*Streptococcus pyogenes*	Microscopy and culture from wound secretion
Trichinellosis (Muscle)	*Trichinella spiralis*	Microscopical detection in muscle biopsy; serology
Cysticercosis (Muscle)	*Taenia solium*	Serology (radiology)
Osteomyelitis/ostitis	***Staphylococcus aureus*** Coagulase-negative staphylococci *Streptococcus* spp. *Enterobacteriaceae* *Pseudomonas* spp. Gram-positive and Gram-negative anaerobes (rare)	Microscopy and culture for bacteria, preferably based on biopsy or surgical material. Swab from fistular duct not useful for diagnosis
Septic arthritis	***Staphylococcus aureus*** *Streptococcus pyogenes* *Streptococcus pneumoniae* *Haemophilus influenzae* *Neisseria gonorrhoeae* *Enterobacteriaceae* *Pseudomonas* spp.	Microscopy and culture from synovial fluid with parallel blood culture

12

Table 12.**12**   Eyes and ears

Infection	Most important pathogens	Laboratory diagnosis
Trachoma	*Chlamydia trachomatis*, serovars A, B, Ba, C	Microscopical detection of inclusions in conjunctival cells (Giemsa stain); direct immuno-fluorescence; cell culture; antigen detection using EIA; PCR. Serology: recombinant immunoassay for antibodies to genus-specific antigen (LPS or MOMP). Microimmuno-fluorescence for antibodies to species- and var-specific anti-bodies.
Conjunctivitis/scleritis		
Viruses	Adenoviruses Enteroviruses Influenzaviruses Measles virus	Isolation from swab
Bacteria	*Neisseria* spp. *Streptococcus* spp. *Staphylococcus aureus* *Haemophilus* spp. Enterobacteriaceae *Pseudomonas* spp. *Mycobacterium* spp. *Moraxella lacunata*	Microscopy and culture for bacteria in conjunctival secre-tion or in scrapings
	Chlamydia trachomatis (inclusion conjunctivitis)	See at "trachoma" (this table)
	Treponema pallidum	Serology (basic diagnostics)
Fungi	*Candida* spp. *Sporothrix schenckii*	Microscopy and culture for fungi in conjunctival secretion or in corneal scrapings
Helminths	*Onchocerca volvulus*	Microscopy for microfilariae in skin snips (or conjunctival) biopsy; serology
	Loa loa	Microscopy for microfilariae in diurnal blood; serology

12

Table 12.**12** *Continued: Eyes and ears*

Infection	Most important pathogens	Laboratory diagnosis
Keratitis		
Viruses	Herpes simplex virus Adenoviruses Varicella zoster virus	Cell culture and PCR from swab or corneal scrapings
Bacteria	*Staphylococcus* spp. *Streptococcus* spp. *Neisseria gonorrheae* *Enterobacteriaceae* *Pseudomonas* spp. *Bacillus* spp. *Mycobacterium* spp. *Moraxella lacunata* *Actinomyces* spp. *Nocardia* spp.	Microscopy and culture for bacteria swab or corneal scrapings
	Chlamydia trachomatis	Diagnostic procedures with corneal swab or scrapings see at "trachoma" (this table)
	Treponema pallidum	Serology (basic diagnostics)
Fungi	*Candida* spp. *Aspergillus* spp. *Fusarium solani*	Microscopy and culture for fungi in swab or corneal scrapings
Protozoa	*Acanthamoeba* spp.	Culture and microscopy from conjunctival lavage and contact lens washing fluid, DNA detection
Endophthalmitis		
Viruses	Herpes simplex viruses Varicella zoster virus Measles virus Rubella virus (german measles)	Cell culture and PCR in aqueous and vitreous aspiration; serology with aqueous humor as required

12

Table 12.**12**   *Continued: Eyes and ears*

Infection	Most important pathogens	Laboratory diagnosis
Bacteria	*Staphylococcus* spp. *Streptococcus* spp. *Neisseria gonorrhoeae* *Enterobacteriaceae* *Pseudomonas* spp. *Bacillus* spp. *Mycobacterium* spp. *Moraxella lacunata* *Actinomyces* spp. *Nocardia* spp.	Microscopy (gram) and culture for aerobic and anaerobic bacteria and mycobacteria in aqueous and vitreous aspiration.
	Chlamydia trachomatis	Cell culture or PCR in aqueous and vitreous aspiration; serology with aqueous humor as required; antibodies in blood
	Treponema pallidum	Serology (basic diagnostics)
Fungi	*Candida* spp. *Aspergillus* spp. *Blastomyces dermatitidis* *Histoplasma capsulatum* *Mucorales* *Sporothrix schenckii* *Fusarium* spp. *Trichosporon* spp.	Microscopy (Gram, Giemsa) and culture for fungi in aqueous and vitreous aspiration.
Protozoa	*Acanthamoeba* spp.	Microscopy and culturing (conjunctival fluid and contact lens washing fluid), DNA detection
	Toxoplasma gondii	Serology
Helminths	*Onchocerca volvulus*	Direct detection of microfilariae in aqueous humor with slit lamp; serology
	Toxocara canis	Serology
	Taenia solium (ocular cysticercosis)	Serology

12

Table 12.**12**   *Continued: Eyes and ears*

Infection	Most important pathogens	Laboratory diagnosis
Otitis externa	***Pseudomonas aeruginosa*** *Staphylococcus aureus* *Streptococcus pyogenes*	Microscopy and culture for bacteria of swab material
	Aspergillus spp. *Candida* spp.	Microscopy and culture for fungi of swab material
Otitis media	***Streptococcus pneumoniae*** ***Haemophilus influenzae*** *Streptococcus pyogenes* *Staphylococcus aureus* *Moraxella catarrhalis* (children) Respiratory viruses (25%)	Microscopy and culture for bacteria of middle ear punctate as required

Literature

Medical Microbiology and Infectious Diseases

Chin J. *Control of Communicable Diseases Manual.* 17th ed. Washington, DC: American Public Health Association; 2000.

Collier L, Balows A, Sussman M. *Topley & Wilson's Microbiology and Microbial Infections.* Bd. 1–6. 9th ed. London: Arnold; 1998.

Joklik WK, Willett HP, Amos DB. *Zinsser's Microbiology.* McCraw Hill; 1995.

Mandell GL, Bennett JE, Dolin, R. *Principles and Practice of Infectious Diseases.* Bd 1–2. 5th ed. Churchill Livingstone; 2000.

Mayhall CG. *Hospital Epidemiology and Infection Control.* 2nd ed. Baltimore: Lippincott, Williams & Wilkins; 1999.

Murray PR, Baron EJ, Jorgensen JH, Pfaller MA, Yolken RH. *Manual of Clinical Microbiology.* 8th ed. Washington DC: American Society of Microbiology; 2003.

Immunology

Goldsby RA, Kindt TJ, Osborne BA, Kuby J. *Immunology.* 5th ed. New York: Freeman; 2003.

Janeway CA, Travers P, Walport M, Shlomchik M. *Immunobiology.* 6th ed. New York: Garland Science Publishing; 2004.

Paul WE. *Fundamental Immunology.* 5th ed. Philadelphia: Lippincott Williams & Wilkins, 2003.

Roitt IM, Brostoff J, Male DK, *Immunology,* 6th ed. London: Elsevier; 2001.

Rose NR, Hamilton RG, Detrick B. *Manual of Cllinical Laboratory Immunology,* 6th ed. Washington, D.C.: ASM Press; 2002.

Bacteriology

Burns DL, Barbieri JT, Iglewski BH, Rappuoli R (eds). *Bacterial Protein Toxins.* Washington DC: American Society of Microbiology; 2003.

Cossart P, Boquetz P, Normark S, Rappuoli R. *Cellular Microbiology.* 1st ed. Washington DC: American Society of Microbiology; 2000.

Garrity GM (editor in chief). *Bergey's Manual of Systematic Bacteriology.* 2nd ed. Vol. 1, *Taxonomic Outline of the Archaea and Bacteria.* New York, Berlin, Heidelberg: Springer; 2001.

Glick BR, Pasternack JJ. *Molecular Biotechnology. Principles and Applications of Recombinant DNA.* 3rd ed. Washington/D.C.: American Society of Microbiology; 2003.

Lengeler JW, Drews G, Schlegel HG. *Biology of the Procaryotes.* Stuttgart: Thieme; 1999.

Lorian V. *Antibiotics in Laboratory Medicine.* 4th ed. Baltimore: Williams & Wilkins; 1996.

Salyers AA, Whitt DD. *Bacterial Pathogenesis. A Molecular Approach.* 2nd ed. Washington/D.C.: American Society of Microbiology; 2002.

Snyder L, Champness W. *Molecular Genetics of Bacteria*. Washington/DC: American Society of Microbiology; 1997.

Mycology

De Hoog GS, Guarro J (eds.). *Atlas of Clinical Fungi*. 2nd ed. Washington D.C.: American Society of Microbiology; 2001.

Larone DH. *Medically Important Fungi: A Guide to Identification*. 4th ed. Washington/D.C.: American Society of Microbiology; 2002.

Richardson MD, Warnock DW. *Fungal Infection: Diagnosis and Management*. 3rd ed. London: Blackwell Scientific Publications; 2003.

Virology

Burkhardt F. *Mikrobiologische Diagnostik*. Stuttgart: Thieme; 1992.

Evans AS, Kaslow RA. *Viral Infections of Humans: Epidemiology and Control*. 4th ed. New Haven, CT: Plenum Publishing; 1997.

Knipe DM, Howley PM, Griffin DE. *Fields Virology*. 4th ed. Philadelphia: Lippincott Williams & Wiking; 2001.

Flint SJ, Enquist LW, Racaniello VR. *Principles of Virology: Molecular Biology, Pathogenesis, and Control*. 2nd ed. Washington/D.C.: American Society of Microbiology; 2004

Parasitology

Acha PN, Szyfres B. *Zoonoses and Communicable Diseases Common to Man and Animals*. 3rd ed. Vol. III: *Parasitic Zoonoses*. Washington D.C.: Pan American Health Organization; 2003.

Aspöck H. Prevention of congenital toxoplasmosis in Austria: experience of 25 years. In: Ambroise-Thomas P, Petersen E (eds.). *Congenital Toxoplasmosis*. Berlin: Springer (France), 277–292, 2000.

Cook G, Zumla A (eds.). *Manson's Tropical Diseases*. 21st ed. London: Saunders; 2002.

Cox FEG, Kreier JP, Wakelin D (eds.). *Topley & Wilson's Microbiology and Microbial Infections*. 9th ed. Vol. 5: Parasitology. London: Arnold; 1998.

Gillepsie S, Perason R (eds.). *Principles and Practice of Clinical Parasitology*. Baffins Lane, Chichester: Wiley Interscience; 2001.

Kettle, DS. *Medical and Veterinary Entomology*. 2nd ed. CAB International, Wallingford, Oxon, UK; 1995.

Lang W, Löscher T (eds.). *Tropenmedizin in Klinik und Praxis*. 3rd ed. Stuttgart: Thieme; 1999.

Mehlhorn H (ed.). *Encyclopedic Reference of Parasitology*. Sec. Edit. Vol. I: *Biology, Structure, Function*. Vol. II: *Diseases, Treatment, Therapy*. Berlin: Springer; 2001.

Palmer SR, Soulsby EJL, Simpson DIH (eds.). *Zoonoses*. Oxford: Oxford University Press; 1998.

Medical Microbiology and the Internet

An ever-growing number of websites specific to problems in microbiology, infection, and communicable disease are today available on the Internet. Below is a compilation of the most important addresses.

Institution	Internet address	Description
World Health Organization	http://www.who.ch/	Home page for the WHO
	http://www.who.int/emc/	WHO subsite providing weekly infectious disease news, prevention, and travel information worldwide
Centers for Disease Control and Prevention (CDC)	http://www.cdc.gov/	Home page for the CDC
	http://www.cdc.gov/travel/index.htm	CDC subsite providing information for travelers
	http://www.cdc.gov/ncidod/id_links.htm	CDC subsite with links related to infectious diseases
	http://www.cdc.gov/nip	CDC subsite recommending childhood and adolescent immunization schedules—USA
American Society of Microbiology (ASM)	http://www.asm.org/search	Homepage of the ASM. Links to medical microbiology and infectious diseases
Infectious Disease Society of America (IDSA)	http://www.idsociety.org/index.html	Homepage of IDSA providing links to infectious diseases
International Society for Infectious Diseases (ISID)	http://idis.org	Homepage of ISID providing links to infectious diseases
Public Health Laboratory Service (PHLS), equivalent to CDC for Great Britain	http://www.co.uk	Homepage of the PHLS. Links to clinical microbiology and infectious diseases, GB

Institution	Internet address	Description
Robert Koch Institut (RKI), equivalent to CDC for Germany	http://www.rki.de	Homepage of the RKI. Links to clinical microbiology and infectious diseases. Health laws and regulations valid for Germany
Society for Systematic and Veterinary Bacteriology (F)	htpp://bacterio.cict.fr	List of bacterial names with standing in nomenclature (LBSN)

Index

■ E

Quinopristin 194
Quorum sensing 19–20

R

Rabies 28, 468–470
  clinical course 468
  diagnosis 645
  epidemiology 469
  prevention 469–470
    postexposure prophy-
    laxis 469–470
  see also Rhabdoviruses
Radial immunodiffusion
technique 122, 123
Radiation
  as disinfection/steriliza-
  tion method 38
  ionizing 38
  nonionizing 38
Radioallergosorbent test
(RAST) 131
Radioimmunoassay (RIA)
128–129
Radioimmunosorbent test
(RIST) 130
RANTES 82, 143
Rat bite fever 648
Rearrangement 143
  B-cell receptor 55
  IgG heavy chain 54
  T-cell receptor 54, 55
Receptors 384
  B-cell receptor 45–46,
  48–50
    genetic rearrange-
    ment 55
  CCR chemokine receptor
  139
  CXCR chemokine recep-
  tor 140
  Duffy antigen receptor
  for chemokines (DARC)
  85, 140
  T-cell receptor (TCR) 45,
  57–58, 62
    genetic rearrange-
    ment 53, 54, 55
Recombination
  bacteria 143, 170,
  171–173, 180–181
  homologous (legitimate)
  171, 180
  illegitimate 181
  site-specific 172, 181
  somatic 144
  transposition 172

viruses 390
Reduviidae 616
Regulator 180
Regulon 170, 180
  virulence regulon 19
Reinfection 10
Rejection see Transplants
Relapses 10
Relapsing fever 324–326,
613
  clinical picture 325
  diagnosis 649
  epidemiology 325–326
  prevention 325–326
  therapy 325
  see also Borrelia
Reoviruses 383, 455–457
  clinical picture 456
  diagnosis 455, 456
  epidemiology 456–457
  pathogenesis 456
  pathogens 456
Replication
  DNA 168, 181
    semiconservative 181
  viruses 381–386, 387
    adsorption 384
    nucleic acid replica-
    tion 384–385, 387
    penetration and un-
    coating 384
Replicon 181
Resistance plasmids 167,
168, 176, 177
Respiration 161
Respiratory chain enzymes
151
Respiratory syncytial (RS)
virus 465, 467
  diagnosis 630, 631, 632
Respiratory tract infec-
tions 295
  adenoviruses 416
  aspergillosis 365
  bronchiolitis 467, 632
  bronchitis 632
  chronic obstructive pulmonary disease (COPD)
  632
  empyema 634
  influenza viruses
  458–460
  laboratory diagnosis
  209, 623, 630–634
    lower respiratory tract
    632–634
    upper respiratory tract
    630–631

mucormycosis 368
mycoplasmas 341
nosocomial infections
344
parainfluenza virus 466
pertussis 632
pharyngitis 630
rhinitis (common cold)
438, 447, 630
severe acute respiratory
syndrome (SARS) 446,
447–448, 634
sinusitis 630
tonsillitis 630
  see also Pneumonia;
  specific infections
Restriction 171, 177–178
Restriction endonucleases
181
Reticuloendothelial sys-
tem (RES) 143
Retroviruses 383,
448–450
  carcinogenic 394–396
    genome structure
    394–395
    replication 394–395
    tumor induction
    395–396
  pathogens 448–449
  release from infected
  cell 389
  replication 385, 387
  see also Human immu-
  nodeficiency virus
  (HIV); Human T-cell
  leukemia virus (HTLV)
rev gene 449
Reverse transcriptase 448
Rhabditida 545
Rhabdoviruses 383,
467–470
  clinical picture 468
  diagnosis 467, 468–469
  epidemiology 28, 469
  pathogenesis 468
  pathogens 468
  prevention 467,
  469–470
Rhesus factor 112, 143
Rheumatoid factor (RF)
143
Rhinitis
  allergic 352
  common cold 438, 447,
  630
Rhinoviruses 434, 438
  clinical picture 438

■S

■W